Nuclear Cardiology

Notice

Medicine is an ever-changing science. As new research and clinical experience broaden our knowledge, changes in treatment and drug therapy are required. The authors and the publisher of this work have checked with sources believed to be reliable in their efforts to provide information that is complete and generally in accord with the standards accepted at the time of publication. However, in view of the possibility of human error or changes in medical sciences, neither the authors nor the publisher nor any other party who has been involved in the preparation or publication of this work warrants that the information contained herein is in every respect accurate or complete, and they disclaim all responsibility for any errors or omissions or for the results obtained from use of the information contained in this work. Readers are encouraged to confirm the information contained herein with other sources. For example and in particular, readers are advised to check the product information sheet included in the package of each drug they plan to administer to be certain that the information contained in this work is accurate and that changes have not been made in the recommended dose or in the contraindications for administration. This recommendation is of particular importance in connection with new or infrequently used drugs.

Nuclear Cardiology
Practical Applications

Third Edition

Gary V. Heller, MD, PhD, FACC, MASNC
Gagnon Cardiovascular Institute
Morristown Medical Center
Morristown, New Jersey

Robert C. Hendel, MD, FACC, FAHA, MASNC
Sidney W. and Marilyn S. Lassen Chair in Cardiovascular Medicine
Chief, Section of Cardiology
Tulane University School of Medicine
Director, Tulane University Heart & Vascular Institute
New Orleans, Louisiana

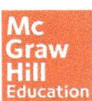

New York   Chicago   San Francisco   Athens   London   Madrid   Mexico City
Milan   New Delhi   Singapore   Sydney   Toronto

Nuclear Cardiology: Practical Applications, Third Edition

Copyright © 2018 by McGraw-Hill Education. All rights reserved. Printed in The United States of America. Except as permitted under the United States Copyright Act of 1976, no part of this publication may be reproduced or distributed in any form or by any means, or stored in a data base or retrieval system, without the prior written permission of the publisher.

Previous editions copyright © 2011, 2004 by The McGraw-Hill Companies, Inc.

1 2 3 4 5 6 7 8 9   LSI   23 22 21 20 19 18

ISBN 978-1-260-12177-3
MHID 1-260-12177-1

This book was set in Minion Pro by Aptara, Inc.
The editors were Karen G. Edmonson and Robert Pancotti.
The production supervisor was Richard Ruzycka.
Project management was provided by Dinesh Pokhriyal, Aptara, Inc.
The text designer was Eve Siegel; the cover designer was Randomatrix.

McGraw-Hill Education books are available at special quantity discounts to use as premiums and sales promotions or for use in corporate training programs. To contact a representative, please visit the Contact Us pages at www.mhprofessional.com.

For Susan, who is as important in my life as breath itself and my brother Steve: I was your wingman and you were my rock.

G.V.H.

To my many mentors, who taught me not only the essence of nuclear cardiology as a subspecialty, but guided me in my professional growth. Additionally, I am so grateful to my family and friends who have supported me on this wonderful journey.

R.C.H.

CONTENTS

Contributors ix

Preface xiii

Section 1. Fundamentals of Nuclear Cardiology 1

1. **Fundamentals of Nuclear Cardiology Physics** 3
   E. Lindsey Tauxe

2. **Radiation Safety and Protection** 15
   Jason S. Tavel

3. **Radiopharmaceuticals for Cardiac Imaging** 27
   Raymond Taillefer

4. **Cardiac SPECT and PET Instrumentation** .. 43
   James A. Case

5. **Quality Control in SPECT and PET Imaging** 63
   Sue Miller, Frank DiGregorio, and Sunil Selvin

6. **Quality Performance in Nuclear Cardiology: A Global Perspective** 81
   Peter L. Tilkemeier

7. **Radiation Reduction Strategies in Myocardial Perfusion Imaging** 91
   Michael C. Desiderio and Gary V. Heller

Section 2. Radionuclide Myocardial Perfusion Imaging (MPI) 101

8. **Exercise and Pharmacologic Stress Testing** 103
   Robert C. Hendel and Archana Ramireddy

9. **SPECT Myocardial Perfusion Imaging Protocols** 121
   Milena J. Henzlova

10. **Cardiovascular Positron Emission Tomography** 131
    Justin B. Lundbye and Gary V. Heller

11. **ECG-Gated SPECT Imaging for Assessment of Ventricular Function and Dyssynchrony** ... 147
    Prem Soman and Saurabh Malhotra

12. **Interpretation and Reporting of SPECT Myocardial Perfusion Imaging** 163
    Eve Vasutakarn Chongthammakun and Robert C. Hendel

Section 3. Indications and Applications of MPI 191

13. **The Appropriate Use of Nuclear Cardiology Techniques** 193
    Camilo A. Gomez and Robert C. Hendel

14. **Evaluation of Patients with Suspected Coronary Artery Disease Using Nuclear Myocardial Perfusion Imaging** 209
    Sanjeev U. Nair and Gary V. Heller

15. **Risk Stratification with Myocardial Perfusion Imaging** 223
    Javier Gomez and Rami Doukky

16. **Preoperative Risk Assessment for Noncardiac Surgery** 245
    Sumeet S. Mitter and Thomas A. Holly

17. **Evaluation of Patients with Known Coronary Artery Disease** 257
    Javier Gomez and Rami Doukky

18. **Radionuclide Imaging in Heart Failure** ... 271
    Gautam V. Ramani and Prem Soman

19. **Myocardial Perfusion Imaging in Special Populations** ... 279
    Upamanyu Rampal and Raja C. Pullatt

20. **Cost-Effectiveness of Nuclear Cardiology** ... 297
    Lawrence M. Phillips, Joe X. Xie, and Leslee J. Shaw

Section 4. Nuclear Cardiology Beyond Myocardial Perfusion ... 307

21. **Nuclear Cardiology Procedures in the Evaluation of Myocardial Viability** ... 309
    Fernanda Erthal, Benjamin Chow, Gary V. Heller, and Rob S.B. Beanlands

22. **Radionuclide Angiography: Equilibrium and First Pass** ... 331
    Rupa M. Sanghani and Kim A. Williams

23. **Radionuclide Imaging of Cardiac Innervation** ... 345
    Mark I. Travin

24. **Cardiac Amyloid Imaging and ^{18}F-FDG PET/CT for Imaging Sarcoidosis and Cardiovascular Infection** ... 365
    Dillenia Rosica and Sharmila Dorbala

Section 5. Alternative Noninvasive Testing ... 385

25. **Hybrid Imaging: SPECT–CT and PET–CT** ... 387
    Patrycja Galazka, Sanjeev A. Francis, and Sharmila Dorbala

26. **ECG Exercise Testing** ... 401
    J. Wells Askew and Todd D. Miller

27. **Echocardiography** ... 411
    Zeina Ibrahim, Elizabeth A. Grier, and Vera H. Rigolin

28. **Coronary Calcium Scoring and Coronary CT Angiography** ... 431
    Subhi J. Al'Aref, Khalil Anchouche, Sarah J. Rinehart, Fay Y. Lin, and James K. Min

29. **Cardiovascular Magnetic Resonance** ... 449
    Jamieson M. Bourque and Christopher M. Kramer

Section 6. Review Questions ... 463

Answers and Explanations for Review Questions ... 483

Index ... 497

CONTRIBUTORS

Subhi J. Al'Aref, MD
Instructor of Medicine and Radiology
Weill Cornell Medicine
Dalio Institute of Cardiovascular Imaging
New York, New York

Khalil Anchouche, BA
Medical Student
Weill Cornell Medicine
Dalio Institute of Cardiovascular Imaging
New York, New York

J. Wells Askew, MD
Assistant Professor of Medicine
Mayo Clinic
Rochester, Minnesota

Rob S.B. Beanlands, MD, FRCPC, FCCS, FACC, FASNC
Vered Chair and Head, Division of Cardiology
Professor, Medicine (Cardiology)/Radiology
Tier 1 University of Ottawa Cardiovascular
  Research Chair
Director, National Cardiac PET Centre
University of Ottawa Heart Institute
Ottawa, Ontario, Canada

Jamieson M. Bourque, MD, MHS
Associate Professor of Medicine and Radiology
Division of Cardiovascular Medicine,
  Department of Medicine
University of Virginia Health System
Charlottesville, Virginia

James A. Case, PhD
University of Missouri, Columbia
Cardiovascular Imaging Technologies
Kansas City, Missouri

Eve Vasutakarn Chongthammakun, MD, PhD
Cardiology Fellow
Cardiovascular Division
University of Miami Miller School of Medicine
Miami, Florida

Benjamin Chow, MD, FRCPC, FACC, FASNC, FSCCT
Professor (Medicine and Radiology)
Cardiologist
Saul and Edna Goldfarb Chair in Cardiac Imaging
Director of Cardiac Imaging
Co-Director of Cardiac Radiology
Director of Postgraduate Cardiac Imaging Training
University of Ottawa Heart Institute
Ottawa, Ontario, Canada

Michael C. Desiderio, DO
Cardiology Fellow
Department of Cardiovascular Medicine
Morristown Medical Center/Atlantic Health System
Morristown, New Jersey

Frank DiGregorio, CNMT, RDMS, CAPPM
President and CEO
Molecular Imaging Services, Inc.
Newark, Delaware

Sharmila Dorbala, MD, MPH, FACC, FASNC
Director of Nuclear Cardiology
Associate Professor, Department of Radiology
Division of Nuclear Medicine and Molecular Imaging and
  the Noninvasive Cardiovascular Imaging Program
Heart and Vascular Center
Departments of Radiology and Medicine (Cardiology)
Brigham and Women's Hospital
Harvard Medical School
Boston, Massachusetts

Rami Doukky, MD, FACC, FASNC
Professor of Medicine and Radiology
Chairman, Division of Cardiology
Cook County Health and Hospitals System
Chicago, Illinois

Fernanda Erthal, MD
Cardiac Imaging Clinical Fellow
Division of Cardiology
Department of Medicine
University of Ottawa Heart Institute
Ottawa, Ontario, Canada
Cardiac Imaging Staff
Department of Cardiac Imagem
Fonte Imagem Medicina Diagnostica, Rio de Janeiro
Rio de Janeiro, Brazil

Sanjeev A. Francis, MD
Director of Education, Cardiovascular Institute Director, Cardiovascular Medicine Fellowship Program
Maine Medical Center, Maine Health Cardiology
Assistant Professor of Medicine
Tufts University School of Medicine
Portland, Maine

Patrycja Galazka, MD
Fellow, Noninvasive Cardiovascular Imaging
The Noninvasive Cardiovascular Imaging Program
Heart and Vascular Center
Departments of Radiology and Medicine (Cardiology)
Brigham and Women's Hospital
Harvard Medical School
Boston, Massachusetts

Camilo A. Gomez, MD
Cardiology Fellow
Cardiovascular Division
University of Miami Miller School of Medicine
Miami, Florida

Javier Gomez, MD, FACC
Assistant Professor of Medicine
Director, Stress Testing and Nuclear Cardiology
Division of Cardiology
Cook County Health and Hospitals System
Chicago, Illinois

Elizabeth A. Grier, MD
Internal Medicine Resident
Division of Cardiology, Department of Medicine
Northwestern University Feinberg School of Medicine
Bluhm Cardiovascular Institute
Chicago, Illinois

Gary V. Heller, MD, PhD, FACC, MASNC
Gagnon Cardiovascular Institute
Morristown Medical Center
Morristown, New Jersey

Robert C. Hendel, MD, FACC, FAHA, MASNC
Sidney W. and Marilyn S. Lassen Chair in Cardiovascular Medicine
Chief, Section of Cardiology
Tulane University School of Medicine
Director, Tulane University Heart & Vascular Institute
New Orleans, Louisiana

Milena J. Henzlova, MD
Professor of Medicine
Mount Sinai School of Medicine
New York, New York

Thomas A. Holly, MD
Professor of Medicine, Radiology, and Medical Education
Program Director, Cardiovascular Disease Fellowship
Northwestern University Feinberg School of Medicine
Medical Director, Nuclear Cardiology
Northwestern Memorial Hospital
Chicago, Illinois

Zeina Ibrahim, MD
Advanced Imaging Cardiovascular Fellow
Division of Cardiology
Department of Medicine
Northwestern University Feinberg School of Medicine
Bluhm Cardiovascular Institute
Chicago, Illinois

Christopher M. Kramer, MD
Ruth C. Heede Professor of Cardiology
Professor of Radiology
Director, Cardiovascular Imaging Center
University of Virginia Health System
Charlottesville, Virginia

Fay Y. Lin, MD
Assistant Professor of Research in Radiology
Director of Clinical Research at Dalio Institute of Cardiovascular Imaging
Weill Cornell Medicine
Dalio Institute of Cardiovascular Imaging
New York, New York

Justin B. Lundbye, MD, FACC, FASNC
Senior Vice President and Chief Medical Officer
The Greater Waterbury Health Network
Waterbury, Connecticut

Saurabh Malhotra, MD, MPH, FACC, FASNC
Assistant Professor of Medicine
Division of Cardiovascular Medicine
Jacobs School of Medicine and Biomedical Sciences
University at Buffalo
Clinical & Translational Research Center
Buffalo, New York

Sue Miller, CNMT
Chief Operating Officer
Molecular Imaging Services, Inc.
Newark, Delaware

Todd D. Miller, MD
Professor of Medicine
Mayo Clinic
Rochester, Minnesota

James K. Min, MD
Professor of Radiology and Medicine
Weill Cornell Medical College
Director, Dalio Institute of Cardiovascular Imaging
New York-Presbyterian Hospital
New York, New York

Sumeet S. Mitter, MD, MS
Cardiology Fellow
Division of Cardiology
Northwestern University Feinberg School of Medicine
Chicago, Illinois

Sanjeev U. Nair, MBBS, MD, FACP
Interventional Cardiology Fellow
Borgess Heart Institute
Michigan State University
Kalamazoo, Michigan

Lawrence M. Phillips, MD
Assistant Professor of Medicine, Division of Cardiology
Director, Nuclear Cardiology
New York University Langone Medical Center
New York, New York

Raja C. Pullatt, MD, FACC, FASNC
Associate Program Director
Clinical Assistant Professor of Medicine
Seton Hall University
Trinitas Regional Medical Center
Elizabeth, New Jersey

Gautam V. Ramani, MD
Assistant Professor of Medicine
Division of Cardiology
University of Maryland
Baltimore, Maryland

Archana Ramireddy, MD
Cardiology Fellow
Cardiovascular Division
University of Miami Miller School of Medicine
Miami, Florida

Upamanyu Rampal, MD
Cardiology Fellow
New York Medical College
Saint Joseph's Regional Medical Center
Paterson, New Jersey

Vera H. Rigolin, MD, FASE, FACC, FAHA
Professor of Medicine
Northwestern University Feinberg School of Medicine
Medical Director, Echocardiography Laboratory
Northwestern Memorial Hospital
Chicago, Illinois

Sarah J. Rinehart, MD
Clinical Assistant Professor
Director for Cardiovascular CT-MR Training at Piedmont Hospital
Fuqua Heart Center—Piedmont Hospital
Atlanta, Georgia

Dillenia Rosica, MD
Associate Professor
Department of Radiology
Geisinger Medical Center
Danville, Pennsylvania

Rupa M. Sanghani, MD, FACC, FASNC
Associate Professor of Medicine
Division of Cardiology
Rush University Medical Center
Chicago, Illinois

Sunil Selvin, CNMT
Vice President, Operations and Clinical Education
Molecular Imaging Services, Inc.
Newark, Delaware

Leslee J. Shaw, PhD
R. Bruce Logue Professor of Medicine
Co-Director, Emory Clinical Cardiovascular Research Institute
Emory University School of Medicine
Atlanta, Georgia

Prem Soman, MD, PhD, FRCP (UK)
Associate Professor of Medicine (Cardiology), and Clinical & Translational Science
Director, Nuclear Cardiology
Director, Advanced Cardiac Imaging Fellowship
University of Pittsburgh Medical Center
Pittsburgh, Pennsylvania

Raymond Taillefer, MD, FRCP, ABNM
Professor of Nuclear Medicine
Department of Radiology
Université de Montréal
Department of Nuclear Medicine
Hôpital du Haut-Richelieu
CISSS de la Montérégie-Centre
Saint-Jean-sur-Richelieu
Québec, Canada

E. Lindsey Tauxe, MEd, CNMT, FASNC
Operations Director
Medicine-Cardiovascular Disease
University of Alabama at Birmingham
Birmingham, Alabama

Jason S. Tavel, PhD, DABR
Medical Physicist
Astarita Associates, Inc.
Smithtown, New York

Peter L. Tilkemeier, MD, MMM
Chair, Department of Medicine, Greenville Health System
Professor, University of South Carolina School of Medicine Greenville
Professor, Clemson University School of Health Research
Department of Medicine
Greenville, South Carolina

Mark I. Travin, MD, FACC, FASNC
Department of Radiology/Division of Nuclear Medicine
Director of Cardiovascular Nuclear Medicine
Montefiore Medical Center
Professor of Clinical Radiology and Clinical Medicine
Albert Einstein College of Medicine
Bronx, New York

Kim A. Williams, MD, MACC, FAHA, MASNC, FESC
James B. Herrick Professor
Chief, Division of Cardiology
Rush University School of Medicine
Chicago, Illinois

Joe X. Xie, MD
Fellow, Department of Cardiology
Emory University School of Medicine
Atlanta, Georgia

PREFACE

Welcome to the third edition of *Nuclear Cardiology: Practical Applications*. This third edition reflects a substantial revision of our first two editions. A greatly expanded section on PET imaging is now present and additional chapters have been added to enhance many of the basic principles of nuclear cardiology, including radiopharmaceuticals, instrumentation, quality imaging, and radiation exposure. Most chapters have been reorganized and several topics combined to provide maximum understanding and clarity. Throughout the book, focus is placed on the clinical applications of imaging technology and a separate chapter on the appropriate use of radionuclide imaging has been added. Once again, this text features considerable graphic content and case illustrations.

Although this book is primarily intended to be practical and clinically useful, we have included chapters that delve in greater detail into the procedural aspects of contemporary nuclear cardiology. Chapters dealing with clinical disease states and the use of radionuclide cardiac imaging focus on diagnosis and risk stratification of patients with known or suspected coronary artery disease, evaluation of therapy, acute chest pain, and heart failure are all revised. This edition also presents newer and emerging techniques in nuclear cardiology, which are currently available or are anticipated shortly, such as neurohumoral imaging, the use of hybrid technology, and cardiac inflammatory and infection imaging. Alternative cardiac imaging modalities are presented in extensively revised chapters in order to provide a perspective of the role of nuclear cardiology in patient management in relation to other options.

While this textbook is useful for all practitioners of nuclear cardiology and for health care providers who refer for these procedures, we believe that it is ideally suited for trainees, including cardiology fellows and radiology residents who seek information that is easy to understand and readily usable. In addition, the book should be useful for examination review. To this end, we have included more than 100 questions to aid in board review preparation, with the in-depth answers and explanations.

We thank our many colleagues who have provided vital material for this book, which will once again allow *Nuclear Cardiology: Practical Applications* to be critically important for readers and one of the most useful educational products in the field of cardiac imaging. As authors and editors, we are proud of our offering and we hope that our readers find true value in this book for optimizing the clinical practice of nuclear cardiology.

Gary V. Heller
Robert C. Hendel

SECTION 1

FUNDAMENTALS OF NUCLEAR CARDIOLOGY

Fundamentals of Nuclear Cardiology Physics

CHAPTER 1

E. Lindsey Tauxe

INTRODUCTION

A practical review of basic atomic and nuclear physics is essential to understand the origins of radiations, as well as their interactions with matter. The nature and type of emissions are determined by the structural character of the atom and nucleus. The ways in which radiation interacts with matter have a direct relationship with imaging and radiation safety. The types of radiation and how they interact with matter are the foundation of radionuclide imaging and radiation safety. This chapter will focus on atomic and nuclear structure and the interaction of radiations with matter as they relate to radionuclide imaging.

ATOMIC AND NUCLEAR STRUCTURE

Matter is composed of atoms and the characteristics of a specific form of matter are determined by the number and type of atoms that make it up. How atoms combine is a function of their electron structure. The electron structure is determined by the nuclear architecture. As we have yet to image the atom, its structure is based on a "most-probable" model that fits physical behaviors we observe. The probabilistic approach is based on the model of the atom proposed by Niels Bohr in 1913. The Bohr atom proposed a positively charged nucleus, surrounded by negatively charged electrons. A neutral atom is one in which the positive and negative charges are matched. A mismatch in these charges determines the ionic character of the atom, which is the basis for its chemistry. The electron configuration is also a source for emissions used in radionuclide imaging.

These emissions, or *radiations*, may be in either of the two forms: particulate or electromagnetic. The origins of either type of radiation may be from the nucleus or the electron structure.

▶ Electron Configuration

Electrons are arranged around the nucleus in shells. The number of shells is determined by the number of electrons, which is, in turn, determined by the number of protons in the nucleus. The force exerted on these shells, called *binding energy*, is determined by the proximity of the shell to the nucleus. Higher binding energies are exerted on shells closest to the nucleus and conversely, lower binding energy for those more distant from the nucleus. The innermost shell is named the "K" shell and electrons in this shell are subject to the highest binding energy. The magnitude of that energy is dependent on the positive forces, which is determined by the number of protons in the nucleus. The shells more distant from the nucleus are named L, M, N, and so on. Each of these shells has lower binding energies as a result of their distance from the nucleus (Fig. 1-1).

The radii of each of these shells increase as a function of their distance from the nucleus. An expression of this is given by assigning an integer value (1, 2, 3, …) to each shell. The lower values represent smaller radii. These integer values are called *quantum numbers*. Therefore, the K shell has a quantum

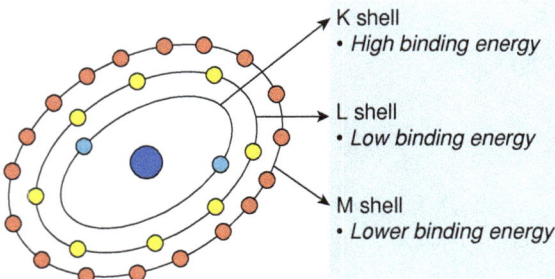

FIGURE 1-1 Atomic structure. The nucleus is surrounded by electron shells. The binding energy decreases as the distance from the nucleus increases (K > L > M).

number of 1, L = 2, M = 3, etc. This pattern continues until all available electrons are bound to a shell. The innermost shells are filled with electrons preferentially. The maximum number of electrons is specific to each shell and is calculated by $2n^2$, where *n* is the *quantum number*. Therefore, the maximum number of electrons for each shell is:

K = quantum #1 = $2(1)^2$ = 2 electrons
L = quantum #2 = $2(2)^2$ + 8 electrons
M = quantum #3 = $2(3)^2$ + 18 electrons…

These shells are further subdivided into *substates*. The number of *substates* for each shell can be calculated by $2n - 1$; therefore:

K shell = 2(1) − 1 = 1 substate
L shell = 2(2) − 1 = 3 substates
M shell = 2(3) − 1 = 5 substates

Each substate for a given shell will have a unique binding energy. For instance, the L shell has 3 substates, L_I, L_{II}, and L_{III}.[1] Each of these has slightly different distances from the nucleus, and therefore slightly different binding energies (Fig. 1-2).[2]

Atomic Radiations

Electrons in inner shells being under high binding energy and thus tightly bound to the nucleus are in an inherently low-energy state. Outer shell and free electrons are in an inherently higher-energy state. Therefore, to move an inner shell electron to an outer shell *requires* energy. The amount of energy required is simply the difference between binding energies.

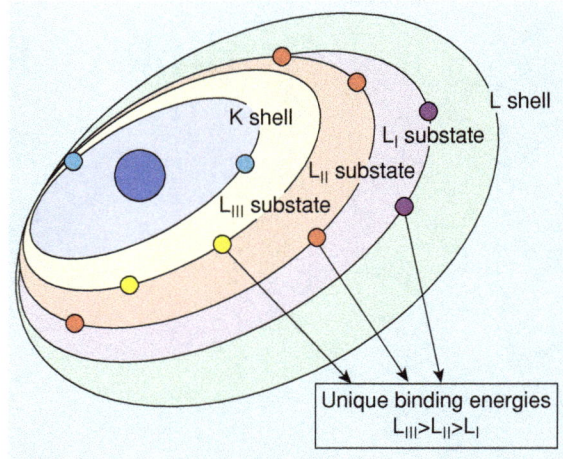

FIGURE 1-2 Electron configuration. Electrons are arranged in subshells, as illustrated for the L shell. Each subshell has a unique binding energy.

Example: Binding energy for a hypothetical "K" shell = 100 keV and "L" = 50 keV. $K_{100} - L_{50}$ = 50 keV of energy *input* to move the electron.

Conversely, the movement of an electron from an outer shell to an inner shell, L → K, yields energy. This energy yield results in the emission of radiation. The energy of the radiation is equal to the differences in binding energies of the shells. The radiation may take on two different forms: characteristic x-ray or Auger (oh-zhay) effect.

Example: Binding energy for a hypothetical "K" shell = 100 keV and "L" = 50 keV. $K_{100} - L_{50}$ = 50 keV of energy *given* to the electron.

Characteristic x-rays are electromagnetic radiations (photons) that are created when an outer shell electron moves to fill an inner shell vacancy. This vacancy may occur for several reasons—to be discussed later. The energy of this photon is equal to the difference between binding energies. Since binding energies are determined by, or characteristic of, the number of protons in the nucleus, and it is the number of protons that determines an element's identity, the characteristic x-ray energies are specific to each element and the electron shells from which they originate. X-radiation is defined as an electromagnetic radiation originating outside the nucleus, therefore the term characteristic x-ray.

The Auger effect occurs under the same conditions as characteristic x-ray, that is, an inner shell vacancy being filled by an outer shell electron. The difference is that the excess energy from the cascading electron is radiated to another electron. This ejects that electron from its shell. This free electron will have kinetic energy equal to the difference in the binding energies less the binding energy of the shell of the free electron. The Auger effect is more common in elements with lower numbers of protons (Z number).[1-3]

Nuclear Structure

The nucleus is composed mainly of neutrons and protons. Any particle contributing to the structure of the nucleus is called a *nucleon*. The conventional nomenclature to describe the nucleons is: $^A_Z X_N$.

$$(P + N) = A$$
$$(\# \text{ of } P) = Z \quad N = (\# \text{ of } N)$$

The total mass of an atom is essentially the combined masses of the nucleons. Electrons contribute less than 1% to the total mass.[1]

Nuclides having the same number of protons (Z number) are called *isotopes*. Isotopes may exhibit different atomic masses (A number) and therefore have different numbers of neutrons (N number). Nuclides with the same N are called *isotones* and will be different elements, since the Z numbers are different. Nuclides with the same A number are called *isobars* and different elements as well.

Isotopes having different N numbers are of particular interest to imagers because they have the same chemistry, since their Z numbers and, therefore, electron numbers are the same.[1-5] Some isotopes exhibit the emission of radiations, which is due to the differences in the number of neutrons. These isotopes are called *unstable*. If all the stable isotopes of all elements are plotted, comparing proton number to neutron number, a pattern emerges as illustrated in Figure 1-3.

Elements with low Z numbers have proton to neutron ratios that are 1:1. As Z numbers increase, this ratio increases to as high as 1.5. This distribution of stable elements is called the *line of stability*. By definition, an element with a proton to neutron ratio that falls to either the left or right of the line of *line of stability* is unstable. The unstable isotopes, *radioisotopes*, are unstable because their nuclear configurations are either proton rich or neutron rich relative to stable configurations. These radioactive elements

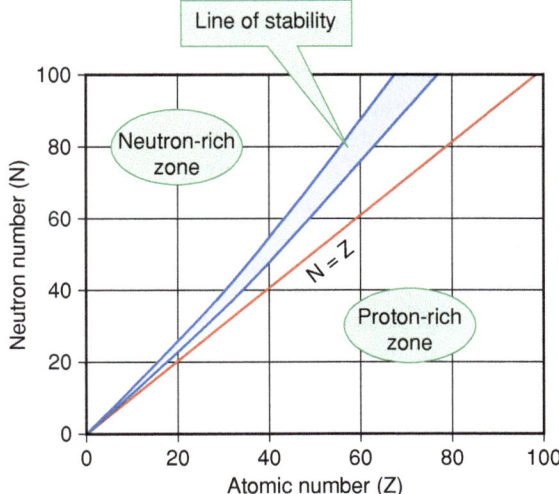

FIGURE 1-3 Line of stability. All naturally occurring stable nuclides fall along a distribution known as the line of stability (LOS). As illustrated, for light elements (Z < 20) N ~ Z and for heavier elements N ~ 1.5Z. Unstable elements, lying to the left of the LOS, are neutron rich; those lying to the right of the LOS are proton rich.

seek stability by undergoing transformations in their nuclear configurations to a more stable P ↔ N ratio. The type of transformation will be a result of P ↔ N ratio, that is, proton rich versus neutron rich. This type of transition is called the mode of decay.[1-4]

Modes of Decay

The goal of nuclear decay is to equate the balance of forces in the nucleus. The repelling forces originating from the positive charge (*coulombic forces*) of the protons, when matched by the attractive forces from within the nucleus (*exchange forces*), define **stability**. When these forces are mismatched, nuclear transformations (*radioactive decay*) result. The mode of decay will produce unique emissions and lead to a more stable nuclear configuration. In radionuclide imaging, the ideal mode of decay would result in a high yield of photons, at an energy that is efficiently detected by our imaging instrumentation. Photon emission is also desirable from the radiation safety and dosimetry perspectives, due to their lower probability of creating potentially damaging interactions as compared to particles. With these considerations, it is important to understand the modes of decay of ^{99m}Technetium, ^{201}Thallium, and ^{82}Rubidium—the most commonly used radionuclides used in nuclear cardiology.[1,2,6]

β⁻ Decay

In an unstable nuclear configuration where the nucleus is neutron rich, β⁻ decay occurs. To decrease the neutron–proton ratio, a neutron is converted to a proton and an energized electron is emitted. The expression of this nuclear transition is:

$$n \rightarrow p + e^- + \nu + \text{energy}$$

where n is the neutron, p the proton, e the electron, and ν the neutrino.

The neutrino (ν) behaves like a particle with no mass and is not critical to imaging considerations. The primary emission is the energized electron (e^-). The nuclear configuration that results from β⁻ decay is a *daughter* with a stable or more stable energy state and an additional proton in its nucleus.

Example: $^X_Z A_N \rightarrow ^X_{Z+1} B_{N-1}$

Since the number of protons is changed, the elemental identity changes. This is called a *transmutation*. The *daughter* atomic mass (X) remains the same as the *parent* nucleus, and the energy carried off by the ejected electron called *transition energy*. This leads to a more balanced relationship of *coulombic* force (repelling forces due to the protons) and *exchange force* (attractive nuclear forces). The resulting emission of the energized electron, a β⁻ particle, is of no use in imaging and contributes to an increase in radiation dose in a biologic system. This decay process may lead to a *daughter* that is not fully stable, but more stable than the *parent*.[1,2]

β⁺ Decay

In nuclear configurations where the *parent* is proton rich, β⁺ decay may occur. In this mode of decay, a proton is converted to a neutron and the emission of an energized, positively charged electron (β⁺) results. The nuclear equation is:

$$p \rightarrow n + e^+ + \nu + \text{energy}$$

The energy of the β⁺ particle contributes to resolving the *transition energy* between the unstable parent and more stable daughter, as in β⁻ decay.

An important secondary emission will result from the formation of the β⁺ particle. Since there is an abundance of negatively charged electrons in nature, the resulting positively charged electron (β⁺) will be attracted to, and collide with, a free negatively charged electron. This collision results in the *annihilation* of both particles. The annihilation leads to the conversion of the mass of these particles to their equivalent energy state. This is expressed by Einstein's equation $E = mc^2$, where E is energy, m the mass, and c the speed of light. This essentially states that energy and mass are simply two physical forms of the same thing. Therefore, two photons (E) are emitted, each with the energy equivalent to the mass (m) of an electron, which is 511 keV. Unique to this annihilation is that these photons are emitted in a 180-degree trajectory from each other. It is these photons that are detected and registered into an image in positron imaging. The change in nuclear configuration is a decrease in Z and increase in N.

Example: $^X_Z A_N \rightarrow ^X_{Z} B_{N+1}$

Electron Capture

An alternative to β⁺ decay in proton-rich nuclear configuration, is *electron capture*. This mode of decay is defined as the capture of a K-shell electron by the nucleus, the subsequent combination with a proton, and creation of a neutron. The nuclear expression is therefore:

$$p + e^- \rightarrow n + \nu + \text{energy}$$

The vacancy left by the captured electron would then be filled by an outer shell electron. A cascade of an electron, filling subsequent vacancies, creates secondary emissions called, *characteristic x-rays* and *Auger electrons*. The energies of these emissions will be characteristic of the binding energy of the daughter, since the nuclear transition occurred prior to the production of the x-rays and Auger electrons. It is the *characteristic x-rays* that are imaged in ^{201}Tl myocardial perfusion imaging. The energy of the x-rays is determined by the binding energy of ^{201}Hg, the daughter of the decay of ^{201}Tl. Electron capture decreases proton–neutron ratio.[1]

Example: $^X_Z A_N \rightarrow ^X_{Z-1} B_{N+1}$

Isometric Transitions and Internal Conversions

The daughter of the decay of a radioactive parent will ideally be in its most stable energy configuration or *ground state*. This does not always occur, leading to either of two unstable states; *excited state* or *metastable state*. Excited states are very unstable and exist for very short time periods, usually less than 10^{-12} seconds. Metastable states, however, may exist for several hours. These metastable states lead to the release of energy in the form of radiation, without changing the proton–neutron ratios. The parent nucleus has the same nuclear structure as the daughter, but in a more stable energy configuration. This form of decay is called an *isometric transition* and results in electromagnetic emissions called γ-*rays*. These radiations are the same as x-rays, differing only by their location of origin, that is, the nucleus. As noted with the production of characteristic x-rays, there is a competing process, resulting in a particulate radiation. This process is called *internal conversion*. For any given metastable state, there is a specific ratio of *isometric transitions* to *internal conversions*. In imaging, the higher percentage of isometric transitions compared to internal conversions is preferred due to the resulting higher yield of photons. The decay of ^{99m}Tc to ^{99}Tc is an example of an isometric transition of the metastable state (^{99m}Tc). The percent occurrence of isometric transitions of a population of ^{99m}Tc nuclei is approximately 87%. For example, for every 100 decays of ^{99m}Tc nuclei, there is a yield of 87 γ photons and 13 internal conversion electrons.

For any given mode of decay, should the daughter be metastable, there will be the emission of γ-photons and internal conversion electrons as secondary emissions. This will be indicated as [B$^-$, γ], [B$^+$, γ], [EC, γ], and so forth. The internal conversion electron yield, in ratio to γ-photon yield, is specific to a given radionuclide.[1,2,5]

Alpha (α) Decay

In unstable nuclei with very high atomic masses, the most probable mode of decay is α decay. An alpha particle consists of two protons and two neurons, which is essentially a helium nucleus. Alpha decay results in a daughter with a Z number of 2 less than the parent and an atomic mass less by 4 relative to the parent.

Example: $^{X}_{Z}A_{N} \xrightarrow{\alpha} {}^{X-4}_{Z-2}B_{N-2}$

Due to its high charges and heavy mass, the alpha particle has a very short travel distance in matter and deposits its energy very quickly. It has no application in diagnostic imaging and induces significant potential for biologic damage.[1,3]

Decay Schemes

The modes of decay may be expressed graphically, called *decay schemes*. Decay schemes graphically illustrate all possible nuclear transitions that unstable nuclei undergo. They are often accompanied by tables with detailed information about the transitions such as the percentage occurrence, isomeric transitions, internal conversions, characteristic x-rays, Auger electrons, and biologic dose information.

In decay schemes, the nuclear energy levels are expressed as horizontal lines. The space between these lines represents the *transition energy (Q)*.

The types of emissions are depicted by a unique direction of a line (Fig. 1-4).

Note the arrows may be angled to either the right or left. In neutron-rich parents, the mode of decay "shifts" the daughter to the right, corresponding to the shift on to the line of stability graph. Conversely, a mode of decay for a proton-rich parent moves to the left, toward the line of stability.

The tables that accompany decay schemes provide additional detail including the secondary emissions, as mentioned earlier. Since many of the secondary emissions are particulate, that is, electrons, these data are of particular interest in radiation dosimetry.

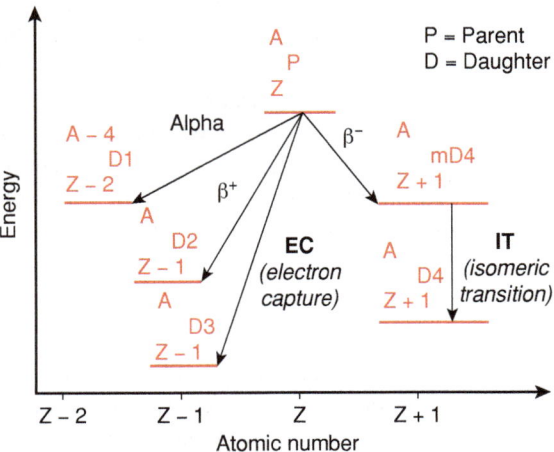

FIGURE 1-4 Decay schemes. This figure illustrates the configurations of decay schemes for the different modes of decay. The schemes move to the left for proton-rich radionuclides and to the right for radionuclides that are neutron rich.

In the decay scheme for ^{201}Tl, the data regarding the characteristic x-rays of ^{201}Hg are in these tables.

Parent–Daughter Equilibrium

Not all nuclear transitions lead to a stable daughter. The β$^-$ decay of ^{99}Mo yields ^{99m}Tc, which then decays to ^{99m}Tc by *isometric transitions* and *internal conversions*. ^{99m}Tc decays to ^{99}Tc with an 87% frequency through isometric transitions. Therefore, for every 100 decays of ^{99m}Tc, we observe 87 γ-rays and 13 internal conversion electrons, as stated earlier. This higher yield of photons makes ^{99m}Tc a very desirable radionuclide for imaging. A sample of ^{99}Mo would always contain some proportion of ^{99m}Tc and ^{99}Tc. Since both parent and daughter are decaying, the relative activities would reach equilibrium, based on their half-lives. These states of equilibrium are employed when using both technetium and rubidium generators. When the parent half-life is marginally longer than that of the daughter, the amount of the daughter in the mixture will reach a maximum over a period of time. That elapsed time will be a multiple of half-lives of the daughter. If the daughter radionuclide is removed from the mixture, the same multiple of half-lives will have to occur, before the maximum amount of the daughter is subsequently reached. This equilibrium state is called *transient equilibrium*.[2,4] It is this transient state that is the basis of ^{99m}Tc production from ^{99}Mo–^{99m}Tc generators (Fig. 1-5).

In parent–daughter mixtures where the half-life of the parent is markedly longer than that of the daughter, *secular equilibrium* is reached. In this state of equilibrium, the concentration of the parent is decreasing so slowly relative to the daughter that the mixture appears to have the half-life of the parent. It is this equilibrium that is the basis for the ^{82}Sr–^{82}Rb generators used in ^{82}Rb PET imaging (Fig. 1-6).[1]

RADIOACTIVITY

The specific time that an unstable nucleus will undergo a transition cannot be determined, only *predicted*. Nuclear transitions are spontaneous and random, so the mathematics of radioactive are based on probabilities and rates, not specific nuclear events. If a population of radioactive atoms, N, is considered, the rate of nuclear transitions would be expressed as

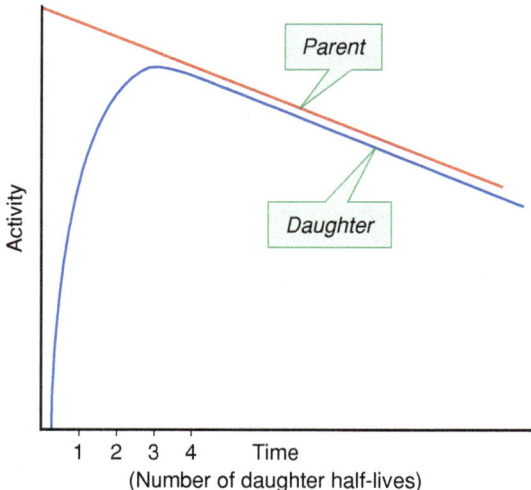

FIGURE 1-5 Transient equilibrium. When the parent half-life is marginally longer than that of the daughter, the amount of daughter activity will reach a maximum after relatively few daughter half-lives have passed. ^{99}Mo and ^{99m}Tc typically reach transient equilibrium after approximately four ^{99m}Tc half-lives.

$\Delta N/\Delta t$. The rate implies that a constant would express the average number of transitions that occur per unit time. This constant is called the *decay constant*; which is specific to a given radionuclide and is expressed

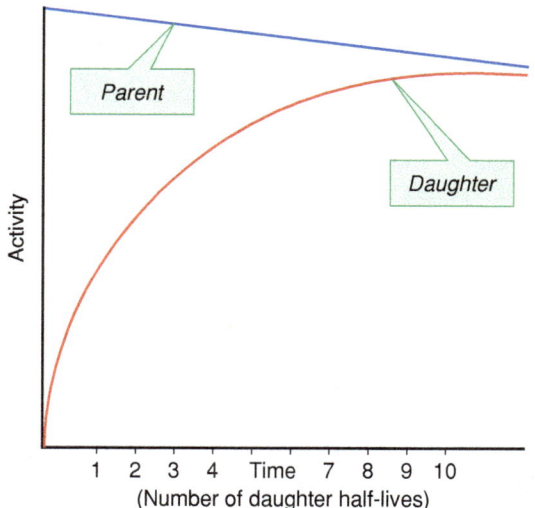

FIGURE 1-6 Secular equilibrium. When the parent half-life is considerably longer than that of the daughter, the amount of parent activity will decrease very little over time. Therefore, many more daughter half-lives must pass before equilibrium is reached. An example is ^{82}Sr with a half-life of 25 days and ^{82}Rb with a 1.2-minute half-life.

as λ. The mathematical relationship is: $\Delta N/\Delta t = -\lambda N$, where N is the total number of radioactive nuclei and λ the decay constant. Since the total N decreases with time (t), the decay constant (λ) is a negative value.[1,2,4] The number of transitions per unit time ($\Delta N/\Delta t$) is called *activity*. Activity is measured in curies (Ci), which is defined as 3.7×10^{10} disintegrations per second (dps). The International System of Units (SI) unit equivalent is the becquerel (Bq), which is defined as $Bq = 1$ dps. So 1 Ci $= 3.7 \times 10^{10}$ Bq. The most commonly used units are in the mCi (MBq) range for nuclear cardiology procedures.

In nuclear decay, the number of radioactive nuclei (N) is always decreasing as time passes at an average rate defined by the decay constant (λ). Decay is expressed, therefore, as exponential function; that is, the number of radioactive nuclei available is affected by both the number of unstable nuclei and its average rate of decay. To calculate the specific number of decays for a given time, we have the following expression:

$$N_{(t)} = N_{(0)}\, e^{-\lambda t}$$

where $N_{(t)}$ is the number of unstable nuclei remaining after elapsed time (t) can be used. The expression $e^{-\lambda t}$ is called the *decay factor* (DF) and is unique to the time (t) and the decay constant (λ). The "e" is the base of natural logs, which is 2.718, so, when raised to the power of $-\lambda t$, it determines the specific fraction of remaining radioactive nuclei after time (t) has elapsed.

When the elapsed time (t) is the time required for half of the total number of radioactive nuclei to decay, it is termed the *half-life*. Half-life ($T_{1/2}$) and decay constant (λ) are related as:

$$T_{1/2} = \frac{\ln 2}{\lambda}$$

Since $\ln 2$ is equal to 0.693, we have

$$T_{1/2} = \frac{0.693}{\lambda}$$

The activity (Ci) is dependent on the number of unstable nuclei and the decay constant. Therefore, units of activity (A) can be substituted for the number of radioactive nuclei (N), in the decay equation, yielding the following expression:

$$A_{(t)} = A_{(0)}\, e^{-\lambda t}$$

where $A_{(t)}$ is the activity at elapsed time t, $A_{(0)}$ the activity at $t = 0$, and $e^{-\lambda t}$ the decay factor for the specific time (t).

As an example of practical use, consider a 30-mCi syringe of a ^{99m}Tc-labeled myocardial perfusion agent. The calibration time for the 30 mCi is 8:00 AM. What will be the activity at 9:45 AM?

$$A_{(0)} = 30 \text{ mCi}$$
$$A_{(t)} = ?$$
$$t = 1 \text{ h, } 45 \text{ min or } 1.75 \text{ h}$$
$$\lambda = \frac{0.693}{T_{1/2}} = \frac{0.693}{6 \text{ h}} = 0.1155$$
$$30 = A_{(t)}^{-(0.1155)(1.75)}$$
$$30 = A_{(t)} \times 0.817$$
$$A_{(t)} = 24.51 \text{ mCi}$$

The same principles apply in the situation where an activity determination is required for a time (t) in the past, the *precalibrated* value. In this case, the DF would be the reciprocal of the elapsed time decay factor[1,2]:

$$DF = \frac{1}{0.817}$$
$$DF = 1.22$$

So, we have:

$$A_{(0)} = (24.51)(1.22) = 30 \text{ mCi}$$

INTERACTIONS OF RADIATION WITH MATTER

As discussed earlier, there are distinct types of radiations; particulate and electromagnetic. These radiations have distinct interactions with matter. Interactions of radiations with matter are processes that absorb or degrade the energy of the radiation and, in some cases, change its fundamental characteristics. The energy of the radiation and the Z number of the matter determine the type of interaction or multiple interactions that occur. Depending on the energy, radiations may be *nonionizing*; that is, the energy is not sufficient to free electrons from their orbit. If the energy is sufficient to free electrons from their binding energy, the radiation is *ionizing*. The energy of the ultrasound radiations in echocardiography does not cause ionization in tissues, and thus are labeled "nonionizing." The photons used in cardiac catheterization and nuclear cardiology are classified as ionizing, implying that their interaction with tissue creates ion pairs. This interaction in tissue forms the basis for radiation biology as applied in radiation safety practices. Further, these interactions form the physical bases for detecting radiation and creating images in our instrumentation.

▶ Particle Interactions with Matter

As we have stated, radionuclide images are created through the detection of photons, γ-rays for ^{99m}Tc, characteristic x-rays for ^{201}Tl, and annihilation photons for ^{82}Rb and other PET radiopharmaceuticals. When photons undergo interactions in matter, either tissue or imaging detectors, energized charged particles, that is, electrons, are produced. Particles, either β or α, interact with matter through electrical collisions. These collisions result in excitation, ionization, or bremsstrahlung. In excitation, energy from the incident particle is transferred to an outer shell electron. The electron is energized but does not exceed its binding energy. That increased energy is dissipated generally as heat radiation. Excitation is a low-energy interaction.

A higher-energy interaction occurs when the incident particle transfers enough energy to exceed the binding energy of the electron. An ion pair, an energized free electron and a positive ion, results. These ionizing interactions represent higher-energy level interactions and contribute to the specific exposure rate when applied to tissue, discussed in detail in a later chapter.

The third type of particulate interaction results when the incident particle penetrates the electron cloud and interacts with the charge field of the nucleus. The trajectory of the incident particle is markedly changed, resulting in a decrease in velocity. The decrease in velocity represents an energy loss. That energy loss produces photons of x-rays called *bremsstrahlung*, German for breaking radiation. Bremsstrahlung interactions are high-energy interactions more typical of high-energy particles interacting with high Z number matter.

Since any of these interactions may lead to partial dissipation of the energy of the incident particle, multiple interactions are required for the full energy of the particle to be absorbed in matter. These multiple interactions occur along a path that is determined by the energy, charge and mass of the particle, as well as the Z number of the matter. A highly charged massive particle will undergo many high-energy interactions over a very short path length. Alternately, a lower energy, less massive particle will undergo several low-energy interactions over a long path length. The difference in the degree of penetrability of the particle is called *linear energy transfer* (LET). A heavy highly charged particle would have a high LET, since the density of interactions is high over a short path length. An alpha particle because of its high charge (two protons) and heavy mass ($Z = 2$; $A = 4$) has high LET where dense levels of excitation, ionization, and bremsstrahlung are created in a very short distance. In contrast, a β particle, having little charge and mass, will lose its energy over a longer path length, and is thus characterized as low-LET particle. The LET may also be expressed in terms of the relative number of ionizations that are produced. This is termed *specific ionization*. Particles with high LET have high SI values; particles with low LET have low SI values. LET and SI characteristics have profound impact on the type of damage done to tissue.

▶ Photon Interactions with Matter

The interactions of photons in matter are energy-degrading processes, just as in particle interactions. There are three mechanisms of photon interaction in matter; *photoelectric absorption*, *Compton scatter*, and *pair production*. The probability of occurrence for each of these mechanisms is a function of the energy of the photon and the atomic number of the matter (Fig. 1-7).

Photoelectric absorption occurs when the photon transfers all of its energy to an inner shell electron. The photon is completely absorbed and the electron, called a *photoelectron*, is ejected from its shell. The energy of the photoelectron is equal to the incident photon energy, minus the binding energy of its shell. It is key to remember that the photon no longer exists (it has been absorbed) and its energy is converted from electromagnetic energy to kinetic energy of the photoelectron. The kinetic energy of the photoelectron is dissipated by the mechanisms previously discussed: excitation, ionization, and bremsstrahlung.

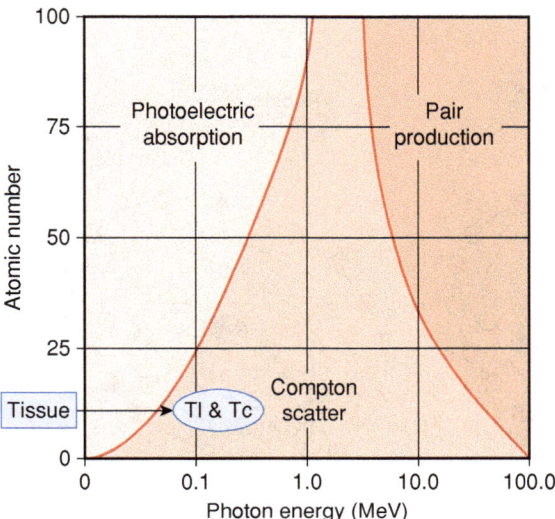

FIGURE 1-7 Probability of interaction. The probability of the interaction of a photon in matter as a function of photon energy and *Z* number is illustrated. Note the most probable interaction of photon from either ^{99m}Tc or ^{201}Tl, in tissue, is Compton scatter.

The vacancy left by the ejected electron is quickly filled by an outer shell electron. Characteristic x-rays and Auger electrons are then emitted, as described earlier. Photoelectric absorption is most probable in interactions of low- to medium-energy photons in matter with high atomic numbers.

The second mode of interaction is Compton scatter. It occurs when a photon interacts with an outer shell electron, that is, an electron with low binding energy. Contrary to photoelectric absorption, the photon is not completely absorbed. It transfers a *portion* of its energy to the electron, which is subsequently ejected, and called a *Compton electron*. The resultant Compton scattered photon is in an energy-degraded state and in an altered trajectory relative to the incident photon. The angle of the scattered photon is related to the amount of energy transferred to the electron. The greater the amount of energy transferred to the electron, the greater the angle of scatter. Compton scatter is most probable in low- to medium-energy photons, interacting in matter with low atomic masses. This is of particular interest in imaging, since it is the most probable interaction of ^{201}Tl (Hg x-rays) and ^{99m}Tc γ-rays in tissues. As the photons are scattered, not absorbed, they still exist, but have lost their association with the point of origin through the scattering process. These photons are the source of image degradation, but can be identified by their lower-energy values. The identification of these photons and their rejection from an image is a critical function of imaging equipment.[1-5]

The third interaction of photons in matter is pair production. High-energy photons may completely avoid interacting with orbital electrons and interact in the magnetic field of the nucleus. This interaction results in the creation of a pair of electrons, one positive and one negative. The positive electron immediately combines with a negative electron, creating two 511-keV annihilation photons. The energy of the incident photon must be at least two times the mass energy equivalency of an electron (511 keV) or 1.022 MeV. Since energies in this range are not used in imaging, pair production is not relevant to this discussion.[2]

In all three mechanisms, there are probabilities of occurrence based on photon energy and atomic number. The distribution of the probabilities is shown in Figure 1-8.

Attenuation

These interactive processes, in addition to photon energy and atomic number, are affected by the thickness of the absorber. For a given thickness, a number of photons will not interact and therefore be transmitted. As the thickness of the absorber *increases*, the fraction of transmitted photons will *decrease*. The fraction of absorbed photons is a function of photon energy and atomic number, but the *total* number of photons absorbed is a function of the *thickness* of the absorber.[1] For any given relationship of photon energy and atomic number, there is an *average rate* of absorption. The rate is called the *linear attenuation coefficient* and is symbolized by μ. Since the linear attenuation coefficient is a fixed rate, the rate of transmitted photons is also fixed. If the thickness of a given absorber is doubled, those transmitted photons will be subject to further absorption. The mathematical relationship of incident beam intensity, transmitted beam intensity, and linear attenuation is exponential.

The mathematical expression is:

$$I_{(x)} = I_{(0)} e^{-\mu x}$$

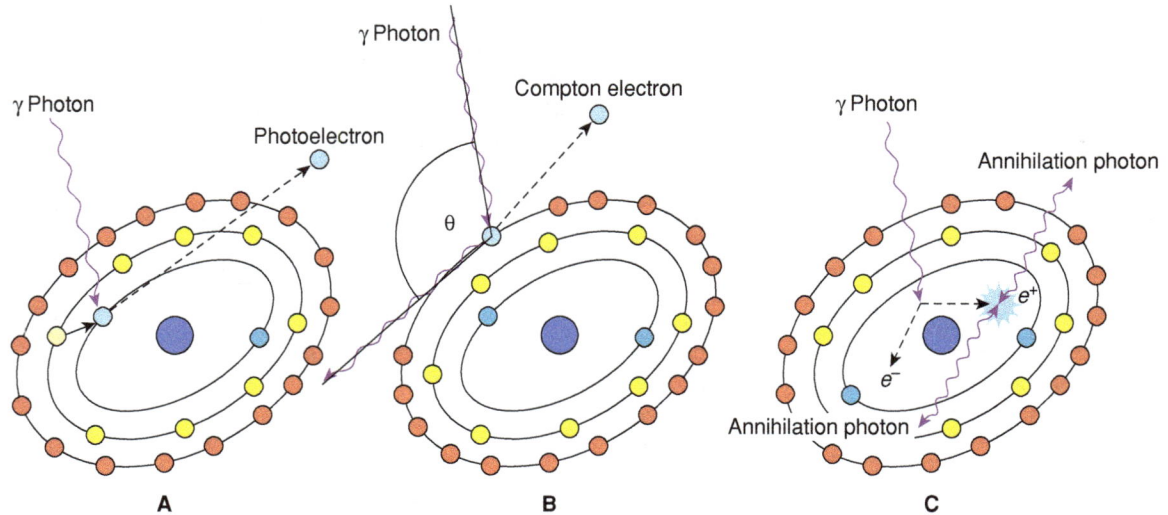

FIGURE 1-8 **(A)** Photoelectric absorption. All photon energy is transferred to the ejected photoelectron. **(B)** Compton scatter. Partial energy transfer, incident photon scattered by angle θ. **(C)** Pair production. Photon converts to an electron pair (e⁻, e⁺); annihilation photon results.

where $I_{(x)}$ is the beam intensity after interacting with an absorber of thickness x and a linear attenuation coefficient of μ, from an initial intensity $I_{(0)}$.[7] This mathematical expression is the same as used in predicting the reduction in activity over time. Therefore, the expression $e^{-\mu x}$ is the specific fraction of absorbed photons by a specific thickness of matter. The thickness of a given absorber that results in a reduction of initial beam intensity of 50% is called the half-value thickness (HVT) or half-value layer (HVL). The HVT can be calculated by,

$$\mathrm{HVT} = \frac{0.693}{\mu}$$

where μ is the linear attenuation coefficient and 0.693 is the ln 2. Note that this is the same equation as used in calculating the half-life of a radionuclide. The absorption characteristics of tissue are essentially the same as water, since the linear attenuation values are similar. Table 1-1 illustrates the differences in HVTs for lead, a common material used in shielding, water (tissue), and NaI, a common detector material in imaging equipment.

Note that the HVT for Tl (80 keV) and Tc (140 keV) are 39.6 and 46.2 mm, respectively. It is typical to have these thicknesses of tissue overlaying the heart. If these thicknesses reduce the beam intensity by 50%, the imaging effects would be a reduction in count density of 50%, as well. It is critical, therefore, to differentiate these tissue attenuation effects, from reductions in biodistributions of tracers in interpreting radionuclide images.

Table 1-1
Half-Value Thickness for Tl, Tc, and Rb

		Half-Value Thickness (mm)[a]		
Matter	Z Number	²⁰¹Tl	⁹⁹ᵐTc	⁸²Rb
Pb	82	0.25	0.30	3.80
Tissue (H₂O)	8	38.0	46.0	73.0
NaI	53	0.67	2.40	21.0

[a]Approximate values.

CONCLUSION

In summary, the photons we use to construct cardiac radionuclide images come from both nuclear and atomic sources, as demonstrated by the emissions from ^{99m}Tc and ^{201}Tl, respectively. The emissions used may also be the result of processes that are secondary to the primary emission, as seen with the annihilation photons from the decay of ^{82}Rb. The principles of the detectors used in imaging equipment, as well as those used in radiation safety, are based on characteristics of photons and the matter in which they interact. Those characteristics are defined by the physics of nuclear structure, mass–energy relationships, and radiation interactions in matter.

As a practical consideration, it is important to note that radionuclide image quality is directly related to the type, energy, and the behavior in matter of photons. The three mainstream radionuclides used in nuclear cardiology, ^{99m}Tc, ^{201}Tl, and ^{82}Rb, exhibit all of these physical differences, therefore familiarity with the physical basis of radiation physics is essential.

REFERENCES

1. Cherry SR, Sorenson JA, Phelps ME. *Physics in Nuclear Medicine*. 3rd ed. Philadelphia, PA: Saunders/Elsevier Science; 2003:7–16, 19–30, 31–43.
2. Chandra R. *Nuclear Medicine Physics*. 6th ed. Philadelphia, PA: Lippincott Williams and Wilkins; 2004:1–5, 7–13, 20–29.
3. Cook SE. *Moderate Atomic and Nuclear Physics*. Princeton, NJ: D. Van Nostrand Company, Inc.; 1961.
4. Murphy PH. Radiation physics and radiation safety. In: Iskandrian AE, Garcia EV, eds. *Nuclear Cardiac Imaging*. 4th ed. New York, NY: Oxford University Press; 2009:10–30.
5. Jelley NA. *Fundamentals of Nuclear Physics*. Cambridge, United Kingdom: Cambridge University Press; 1990:26–31, 140–158.
6. Heller GV, Hendel RC, eds. *Nuclear Cardiology Practical Applications*. 2nd ed. New York: McGraw-Hill; 2011:292–294.
7. Saha GB. *Basics of Pet Imaging*. New York: Springer Science + Business Media; 2005:1–14, 111–121.

Radiation Safety and Protection

CHAPTER 2

Jason S. Tavel

INTRODUCTION

The Health Physics Society defines radiation as "energy that comes from a source and travels through space."[1] The source could be atomic particles such as alpha and beta emissions as well as electromagnetic energy associated with AM/FM radio, radar, visible light, ultraviolet light, x-rays, and gamma rays. Radiation with enough energy to remove an electron from an atom is termed ionizing radiation.[2] A characteristic of x-rays, gamma rays, alpha and beta particles, radiation having this ability can lead to biological damage when absorbed in human tissue.

This chapter will introduce the common units to describe radiation, sources of radiation exposure, radiation dose limits, and an introduction to radiation biology. The chapter will further focus on radiation safety and protection regulations pertinent to the practice of Nuclear Cardiology. These regulations are governed by the Nuclear Regulatory Commission (NRC) and are found in Title 10, Parts 19, 20, and 35 of the Code of Federal Regulations (CFR). NRC NUREG 1556 Volume 9, Revision 2 provides guidance specific to radioactive materials licensing and offers suggested policies and procedures for radiation safety compliance.

RADIOLOGICAL UNITS

There are several conventional terms used when describing radiation. These include exposure, absorbed dose, and dose equivalent. Named after Wilhelm Roentgen, the scientist who discovered x-rays in 1895, the Roentgen (R) is the unit of radiation exposure in air.[3] In comparison to the International System of Units (SI), one Roentgen corresponds to the amount of radiation required to liberate 2.58×10^{-4} Coulombs per kilogram of air.

The Rad, or Radiation Absorbed Dose, is the measure of the amount of energy absorbed by an object as radiation passes through.[4] The amount of energy absorbed is dependent on the energy of the incident photon and the composition of the material. The f-factor is a tissue weighting factor used to convert exposure in air (R) to absorbed dose (rad) in tissue taking into account the x-ray or gamma ray energy and effective atomic number of the tissue exposed. For example, a 100-keV gamma photon incident on fat will transfer 91% of its energy, whereas the same photon will deliver 96% of its energy to muscle tissue. Therefore, a source of radiation exposing a point in air to 100 R will deliver a dose of 91 rad to fat tissue and 96 rad to muscle tissue at the same reference point.

Dose equivalent is a term used to quantify the amount of energy deposited in tissue along with the associated biological risk from the type of radiation.[5] The conventional unit for dose equivalent is rem which is calculated by multiplying the radiation absorbed dose (rad) by a radiation quality factor or QF.[6] Table 2-1 illustrates that the QF for x-rays, gamma rays, and beta particles is equal to 1 whereas the QF for alpha particles is 20.[7] This means that an absorbed dose of 10 rads from an

Table 2-1		
Quality Factors for Different Types of Ionizing Radiation		
Type of Radiation	Radiation Quality Factor (for Converting Absorbed Dose to Dose Equivalent)
X-ray and gamma rays	1
Beta particles	1
Neutrons	5–10
Alpha particles	20

x-ray, gamma ray, or beta particle equates to 10 rem (10 rad × 1), whereas the dose equivalent would be 200 rem (10 rad × 20) if originating from alpha particulates.

Although the conventional unit to describe absorbed dose and dose equivalent is the rad and rem, the international community now uses the term Gray (Gy) and Sievert (Sv), respectively. 1 Gy = 100 rad and 1 Sv = 100 rem. Table 2-2 provides a summary of the units of radiation exposure, absorbed dose, and dose equivalent.

SOURCES OF IONIZING RADIATION EXPOSURE

Ionizing radiation occurs naturally in the earth's soil and rock, in the cosmic rays descending from the sun and stars, as well as in our own body.[8] This ubiquitous background radiation in the United States totals approximately 3.1 mSv/yr across the population.[9] Exposure to Radon and its decay products accounts for the majority of the natural background radiation.

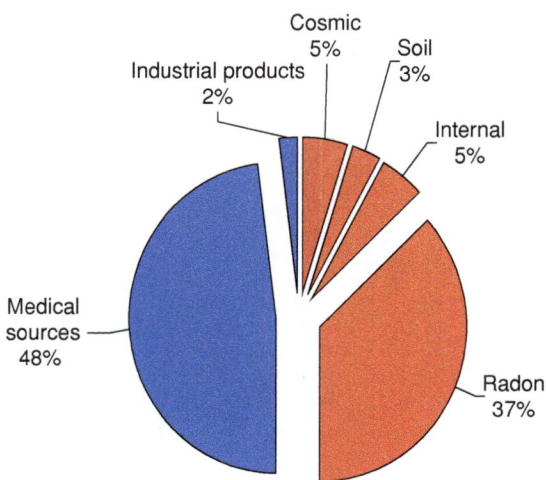

FIGURE 2-1 Background radiation in the United States. The U.S. population receives approximately 620 mrem (6.2 mSv) annually, with 50% from manmade sources and 50% from background radiation.

In addition to natural background, people are exposed to radiation in manufactured products such as smoke detectors, ceramics, and building materials, as well as from medical sources including diagnostic x-rays and nuclear medicine procedures.[10] The effective radiation dose from these products accounts for an additional 3.1 mSv/yr (Fig. 2-1). It is important to note that these estimates are population based and not all individuals are exposed to radiation from manufactured products and radiological examinations.

The term BERT, or Background Equivalent Radiation Time, has recently been introduced to explain levels of radiation dose to patients relative to natural background radiation exposure. Table 2-3 illustrates

Table 2-2			
Units of Radiation Exposure and Dose			
Quantity	Classical Unit	International Unit (SI)	Relationship
Exposure (in air)	Roentgen (R)	C/kg	1 R = 2.58 × 10⁻⁴ C/kg
Dose (in tissue)	Radiation absorbed dose (Rad = R × f)	Gray (Gy)	1 Gy = 100 rad 1 mGy = 0.1 rad
Dose equivalent (risk adjusted dose)	Roentgen equivalent in man (Rem = Rad × QF)	Sievert (Sv)	1 Sv = 100 rem 1 mSv = 0.1 rem

Table 2-3

Effective Radiation Dose from Common Examinations in Terms of Background Radiation

Examination	Effective Dose (mSv)	Background Equivalent Radiation Time (BERT)
^{99m}Tc—Tetrofosmin 40 mCi Stress/rest	10.2	3.3 years
^{201}Tl—Thallous Chloride	15.5	5 years
^{18}F-FDG[1]	7.0	2.3 years
Airplane round trip (NY to LA)	0.05	6 days

Data from ICRP: Radiation dose to patients from radiopharmaceuticals. Addendum 3 to ICRP Publication 53. ICRP Publication 106. Approved by the Commission in October 2007. *Ann ICRP.* 2008;38(1-2):1–197.

radiation doses to patients from Nuclear Cardiology procedures and their associated BERT.

RADIATION DOSE LIMITS AND INVESTIGATIONAL LEVELS

The regulations for dose limits in the United States can be found in Title 10, Part 20 of the Code of Federal Regulations (10 CFR 20). Table 2-4 illustrates these limits, which include limiting radiation to occupational workers, the embryo/fetus of an occupational worker, and the public. Both occupational and public dose limits exclude exposure to natural background radiation.

While the dose limit to the public from sources of ionizing radiation is 1 mSv (0.1 rem) per year, this limit may be increased to 5 mSv (0.5 rem) from an infrequent exposure related to another person's medical procedure providing the authorized user determines the exposure is appropriate.

Because it is impractical to set occupational worker dose limits to that of the public, regulators rely on the Linear Non-Threshold risk model to set limits at a point below which the threshold for radiation effects are known and at a point to minimize the theoretical effects from the stochastic risks from ionizing radiation exposure. The dose limits are established at levels of risk already assumed by occupational workers.[11] To this point, radiation dose limits are established at a level where the risk of a fatal cancer from occupational exposure to ionizing radiation is similar to the assumed risk of a fatal work accident, which is 1 in 10,000 annually.[12]

In addition to ensuring dose limits are not exceeded, an institution must adopt investigational levels in order to maintain radiation levels consistent

Table 2-4

Radiation Dose Limits in the United States

Area	Dose Limit
Occupational worker Whole-body total effective dose	0.05 Sv (5 rem) per year
Occupational worker Lens of the eye	0.15 Sv (15 rem) per year
Occupational worker Shallow dose to skin or extremity	0.5 Sv (50 rem) per year
Embryo/fetus of a declared pregnant Occupational worker	5 mSv (0.5 rem) over the gestation period
Individual member of the public	1 mSv (0.1 rem) per year
Individual member of the public—special circumstance	5 mSv (0.5 rem) per year

Data from Standards for Protection Against Radiation, 10 CFR §20.1201–1208, 1301. (2004).

Table 2-5
ALARA Investigational Levels

Area	ALARA Investigational Level I (Per Calendar Quarter)	ALARA Investigational Level II (Per Calendar Quarter)
Whole body	1.25 mSv (125 mrem)	3.75 mSv (375 mrem)
Extremity and skin	12.5 mSv (1250 mrem)	37.5 mSv (3750 mrem)
Lens of the eye	3.75 mSv (375 mrem)	11.25 mSv (1125 mrem)

Data from Howe DB, Beardsley M, Bakhsh SR: Consolidated guidance about materials licenses. Program-specific guidance about medical uses licenses (NUREG-1556, volume 9, revision 2). 2014.

with the As Low As Reasonably Achievable (ALARA) philosophy. These quarterly investigational levels may be established by the institution, or the facility may adopt those recommended by the NRC. As illustrated in Table 2-5, there are two investigational levels associated with various monitoring points on the body. An ALARA Level I is a dose equal to 10% of the annual dose limit whereas an ALARA Level II is triggered at 30% of the annual dose limit. To help ensure annual dose limits are not exceeded, these ALARA investigational levels are routinely checked on a quarterly basis.

The NRC recommends the following actions must be taken when an employee exceeds ALARA investigational levels:

▶ **ALARA I Exceeded**

The RSO or designee should investigate and review actions that might be taken to reduce a recurrence. No further action is necessary unless determined otherwise by the RSO.

▶ **ALARA II Exceeded**

The RSO should perform a timely investigation into the cause, take action to reduce the recurrence, and submit a report to the institution's Radiation Safety Committee.

RELEASE OF PATIENTS ADMINISTERED WITH RADIOACTIVE MATERIAL

Patients administered with radioactive material may be released into the public providing they are not likely to expose any individual to a point where their dose equivalent could exceed 5 mSv (0.5 rem).[13] Furthermore, the patient or patient's guardian must be provided with a set of instructions to maintain doses to as low as reasonably achievable if the total effective dose equivalent to any other individual is likely to exceed 1 mSv (0.1 rem). Breast-feeding cessation guidelines must also be provided if the dose equivalent to a nursing child could exceed 1 mSv (0.1 rem).

NRC Radiation Guide 8.39, "Release of Patients Administered Radioactive Material"[14] provides guidance for the release of patients, administered activities of radiopharmaceuticals requiring instructions, and breast-feeding cessation recommendations. As illustrated in Table 2-6, patients administered with diagnostic activities of ^{99m}Tc-Sestamibi may be immediately released without radiation safety instructions and do not require stoppage of breast-feeding.

RADIATION BIOLOGY

The deleterious risks from ionizing radiation exposure are similar to exposure from other hazards encounter by employees in the workplace, which include both chemical and biological agents.[15] Moreover, the resulting damage to cells from ionizing radiation cannot be distinguished from cellular injury due to these other harmful factors.[16] The killing of cells directly and/or damage to the DNA are dependent on several variables including the caustic agent source and strength, duration of exposure, and stage of cell growth.[17,18] The effects are classified as either stochastic, where the probability of the effect increases with dose, or deterministic, in which the severity increases with dose, after a threshold is exceeded (Fig. 2-2).[19] Stochastic effects include

Table 2-6

Activity Limits for the Release of Patients, Radiation Safety Instructions, and Breast-Feeding Cessation Times for ^{99m}Tc and ^{201}Tl

Radiopharmaceutical	Maximum Activity to Release Patient	Activities above Which Radiation Safety Instructions Are Required	Recommended Breast Feeding Cessation Time
^{99m}Tc Sestamibi	760	150	None listed
^{201}Tl Thallous chloride	430	85	2 weeks

Note: NRC Guide 8.39 does not list breast-feeding cessation guidelines for ^{99m}Tc—Sestamibi. Administered activities will result in an effective dose below the threshold of 1 mSv.

cancer and genetic manifestations whereas deterministic effects include reddening of the skin (erythema), and development of cataracts.

The source of radiation and its strength play a particular role in assessing risks from exposure. While both stochastic and deterministic risk effects are dose dependent, meaning risk increases with radiation energy and duration of exposure, these effects are heightened by the type of radiation. X-rays and gamma rays are high-energy quanta of electromagnetic radiation characterized by short wavelengths and high frequencies that have the ability to ionize an exposed atom. The biological effectiveness, or the risk adjusted for radiation quality, for x-rays, gamma rays, and beta particles are the same (Table 2-1). On the other hand, alpha emissions are high-energy particulate radiation that deposit significantly more energy as it passes through tissue. Because of this increased transfer of energy, alpha particles bear a higher biological risk than x-rays, gamma rays, and beta particles. At equivalent doses of radiation, the associated biological risk from alpha emissions is 20 times that of x-rays, gamma rays, and beta particles.

When exposed to radiation, cells can be affected directly by energy deposited into the atom/molecule or indirectly through ionization of the surrounding medium, which then interacts with the target cells. Whether directly or indirectly via free radical production in cellular water, the toxic effects from radiation exposure include the removal of an electron from DNA molecules causing single- or double-strand breaks. Double DNA strand breaks are overly traumatic and often lead to cellular death. Although single-strand breaks frequently repair themselves correctly, incorrect or mutagenic repairs do occur. A mutagenic repair represents a change in the cellular DNA. This may leave the cell modified yet still viable.[16]

RADIATION PROTECTION PRINCIPLES

Occupational workers exposed to ionizing radiation must practice radiation safety techniques on a daily basis to maintain levels of exposure below federal dose limits. To assess the levels of cumulative exposure, occupational workers are issued personal

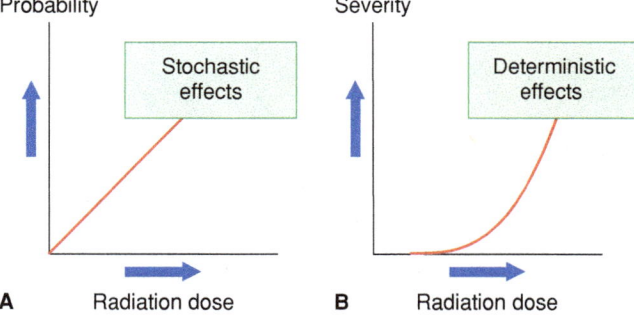

FIGURE 2-2 Stochastic and deterministic effects from exposure to radiation. The effects from radiation exposure are classified as either **(A)** Stochastic—the probability for the effect to appear increases with radiation dose, or **(B)** Deterministic—the severity of the effect increases with radiation dose only after a dose threshold is exceeded.

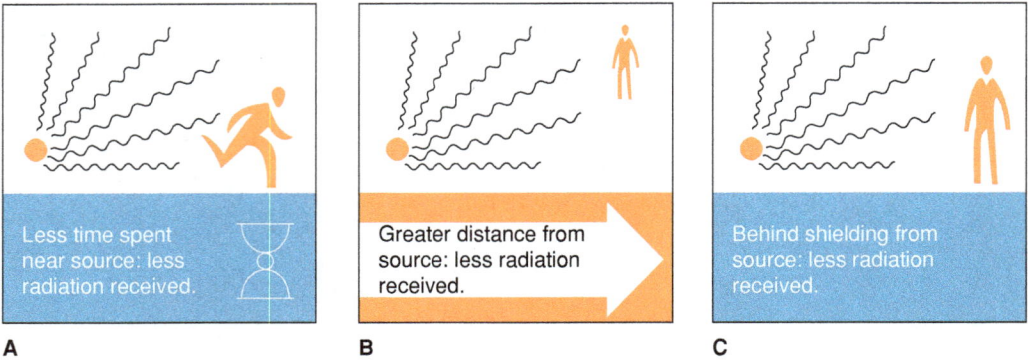

FIGURE 2-3 Principles of radiation protection. From http://www.nrc.gov/about-nrc/radiation/protects-you/protection-principles.html. The three rules for protection from radiation are **(A)** reduce your **time** around a source, **(B)** increase your **distance** from the source, and **(C)** use appropriate **shielding** devices.

radiation monitors. When a pregnant worker declares her pregnancy status, an additional monitor is provided to be worn at the waist level for assessing the radiation dose to the fetus.

Over and above the universal precautions common to the healthcare environment, there are three cardinal rules in the protection against ionizing radiation. These are time, distance, and shielding (Fig. 2-3).[20]

Time

Radiation is emitted as a rate. A radiation source emitting photons or particles at a rate of 80 mGy/hr would expose a particular area to 80 mGy in 1 hour. Understanding this principle, occupational workers limit their time around known radiation sources, which in turn limits their cumulative exposure. In the example above, a worker exposed to an 80 mGy/hr source would only receive 40 mGy of exposure if their time around the source were limited to 30 minutes.

Distance

Like a source of visible light that appears dimmer at increased distances, ionizing radiation decreases in intensity as well. The inverse square law states that the intensity of radiation decreases with the inverse of the square of the distance, or $I_1(d_1)^2 = I_2(d_2)^2$, where I = intensity and d = distance. Radiation is emitted in an isotropic manner. As distance increases, the same fluence of radiation covers a larger surface area, thereby decreasing the exposure to a finite object in the path (Fig. 2-4). Continuing the previous example, a worker exposed to 40 mGy at 1 m from a radiation source will reduce their exposure to 10 mGy at a distance of 2 m.

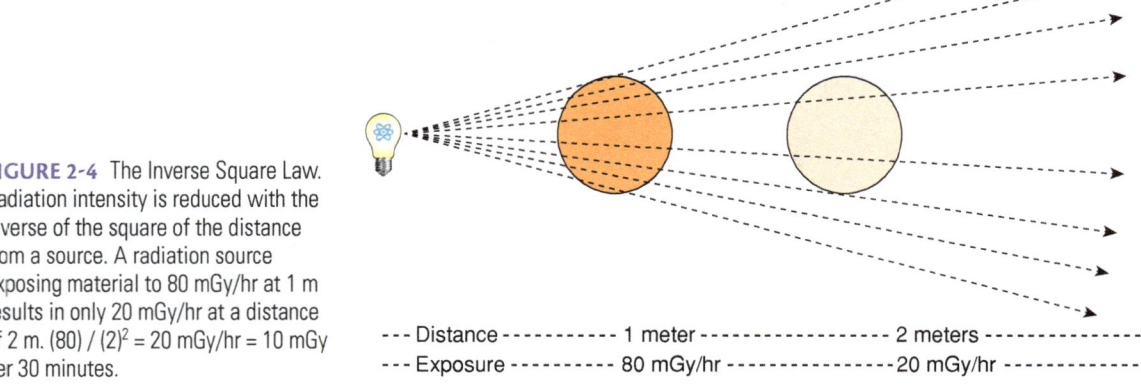

FIGURE 2-4 The Inverse Square Law. Radiation intensity is reduced with the inverse of the square of the distance from a source. A radiation source exposing material to 80 mGy/hr at 1 m results in only 20 mGy/hr at a distance of 2 m. $(80) / (2)^2 = 20$ mGy/hr = 10 mGy per 30 minutes.

Example:

$$I_1 \times (d_1)^2 = I_2 \times (d_2)^2$$
$$40 \text{ mGy} \times (1 \text{ m})^2 = I_2 \times (2 \text{ m})^2$$
$$40 \text{ mGy} = I_2 \times 4$$
$$I_2 = 10 \text{ mGy}$$

▶ Shielding

Shielding is often used to provide a protective barrier between a worker and a radiation source. The shielding material and thickness is dependent upon the radiation source and strength. Inches of concrete or fractions of an inch of lead are commonly used in barriers to provide structural protection to occupational workers and the general public. Partial barriers, lead-lined transport containers, and lead-lined syringe shields are also used to protect radioisotope workers during the preparation and administration of radiopharmaceuticals.

PERSONNEL MONITORING

Occupational radiation workers are required to be monitored for radiation exposure if they are likely to enter a high or very high radiation area, are likely to exceed 10% of the annual dose limits, or are a declared pregnant woman likely to receive an annual dose in excess of 1 mSv (0.1 rem).[21]

There are several types of personnel monitors used in Nuclear Cardiology facilities. These include the film badge, a thermo luminescent dosimeter (TLD), and an optically stimulated luminescence (OSL) device. The NRC requires evaluation of these devices by a laboratory that is accredited by the National Voluntary Laboratory Accreditation Program (NVLAP).

Film badges utilize a strip of photographic film contained in a plastic holder. Exposure to radiation will increase the darkening in the developed film. The degree of darkening is proportional to the radiation exposure received. Incorporated into the badge holder are filters such as lead, copper, aluminum, and plastic. The degree of darkening behind each filter helps determine the quality of the radiation received, such as high-energy photons, low-energy photons, and particulate radiation. Film badges are commonly used to measure whole-body irradiation and are comparatively inexpensive. However, they are affected by heat, moisture, and sunlight and must be utilized with care.

TLDs use inorganic crystals such as Lithium Fluoride to measure radiation exposure. When exposed to ionizing radiation, excitation of atoms causes electrons to elevate from their valence band to become trapped in the forbidden band. When heated with high temperatures (annealing), the electrons are released back into the valence band emitting light proportional to the radiation received. By returning to their stable state, the annealing process allows the TLD to be re-used. TLDs do not have the ability to distinguish radiation quality and are commonly used as extremity monitors, such as the ring badge.

OSL combines the benefits of film badge and TLD technology. An aluminum oxide crystalline structure is manufactured into a thin strip and placed between a filter pack. Irradiated atoms in the structure liberate electrons that become trapped and these electrons release light when stimulated by a laser. The release of light is proportional to the radiation received. Similar to that in film badge technology, plastic and metal filters are used to assess the incident radiation quality. OSL devices are commonly used for whole-body radiation monitoring. The devices are sealed in a blister pack and are unaffected by light, heat, and moisture.

MEDICAL EVENTS

Formally known as misadministrations, medical events are defined by the NRC. The NRC must be notified of a reportable medical event no later than the next calendar day after occurrence. The telephone notification must be followed by a written report within 15 days. Pertinent to Nuclear Cardiology, the following events must be reported to the NRC if they result in a dose equivalent to the patient that exceeds 0.05 Sv (5 rem) or a dose to the skin or an organ that exceeds 0.5 Sv (50 rem). Events meeting these definitions but not exceeding the reportable dose limits need only be reported to the facility's administrators.

a. An administration of a dose that is greater than 20% difference from the prescribed dose
b. An administration of the wrong radiopharmaceutical
c. An administration of a radiopharmaceutical to the wrong person

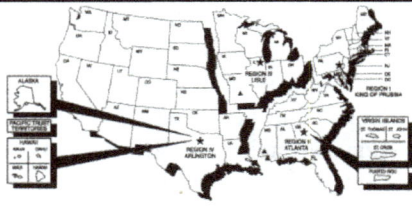

FIGURE 2-5 NRC Form 3—Notice to employees.

d. An administration of a radiopharmaceutical by the wrong route (i.e., oral vs. intravenous)

POSTINGS

There are several postings required in a Nuclear Cardiology laboratory. These include the "Notice To Employees" (NRC Form 3) and appropriate radiation caution signage.[22-24] NRC Form 3 (Fig. 2-5) is required to be posted in a conspicuous manner and replaced if defaced or altered. This form should be posted in an area frequented by workers either to or from the area where radiation is used or stored. This form is commonly found in employee lounges and entrance doors to radiation areas.

A "Caution Radioactive Materials" sign (Fig. 2-6) is required to be posted in any area where radioactive materials are used or stored that exceed 10 times the quantity listed in Appendix C of Title 10, Part 20 of the Code of Federal Regulation. This equates to 1 mCi of ^{57}Co, 0.1 mCi of ^{137}Cs, and 10 mCi of ^{99m}Tc and ^{201}Tl. A "Caution Radiation Area" sign is required to be posted in each area where radiation levels could result in an individual receiving 0.05 mSv (5 mrem) in 1 hour at 30 cm from a radiation source. Caution signs are commonly located on the entrance doors to the hot lab, imaging room, and injections areas such as the treadmill room. If a radioactive material

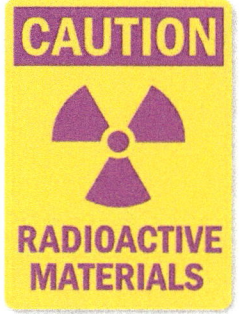 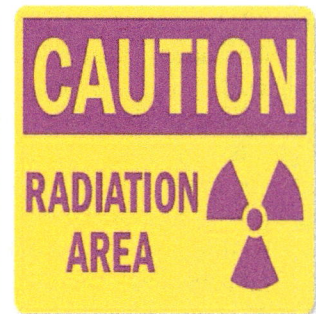

FIGURE 2-6 Radiation caution signs found in Nuclear Cardiology laboratories.

is used in a room for less than 8 hours per day and is under constant supervision, the area is not required to be posted with the caution sign. Furthermore, a radiation area sign is not needed if the source of the exposure is from a patient meeting the criteria to be released into the public.

AREA SURVEYS AND SPILL PROCEDURES

Ambient radiation level surveys must be performed at the end of each working day in areas where radioactive materials are used and stored. The most common instrument for performing ambient radiation surveys in the Nuclear Cardiology department is the Geiger–Müller (GM) meter, a gas-filled detector that produces and collects ion pairs when ionizing radiation passes through the detector and deposits energy. The NRC recommends an ambient exposure trigger limit of 5 mR/hr in restricted areas and 0.1 mR/hr in unrestricted areas.[25]

Removable contamination surveys (wipe tests) should be performed weekly using an appropriate gamma-counting device such as sodium iodide (NaI) well counter. While Appendix R of NRC NUREG 1556 Volume 9,[25] suggests an action level of 20,000 dpm/100 cm^2 for ^{99m}Tc and ^{201}Tl, many Nuclear Cardiology facilities use the 2000 dpm/100 cm^2 action level required for other isotopes common in general nuclear medicine departments. It is also important to verify ambient radiation and contamination limits in your individual area of practice as many states have more restrictive requirements.

When ambient radiation levels or contamination surveys exceed limits, a radiation spill has occurred requiring action. The NRC recommends establishing an activity threshold for a major and minor spill and provides guidance in Appendix N of NRC NUREG 1556 Volume 9.[25] The suggested procedures are as follows:

Minor Spill (less than 100 mCi of ^{99m}Tc/^{201}Tl)

1. Notify persons in the area that a spill has occurred.
2. Prevent the spread of contamination by covering the spill with absorbent paper.
3. Wear gloves and protective clothing and clean up the spill using absorbent paper.
4. Survey the area with an appropriate radiation detection instruments.
5. Report the incident to the RSO.

Major Spill (greater than 100 mCi of ^{99m}Tc/^{201}Tl)

1. Clear the area. Notify all persons not involved in the spill to vacate the room.
2. Prevent the spread of contamination by covering the spill with absorbent paper labeled "caution radioactive material," but do not attempt to clean it up.
3. Shield the source if possible. Do this only if it can be done without further contamination or a significant increase in radiation exposure.
4. Close the room and lock or otherwise secure the area to prevent entry.
5. Notify the RSO immediately.
6. Decontaminate personnel by removing contaminated clothing and flushing contaminated skin with lukewarm water, then washing with mild soap. If contamination remains, the RSO may consider inducing perspiration. Then wash the affected area again to remove any contamination that was released by the perspiration.

WASTE DISPOSAL

Radioactive waste generated in the Nuclear Cardiology department may be disposed by various methods. The two most common are decay-in-storage and return to an authorized recipient. Decay-in-storage is allowed for isotopes with a half-life of 120 days or less.[26] Storage of waste for decay requires that the waste to be held for a minimum of 10 half-lives in a shielded container and prior to final disposal the waste must be surveyed to ensure it is consistent with background radiation. All radioactive labels must be removed or defaced, and a record of the waste disposal must be maintained for 3 years. A summary of the minimum length of time radioactive waste must be held in storage for isotopes common to Nuclear Cardiology is summarized in Table 2-7.

Table 2-7

Minimum Time Required for Decay-in-Storage

Isotope	Half-Life (hours)	Minimum Time in Storage (10 half-lives)[1]
^{99m}Tc	6.01	61 hours
^{201}Tl	72.9	31 days
^{18}F	1.83	19 hours

Note: Decay-in-storage time rounded up to the nearest larger whole number.

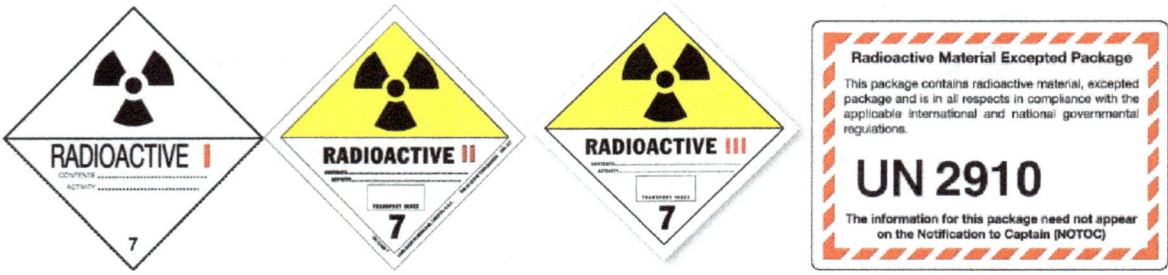

FIGURE 2-7 DOT labels for shipping radioactive packages. From left to right: The Radioactive I "White," Radioactive II "Yellow," Radioactive III "Yellow," and the Excepted Package Limited Quantity.

Radioactive waste, including used and unused doses, may also be transferred to an authorized recipient. Transfer of the waste requires verification the recipient is licensed to receive the specified radioactive material. Furthermore, when transferring this radioactive material the facility must follow Department of Transportation (DOT) shipping guidelines. A summary of these requirements is outlined in the "Shipping of Radioactive Packages" section.

RECEIVING

Receipt of radioactive packages is outlined in Title 10, Part 20.1906 of the Code of Federal Regulations. Radioactive packages must be monitored within 3 hours of delivery if received during normal working hours and no later than 3 hours from the beginning of the next working day if received after normal hours. Proper monitoring requires surveying the package for external radiation exposure and wipe testing for removable contamination. Radiation surveys must be less than 10 mR/hr at 1 m and less than 200 mR/hr at the package surface. Contamination wipe testing must be performed if there is suspicion the package is damaged or the integrity is degraded in any manner. The wipe test results must be less than 6600 dpm/300 cm². Should the wipe test or survey results exceed limits, the delivery carrier and the NRC must be notified immediately.[27]

SHIPPING OF RADIOACTIVE PACKAGES

In addition to receiving radioactive materials, the Nuclear Cardiology department must routinely ship radioactive materials. These shipments include the return of spent and unused patient radiopharmaceutical doses as well as the return of sealed calibration sources. Shipping of radioactive materials is regulated by the DOT under Title 49 of the Code of Federal Regulations (49CFR).

There are four DOT labels used for shipping radioactive materials (Fig. 2-7). The use of each label is determined by the quantity of material in the package and the radiation exposure at the surface and 1 m from the package.

The most common radioactive package shipped from the Nuclear Cardiology department is the "UN2910—Excepted Package, Limited Quantity." For a package to ship under the specifications of UN2910, the maximum quantity in the package cannot exceed the limits derived from the table in 49CFR173.425. Furthermore, the following criteria must be met:

a. The surface of the package must not exceed 0.5 mR/hr
b. A wipe test of the package must not exceed 6600 dpm/300 cm²

The limited quantity package limits for common isotopes derived from 49CFR173.425 are illustrated in Table 2-8. The limits apply to radioactive material in both solid and liquid forms. For packages

Table 2-8

"Excepted Package Limited Quantity" Limits for Common Isotopes Used in Nuclear Cardiology

Isotope	Form	Limit
^{99m}Tc	Liquid	11 mCi
^{201}Tl	Liquid	11 mCi
^{18}F	Liquid	1.6 mCi
^{57}Co	Liquid	27 mCi
^{137}Cs	Liquid	1.6 mCi
^{68}Ge	Solid	14 mCi

Table 2-9
DOT Label Radiation Exposure Limits

DOT Label	Surface Exposure (mR/hr)	1 M Exposure (mR/hr)	Wipe Test Limit
Excepted Package Limited Quantity[a]	≤0.5	Background	6600 dpm/300 cm^2
White I	≤0.5	Background	6600 dpm/300 cm^2
Yellow II	> 0.5 ≤50	1.0	6600 dpm/300 cm^2
Yellow III	>50 ≤200	10	6600 dpm/300 cm^2

[a]The Excepted Package Limited Quantity label conforms to White I limits and the contents of the package meet the specifications of 49CFR173.425.

containing more than one isotope, the lower limit applies to the entire contents of the package.

A radioactive package that exceeds the excepted package quantities, has a surface exposure of less than 0.5 mR/hr, an exposure at 1 m that is indistinguishable from background, and a wipe test of less than 6600 dpm/300 cm^2 receives a Radioactive I "White" label.

Model Procedure for the Safe use of Unsealed Licensed Material
NRC NUREG 1556 Volume 9, Revision 2, Appendix T[15]

1. Wear laboratory coats or other protective clothing at all times in areas where radioactive materials are used
2. Wear disposable gloves at all times while handling radioactive materials
3. Either after each procedure or before leaving the area, monitor hands for contamination in a low-background area using an appropriate survey instrument
4. Use syringe shields for reconstitution of radiopharmaceutical kits and administration of radiopharmaceuticals to patients, except when their use is contraindicated
5. Do not eat, store food, drink, smoke, or apply cosmetics in any area where licensed material is stored or used
6. Wear personnel monitoring devices, if required, at all times while in areas where radioactive materials are used or stored. These devices shall be worn as prescribed by the RSO. When not being worn to monitor occupational exposures, personnel monitoring devices shall be stored in the work place in a designated low-background area
7. Wear extremity dosimeters, if required, when handling radioactive material
8. Dispose of radioactive waste only in designated, labeled, and properly shielded receptacles
9. Never pipette by mouth
10. Wipe-test unsealed byproduct material storage, preparation, and administration areas weekly for contamination. If necessary, decontaminate the area
11. Survey with a radiation detection survey meter all areas of licensed material use
12. Store radioactive solutions in shielded containers that are clearly labeled
13. Radiopharmaceutical multi-dose diagnostic vials must be labeled in accordance with 10 CFR 35.69 and 10 CFR 20.1904
14. Syringes and unit dosages must be labeled in accordance with 10 CFR 35.69 and 10 CFR 20.1904. Mark the label with the radionuclide, the activity, the date for which the activity is estimated, and the kind of materials. To avoid mistaking patient dosages, label the syringe with the type of study and the patient's name.
15. For prepared dosages, assay each patient dosage in the dose calibrator before administration
16. Do not use a dosage if it does not fall within the prescribed dosage range or if it varies more than ±20% from the prescribed dosage, except as approved by an AU
17. When measuring the dosage, licensees need not consider the radioactivity that adheres to the syringe wall or remains in the needle
18. Check the patient's name and identification number and the prescribed radionuclide, chemical form, and dosage before administering.
19. Always keep flood sources, syringes, waste, and other radioactive material in shielded containers
20. Secure all licensed material when not under the constant surveillance and immediate control of an authorized individual

FIGURE 2-8 NRC recommended policy for the safe use of radioactive materials.

A Radioactive II "Yellow" label is used for packages with a surface exposure of 0.5 to 50 mR/hr, a 1 m exposure of less than 1 mR/hr and a wipe test of less than 6600 dpm/300 cm^2. The Radioactive II labeled is commonly used when shipping calibration sources back to the vendor for disposal.

Packages with a surface exposure of 50 to 200 mR/hr, a 1 m exposure of less than 10 mR/hr and a wipe test of less than 6600 dpm/300 cm^2 must be labeled with a Radioactive III "Yellow" label.

Radioactive labels must be placed onto two sides of the package and packages requiring the Radioactive I, II, or III label must be a classified as a "Type A" shipping container. A "Type A" shipping container is a strong package that has met certain criteria including a water spray test, drop test, compression test, and penetration test. A summary of the radiation exposure limits for each DOT label is illustrated in Table 2-9.

SAFE USE OF RADIOACTIVE MATERIAL

The NRC requires licensees to develop a policy for the safe use of radioactive materials. Appendix T of NRC NUREG 1556 Volume 9 Revision 2 provides a sample policy that facilities may choose to adopt in lieu of developing their own. The NRC policy for the safe use of radioactive materials illustrated in Figure 2-8 provides a basis for establishing a safe working environment.

REFERENCES

1. The Health Physics Society. 2014. http://hps.org/publicinformation/ate/faqs/whatisradiation.html. Accessed October 29, 2014.
2. United States Nuclear Regulatory Commission. 2014. http://www.nrc.gov/reading-rm/basic-ref/glossary/ionizing-radiation.html. Accessed September 9, 2014.
3. United States Nuclear Regulatory Commission. 2014. http://www.nrc.gov/reading-rm/basic-ref/glossary/roentgen-r.html. Accessed October 28, 2014.
4. United States Nuclear Regulatory Commission. 2014. http://www.nrc.gov/reading-rm/basic-ref/glossary/rad-radiation-absorbed-dose.html. Accessed October 28, 2014.
5. United States Nuclear Regulatory Commission. 2014. http://www.nrc.gov/reading-rm/basic-ref/glossary/dose-equivalent.html. Accessed September 9, 2014.
6. United States Nuclear Regulatory Commission. 2014. http://www.nrc.gov/reading-rm/basic-ref/glossary/rem-roentgen-equivalent-man.html. Accessed September 9, 2014.
7. Standards for Protection Against Radiation, 10 CFR § 20.1004 (2004).
8. United States Nuclear Regulatory Commission. 2014. http://www.nrc.gov/about-nrc/radiation/around-us/sources/nat-bg-sources.html. Accessed October 28, 2014.
9. United States Nuclear Regulatory Commission. 2014. http://www.nrc.gov/about-nrc/radiation/around-us/sources.html. Accessed October 28, 2014.
10. United States Nuclear Regulatory Commission. 2014. http://www.nrc.gov/about-nrc/radiation/around-us/sources/man-made-sources.html. Accessed October 28, 2014.
11. Kase KR. Radiation protection principles of NCRP. *Health Phys.* 2004;87(3):251–257.
12. NCRP 116. 1993. National Council on Radiation Protection and Measurements. Limitation of Exposure to Ionizing Radiation, NCRP Report No. 116. http://app.knovel.com/hotlink/toc/id:kpLEIRRN04/limitation-exposure-ionizing/limitation-exposure-ionizing. Accessed November 26, 2014.
13. Standards for Protection Against Radiation, 10 CFR § 35.75 (2004).
14. U.S. Nuclear Regulatory Commission. Release of patients administered radioactive materials. Washington, DC: U.S. Nuclear Regulatory Commission; Regulatory Guide 8.39; 1997.
15. Salihu HM, Myers J, August EM. Pregnancy in the workplace. *Occup Med (Lond).* 2012;62(2):88–97.
16. Travis EL. Basic biologic interactions of radiation. In Kelly KM, ed. *Primer of Medical Radiobiology.* St. Louis, MO: Mosby-Yearbook, Inc.; 1989:25–44.
17. Bushberg JT, Boone JM. Radiation biology. In Mitchell CW, ed. *The Essential Physics of Medical Imaging.* Baltimore, MD: Lippincott Williams & Wilkins; 2011:600, 751–836.
18. Valentin J. ICRP publication 84: Pregnancy and medical radiation. *Ann ICRP.* 2000;30, 7–67.
19. Adriaens I, Smitz J, Jacquet P. The current knowledge on radiosensitivity of ovarian follicle development stages. *Hum Reprod Update.* 2009;15(3):359–377.
20. United States Nuclear Regulatory Commission. 2014. http://www.nrc.gov/about-nrc/radiation/protects-you/protection-principles.html. Accessed November 26, 2014.
21. Standards for Protection Against Radiation, 10 CFR § 20.1502 (2004).
22. Standards for Protection Against Radiation, 10 CFR § 19.11 (2004).
23. Standards for Protection Against Radiation, 10 CFR § 20.1901 (2004).
24. Standards for Protection Against Radiation, 10 CFR § 20.1902 (2004).
25. Howe DB, Beardsley M, Bakhsh SR. Consolidated guidance about materials licenses. Program-specific guidance about medical uses licenses (NUREG-1556, volume 9, revision 2). 2014.
26. Standards for Protection Against Radiation, 10 CFR § 35.92 (2004).
27. Standards for Protection Against Radiation, 10 CFR § 20.1906 (2004).

Radiopharmaceuticals for Cardiac Imaging

CHAPTER 3

Raymond Taillefer

INTRODUCTION

This chapter reviews the most important characteristics of the various single-photon emission computed tomography (SPECT) and positron emission tomography (PET) radiopharmaceuticals that are currently used in clinical practice. Myocardial perfusion scintigraphy has significantly evolved[1] since its introduction more than four decades ago. Three major factors have specifically contributed to this evolution: (1) technical improvements in scintigraphic data acquisition and analysis, (2) introduction of new technetium-99m (Tc-99m)-labeled MPI radiopharmaceuticals with different properties than thallium-201 (Tl-201), and (3) availability of PET radiotracers and PET-dedicated cameras. This chapter reviews the most important characteristics of the various SPECT and PET MPI radioactive agents that are currently used in clinical practice. The knowledge of the characteristics and kinetics of the various radiotracers is clinically relevant and essential for designing and implementing optimized imaging protocols.[2] The optimal timing of imaging after injection either at stress or at rest is determined by rate of uptake in the heart and adjacent organs, as well as the residence time of radiotracers within the myocytes. The efficiency of myocardial extraction over a wide range myocardial blood flows is relevant for reliable detection of obstructive coronary artery disease and absolute quantification of regional myocardial blood flow. Therefore, knowledge of the basic characteristics of MPI radiotracers is essential for optimal clinical use of these agents. In addition, a section on ^{99m}Tc-pyrophosphate cardiac imaging is included, given its role in the diagnosis of cardiac amyloidosis, while other more specific agents such as ^{123}I-MIBG and ^{123}I-IPPA are covered in another chapter (Chapter 23). Radiation safety has become a more sensitive concern more recently. Therefore, data on radiation dosimetry are also discussed for each radiopharmaceutical.

SPECT RADIOPHARMACEUTICALS

▶ General Physiologic Characteristics of Perfusion Imaging Agents

Although many different classes of radioactive MPI agents exist, they should all present a minimum of common basic characteristics.[4]

1. The myocardial uptake of the radiotracer must be proportional to the regional myocardial blood flow over a relatively wide range of blood flows.
2. The myocardial uptake should be high enough to allow for detection of regional inhomogeneity by external gamma scintigraphy.
3. The initial myocardial distribution of the radiotracer at the time of injection must remain stable during the acquisition time of the images.
4. The effect of blood flow on myocardial transport of the radiotracer must be predominant to the effect of metabolic cellular alterations.
5. Finally, the agent should be labeled to a radionuclide having adequate physical characteristics to provide high photon flux and optimal counting statistics.

Table 3-1			
Comparative Characteristics of Radiopharmaceuticals for Myocardial Perfusion Imaging			
	Tl–201	Tc-99m-Sestamibi	Tc-99m-Tetrofosmin
Class	Element	Isonitrile	Diphosphine
Charge	Cation	Cation	Cation
Emax	0.73 ± 0.10	0.38 ± 0.09	0.32 ± 0.07
Enet	0.57 ± 0.13	0.41 ± 0.15	0.23
PS cap (mL/mg)	1.30 ± 0.45	0.44 ± 0.23	0.40
Myocardial redistribution	Yes	Very partial	No
Myocardial uptake (%ID)	3.0–4.0	1.4 ± 0.3	1.0–1.2
IV imaging interval	5–10 minutes	15–60 minutes	15 minutes
Target organ	Kidney	Upper large intestine	Gallbladder wall

Emax, maximum radiotracer extraction; Enet, net radiotracer extraction; PS cap, radiotracer permeability-surface area product; %ID, percentage of injected dose.

Information on basic properties of radionuclide MPI agents is generally obtained from cultured myocardial cells, isolated perfused hearts, or in vivo animal models.[5] Precise measurements of cellular or capillary-tissue tracer kinetics are usually obtained from cell cultures and isolated perfused heart models, whereas regional tracer distribution and uptake in other organs are studied with in vivo animal models. The two most important physiologic factors that affect the myocardial uptake of an MPI agent are the variations in regional myocardial blood flow and the myocardial extraction of the radiotracer. Three major parameters (Enet, Emax, and PS cap) can be determined using indicator-dilution techniques and radiolabeled albumin used as an intravascular reference. The difference between the intravascular albumin reference and the radiopharmaceutical that is evaluated (i.e., a diffusible perfusion agent) on a venous dilution curve is used to calculate its instantaneous cardiac extraction. The early peak of the curve, or Emax, represents the maximum fractional tissue extraction of the diffusible agent. This value is used to calculate the capillary permeability surface area product, PS cap. The net extraction (Enet) is the integral of the curve and is used as a measure of myocardial radiotracer retention, including both initial extraction and subsequent back-diffusion. A high value for Emax and PS cap indicates a rapid blood-tissue exchange and suggests that the diffusible radiotracer will be able to assess high levels of hyperemic flow accurately. Table 3-1 summarizes and compares these values for the commonly used radiopharmaceuticals.

THALLIUM-201

The criteria necessary for a radiopharmaceutical to be used to determine regional perfusion were elaborated by Saperstein in the mid-1950s.[3] As described by the Saperstein principle, a given type of radiopharmaceutical will be distributed in proportion to regional perfusion if its extraction by the organ of interest is high and if its clearance from the blood is rapid. One of the first classes of radiopharmaceuticals used to image myocardial perfusion was the potassium analogs—cesium, rubidium, and thallium, which enter the myocardium by the sodium–potassium–ATPase pump mechanism. Although different radioisotopes of these cations have been evaluated, Tl-201 was found to have the best physical and biological characteristics for imaging and has been the most popular radionuclide MPI agent used in noninvasive detection and evaluation of patients with known or suspected coronary artery disease for more than two decades.

Thallium-201 is a cyclotron-produced monovalent cation with a physical half-life of 73.1 hours. It decays by electron capture to mercury-201. Thallium-201 is a low-energy gamma emitter with principal photopeaks at 135.3 keV (2.7% abundance) and 167.4 keV (10% abundance) and x-rays emitted from the mercury daughter at 68 to 80.3 keV (95% abundance). Some contaminants such as Tl-200 (<0.3%), Tl-202 (<1.2%), and Pb-202 (<0.2%) can be present, but that usually represents less than 2% of the total Tl-201 activity at the time of calibration. Contrary to the Tc-99m-labeled MPI agents, there is no in-house preparation and no quality control procedure required before injection in humans.

▶ Physiologic Characteristics

The myocardial transmicrovascular transport of Tl-201 was evaluated by Leppo and Meerdink[6] in a blood-perfused, isolated rabbit heart model. The averaged myocardial extraction (Emax) of Tl-201 was 0.73 ± 0.10. The net myocardial extraction measured over a 2- to 5-minute period was 0.57 ± 0.13. The mean PS cap of Tl-201 was 1.30 ± 0.45 mL/g/min. Although Tl-201 is considered biologically similar to potassium, its myocardial uptake is greater than that of potassium. The myocardial extraction fraction of Tl-201 in in vivo model is approximately 87% at normal flow rates.[7] Studies on the relationship of myocardial uptake of Tl-201 to regional coronary blood flow as determined by radiolabeled microspheres showed that there is a nearly linear correlation over a wide range of coronary blood flows (Fig. 3-1). However, at high flow rates (at approximately 2.5 mL/min/g), there is a diffusion limitation and a fall in tracer extraction fraction and also an increased cellular washout, resulting in a plateau in myocardial uptake. This results in an overall underestimation of higher levels of coronary blood flows. Conversely, at very low flow rates (usually less than 10% of the baseline blood flow), there is an increased myocardial extraction fraction of Tl-201 relative to blood flow, resulting in an overestimation of coronary blood flow.

One of the most clinically important characteristics of Tl-201 is its myocardial redistribution. Myocardial uptake of Tl-201 is not static over time. This property forms the basis of the stress-redistribution imaging protocol used to diagnose the presence of coronary artery disease with Tl-201. The redistribution or the filling in of a myocardial perfusion defect generally occurs between 3 and 5 hours after the injection of Tl-201 at peak stress and is related to two factors: the rate of influx of Tl-201 into the

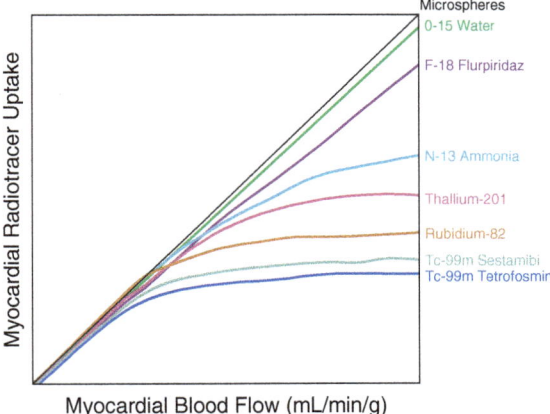

FIGURE 3-1 Schematic representation of the relationship between myocardial blood flow levels and net myocardial radiotracer extraction for commonly used SPECT and PET myocardial perfusion imaging agents. The line of identity indicates the experimental gold standard for measuring blood flow, that is, trapped radiolabeled microspheres with a linear relationship between coronary blood flow and radiotracer uptake at various levels of blood flows.

myocardium from whole-body blood pool activity and the rate of clearance or washout of Tl-201 from the myocardium. A myocardial perfusion defect related to ischemic disease will show a normalization of the Tl-201 uptake at 3 to 4 hours after the injection at stress because of a delayed accumulation into the ischemic segment and a more rapid washout from normal myocardial segments than from hypoperfused segments.

▶ Biodistribution and Dosimetry

The greatest concentration of Tl-201 is found in kidneys, heart, and liver. The activity in these organs remains high for few hours after the injection. Maximal myocardial uptake, which is approximately 3.7% to 4.0% of the injected dose, is achieved by 10 to 15 minutes after the administration of the radiopharmaceutical. Tl-201 myocardial uptake has two components: an early component with a half-life of approximately 4 hours (80%) and a delayed component with a half-life of 40 hours (20%). Disappearance of Tl-201 from the blood compartment is rapid with two components: 92% of the blood activity disappears with a half-life of 5 minutes, and the other 8% will be cleared from the blood with a half-life

Table 3-2
Radiation Dose Estimate for Myocardial Perfusion Imaging Agents (Rads/30 mCi)

	Tl-201 Stress (Rads/3 mCi)	Tc-99m-Sestamibi		Tc-99m-Tetrofosmin	
		Rest	Stress	Rest	Stress
Adrenals	0.7	—	—	0.5	0.5
Brain	0.7	—	—	0.2	0.3
Breasts	0.4	0.2	0.2	0.2	0.2
Gallbladder wall	0.9	2.0	2.8	5.4	3.7
LLI	1.60	3.9	3.3	2.5	1.7
ULI	0.80	5.4	4.5	3.4	2.2
Small intestine	0.20	3.0	2.4	1.9	1.3
Stomach	0.3	0.6	0.5	0.5	0.5
Heart wall	0.3	0.5	0.5	0.4	0.5
Kidneys	5.1	2.0	1.7	1.4	1.2
Liver	1.1	0.6	0.4	0.5	0.4
Lungs	0.5	0.3	0.3	0.2	0.2
Muscles	0.5	—	—	0.4	0.4
Ovaries	1.1	1.5	1.2	1.1	0.9
Pancreas	0.8	—	—	0.5	0.6
Red marrow	0.6	0.5	0.5	0.4	0.5
Bone surface	1.0	0.7	0.6	0.6	0.7
Spleen	2.0	—	—	0.4	0.5
Testes	0.9	0.3	0.3	0.3	0.4
Thymus	0.5	—	—	0.3	0.3
Thyroid	3.0	0.7	0.3	0.6	0.5
Bladder wall	0.6	2.0	1.5	2.1	1.7
Uterus	1.0	—	—	0.9	0.2
Total body	—	0.5	0.4	0.4	0.4
Effective dose equivalent (rem/30 mCi)	3.9 (rem/3 mCi)	1.5	1.3	1.0	0.8

LLI, lower large intestine; ULI, upper large intestine.

of approximately 40 hours. This rapid clearance of Tl-201 from the blood results in a decreased blood pool background when MPI is performed. Table 3-2 summarizes the radiation dose estimates for Tl-201 along with the two Tc-99m-labeled MPI agents. Kidneys are the target organs.[8] Based on the dosimetric data, the recommended adult dose of intravenous Tl-201 for SPECT MPI is 74 to 111 MBq (2–3 mCi), although several authors are using doses up to 4.0 mCi.

Tc-99m PERFUSION AGENTS

Thallium-201 was the major radiopharmaceutical in nuclear cardiology for almost two decades. Although hundreds of studies have demonstrated the clinical value of Tl-201 myocardial perfusion scintigraphy, the physical characteristics of this radionuclide are suboptimal for scintillation camera imaging. Therefore, in the late 1970s and early 1980s, many investigators attempted to develop an MPI agent labeled with Tc-99m to circumvent the physical limitations of Tl-201. The potential advantages of a Tc-99m-labeled agent over Tl-201 are significant and include the following:

1. The 140-keV photon energy of Tc-99m, which is optimal for standard gamma camera imaging, results in an improved resolution due to less Compton scatter and less tissue attenuation in the patient (in comparison to the low photon energy of 68–80 keV for Tl-201).
2. The much shorter physical half-life of Tc-99m (6 hours vs. 73 hours for Tl-201) and the better radiation dosimetry permit the administration of a 10 times higher dose of a Tc-99m-labeled compound than Tl-201. This yields better image quality, and images can be performed in a shorter time period.
3. The resulting overall better counting statistics of Tc-99m allows for the perfusion images to be optimally obtained in a gated mode. Simultaneous assessment of perfusion and function (global and regional wall motion) can thus be obtained.
4. It is possible to perform first-pass function studies (if the initial lung transit is rapid enough) with a Tc-99m-labeled radiopharmaceutical agent.
5. Because Tc-99m is constantly available from a molybdenum generator in a nuclear medicine laboratory, special deliveries from a distribution center or a commercial radiopharmacy are not required. A Tc-99m-labeled MPI agent can thus be available almost 24 hours a day.

For the above reasons, Tc-99m-labeled agents have enormous potential to assess myocardial perfusion and could be very useful clinically.[9–11]

Tc-99m-Sestamibi

The first member of the Tc-99m-isonitrile family to be evaluated in humans was the hexakis (t-butyl-isonitrile)-technetium (I), also known as Tc-99m-TBI.[12,13] Although the myocardial uptake of Tc-99m-TBI was proportional to myocardial blood flow and was satisfactory for imaging purposes, its routine clinical use was limited by an increased lung uptake and prominent and persistent liver uptake. The initial lung uptake and subsequent washout of Tc-99m-TBI from the lungs also created significant imaging problems. A subsequently developed Tc-99m-isonitrile compound emerged from intensive search,[14–16] initially known by the coded name of RP-30A (nonlyophilized form) or RP-30 (lyophilized form), and then as either Tc-99m-hexakis 2-methoxyisobutyl isonitrile, Tc-99m-hexakis-2-methoxy-2-methylpropyl-isonitrile, Tc-99m-hexamibi, or Tc-99m-MIBI, and currently by its generic name Tc-99m-sestamibi or Cardiolite™. Tc-99m-sestamibi has favorable biological characteristics for clinical applications with transient liver uptake and rapid hepatobiliary excretion, along with minimal lung uptake. Tc-99m-sestamibi was approved by the U.S. Food and Drug Administration for clinical application in December 1990.

Intravenous injections of Tc-99m-sestamibi have been associated with very few adverse reactions. According to the product monograph, during clinical trials (Phase III study) approximately 5% to 10% of patients experienced transient parosmia and/or taste perversion (metallic or bitter taste) occurring a few seconds after the injection. Usually, this side effect disappears within 15 to 30 seconds. This adverse effect seems to be related to the presence of the copper salt in the kit formulation, and its incidence may be related to the concentration of Tc-99m-sestamibi used.

Physiologic Characteristics

Tc-99m-sestamibi is a cationic complex that is taken up by myocytes in proportion to regional myocardial blood flow. The cationic charge of the compound provides hydrophilic properties, and the six isonitrile groups allow hydrophobic interaction with cell membranes.

Tc-99m-sestamibi, which is retained within cells because of the negative charge generated on the mitochondria, has a high affinity for cytoplasm and shows very little extracellular exchange. Thus, metabolic derangements affecting myocytes' viability would also result in decreased Tc-99m-sestamibi uptake, independently of myocardial blood flow. Using aerobic metabolic blockade, Beanlands et al.[17] showed that an irreversible cellular injury resulted in a marked increase in Tc-99m-sestamibi clearance rate. They concluded that the accumulation and clearance kinetics of Tc-99m-sestamibi were dependent on sarcolemmal integrity and on aerobic metabolism and were significantly affected by cell viability.

Okada et al.[18] investigated the myocardial kinetics of Tc-99m-sestamibi in dogs undergoing a partial occlusion of the left circumflex coronary artery. They showed that Tc-99m-sestamibi was rapidly taken up by nonischemic and ischemic myocardium at rest in proportion to regional myocardial blood flow. There was a good correlation between the initial myocardial flow at normal resting flow rates and the Tc-99m-sestamibi myocardial distribution. Another study from the same group of investigators[19] using the same animal model evaluated the myocardial kinetics of Tc-99m-sestamibi after pharmacologic vasodilation with dipyridamole and showed that the initial myocardial uptake was closely related in a linear fashion to the regional myocardial blood flow at rates up to approximately 2.0 mL/min/g. However, at higher flow rates, there is a plateau in the myocardial distribution versus flow curve, resulting in an underestimation of coronary blood flow. Similar findings have been reported other investigators, which parallel the kinetics of thallium-201.[20,21] There is overestimation of myocardial blood flow at low flows which is probably related to an increased extraction seen with diffusible indicators. Thus myocardial uptake of Tc-99m-sestamibi is proportional to regional myocardial blood flow over the physiological flow range with decreased extraction at hyperemic flows and increased extraction at low flows.

In contrast to Tl-201, Tc-99m-sestamibi shows a very slow myocardial clearance after its initial myocardial uptake. A fractional Tc-99m-sestamibi clearance of 10% to 15% over a period of 4 hours has been measured by Okada et al.[18] in a canine model of partial coronary occlusion. The clearance was similar in the hypoperfused and normal zones. Animal studies have shown that after Tc-99m-sestamibi injection during brief periods (6–15 minutes) of coronary occlusion in dogs, the occluded zone shows a continued myocardial uptake during the reperfusion phase. Thus, following transient ischemia and reperfusion, there is some degree of myocardial redistribution of Tc-99m-sestamibi, although it is slower and less complete than Tl-201.[22]

Sinusas et al.[23] studied the myocardial uptake of Tc-99m-sestamibi and Tl-201 showed that as long as myocardial cells were still viable, the myocardial uptake of the tracer was not affected by an ischemia. These data suggest that the agent can also assess myocardial viability. Tc-99m-sestamibi uptake is maintained in viable myocardium but reduced in necrotic tissue. Using a dog model with coronary occlusion and reperfusion, Verani et al.[24] demonstrated that the size of the perfusion defect during occlusion as detected by scintigraphic images correlated with the amount of myocardium supplied by the occluded vessel, the area at risk. A smaller perfusion defect was detected on Tc-99m-sestamibi imaging during reperfusion. This defect correlated with the amount of infarcted myocardium and the area showing improved perfusion pattern after reflow represented the salvaged myocardium.

Biodistribution and Dosimetry

The blood clearance, biodistribution, dosimetry, and safety of Tc-99m-sestamibi were initially reported by Wackers et al.[15] Both rest and stress blood clearance curves approximate a dual exponential curve with an initial fast and later slow component. The maximal activity at rest was noted at 1 minute after injection (36 ± 18% of injected dose), and the maximal activity after injection during exercise was measured at 0.5 minute. At 1 hour after the intravenous injection of Tc-99m-sestamibi, the blood pool activity progressively decreased to 1.10 ± 0.01% and 0.7 ± 0.1% of the injected dose at rest and after stress, respectively. At 60 minutes after the injection at rest, the uptake in the heart was 1.0 ± 0.4% of injected dose. The 24-hour urinary excretion was 29.5% of injected dose, whereas the 48-hour fecal excretion was 36.9% of injected dose. The study of the upper-body organ distribution showed that the highest initial Tc-99m-sestamibi concentration (counts/pixel) is found in the gallbladder and liver followed by heart, spleen, and lungs. The myocardial activity remained relatively stable over time (27 ± 4% of initial activity has cleared from the heart at 3 hours), whereas activity in the spleen and lung decreased gradually. The maximal accumulation in the gallbladder occurred approximately at 60 minutes after the injection. Similar biodistribution and radiation dosimetry was noted after exercise.

Radiation dose estimates for Tc-99m-sestamibi have been evaluated from whole-body images.[15] The estimated radiation absorbed dose at rest and at stress, assuming a 2.0-hour void, are summarized in Table 3-2. The uptake in the heart is 1.06 ± 0.4% of injected dose at 60 minutes after injection at rest and

$1.4 \pm 0.3\%$ at 60 minutes for the stress study. The upper large intestine wall receives the highest dose of radioactivity, both at rest and at stress. To decrease dosimetry to the urinary bladder, increasing voiding frequency should be encouraged. If patients are administered a total dose of 30 mCi of Tc-99m-sestamibi, no individual organ dose will exceed 5 rads (50 mGy). Although there is accumulation of Tc-99m-sestamibi in the mammary glands, there is a minimal transfer into milk: approximately 0.01% to 0.03% of the injected Tc-99m-sestamibi activity can be excreted in human breast milk of a breastfeeding patient.[25]

Tc-99m-Tetrofosmin

Tc-99m-tetrofosmin, a diphosphine complex of Tc-99m, was the third Tc-99m-labeled MPI FDA-approved agent, following Tc-99m-teboroxime (no longer clinically available) and Tc-99m-sestamibi. Tc-99m-tetrofosmin shows similar myocardial uptake, retention, and blood clearance kinetics to Tc-99m-sestamibi. However, its clearance from both the liver and the lung is faster than that of Tc-99m-sestamibi. These characteristics can have an impact on the injection and imaging protocols. Tetrofosmin is a ligand that forms a lipophilic, cationic complex with Tc-99m. Tc-99m-tetrofosmin is the generic name for 1,2,-bis [bis(2-ethoxyethyl) phosphino] ethane, also called p53 or Myoview™. Tetrofosmin has a molecular weight of 382, and an empirical formula of $C_{18}H_{40}O_4P_2$. The functionalized diphosphine complex of Tc-99m has a molecular weight of 895 and a formula of $[TcO_2 (tetrofosmin)_2]$.[1] There are no known contraindications to intravenous administration.

Physiologic Characteristics

Sinusas et al.[26] tested the hypothesis that Tc-99m-tetrofosmin was a reliable coronary blood flow tracer over a physiologic range of flows seen in ischemia or infarction conditions. Dogs were injected with 30 mCi Tc-99m-tetrofosmin during peak pharmacological stress performed with either adenosine or dipyridamole. Myocardial Tc-99m-tetrofosmin activity at 15 minutes after the injection correlated linearly with radiolabeled microsphere flow during peak stress in each dog. Myocardial Tc-99m-tetrofosmin activity appeared to underestimate flow at flows exceeding 1.5 to 2.0 mL/min/g. The plot of Tc-99m-tetrofosmin activity versus blood flow achieved a plateau at approximately 2.0 mL/min/g (see Fig. 3-1). On the other hand, as with Tc-99m-sestamibi and Tl-201, Tc-99m-tetrofosmin activity overestimated coronary blood flow in low flow ranges, at less than 0.2 mL/min/g. Tc-99m-tetrofosmin activity cleared rapidly from the blood with 2.8% and 0.8% of peak activity remaining in the blood at 5 and 15 minutes, respectively. The myocardial clearance between 3 and 15 minutes was similar in both ischemic and nonischemic regions. The myocardial activity cleared $18 \pm 11\%$ in the ischemic region. Lung activity remained lower than myocardial activity and the liver activity remained elevated over the initial 15-minute period following injection.

Mechanisms of Tc-99m-tetrofosmin myocardial uptake have been studied using different experimental models. Dahlberg and Leppo[27] evaluated the effect of coronary blood flow on the uptake of Tc-99m-tetrofosmin in the isolated rabbit heart model. The Emax of 0.37 for Tc-99m-tetrofosmin suggests a PS cap similar to that of Tc-99m-sestamibi. In comparison, Emax for Tl-201 is 0.73 and for Tc-99m-sestamibi is 0.39. However, Tc-99m-tetrofosmin has the lowest Enet among all perfusion agents. Although this lower value of Enet for Tc-99m-tetrofosmin in rabbits suggests myocardial clearance of this compound, human studies[28] have shown a stable myocardial retention of Tc-99m-tetrofosmin, at least up to 4 hours. This difference between animal and human data is not really surprising, considering that similar interspecies variability has been previously observed for the kinetics of other Tc-99m-labeled phosphine compounds.[29] Platts et al.[30] found that the uptake of Tc-99m-tetrofosmin into rat myocytes was rapid, temperature-dependent and independent of extracellular Tc-99m-tetrofosmin concentration. The lack of effect of ion channel inhibitors on Tc-99m-tetrofosmin uptake is similar to that on uptake of other cations such as Tc-99m-sestamibi. Thus, Tc-99m-tetrofosmin differs from Tl-201 in that it does not appear to act as potassium analog.

Based on experimental studies, mitochondrial membrane potential appears to play a major role in the myocardial uptake and retention of Tc-99m-tetrofosmin, as seen with Tc-99m-sestamibi. Younes et al.[31] demonstrated that Tc-tetrofosmin uptake into myocytes is likely the potential-driven transport of the lipophilic cation and myocardial uptake in vivo was related to the metabolic status of the myocytes.

Biodistribution and Dosimetry

Human biodistribution, dosimetry, and safety of Tc-99m-tetrofosmin administration at rest and during exercise were by Higley et al.[32] By 10 minutes after the injection, there was less than 5% of the injected dose in the whole blood volume and less than 3.5% of the injected dose in the total plasma volume. The blood clearance was initially faster following exercise. At 2 hours after injection, the urinary clearance was $13.1 \pm 2.1\%$ in the resting study and $8.9 \pm 1.7\%$ in the exercise study ($p < 0.001$). At 48 hours postinjection, the rate of urinary clearance was almost identical for both physiological conditions: $39.0 \pm 3.7\%$ at rest and $40.0 \pm 3.7\%$ at exercise. Analysis of whole-body images showed that good quality images of the heart can be obtained as early as 5 minutes after the injection of Tc-99m-tetrofosmin, and this uptake persisted for several hours. Myocardial background clearance resulting from activity in the blood, liver, and lung was rapid. After exercise, there was less Tc-99m-tetrofosmin activity in certain organs, mainly liver, urinary bladder, and salivary glands, in comparison to the rest study. As with Tc-99m-sestamibi, this relatively reduced liver uptake at stress can be explained by an enhanced retention in peripheral muscles as a result of the increased blood flow induced by physical exercise and by splanchnic vasoconstriction during exercise.

After a stress injection, the myocardial uptake of Tc-99m-tetrofosmin, although relatively stable over time, slightly decreases from 1.3% of the injected dose at 5 minutes to 1.0% at 2 hours after the injection. From 5 to 60 minutes after injection, the heart-to-lung ratio increases from 4.0 ± 1.1 to 5.9 ± 1.3 and the heart-to-liver ratio increases from 0.8 ± 0.3 to 3.1 ± 3.0. After a rest injection, similar kinetics were noted, and the heart-to-lung ratio increases from 3.1 ± 1.8 to 7.3 ± 4.4, and the heart-to-liver ratio increases from 0.4 ± 0.1 to 1.2 ± 0.8 from 5 to 60 minutes after injection.

Sridhara et al.[33] compared Tc-99m-tetrofosmin and Tl-201 myocardial imaging in patients with documented coronary artery disease and showed that there was no significant Tc-99m-tetrofosmin myocardial redistribution with a slow myocardial washout of approximately 4% to 5% per hour after exercise and 0.4% to 0.6% per hour after a rest injection. The estimated absorbed radiation doses at rest and at stress are given in Table 3-2. The results show that both at rest and at stress, the gallbladder wall is the target organ, followed by the other excretory organs, such as upper large intestine, lower large intestine, bladder wall, and small intestine. Overall, the radiation dose to most organs is significantly reduced during exercise in comparison to rest study.

▸ ^{99m}Tc-Pyrophosphate

Cardiac amyloidosis, a significantly underdiagnosed cause of heart failure, is usually detected late when the heart is already significantly affected. Differentiating immunoglobulin light-chain (AL) from transthyretin-related (ATTR) cardiac amyloidosis is important given the implications for prognosis, therapy, and genetic counseling.[34]

During the last two decades, noninvasive detection of cardiac amyloidosis using nuclear medicine techniques has gained in popularity.[35-38] ^{99m}Tc-labeled phosphate derivatives, initially developed as bone-seeking radiotracers for bone scintigraphy, were noted to localize to amyloid deposits. Different agents were used to detect myocyte necrosis and calcifications in amyloid deposits (with localized increased tissue calcium deposits) such as ^{99m}Tc-diphosphonate, ^{99m}Tc-pyrophosphate, ^{99m}Tc-MDP (methylene-diphosphonate) and ^{99m}Tc-DPD (diphosphino-propanodicarboxylic acid). The latter radiotracer is extensively used in European countries but is not yet approved by the FDA. Therefore, ^{99m}Tc-pyrophosphate (PYP), approved since more than 30 years for bone scintigraphy, blood pool imaging and detection of myocardial infarction, is currently used in clinical practice. The precise mechanism by which ^{99m}Tc-PYP (and the other bone-seeking radiotracers) accumulates in the myocardium of patients with cardiac amyloidosis remains unclear but is probably related to high calcium levels in amyloidosis. Different studies have shown that ^{99m}Tc-PYP cardiac imaging can distinguish ATTR from AL amyloidosis possibly because ^{99m}Tc-PYP may bind TTR amyloid fibrils more intensely than AL fibrils as a result of higher calcium containing substances in ATTR hearts. Using quantitative ^{99m}Tc-PYP cardiac imaging,

Bokhari et al[39] were able to differentiate light-chain cardiac amyloidosis from the TTR-related familial and senile cardiac amyloidosis. Using a heart-to-contralateral uptake ratio of more than 1.5, they showed a sensitivity of 97% and a specificity of 100% for identifying ATTR cardiac amyloidosis.

Two hours after intravenous injection of ^{99m}Tc-PYP, 40% to 50% of the injected dose is taken up by the skeleton. Within a period of 1 hour, 10% remains in the vascular system. The average urinary excretion is about 40% of the administered dose after 24 hours. The usual injected dose for cardiac scintigraphy is 15 mCi (555 MBq). The target organs are the bladder (1.46 rads/15 mCi with a 2-hour void and 3.45 rads/mCi with a 4-hour void) and the kidneys (2.1 rads/15 mCi).

POSITRON EMITTING RADIOPHARMACEUTICALS

There is general consensus that PET myocardial perfusion imaging is of consistently of better quality than SPECT imaging, particularly in obese patients. Attenuation correction (currently often with x-ray computed tomography) is a standard component of PET imaging. Only two PET radiotracers are currently used in North America for PET myocardial perfusion imaging: Rubidium-82 chloride (^{82}Rb) and nitrogen-13 ammonia (^{13}NH$_3$). ^{18}F-Flurpiridaz is a novel PET MPI radiotracer undergoing Phase III studies and not yet approved by the FDA for clinical use.

Table 3-3 summarizes the criteria for the ideal PET myocardial perfusion imaging radiotracer. High and rapid myocardial uptake followed by long retention in myocytes are among the most important characteristics. Mitochondria are abundant in high energy consuming such as in the heart. Various radiolabeled analogs of mitochondrial complex I inhibitors, including rotenone, have been investigated.[60,61]

▶ Rubidium-82

Rubidium (Rb)-82 is the only one PET radiotracer currently available for MPI produced by a generator. Rb-82 is a monovalent cation potassium analog and is produced by eluting a Strontium-82/Rb-82 generator[40,41] (Table 3-4). Strontium-82 decays to Rb-82 by electron capture. The elution of Rb-82 can be repeated every 8 to 10 minutes. The energy of the Rb-82 positron is relatively high (3.15 MeV) and thus the range of positron travel before annihilation is relatively long. The positron range is approximately 2.6 mm root mean square (this is the distance traveled by the emitted positron before it combines with an electron to produce two 511-keV annihilation photons), resulting in lower spatial imaging resolution than with other PET tracers (e.g., F-18 and N-13). The physical half-life of Rb-82 is 76 seconds, allowing for multiple repeat imaging sequences. The half-life of the parent Strontium-82 is 25.5 days, and therefore the strontium–rubidium generator can be used for approximately 1 month.

Table 3-3

Criteria for the "Ideal" PET Myocardial Perfusion Imaging Radiotracer

1. High myocardial uptake with no or minimal myocardial redistribution.
2. A high target-to-background ratio with low uptake in the adjacent organs (lungs, liver, stomach).
3. Linear relationship between radiotracer myocardial uptake and coronary blood flow: <5 mL/min/g (level seen with pharmacological vasodilation). This requires a high first-pass myocardial extraction fraction and a subsequent very rapid blood clearance.
4. A physical half-life that allows enough time for adequate image acquisition (and repeated acquisition if necessary) with both treadmill stress test and pharmacological intervention.
5. Positron energy that will provide better image quality and high diagnostic accuracy for the detection of CAD.
6. Quantification of absolute myocardial blood flow, enabling identification of diffuse, multivessel, or balanced CAD.
7. Appropriate radiation dosimetry and safety profile.
8. Availability as unit dose, preferably labeled with 18F because of its favorable positron physical characteristics and physical half-life of 110 minutes.

Reproduced with permission from Dilsizian V, Taillefer R: Journey in evolution of nuclear cardiology: will there be another quantum leap with the F-18-labeled myocardial perfusion tracers? *JACC Cardiovasc Imaging*. 2012;5(12):1269–1284.

Table 3-4
Summary of Some Characteristics of PET Radiotracers for Myocardial Imaging

Radiotracer	Physical Half-Life (minutes)	Maximal Energy (MeV)	Positron Range in Water (mm)	Production Method	Extraction Fraction	Retention Fraction	Effective Dose (mSv/mCi)	Typical ED (mSv/Dose)[a]
^{13}N-Ammonia	9.97	1.19	1.4	Cyclotron	92–98%	70–90%	0.074	2/15 mCi
^{15}O-water	2.03	1.70	1.5	Cyclotron	97–100%	0%	0.041	3/70 mCi
^{18}F-FDG	109.8	0.64	1.0	Cyclotron	Plasma glucose dependent	100%	0.7	7/10 mCi
^{18}F-Flurpiridaz	109.8	0.64	1.0	Cyclotron	90–95%	60–90%	0.6	8/14 mCi
^{82}Rb-Chloride	1.26	3.15	1.7	Generator	40–75%	30–60%	0.04	2/50 mCi

[a]Typical ED (effective dose): effective dose in mSv for a typical range of injected dose (average, patient-weight adjusted) for a standard clinical study (in mCi).

Being a potassium analog, Rb-82 enters the myocytes using the sodium/potassium pump, and the biologic behavior is very similar to that of thallium-201.[36,37] The first-pass extraction fraction of Rb-82 is 40% to 75% at resting flow levels, which falls to 25% to 30% at high flow, and therefore also demonstrates "roll-off" at higher blood flow levels (Fig. 3-1).[38,39] However, the roll-off starts at slightly higher blood flow levels than for Tc-99m-Tc-99m-Tc-99m-sestamibi and Tc-99m-tetrofosmin, but at lower flow levels than for Tl-201. However, this is offset by the fact that generally Rb-82 perfusion images have higher count density and are of better quality than those with single-photon imaging agents.

The myocardial extraction fraction of Rb-82 remains reduced in the myocardium recovering from transient ischemia.[42-46] It is retained in the myocardium and shows equilibrium with the potassium pool. Cell membrane disruption may cause rapid tissue loss of the radiotracer. Rubidium-82 myocardial retention can thus be used as a marker of tissue viability.[47] Furthermore, quantitative assessments of relative Rb-82 perfusion defects have correlated well with those obtained from microspheres.[48] Because of the short half-life of Rb-82 it is not practicable to perform imaging after symptom-limited physical treadmill exercise. It is therefore standard to administer coronary vasodilator stress with the patient lying on the imaging table and infuse Rb-82 during the vasodilatory state.

Patient radiation exposure with an injected dose of 50 to 60 mCi of Rb-82 is relatively low because of the short half-life of Rb-82. The estimated effective radiation dose is 0.04 mSv/mCi and total patient dose may range from 4.0 to 6.0 mSv for a complete rest–stress Rb-82 study. Even though myocardial extraction of Rb-82 is not linear at higher flow levels, several investigators have shown that absolute regional myocardial blood flow may be derived from mathematical analysis of tracer kinetics.[49] The kinetic behavior of Rb-82 can be described as a two-compartmental model with a rapid and a slow clearance component.

The arterial input function is measured from serial regions of interest (ROI) over the cardiac blood pool and the myocardial inflow from ROIs over myocardial segments. The generated time–activity curves, corrected for spillover from the blood and decay, are fitted to the two-compartmental kinetic model to derive estimates of myocardial blood flow in mL/min/g.

In practice, quantification of myocardial blood flow with Rb-82 is a challenging task because of the low signal/noise ratio of the time–activity curves. Recently, Prior et al [50] have validated a new method of quantification of myocardial blood flow using a correction methodology for the flow-dependent variable extraction of Rb-82.

▶ N-13 Ammonia

Nitrogen-13 (N-13) ammonia was the first PET radiotracer developed for MPI and the first to be approved by the FDA for this specific clinical indication. N-13 ammonia is a cyclotron-produced cation with a physical half-life of 9.8 minutes (Table 3-4).

The positron range is very short at 0.7 mm (1.4 mm in water). N-13 ammonia is rapidly extracted from the blood and trapped in the myocardium by the glutamine synthesis reaction. Myocardial uptake of N-13 ammonia depends on flow, extraction, and retention. The first-pass extraction fraction is nearly 100%, since N-13 ammonia freely diffuses across membranes.[51,52] In the myocardial tissues, N-13 ammonia is either incorporated into synthesis of N-13 glutamine or back-diffused into the vascular space. The net extraction fraction is approximately 80% (70–90%) at resting coronary blood flow range. Although linearity of myocardial uptake is better than the conventional myocardial perfusion imaging agents, roll-off does occur at higher myocardial blood flow levels (Fig. 3-1). N-13 ammonia crosses the cell membrane by passive diffusion as well as by means of active transport of the ammonium ion by the sodium/potassium pump.

Its relatively long physical half-life, high myocardial extraction fraction, and low liver and low background activity make N-13 ammonia one of the best available PET myocardial perfusion tracers. Different tracer kinetic models were used but the most common is the three-compartmental model that relates the N-13 ammonia activity: 1—in the vascular space, 2—the free interstitial space, and 3—the metabolically trapped space. Comparative studies in the animal model with microsphere measurements suggested that regional myocardial blood flow can be quantitatively assessed over a wide range of blood flow with the three-compartmental N-13 ammonia model.[53-55]

For imaging usually 10 to 20 mCi's are injected as a bolus, followed by dynamic acquisition for 10 to 15 minutes. The dynamic list mode data are then fitted to three-compartmental model. Absolute myocardial blood flow is expressed in mL/min/g. The total effective radiation dose is approximately 2.0 mSv for an injection of 20 mCi of N-13 ammonia. The target organ is the bladder, which receives 6 mSv.

O-15 Water

Oxygen (O)-15 water was one of the first radiopharmaceutical used for PET application.[56] O-15 gas is produced either by $^{14}N (d,n)$ ^{15}O reaction or $^{15}N (p,n)$ ^{15}O method. $^{15}O_2$ gas is combined to hydrogen gas to produced O-15 water.

O-15 water is cyclotron-produced, has a half-life of 2 minutes and a positron range of 1 mm (Table 3-4). After injection it diffuses freely from the blood into myocardial cells. The extraction fraction is very high and not affected by myocardial blood flow rates and is independent of metabolic state of the myocardium. Because of these characteristics, the biologic behavior of O-15 can be modeled with a simple one-compartmental Kety's model. As a consequence myocardial uptake is perfectly linear over a wide range of myocardial blood flows (Fig. 3-1). Therefore, O-15 water is considered the gold standard for clinical noninvasive absolute myocardial blood flow measurements. Cardiac PET imaging with O-15 water is very demanding because of persisting high blood pool activity, requiring subtraction of blood pool activity from the original image to visualize the myocardium. Using advanced processing of dynamic images with dedicated research softwares, relative myocardial blood flow can be estimated. Despite its success in research studies, the clinical use of O-15 water in patients is limited. Although O-15 water is used clinically in some European hospitals, it is not FDA approved yet and still considered investigational in North America.

F-18 Fluorodeoxyglucose (FDG)

The myocardium can choose various energy substrates, including free fatty acids, glucose, lactate, and ketone bodies. In the fasting state, plasma free fatty acid levels are high so that 70% to 80% of the myocardial oxygen consumption is obtained by oxidation of free fatty acid.[57] Conversely, the postprandial state elevates plasma glucose level so that myocardium shifts its fuel selection to glucose.

Fluorodeoxyglucose (FDG) is a glucose analog that enters cardiac myocytes by facilitated diffusion via glucose transporters. Once FDG is in the cell it is phosphorylated by hexokinase to FDG-phosphate. However, this is not further metabolized and FDG is trapped within the myocytes. Myocardial accumulation of FDG therefore parallels exogenous glucose utilization. FDG can be labeled with Fluor-18 (F-18), which has a half-life of 110 minutes and a positron range of 0.6 mm.

The myocardial extraction of FDG from the blood is rapid but only a small percentage of injected dose,

1% to 5%, is taken up by the heart, depending on the nutritional state or insulin stimulation. To enhance FDG uptake in the heart, the patient should be either glucose loaded or undergo the hyperinsulinemic euglycemic clamp; these techniques are beyond the scope of this chapter. These preparations drastically reduce plasma free fatty acid levels and stimulate glucose utilization.

F-18 FDG is cleared via the kidneys and excreted in the urine. The effective dose from the administration of F18-FDG for a PET-CT scan is estimated to be approximately 0.019 mSv/MBq for adults using 370 to 740 MBq (10–20 mCi). The bladder is the organ receiving the highest radiation dose. The effective dose from the CT portion of the PET/CT study can range from approximately 5 to 80 mSv depending on the CT system and protocol being used but is often comparable to the effective dose from the PET portion of the study.

F-18 FDG is predominantly used in cardiac imaging to assess myocardial viability in association to MPI radiotracers.[58,59] For this specific clinical application, glucose metabolism and uptake should maximized by the above-mentioned patient preparation. However, when F-18 FDG imaging is used to detect resting myocardial ischemia, for example, in unstable angina, or to detect active cardiac sarcoid lesions, one may consider to administer FDG in *fasting state* in order to bring out areas with enhanced glucose metabolism adjacent to areas with normal fatty acid myocardial metabolism.

F-18 Flurpiridaz

One of the most promising radiolabeled analogs of these mitochondrial complex I inhibitor is ^{18}F-flurpiridaz with a pyridaben pharmacophore.[62] Initially named RP1012 or BMS747158, the chemical structure of ^{18}F-flurpiridaz is: 2-*tert*-butyl-4-chloro-5-[4-(2-fluoro-ethoxymethyl)-benzyloxy]-2H-pyridazin-3-one. ^{18}F-flurpiridaz can be synthesized by a one-step direct fluorination in a radiopharmacy, using an automated synthesis unit.

In a rat cardiac myocytes kinetics assay, ^{18}F-flurpiridaz showed rapid uptake with a half-life of 35 seconds for maximal uptake and showed washout with a half-life of more than 2 hours.[63] Yu et al.[64] evaluated the tissue biodistribution and first-pass extraction fraction of ^{18}F-flurpiridaz in rat, rabbit, and nonhuman primate models at rest and reported first-pass extraction fraction of more than 90%. The results showed that myocardial uptake of ^{18}F-flurpiridaz was significantly higher than that of ^{99m}Tc-sestamibi not only at normal MBF range in rats but also at high MBF ranges (<5 mL/min/g) in isolated rabbit hearts, suggesting that ^{18}F-flurpiridaz may be less affected by the roll-off phenomena commonly seen with SPECT myocardial perfusion imaging agents. The cardiac uptake of ^{18}F-flurpiridaz at 15 minutes in rats was 3.5 ± 0.3% of injected dose/g in comparison to 1.9 ± 0.1 for ^{99m}Tc-sestamibi. The heart/lung and heart/liver ratio at 60 minutes after injection was 12.7± 1.4 and 3.7 ± 0.2, respectively (5.9 ± 0.5 and 2.4 ± 0.3 for ^{99m}Tc-sestamibi, respectively). Myocardial uptake of ^{18}F-flurpiridaz was shown to be stable for at least 1 hour after injection, and there was no significant myocardial redistribution.

In rat and pig models of myocardial infarction and ischemia, the ^{18}F-flurpiridaz defect area was clearly detected.[65–67] There was a good correlation between the infracted regions detected by ^{18}F-flurpiridaz and the necrotic area identified by ex vivo tissue histology. In comparison to ^{13}N-ammonia, ^{18}F-flurpiridaz showed higher activity ratios between the myocardium and blood, liver, and lungs.[67] Regional myocardial blood flow assessed with 18F-flurpiridaz showed a good correlation ($r = 0.88$, slope = 0.84) and agreement with that measured with radioactive microspheres over a wide flow range from 0.1 to 3.0 mL/min/g. A linear correlation existed between MBF quantified by radiolabeled microspheres and myocardial uptake of F-18 flurpiridaz after adenosine hyperemia.[62,68]

The high spatial resolution of PET imaging, along with high target-to-background ratios achieved with ^{18}F-flurpiridaz, allows the acquisition of very high-quality electrocardiographic-gated PET images in both animal and human studies. Initial studies in humans have shown a very good diagnostic accuracy in detection of significant CAD.[69,70] Early clinical trials have shown that ^{18}F-flurpiridaz intravenous injection is well tolerated and no clinically safety concerns have been raised. In humans, the mean effective dose is 0.02 ± 0.002 mSv/MBq at rest and 0.019 and 0.015 mSv/MBq with adenosine and exercise stress, respectively. This corresponds to that of

^{18}F-FDG (0.019 mSv/MBq). The organ with the highest radiation exposure is the heart with both adenosine and exercise stress.

The longer half-life (110 minutes) of the F-18 label of flurpiridaz makes it possible to administer the radiotracer at peak physical exercise and perform PET imaging immediately thereafter, which represents another potential advantage of ^{18}F-flurpiridaz PET imaging in comparison to all the other PET radiotracers which are suited for pharmacological stress tests and not for treadmill stress test.

CONCLUSIONS

Multiple radionuclide MPI agents are now commercially available, for both SPECT and PET imaging. Although many of their characteristics differ, they all share the same utilization, that is, the diagnostic and evaluation of patients with coronary artery disease. We are still learning how to obtain the best diagnostic results from Tl-201, Tc-99m-MPI agents, and PET radiotracers for myocardial perfusion scintigraphy. It is likely that with the newest agents and constantly evolving technology in data acquisition and analysis, our knowledge will improve and all these agents will be able to fulfill a more specific role in clinical practice.

REFERENCES

1. Dilsizian V, Taillefer R. Journey in evolution of nuclear cardiology: will there be another quantum leap with the F-18-labeled myocardial perfusion tracers. *JACC Cardiovasc Imaging*. 2012; 5:1269–1284.
2. Watson DD, Glover DK. Chapter 1: Overview of tracer kinetics and cellular mechanisms of uptake. In: Zaret BL, Beller GA, eds. *Clinical Nuclear Cardiology: State of the Art and Future Directions*. Philadelphia, PA: Mosby Elsevier; 2010:3–13.
3. Saperstein LA. Regional blood flow by fractional distribution of indicators. *Am J Physiol*. 1958;193:161–166.
4. Beller GA, Watson DD. Physiological basis of myocardial perfusion imaging with the technetium99m agents. *Semin Nucl Med*. 1991;12:173–181.
5. Dahlberg ST, Leppo JA. Myocardial kinetics of radiolabeled perfusion agents: basis for perfusion imaging. *J Nucl Cardiol*. 1994;1:189–197.
6. Leppo JA, Meerdink DJ. Comparison of the myocardial uptake of a technetium-labeled isonitrile analogue and thallium. *Circ Res*. 1989;65:632–639.
7. Weich HF, Strauss HW, Pitt B. The extraction of Tl-201 by the myocardium. *Circulation*. 1977;56:188.
8. Krahwinkel W, Herzog H, Feinendegen LE. Pharmacokinetics of thallium-201 in normal individuals after routine myocardial scintigraphy. *J Nucl Med*. 1988;29:1582.
9. Deutsch E, Bushong W, Glavan KA, et al. Heart imaging with cationic complexes of technetium. *Science*. 1981;214:85–86.
10. Dudczak R, Angelberger P, Homan R, et al. Evaluation of Tc-99m-dichloro bis (1,2-dimethylphosphino)ethane (Tc-99m-DMPE) for myocardial scintigraphy in man. *Eur J Nucl Med*. 1983;8:513–515.
11. Gerson MC, Deutsch EA, Libson KF, et al. Myocardial scintigraphy with Tc-99m-Tris-DMPE in man. *Eur J Nucl Med*. 1984;9:403–407.
12. Holman BL, Jones AG, Lister-James J, et al. A new Tc-99m labelled imaging agent, hexakis (T-butyl-isonitrile)-technetium (I) (Tc-99m-TBI): initial experience in the human. *J Nucl Med*. 1984;25:1350–1355.
13. Sia ST, Holman BL, Campbell S, et al. The utilization of technetium-99m CPI as a myocardial perfusion imaging agent in exercise studies. *Clin Nucl Med*. 1987;12:681–687.
14. Jones AG, Davison A, Abram S, et al. Biological studies of a new class of technetium complexes: the hexakis (alkylisonitrile) technetium (I) cations. *Int J Nucl Med Biol*. 1984;11:225–234.
15. Wackers FJ, Berman DS, Maddahi J, et al. Technetium-99m hexakis-2-methoxyisobutyl isonitrile: human biodistribution, dosimetry, safety and preliminary comparison to thallium-201 for myocardial perfusion imaging. *J Nucl Med*. 1989;30:310–311.
16. Piwnica-Worms D, Kronauge JF, Chiu ML. Uptake and retention of hexakis (2-methoxyisobutyl-isonitrile) technetium (I) in cultured chick myocardial cells. Mitochondrial and plasma membrane potential dependence. *Circulation*. 1990;82:1826–1838.
17. Beanlands RSB, Dawood F, Wen WH, et al. Are the kinetics of technetium-99m methoxyisobutyl isonitrile affected by cell metabolism and viability? *Circulation*. 1990;82:1802–1814.
18. Okada RD, Glover D, Gaffney T, et al. Myocardial kinetics of technetium-99m-hexakis-2-methoxy-2-methylpropyl-isonitrile. *Circulation*. 1988;77:491–498.
19. Glover DK, Okada RD. Myocardial kinetics of Tc-MIBI in canine myocardium after dipyridamole. *Circulation*. 1990;81:628–636.
20. Mousa SA, Cooney JM, Williams SJ. Relationship between regional myocardial blood flow and the distribution of Tc-99m-sestamibi in the presence of total coronary artery occlusion. *Am Heart J*. 1990;119:842–847.
21. Canby RC, Silber S, Pohost GM. Relations of the myocardial imaging agents Tc-99m mibi and Tl-201 to myocardial blood flow in a canine model of myocardial ischemic insult. *Circulation*. 1990;81:289–296.
22. Li QS, Solot G, Frank TL, et al. Myocardial redistribution of technetium-99m-methoxyisobutyl isonitrile (sestamibi). *J Nucl Med*. 1990;31:1069–1076.
23. Sinusas AJ, Bergin JD, Edwards NC, et al. Redistribution of Tc-99m-sestamibi and 201Tl in the presence of a severe coronary artery stenosis. *Circulation*. 1994;89:2332–2341.
24. Verani MS, Jeroudi MO, Mahmarian JJ, et al. Quantification of myocardial infarction during coronary occlusion and myocardial salvage after reperfusion using cardiac imaging with technetium-99m hexakis 2-methoxyisobutyl isonitrile. *J Am Coll Cardiol*. 1988;12:1573–1581.

25. Rubow S, Klopper J, Wasserman H, et al. The excretion of radiopharmaceuticals in human breast milk: additional data and dosimetry. *Eur J Nucl Med.* 1994;21:144–153.
26. Sinusas AJ, Shi QX, Saltzberg MT, et al. Technetium-99m-tetrofosmin to assess myocardial blood flow: experimental validation in an intact canine model of ischemia. *J Nucl Med.* 1994;35:664–671.
27. Dahlberg ST, Leppo JA. Myocardial kinetics of radiolabeled perfusion agents: basis for perfusion imaging. *J Nucl Cardiol.* 1994;1:189–197.
28. Sridhara BS, Braat S, Rigo P, et al. Comparison of myocardial perfusion imaging with technetium-99m tetrofosmin versus thallium-201 in coronary artery disease. *Am J Cardiol.* 1993;72:1015–1019.
29. Deutsch E, Ketring AR, Libson K, et al. The Noah's ark experiment: species dependent biodistributions of cationic Tc-99m complexes. *Nucl Med Biol.* 1989;16:191–232.
30. Platts EA, North TL, Pickett RD, et al. Mechanism of uptake of technetium-tetrofosmin. I: Uptake into isolated adult rat ventricular myocytes and subcellular localization. *J Nucl Cardiol.* 1995;2:317–326.
31. Younes A, Songadele JA, Maublant J, et al. Mechanism of uptake of technetium-tetrofosmin. II: Uptake into isolated adult rat heart mitochondria. *J Nucl Cardiol.* 1995;2:327–333.
32. Higley B, Smith FW, Smith T, et al. Technetium-99m-1, 2-bis[bis(2-ethoxyethyl) phosphino]ethane: human biodistribution, dosimetry and safety of a new myocardial perfusion imaging agent. *J Nucl Med.* 1993;34:30–38.
33. Sridhara B, Sochor H, Rigo P, et al. Myocardial single-photon emission computed tomographic imaging with technetium-99m tetrofosmin: stress-rest imaging with same-day and separate-day rest imaging. *J Nucl Cardiol.* 1994;1:138–143
34. Shah KB, Inoue Y, Mehra MR. Amyloidosis and the heart: a comprehensive review. *Arch Intern Med.* 2006;166:1805–13.
35. de Haro-del Moral FJ, Sanchez-Lajusticia A, Gomez-Bueno M, et al. Role of cardiac scintigraphy with 99mTc-DPD in the differentiation of cardiac amyloidosis subtype. *Rev Esp Cardiol.* 2012;65:440–446.
36. Noordzij W, Glaudemans JM, Longhi S, et al. Nuclear imaging for cardiac amyloidosis. *Heart Fail Rev.* 2015;20:145–154.
37. Puille M, Altland K, Linke RP, et al. 99mTc-DPD scintigraphy in transthyretin-related familial amyloidotic polyneuropathy. *Eur J Nucl Med Mol Imaging.* 2002;29:376–379.
38. Falk RH, Lee VW, Rubinow A, et al. Sensitivity of technetium-99m-pyrophosphate scintigraphy in diagnosing cardiac amyloidosis. *Am J Cardiol.* 1983;51:826–830.
39. Bokhari S, Castano A, Pozniakoff T, et al. 99mTc-pyrophosphate scintigraphy for differentiating light-chain cardiac amyloidosis from the transthyretin-related familial and senile cardiac amyloidosis. *Circ Cardiovasc Imaging.* 2013;6: 195–201.
40. VanTosh A, Garza D, Roberti R, et al. Serial myocardial perfusion imaging with dipyridamole and rubidium-82 to assess restenosis after angioplasty. *J Nucl Med.* 1995;36:1553–1560.
41. Gould K, Goldstein R, Mullani N, et al. Noninvasive assessment of coronary stenoses by myocardial perfusion imaging during pharmacologic coronary vasodilation. VIII. Clinical feasibility of positron cardiac imaging without a cyclotron using generator-produced rubidium-82. *J Am Coll Cardiol.* 1986;7:775–789.
42. Mullani N, Gould K. First pass regional blood flow measurements with external detectors. *J Nucl Med.* 1983;24:577–581.
43. Nishiyama H, Sodd V, Adolph R, et al. Intercomparison of myocardial imaging agents: 201Tl, 129Cs, 43K, and 81Rb. *J Nucl Med.* 1976;17:880–889.
44. Donato L, Bartolomei G, Giordani R. Evaluation of myocardial blood perfusion in man with radioactive potassium or rubidium and precordial counting. *Circulation.* 1964;29:195–203.
45. Mullani N, Goldstein R, Gould K, et al. Myocardial perfusion with rubidium-82. I. Measurement of extraction fraction and flow with external detectors. *J Nucl Med.* 1983;24:898–906.
46. Wilson RA, Shea M, DeLandsheere C, et al. Rubidium-82 myocardial uptake and extraction after transient ischemia: PET characteristics. *J Comput Assist Tomogr.* 1987;11:60–66.
47. Goldstein R. Kinetics of rubidium-82 after coronary occlusion and reperfusion. Assessment of patency and viability in open-chested dogs. *J Clin Invest.* 1985;75:1131–1137.
48. Lautamaki R, George RT, Kitagawa K, et al. Rubidium-82 PET-CT for quantitative assessment of myocardial blood flow: validation in a canine model of coronary artery stenosis. *Eur J Nucl Med Mol Imaging.* 2009;36:576–586.
49. Knuuti J, Kajander S, Maki M, et al. Quantification of myocardial blood flow will reform the detection of CAD. Editorial point of view. *J Nucl Cardiol.* 2009;16:497–506.
50. Prior JO, Allenbach G, Valenta I, et al. Quantification of myocardial blood flow with Rb-82 positron emission tomography: clinical validation with O-15 water. *Eur J Nucl Mol Imaging.* 2012;39:1037–1047.
51. Schelbert HR, Phelps ME, Huang SC, et al. N-13 ammonia as an indicator of myocardial blood flow. *Circulation.* 1981;63:1259–1272.
52. Schelbert HR, Phelps ME, Hottman EJ, et al. Regional myocardial perfusion assessed with N-13 labeled ammonia and positron emission computerized axial tomography. *Am J Cardiol.* 1979;43:209–218.
53. Bol A, Melin JA, Vanoverschelde JL, et al. Direct comparison of 13N ammonia and 15O water estimates of perfusion with quantification of regional myocardial blood flow by microspheres. *Circulation.* 1993;87:512–525.
54. Muzik O, Beanlands RS, Hutchins GD, et al. Validation of nitrogen-13-ammonia tracer kinetic model for quantification of myocardial blood flow using PET. *J Nucl Med.* 1993;34:83–91.
55. Khule WG, Porenta G, Huang SC, et al. Quantification of regional myocardial blood flow using N-13 ammonia and reoriented dynamic positron emission tomographic imaging. *Circulation.* 1993;86:1004–1017.
56. Bergmann SR, Fox KA, Rand AL, et al. Quantification of regional myocardial blood flow in vivo with H215O. *Circulation.* 1984;70:724–733.
57. Bing RJ. *The Metabolism of the Heart. Harvard Lecture Series.* New York: Academic Press; 1954:27–70.
58. Gropler RJ. Recent advances in metabolic imaging. An ASNC 20th anniversary article: Review article. *J Nucl Cardiol.* 2013;20:1147–1172.
59. Camici PG, Prasad SK, Rimoldi OE. Stunning, hibernation, and assessment of myocardial viability. *Circulation.* 2008;117:103–114.
60. Hollingwoth RM, Ahammadsahib KI, Gadelhak G, et al. New inhibitors of complex I of the mitochondrial electron transport chain with activity as pesticides. *Biochem Soc Trans.* 1994;22:230–233.

61. Gurm GS, Danik SB, Shoup TM, et al. 4-(18F)-Tetraphenylphosphonium as a PET tracer for mitochondrial membrane potential. *J Am Coll Cardiol Img.* 2012;5:285–292.
62. Yu M, Nekolla SG, Schwaiger M, et al. The next generation of cardiac positron emission tomography imaging agents: Discovery of Flurpiridaz F-18 for detection of coronary artery disease. *Sem Nucl Med.* 2011;41:305–313.
63. Yalamanchili Y, Wexler E, Hayes M, et al. Mechanism of uptake and retention of F-18 BMS-747158-02 in cardiomyocytes: a novel PET myocardial imaging agent. *J Nucl Cardiol.* 2007;14:782–788.
64. Yu M, Guaraldi MT, Mistry M, et al. BMS-747158-02: a novel PET myocardial perfusion imaging agent. *J Nucl Cardiol.* 2007;14:789–798.
65. Higuchi T, Nekolla SG, Huisman MM, et al. A new 18F-labeled myocardial PET tracer: myocardial uptake after permanent and transient coronary occlusion in rats. *J Nucl Med.* 2008;49:1715–1722.
66. Sherif HM, Saraste A, Weidl E, et al. Evaluation of a novel 18F-labeled positron emission tomography perfusion tracer for the assessment of myocardial infarct size in rats. *Circ Cadiovasc Imaging.* 2009;2:77–84.
67. Nekolla SG, Reder S, Saraste A, et al. Evaluation of a novel myocardial perfusion positron-emission tomography tracer 18F-BMS-747158-02: comparison to 13N-ammonia and validation with microspheres in a pig model. *Circulation.* 2009:2333–2342.
68. Maddahi J. Properties of an ideal PET perfusion tracer: New PET tracer cases and data. *J Nucl Cardiol.* 2012;19:S30–S37.
69. Maddahi J, Czernin J, Lazewatsky J, et al. Phase I, first-in-human study of BMS747158, a novel 18F-labeled tracer for myocardial perfusion PET: dosimetry, biodistribution, safety and imaging characteristics after a single injection at rest. *J Nucl Med.* 2011;52:1490–1498.
70. Berman DS, Maddahi J, Tamarappoo BK, et al. Phase II safety and clinical comparison with single-photon emission computed tomography myocardial perfusion imaging for detection of coronary artery disease. *J Am Coll Cardiol.* 2013;61:469–477.

Cardiac SPECT and PET Instrumentation

CHAPTER 4

James A. Case

INTRODUCTION

The changing needs of cardiologists and patients have led to an unprecedented evolution in nuclear cardiology instrumentation. Modern instrumentation has a wide range of collimation, attenuation correction (AC) options, and many of the newest systems no longer relying on the Anger gamma camera design. Solid-state detector technologies and new aperture designs are commercially available and in widespread use. Hybrid SPECT and PET systems now have transmission imaging options for AC using x-ray CT, radionuclide, or novel fluorescence x-ray sources.

The changes in instrumentation have been driven by *revolutionary changes* in the delivery of health care. In particular, there has been a shift from office-based nuclear cardiology services to hospital-based imaging. According to MedAxiom, respondents reported a dramatic shift in providers from private practices to integrated practices. In 2008, only 11% of MedAxiom respondents reported being in an integrated group (e.g., integrated into a hospital environment). By 2012, almost 60% of respondents reported practicing within an integrated practice.[1] The integration of cardiovascular imaging into the hospital setting has significantly altered the kinds of instrumentation available to the cardiologist. This access has provided clinicians the capability for routine AC, neuronal imaging, absolute blood flood, sarcoid imaging, amyloid imaging, metabolic imaging (glucose and fatty acid tracers) and other advanced molecular imaging techniques. This chapter will describe the instrumentation that is commonly used in nuclear cardiology and explain some of the important advances in instrumentation that can improve image quality and reduce radiation exposure.

SPECT INSTRUMENTATION

▶ Anger Camera

Hal Anger, with his team at the University of California, Berkeley had worked with the rectilinear scanners and pin-hole camera designs. In 1957, this group changed the design to allow for a uniform magnification and resolution across the field of view with increased system sensitivity. The first "Anger" scintillator camera consisted of a 4-in sodium iodine crystal optically coupled to 7 photomultiplier tubes (PMTs).[2,3]

Gamma camera design has evolved significantly since 1957 with improvements in resolution, sensitivity, and energy discrimination, however the conceptual design of the Anger camera is remarkably unchanged. The "Anger" gamma camera consists of (see Fig. 4-1):

- **Focusing, multi-hole collimator:** The focusing collimator is placed in front of the other camera components. The image is formed by excluding photons not traveling along a particular path, for example, perpendicular to the camera face or holes focusing on a point or line.
- **Scintillation crystal:** A material that will luminesce with optical photons when excited by ionizing radiation.

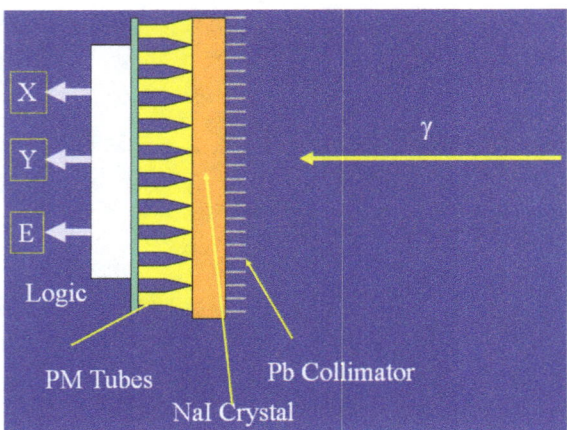

FIGURE 4-1 The Anger camera "focuses" the incident gamma radiation using a collimator. The incident photon is converted to visible light in a scintillator crystal. From there, the light pulse is converted to an electronic signal that is digitized and recorded.

- **PMT array:** Electronics for capturing the photons produced by the scintillator crystal and converting those photons into an electronic pulse.
- **Analog-to-digital conversion hardware:** A digitization board converts the analog pulse-height information into a position and energy for each photon event.

Collimation, Imaging Efficiency, and Image Quality

Unlike optical photons, gamma photons cannot be focused with either reflection or refraction. "Focusing" for gamma rays is typically performed by preferentially accepting only those photons traveling in a particular direction. The use of collimation dramatically reduces photon sensitivity by absorbing almost 99.99% of all photons entering the camera. The most common collimator used in SPECT is a parallel-hole collimator. These collimators function by using an array of parallel holes in a block of attenuating material such as lead or tungsten (see Fig. 4-2). There are some less common geometry collimators that are specific to various cardiac application such as fan beam collimation that focus on a line at a fixed distance from the collimator and variable distance collimator.[4]

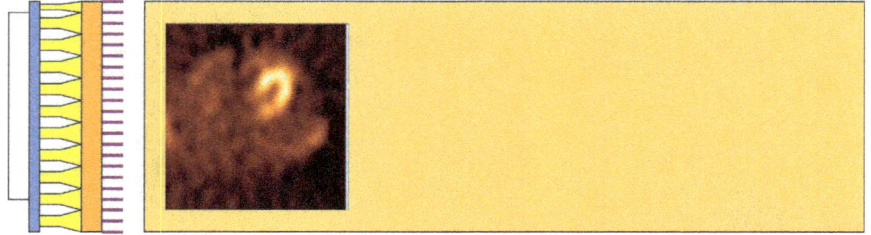

Parallel Hole Geometry: Sensitivity independent of distance

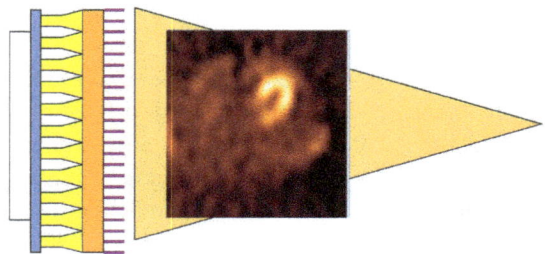

Fan Beam Geometry: FOV changes with distance and concentrates counts

FIGURE 4-2 Collimator designs can be varied to alter the field of view and sensitivity of the imaging system as a functions of distance.

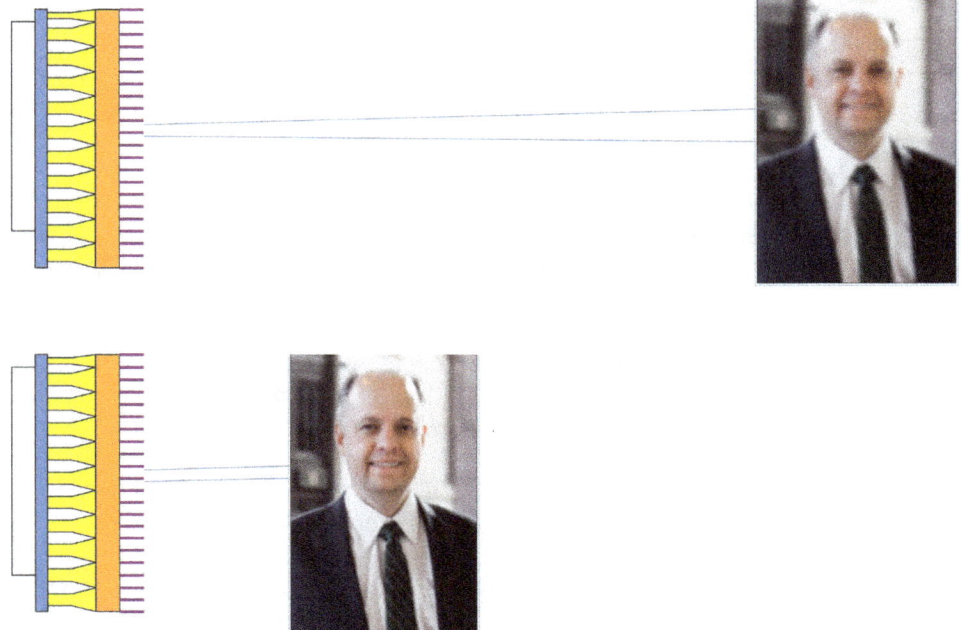

FIGURE 4-3 Illustration of distance-dependent spatial resolution with parallel-hole collimation on SPECT cameras. Larger distances (above) have a larger point spread function (lower resolution) when compared with shorter distances (below).

The use of collimation instead of the lenses that are used in conventional photography, leads to some interesting differences in nuclear imaging:

1. The use of collimation results in a loss of resolution with increasing source distance from the detector surface (see Fig. 4-3).[5]
2. Sensitivity is constant with distance. Specifically, the number of counts/second recorded is independent of distance, so long as the loss of resolutions does not result in counts missing the detector entirely.
3. The field of view for parallel-hole collimation does not change with distance.

The resolution of a gamma camera depends on the diameter and length of the holes in the collimating material. "High-resolution" collimators tend to have a longer hole length, smaller hole diameter, and thinner septa compared with "general-purpose" or "all-purpose" collimators.[6]

Parallel-hole collimation is generally favored but most nuclear laboratories because of the consistency of the resolution with patient positioning, camera rotation, and protocol variation.[7]

Fan-beam geometry allows radiation emitted from a source at a specific distance to pass through the collimator without interaction and reach the crystal surface.[8] A hybrid design combining both fan-beam properties in the center of the field of view and a gradual approach to parallel-hole design toward the edge of the field of view has been implemented on a dual detector Anger-based SPECT system for cardiac SPECT.[4,9] This design improves the geometric component of system sensitivity by a factor of 2 over parallel geometry and minimizes truncation of projections near the edge of the field of view.

▶ **Image Formation**

When a gamma photon is absorbed by the scintillation crystal, a burst of secondary optical photons is then released. An array of PMTs, positioned behind the crystal, detects and converts the light pulse into an electric pulse that is digitized.

The digitization process is a mathematical weighting of the pulses from all PMTs detecting the scintillation produces X, Y (spatial location), and Z

(energy) values. The energy value is tested by a discrimination circuit that will exclude the signal if it is not within the permitted energy range (referred to as the "energy window").

Energy resolution has an important role in differentiating between scatter and photopeak photons. When gamma rays scatter off of electrons in the media, they release some of their energy to the electrons (referred to as the recoil electron). As a result of scattering of the electrons, the energy of the scattered photon is reduced. This process of photons elastically scattering off of electrons in the media is referred to as Compton scattering. Compton scattering degrades the images quality by reducing the contrast resolution and spatial resolution of the image.

System sensitivity is another key imaging performance measure expressed in units of counts/min/μCi (cpm/μCi) of Tc-99m. It is dependent on the length and diameter of the holes in the collimator. Higher system sensitivity collimators allow more photons to pass through the collimator at the expense of spatial resolution. Conversely, higher-resolution collimators allow fewer photons to pass through the collimator by restricting the acceptance angle of the collimator holes. This reduction in acceptance angle improves the spatial resolution of the system.

Tomographic Gantry

To produce tomographic images of a patient, a series of projections around the patient is needed. The most common approach is to mount one or more Anger cameras on a rotating gantry. Early designs for the gantry involved a single camera head that could be rotated around the patient on a fork mount. Because these systems were also used for planar imaging, the camera head could be rotated around two axes.[10] With the increase use of SPECT and the challenge of maintaining an accurate center of rotation led to near universal use of the single axis of rotation gantry for cardiac studies.

The most common design in use today for cardiac SPECT is a dual-headed gamma camera with 90 degrees of separation between each camera head (see Fig. 4-4). To complete a tomographic study, the camera only needs to complete a 90-degree arc, and camera heads rotate simultaneously, thus saving image acquisition time. This geometry offers an excellent combination of a wide field of view, scanning efficiency, and simplicity. Most systems also offer the option to acquire a noncircular orbit to minimize the distance between the camera and the patient. This has the effect of improving the resolution by up to 1.5 to 2.5 mm.[11]

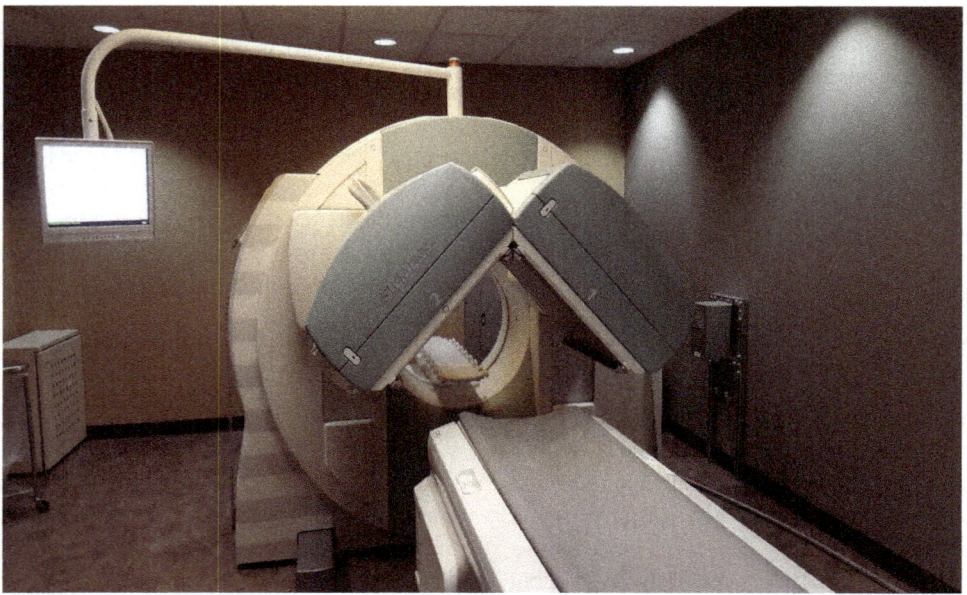

FIGURE 4-4 Picture of an Anger-based SPECT system. The system above displayed also has a 6-slice CT scanner attached (hybrid SPECT/CT system).

Solid State, Non-Anger Imaging

Several solid-state detector-based systems are now available commercially.[12-14] These systems have a crystal layer placed over an array of semiconductor units that collect the scintillation light directly forming a net electronic charge in each unit that is proportional to the incident scintillation light. Because of the more direct coupling of crystal and detectors, the energy and location are more easily determined. Common solid-state crystals are cadmium-zinc telluride (CZT) and cesium-iodide (CsI) due to their physical and optical emission properties.[15] A lead or tungsten collimator is also used over the crystal surface for localization of incident photons as with the Anger approach. In comparison to Anger systems, solid-state detectors have superior energy resolution compared with the NaI(Tl) crystals. Thus, solid-state detectors intrinsically have greater contrast resolution. System sensitivity of the solid-state detectors is modestly (10–15%) lower than Anger systems.[16] However, this decrease in acquisition efficiency is offset by the use of multiarrays of detectors encompassing greater angular range for detection about the patient that improves the efficiency for detection.

Multi-Detector System

More recently, several alternatives to the Anger gamma camera have been introduced. One such system utilizes nine independent scanning detectors to concentrate the imaging on a small field of view, centered on the heart[12] (D-SPECT, Spectrum Dynamics, Haifa, Israel). The advantage of this system is the ability of the scanner to concentrate the acquisition on the myocardium. This has the effect of preferentially improving the system's SPECT sensitivity in the region of the heart (see Fig. 4-5). The D-SPECT system does not have the same quality control procedures as a conventional Anger SPECT system. Daily quality control (QC) consists of three QC steps: (1) global homogeneity, (2) regional homogeneity, and (3) field of view.[17] These must be performed to insure optimal image quality.

Several studies have been performed to investigate the potential for this scanner for ultra–low-dose, stress first imaging.[18] In a study of 284 patients (208 with coronary angiography, 76 low likelihood) populations were split into a 128 standard stress dose

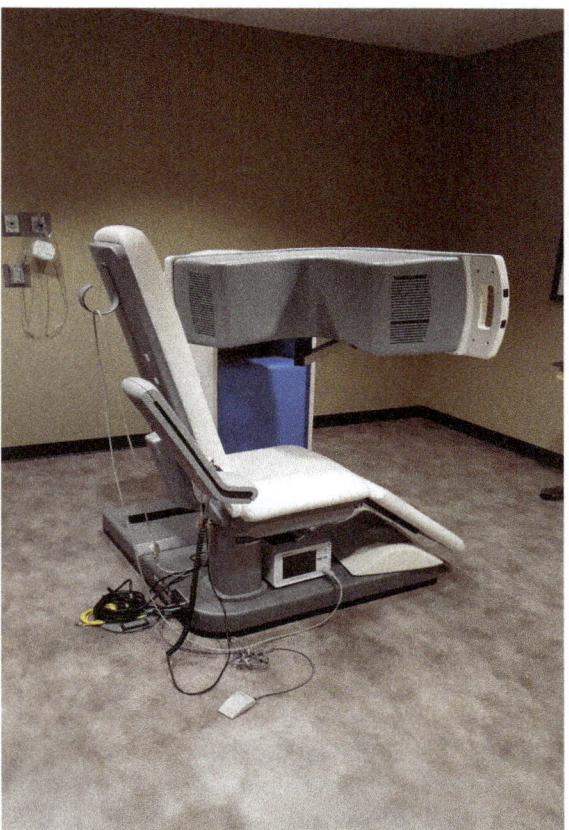

FIGURE 4-5 The D-SPECT system is a cardiac-only system that has the capability of rapid imaging in both the upright and supine positions.

(10.2 ± 0.5 mCi) patients and 156 low stress dose (5.9 ± 1.2 mCi). In that study there was no significant difference between sensitivity, specificity, and accuracy between the low dose and standard dose studies (86.1%, 76.6%, and 81.4%; and 90.6%, 78.1%, and 84.4%, respectively, p = ns). This implied that for those patients that only required a stress study, the radiation dose was as 1.7 ± 0.3 mSv.

Multi Pinhole

In the multipinhole aperture approach,[13,19] individual "pinholes" are placed strategically on the surface of a solid lead structure on each detector such that photons may only pass through the apertures to reach the underlying detectors (see Fig. 4-6). This approach permits the images to be acquired without gantry rotation as with conventional systems. The

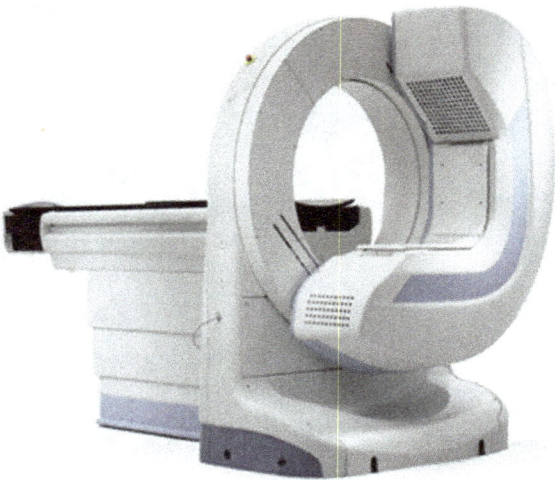

FIGURE 4-6 The Discovery 530 NM systems uses a system of multiple pinholes to focus the incident gamma radiation. This system has the advantage of simultaneously acquiring all of the projections necessary for tomographic imaging, thus enabling the potential of true dynamic imaging.

system sensitivity (per unit activity) compared with conventional Anger-based systems is approximately five times that of conventional SPECT imaging.

One such system consisting of 19 pinholes has become available to cardiologists (Discovery NM 530c, General Electric). This system projects onto 4 solid-state CZT pixilated detector. This system has the advantage that there are no moving parts and is 5 to 10 times more sensitivity than conventional Anger systems.[20]

Sensitivity and specificity of the Discovery NM 530c were studied in a population of 160 patients imaged myocardial perfusion patients using a weight-adjusted rest/stress Tc-99m-sestamibi study. In that study, the automated, computer results showed higher specificity (59–67% vs. 27–60%) and lower sensitivity (71–72% vs. 79–93%) than the visual reads.[21] This would suggest that the appearance of these images may be different than conventional images, however the differences are predictable. It is likely that with experience, visual interpretation should approach computer-generated results.

ATTENUATION CORRECTION AND TRANSMISSION IMAGING

AC is employed in cardiac SPECT to compensate for image artifacts that can result from absorption of photons by the soft tissue of the patient.[22-24] AC requires an anatomical map as additional information for the reconstruction algorithm to compensate for this loss of signal. Two transmission imaging approaches commonly used to measure the patient anatomy are as follows:

- **Radionuclide sources:** These sources can acquire transmission data simultaneously or sequentially with the emission scan while the x-ray–based approaches acquire images only in sequential mode.[8,22] These approaches typically have a very low radiation dose (0.03 mSv).[25]
- **X-ray–based CT systems:** X-ray CT images also have spatial resolution that is on the order of 10 times greater than the emission images. X-ray CT images can be temporally gated with ECG signals for AC while radionuclide source methods are generally not acquired with ECG gating.[23]

Line Source Attenuation Correction

Scanning line sources using Gd-153 (100 keV, $T_{1/2}$ = 273 days) are the most commonly used radionuclide source method for SPECT AC.[8,22] These systems use an external source of radiation to project gamma rays through the patient to the detector on the far side of the patient. To create a transmission reconstruction of the attenuating medium, two scans are needed: a blank scan of the line source without the patient present, and a scan with the patient present. The ratio of the scan divided by the blank scan is then used to create a patient-specific map of the attenuation.

One advantage line source AC has over CT-based AC is that it can be performed simultaneous to the emission study. This improves laboratory efficiency and removes the possibility of misregistration between the transmission and emission datasets. Another advantage of using a line source AC is the elimination of common CT artifacts such as breathing artifacts, metal artifacts, etc.

The greatest challenge of using line source AC is acquiring sufficient counts to perform a transmission reconstruction. It is important for quality of AC imaging to maintain the strength of the radionuclide sources by periodic replenishment as recommended by the manufacturer.[26] As the sources decay, the acquisition time must be extended proportionally to maintain image quality, which can decrease patient convenience and laboratory efficiency. Compromised quality of the attenuation map may result from image noise otherwise, introducing artifacts in the attenuation maps resulting in compromised accuracy or artifacts in the corrected images.[27]

CT-Based Attenuation Correction

The high spatial resolution of x-ray CT images has significant implications for AC quality. CT-based AC is similar to line source AC in that a patient-specific map of the patient's anatomy is used to compensate for the influence of soft tissue attenuation. Though this process on its surface is similar to line source AC, there are several important differences:

1. X-ray CT-based transmission imaging is by necessity performed sequentially to the emission study. This has a negative impact on laboratory efficiency. This also can introduce artifacts that are a result of misregistration between the transmission and emission datasets.
2. X-ray CT-based images are recorded in Hounsfield units. An algorithm is needed to translate these units into attenuation coefficients.
3. X-ray CT-based AC typically has higher radiation dose for the patient.[28] Every effort must be made to minimize the radiation from the CT portion of the study.

Proper AC requires the attenuation map images be aligned in all dimensions with the SPECT images.[29] As the CT images may be acquired over a single phase, and the emission images over multiple phases, this is not always easily performed. As a result, the attenuation map boundaries of the CT images are much sharper compared with the radionuclide images in the same patient. Misalignment by as little as 1 cm may produce artifacts with severity similar to true perfusion defects. The linear attenuation coefficients (or Hounsfield units), which comprise the attenuation map pixel values, vary greatly in the thorax compared with other regions of the body where lung tissue values for 140 keV (Tc-99m) are almost 10 times less than those for the myocardium. Whenever CT-based AC is applied, images must be carefully inspected for misregistration and corrected as necessary.[30]

One application that has been suggested is to use diagnostic quality CT in conjunction with myocardial perfusion to assess the presence of coronary calcium in patients with no known history of CAD. In a study of 1,126 asymptomatic patients with a quantitative coronary calcium score, it was demonstrated that the use of coronary calcium assessment in conjunction with myocardial perfusion assessment independently improved the prediction of future cardiac events.[31] There have also been smaller studies that suggest that the combination of SPECT with CT angiographic result could provide some added clinical value, additional research is needed to establish optimal clinical scenarios and justification for the additional procedure and radiation dose.[32]

TOMOGRAPHIC IMAGE RECONSTRUCTION

In conventional parallel-hole SPECT imaging, multiple projection images of the patient are taken at uniformly spaced angles to obtain a three-dimensional (3D) image. Iterative algorithms, described below, may include additional information about the physics of the imaging process, including spatial resolution, noise, and attenuation properties to improve the accuracy of reconstruction.[33-35]

▶ Filtered Backprojection Reconstruction

The physics of the image formation process is modeled mathematically by a *projector matrix*. A common model for this process is the Radon transform.[36] All the activity along each line of sight is integrated onto a single (ideal) point on the detector surface.

The 3D reconstruction is made by taking the Fourier transform of each projection dataset and filtering that data using a linear filter that suppresses lower-frequency modes when compared to higher frequency modes (the "ramp filter," see Fig. 4-7). Noise filtering can also be applied to the projections prior to reconstruction, during reconstruction, or postreconstruction. ECG-gated projections, separated into bins over the cardiac cycle, are independently reconstructed to produce the dynamic functional representation of the heart over the cardiac cycle.

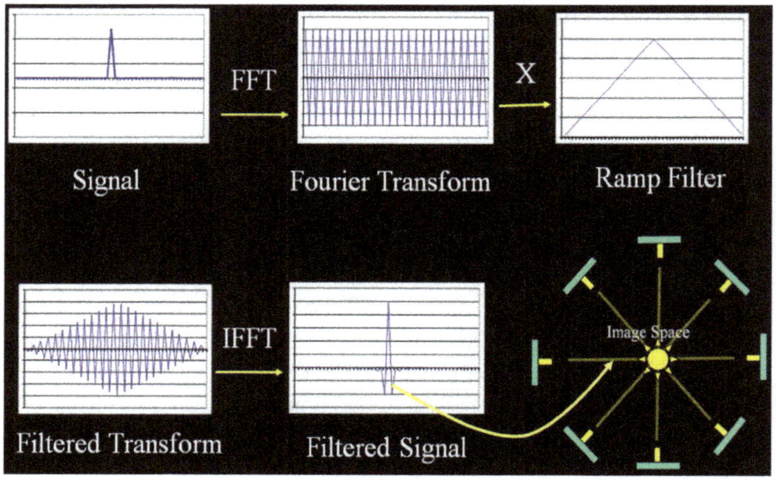

FIGURE 4-7 The ramp filter is a filter that is applied to the Fourier transform of the image to suppress low-frequency artifacts that produce from simple back projection. The result is negative sidelobes to the point spread function that eliminate these artifacts, creating a true tomographic reconstruction from the projection data.

Filtered-backprojection (FBP) reconstruction is being replaced by iterative reconstruction technique. Iterative reconstructions can model the noise in the data, resolution, scatter, and attenuation. For these reasons, FBP reconstruction should be avoided when iterative techniques are available.

Iterative Image Reconstruction

Iterative algorithms use a stepwise approach and have a more comprehensive and mathematically acceptable framework for tomographic imaging.[37,38] They provide a statistically "most probable" image that would produce the projection data, given the projection model including the physics of imaging. Iterative SPECT reconstruction begins with an initial estimate of the activity distribution, usually a uniform map. At each step of the iteration sequence, an update of the present estimate on each transverse plane is calculated. The most common strategy for performing iterative reconstruction are the maximum likelihood expectation–maximization (MLEM) algorithm[37] and the ordered subsets expectation–maximization (OSEM) model[38] (see Fig. 4-8). MLEM reconstruction requires the specification of the number of iterations, while OSEM requires specification of both number of iterations and subsets (a subgroup of the projection images).

Iterative algorithms can be used to reconstruct the attenuation map from transmission images, or to reconstruct attenuation-corrected images where the attenuation map is provided as an input to the MLEM

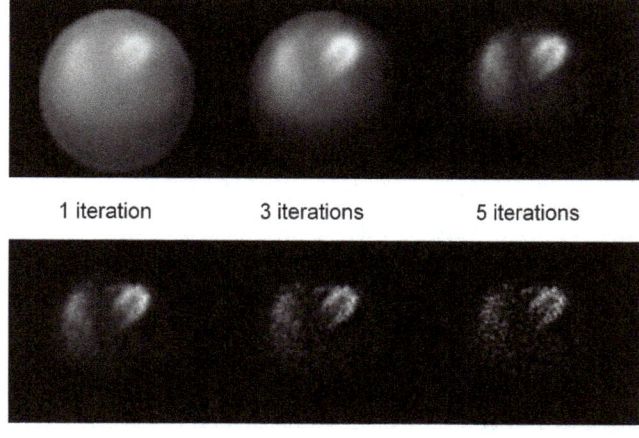

FIGURE 4-8 Iterative reconstruction is a stepwise algorithm for successively improving the estimate of the tracer distribution base on the projection data and a model the photon transport to the imaging system. This model can include attenuation, scatter, blur, etc.

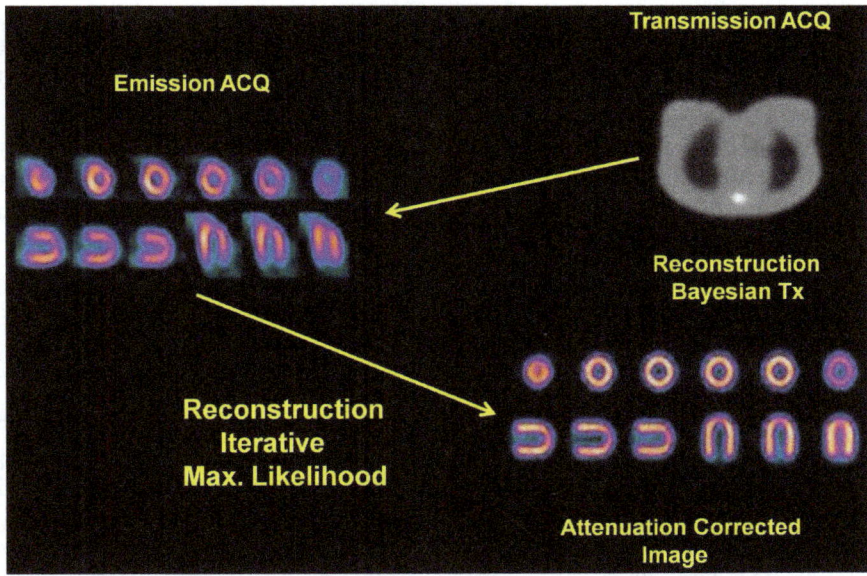

FIGURE 4-9 Attenuation correction of SPECT is performed by building the attenuation map into an iterative reconstruction algorithm. This way the attenuation artifacts can be stepwise removed from the final reconstruction.

or OSEM algorithm. The attenuation information is integrated into the reconstruction and creates a set of weights for compensating for the attenuation in the image (see Fig. 4-9). When applied to x-ray CT acquisitions, this approach removes the severe artifacts that result from metals or other highly dense materials used in devices such as ICDs for CT.[39,40]

Reconstruction Algorithms for Rapid SPECT Acquisitions

Software approaches for image reconstruction have been recently described and clinically validated for "fast" image acquisition protocols with "one-half" to "one-fourth" the time of conventional acquisitions.[33-35] These algorithms differ somewhat in modeling detail by manufacturer, but they are based on the principle described by Muehllehner that when system resolution improves, the signal-to-noise value increases at each point, as the blur is reduced and the counts are more efficiently utilized.[41] The various methods have the common attributes of combined distance-dependent spatial resolution compensation and optimized statistical noise modeling internal to the iterative reconstruction algorithm. These new algorithms offer an opportunity to reduce radiation dose to the patient and/or decrease image acquisition time.

Photopeak Scatter and Nonstationary Spatial Resolution

AC for SPECT is performed using iterative reconstruction, but it does not correct for all of the artifacts that are present in SPECT. The different commercial approaches differ by what processes are included, and how they are balanced in the modeling of the image formation process. Compton scattering of photons, partial volume effects, and depth-dependent spatial resolution are factors that are also important to correct for physical limitations of SPECT.[42] Compton-scattered photons detected in the photopeak window reduce the contrast resolution or "blur" the image as a result of redirection by the scattering process. This increases the "background" or surrounding pixel values locally, but may actually lead to false-negative regions depending on the management by the reconstruction algorithm. Tracer uptake in the liver and other sub diaphragmatic structures can significantly influence the image values in the heart, typically the inferior regions where blurring into surrounding pixels occurs.[43] Using techniques to minimize uptake prior to imaging is important for Tc-99m–based agents because of the affinity of sub diaphragmatic structures.[44] Extracardiac activity adjacent to the myocardium can cause improper scaling of the image suppressing the other regions of the myocardial image. This has the potential for an artifactual decrease in anterior wall intensity.[45] Information for estimating the amount of scatter in the photopeak can be collected in a separate energy window simultaneously to subtract a fraction of these data from the photopeak image. Most scatter correction methods with conventional cardiac SPECT are implemented in combination with AC methods utilizing the attenuation map or modeling to estimate scatter interaction and perform the corrections during image reconstruction.[46]

PET INSTRUMENTATION

Basics of PET

The first application of positron annihilation medical imaging was first explored in by Brownell et al. for imaging brain tumors.[47] This technique was later expanded to tomographic imaging in 1971.[48] Myocardial perfusion PET with ^{13}N ammonia was one of the first practical implementations of PET in the myocardium.[49] ^{13}N ammonia produces high-quality myocardial perfusion images with favorable responses to changes in blood flow.[49-50] The short half-life of ^{13}N requires a nearby cyclotron for production, thereby limiting the number of sites that can use it. A more practical approach employs a generator to produce the radionuclide. ^{82}Rb was studied in 1986 as a generator-produced potassium analog for the detection of myocardial infarction.[51-52] Using an ^{82}Sr generator ($T_{1/2}$ = 28 days), a user could be provided with an on-site generator every 4 weeks. More recently, these generators can be supplied for up to 6 weeks, depending upon available camera technology.[53,54]

Metabolic cardiac imaging with PET has been of great interest because of the relative simplicity of using PET radionuclides with metabolically active molecules. ^{18}F-labeled deoxyglucose (FDG) (a glucose analog) has long been used for imaging myocardial viability[55,56] and has been also used for imaging of ischemic activation[57] and sarcoid imaging.[58] As a metabolic agent, FDG is trapped in cells that utilizes predominately glucose metabolism. This can be present in hibernating myocardium, severely ischemic myocardium, infections and inflammation as well as in tumors. In addition, metabolic agents have been explored for fatty acid metabolism, cardiac denervation, and the detection of amyloid plaques.[59-61]

PET Scanners

PET photon events consist of the following[62]:

- True pairs: Actual coincidence events where two unscattered 511-MeV photons produced by the same positron annihilation and are detected by the system. These events are used for producing the tomographic images.
- Photon scatter events: Coincidence events where two photons produced by the same positron annihilation are recorded by the system, but at least one of the photons has been scattered by electrons in the patient. These events degrade image contrast.
- Random events: Coincidence events where two photons produced by different positron annihilations are recorded by the system within the timing gate of the system. These events degrade image contrast.
- Prompt gamma: Additional photons that are produced during the nuclear decay that produces the positron. Given the timing, these photons can appear as coincidence photons. With Rb-82, 13% of all decays produce and additional 776-keV prompt gamma. When these photons are not accounted for, the over-correction for scatter can reduce specificity from 90% to 22%.[63]

A coincidence "event" occurs when two 511-keV photons resulting from positron decay and annihilation, emitted nearly 180 degrees apart, are detected "simultaneously" within a small (4–12 nanoseconds) timing window.[62] Most PET scanners consist of a system of concentric rings of multiple-detector blocks around a central axis (see Fig. 4-10). Each of these detectors contains a scintillator crystal and a small array of photo-multiplier tubes. The physical properties of the scintillator crystal determine much of the performance of the PET scanner. Ideally, a

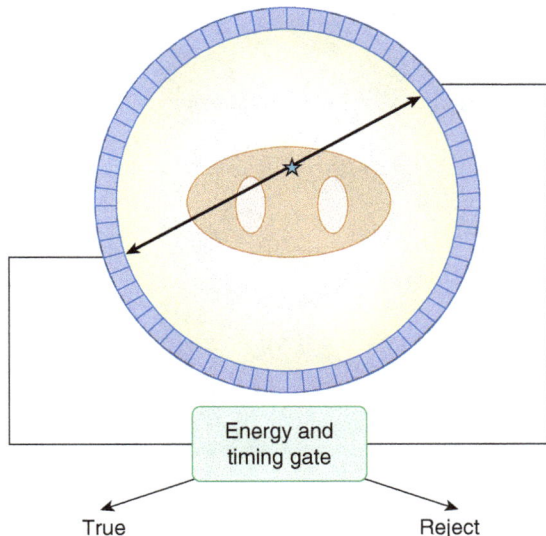

FIGURE 4-10 A PET scanner consists of a concentric ring of detector design to detect the coincidence of photon received by the scanner. A timing gate is used to identify photon events that fall in the correct timing range, approximately 5 to 10 nanoseconds. The logic also determines if the events are within an acceptable energy range.

scintillator crystal has a high stopping power (to reduce the depth the gamma rays penetrate before being recorded), high light output per event (needed to differentiate photon energies), and a rapid light curve decay (to minimize the time needed to record the photon event and have the crystal ready to receive the next event). Response time of the system describes how effective a system can differentiate random events from true coincidence. To accomplish this, a coincidence timing window of <10 nanoseconds is needed to differentiate true pairs from random coincidence event. As challenging as that may appear, most modern PET scanners have coincidence windows of <5 nanoseconds, making it possible to not only differentiate the difference between randoms and trues, but utilize the differences in the arrival times of the two annihilation photons to localize the annihilation event along the line of site.

The intrinsic sensitivity of PET is typically much higher than SPECT due to the fact that localization of the annihilation event does not require the use of collimation. Despite this fact, a large number of PET imaging systems use a system of septa to reduce scatter and randoms and thereby improve the image quality of the final reconstructed images.

Recent enhancements in processing techniques have enabled fully 3D imaging (septa removed) with Rb-82.[64] Removing the septa significantly improves the sensitivity of the imaging system, potentially increasing system sensitivity by a factor of two to five times.[65] The American Society of Nuclear Cardiology recommends reducing the infused dose of Rb-82 from 50 mCi using two-dimensional (2D) imaging to 30 mCi in 3D. Similar dose reduction is also recommended for FDG imaging.[66]

▶ **Attenuation Correction of PET**

In contrast with SPECT, AC is almost always applied in the processing of cardiac PET. The geometry of PET makes it possible to estimate attenuation without knowing the depth of the annihilation event in the patient. Unlike SPECT, the attenuation of a true event is the sum of the attenuation both 511-keV photons; specifically the total attenuation along the line of response (see Fig. 4-11). Therefore, the correction that is applied is independent of where the annihilation event took place along a line of response. The result is a high-resolution final image with greatly reduced attenuation and scatter artifacts (see Fig. 4-12).

▶ **Radionuclide Source for Attenuation Correction**

Radionuclide sources for transmission imaging used for AC are Germanium-68 (Ge-68, 511 keV) or Cesium-167 (Cs-137, 630 keV). Both are contained in rotating rod sources that can be extended and retracted for image acquisition as needed throughout the study. Such cameras that utilize radioactive line sources are called "dedicated" PET systems. Because the source photons are positrons, there is no need to translate the attenuation coefficients from the transmission energy to the emission energy. Another advantage of dedicated PET is the attenuation map is acquired while the patient is free breathing. This reduces misregistration and breathing artifacts when compared to PET/CT.[67,68] Finally, the radiation dosage from a dedicated PET scanner is typically less than an x-ray–based CT

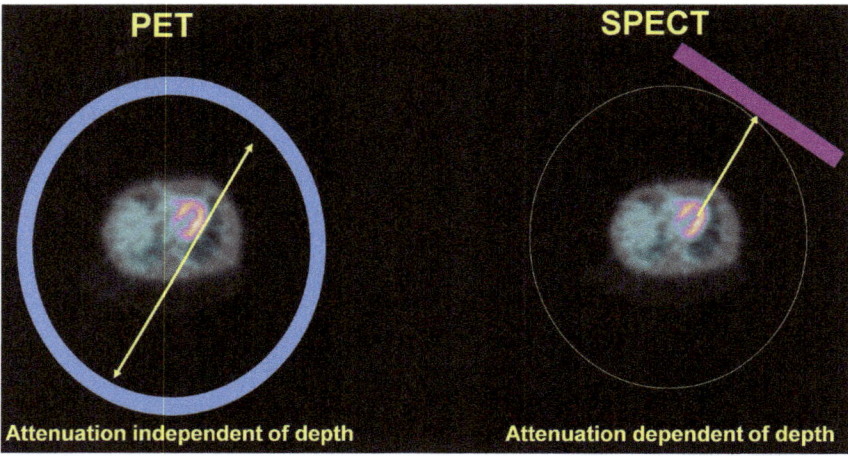

FIGURE 4-11 Attenuation in PET is different than SPECT because the attenuation experienced by a true pair is the sum of the attenuation of both photons, for example, the total line of response. Because of this, it is not necessary to know the depth of the annihilation in the patient to correct the attenuation.

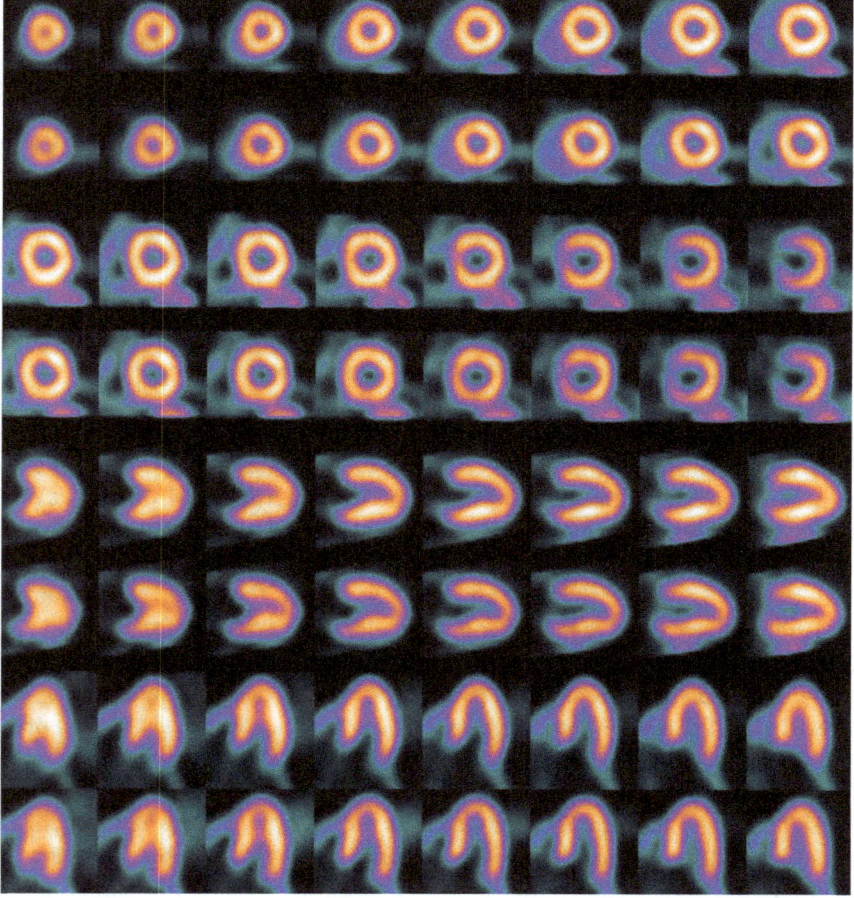

FIGURE 4-12 A high-quality PET perfusion study has a nearly uniform uptake appearance.

(though dosage-reducing strategies can be employed to minimize x-ray radiation dosage). One possible limitation of dedicated PET is some systems require long transmission acquisition scans (4–8 minutes). Newer reconstruction methods with newer instrumentation reduce the number of counts required for image reconstruction, reducing the acquisition time to 60 to 90 seconds.[40]

CT Source for Attenuation Correction

PET-CT systems can employ a conventional multi-slice CT system, capable of acquiring high-resolution, diagnostic quality data and/or low dose, AC specific x-ray tubes. CT-derived attenuation maps have the advantage of being able to acquire a high signal-to-noise transmission image in a short period of time. Despite this, CT-specific artifacts can make PET/CT more challenging than line source AC (see Fig. 4-13).[67] Patient motion and breathing introduce the greatest challenges. Several approaches have been proposed such as end expiration breath holding[68] and shallow free breathing. Cine/CT has been demonstrated to be both robust and easy to implement.[69] By using several passes over the diaphragm, an average position for the diaphragm can be obtained. Though this does reduce breathing artifacts, it requires rescanning the same tissue areas several times to cover the entire respiratory cycle, thus increasing potential radiation dose. Lowering kVp and tube current can help reduce the dose, however these improvements still result in CTAC scans of over 2 mSv.

Radiation exposure for the CT portion of a PET/CT scan can be a significant contributor to the overall radiation of the patient study and can be as high as 8 mSv when dose optimization is not used.[70] Optimizing the acquisition setting is crucial for obtaining the best transmission study at the lowest possible radiation exposure[71]:

- Optimize the CT scanner acquisition parameters. The x-ray tube voltage (kVp, which determines the mean energy of the x-rays produced by the x-ray tube) and tube current (mA which is proportional to the photon output of the x-ray tube). These should be less than 100 kVP and 10 mAs for most applications
- When possible, prospective ECG triggering should be used.
- If helical scanning is required, dose modulation should be employed.

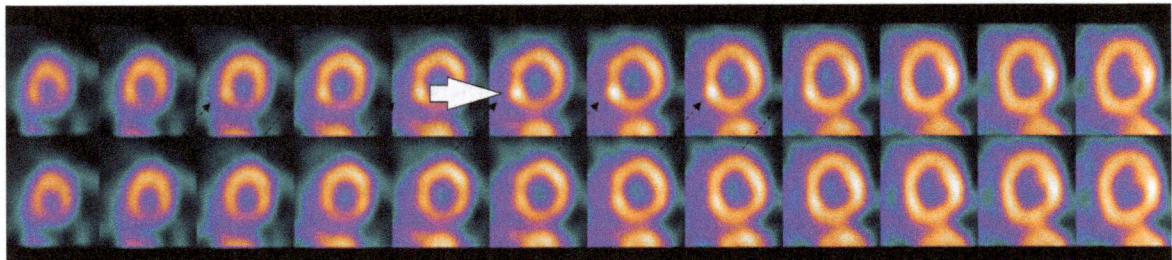

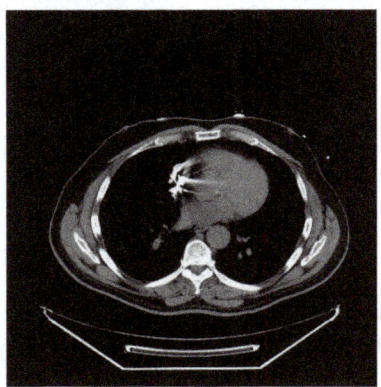

FIGURE 4-13 Attenuation correction of PET using CT can be complicated in the presence of metal artifacts. Though this is not a contraindication for cardiac PET, corrections must be applied to minimize the influence of metal beam hardening artifacts.

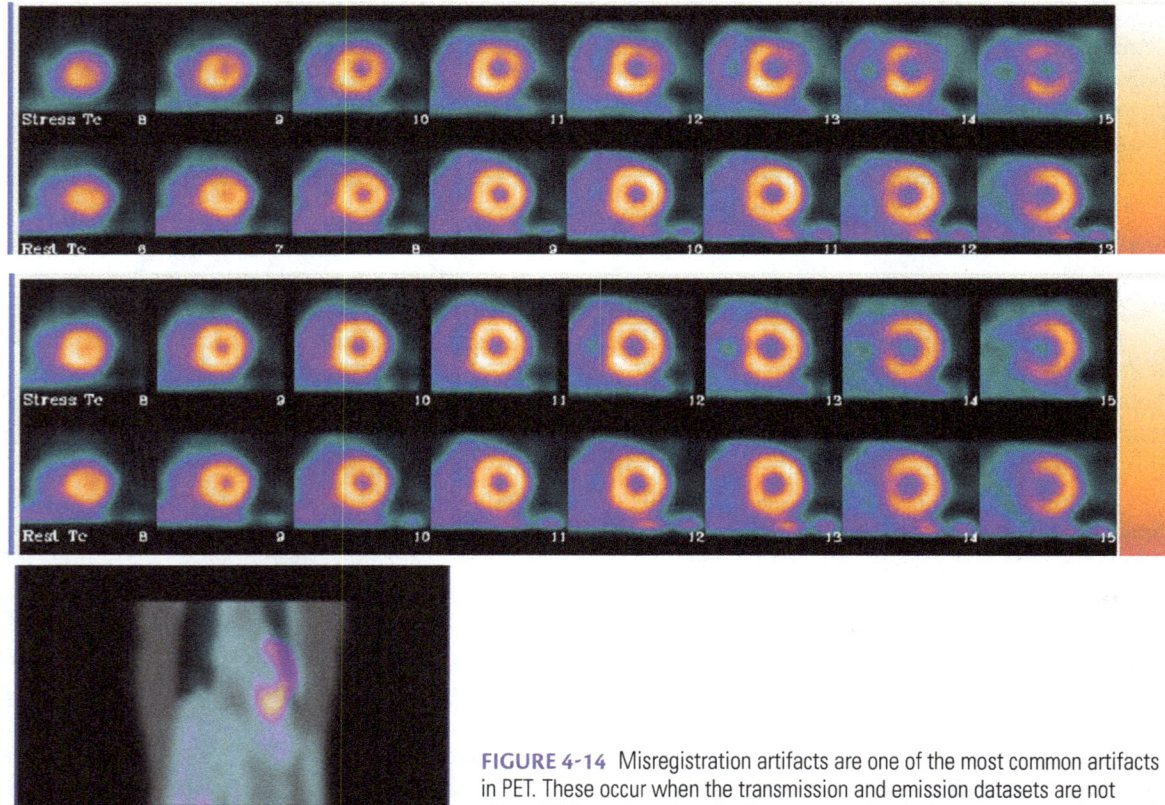

FIGURE 4-14 Misregistration artifacts are one of the most common artifacts in PET. These occur when the transmission and emission datasets are not aligned. When misregistration is present, technologists must correct images for these artifacts before proceeding.

- Field-of-view settings for obtaining the AC scan should be confined to the cardiac region only without truncating the heart.
- Cine-CT free breathing protocols should be avoided unless the PET/CT system is designed by the manufacturer to perform this scan at radiation dose comparable to either ECG triggering or helical scanning with dose modulation.

One of the most significant sources of artifact in cardiac PET is misregistration of the transmission and emission datasets in space. When a patient moves between these two scans, the AC cannot be properly applied without adjusting for the patient movement (Fig. 4-14). This artifact is thought to be significant in as many as 40% of all PET/CT studies, thus if software is not available to align the images, a substantially lower specificity will occur.[72] Imaging guidelines recommended that all cardiac PET studies be routinely examined for misregistration and corrected whenever possible.[2]

By far the most common technique for misregistration correction is a rigid shift of the transmission and emission datasets.[73] The user can interactively visualize an overlay of the transmission and emission data and move one of the datasets relative to the other until a satisfactory positioning is obtained. These offsets can then be used to re-reconstruct the tomographic data.

Scatter Correction

When the sinogram data are acquired in the 2D mode (septa extended), the scatter fraction defined as the ratio between the number of scatter events and the total number of coincidence events (scattered and unscattered) is from 10% to 15%, depending on the scanner geometry, the energy window, and the patient sizes.[74] With septa retracted (no septa in the 3D mode), the scatter fraction can even increase to 30% to 50%, additionally depending on the maximum ring difference and span of the 3D data acquisition. Currently, most commercialized PET scanners offer options for scatter correction for the demand of imaging accuracy. For 2D PET imaging, implementation of nonstationary convolution–subtraction method has been used.[74] The methods for 3D scatter correction are primarily relied on physical models for simulating the scatter process of the entire images.[74-76] The 3D scatter simulation uses the activity images obtained from reconstructing uncorrected emission sinogram as the initial input of activity distribution to estimate the scatter component. The attenuation map functions to produce 3D scattering probabilities for each LOR of scatter events, based on the Klein–Nishina formula.[77,78]

Randoms Corrections

Random events (randoms) are a result of unrelated photon events being recorded within the timing acceptance window of the system. Random events degrade image contrast, however because random photons are from unrelated annihilation events they only reduce overall image contrast. Hence, most randoms correction algorithm are implemented by subtracting a constant from the entire image.[79]

Protocols for Cardiac PET Perfusion Acquisition

The American Society of Nuclear Cardiology has developed imaging guidelines for the development of cardiac PET imaging protocols and should be consulted when developing clinical protocols.[66] For a detailed explanation of protocols, see Chapter 10. Almost all cardiac PET perfusion studies are performed using vasodilator stress (although dobutamine may also be used). Patients should refrain from using of any product containing caffeine and other substance that could interfere with the vasodilator. For specific requirements, practitioners should refer the package insert of the vasodilator and national guidelines.[80]

For most studies, this single infusion site can be used for both the vasodilator and the ^{82}Rb, particularly dipyridamole or regadenoson. A notable exception is when adenosine is used as the vasodilator. Because of the short half-life of adenosine, it is impractical to switch between the low flow rate adenosine to the high flow rate ^{82}Rb without bolusing the adenosine into the heart or interrupting the flow of adenosine. Stress testing using ^{13}N ammonia is considerably less restrictive than Rb-82, allowing for vasodilator and exercise testing.

Prior to the study, technologists will need to apply ECG patches for both the 12-lead cardiac monitoring system and 3-lead ECG triggering system for the scanner. Once patients have been prepared, they are positioned supine in the scanner system. Because AC is applied in all cardiac PET studies, it is possible to image patients with an arm down, however, it is important that the arm is immobilized and is free from the infusion activity.

The first stage of imaging is the transmission study, either acquired using CT or line source. For PET/CT systems, a low dosage chest planar image for positioning followed by a low dosage chest CT for AC will then be acquired of the mediastinal region. Can you explain how you use the map for positioning? For dedicated PET systems, a line source transmission study is acquired for both positioning and AC. How do you position? The transmission studies must be repeated if patient positioning is not correct.

The most common PET radiotracer for perfusion studies is Rubidium-82. Generally for this tracer, the resting perfusion study typically follows the transmission study. Delivery of the ^{82}Rb using a generator cart requires strict adherence to the manufacturer's recommendations for dose delivery, QC, and general operations. Laboratories using an ^{82}Rb generator should obtain training from the manufacturer prior to using the generator cart. To minimize the chance of patient motion between the emission and transmission study, it is important to begin the emission study as soon as practical. Most imaging protocols recommend a delay between the end of the infusion to the start of imaging of 90 to 120 seconds. Studies that measure flow however, require that the dynamic flow study be started prior to the infusion.[81-83] The stress protocol immediately follows the rest acquisition.

These imaging studies can be acquired either using a list mode (inclusion of all photon pair events) or a frame mode. In principle, these two modes will yield similar results, however list mode acquisitions do offer some additional flexibility to create multiple studies from a single data acquisition. Practically, frame mode and list mode acquisitions do not appear to be different either quantitatively or visually.[84]

Reconstruction

Because AC is applied prior to reconstruction, either FBP or iterative reconstruction can be used for creating 3D tomograms. Early PET systems utilized an FBP algorithm for reconstruction. More recently modern reconstruction algorithms for PET utilize an iterative, ordered subsets/expectation maximization algorithm because of the improved noise and image quality properties of the final reconstructed volumes.[37,38]

Iterative reconstruction algorithms use a stepwise updating algorithm to "search" for a source distribution that could produce the projection data observed. It relies on a model (the projector), of the transport of photons through the patient to the camera. In principle, this projector can be used to model any physical process in the photon transport, thus giving it considerably more flexibility than the FBP algorithm.

The iterative reconstructions PET in principle are similar to the reconstruction algorithms used in SPECT except the projection model is different. For a standard 2D acquisition, straight forward application of MLEM or OSEM is sufficient. If data are acquired in 3D, additional steps must be applied to take into account the oblique planes of data.

The simplest technique for reconstructing 3D data is to use the Fourier rebinning algorithm.[85] This algorithm uses the geometric properties of the oblique planes to create a translation of the 3D data into traditional 2D planes.

Time-of-Flight PET

Localization of the point of annihilation using the 511-keV photon pair to a line through the patient is improved upon by using "time-of-flight" (TOF) measurement capabilities.[51] In this approach, additional information about the location of the annihilation event is obtained by measuring the (very small) difference in arrival times of the two coincidence photons. With conventional coincidence detection, the small difference in arrival times is ignored. TOF imaging requires very precise detector and electronic circuitry and calibration given the speed of light and the very short distances that the photons travel. Information provided by the difference in arrival times is included in reconstruction algorithms that model this modified probability information to improve spatial resolution and system sensitivity compared with conventional coincidence detection.[86] It may also be used to improve separation of scattered photons from true coincidence events and system contrast resolution.

CONCLUSIONS

An understanding of the physics and related technical principles for conventional and evolving SPECT is essential for obtaining the highest-quality clinical utilization in nuclear cardiology. From image interpretation to laboratory management, the clinician will be called upon to understand these principles in daily routine. Basic physics, statistics, mathematics, and radiation physics all play a vital role in daily service that provides the optimal patient care, provides the required and regulatory requirements for accreditation as regionally required, and sustains the competitiveness of the specialty.

Nuclear cardiology imaging instrumentation currently offers a great diversity of options. Current systems are the result of continued efforts to develop hardware/detector configurations and reconstruction software that have addressed specific challenges to imaging the heart. The integration of CT options has enhanced conventional perfusion imaging, permitted new protocols through AC, and broadened the scope of services for diagnosing and managing cardiovascular disease with noninvasive techniques. Notably, PET myocardial perfusion imaging is poised to leverage its strengths in nontraditional laboratory environments also in response to pressure for improved efficiency and accuracy of performing studies.

REFERENCES

1. 2013 Nuclear Cardiology Trends. *J Nucl Cardiol*. 2014;21: S5–88.
2. Anger HO. A new instrument for mapping gamma ray emitters. *Biol Med Q Rep*. 1957;UCRL-3653:38.
3. Wagner HN. Hal Anger: Nuclear medicone's quiet genius. *J Nucl Med*. 2003;44(11):26N–34N.
4. Hawman PC, Haines EJ. The cardiofocal collimator: a variable-focus collimator for cardiac SPECT. *Phys Med Biol*. 1994;39(3):439–450.
5. Case JA, Bateman TM. Taking the perfect nuclear image: Quality control, acquisition, and processing techniques for cardiac SPECT, PET, and hybrid imaging *J Nucl Cardiol*. 2013, 20(5): 891–907.
6. Sorenson JA, Phelps ME. *Physics in Nuclear Medicine*. 2nd ed. New York: WB Saunders Company; 1987: Chapter 15.
7. Holly TA, Abbott BG, Al-Mallah M, et al. ASNC imaging guidelines for nuclear cardiology procedures: single photon-emission computed tomography. *J Nucl Cardiol*. 2010;17(5): 941–973.
8. Tung C-H, Gullberg GT, Zeng GL, et al. Nonuniform attenuation correction using simultaneous transmission and emission converging tomography. *IEEE Trans Nucl Sci*. 1992;39: 1134–1114.
9. IQ-SPECT. http://www.medical.siemens.com/siemens/en_INT/gg_nm_FBAs/files/brochures/2008/IQ_SPECT_Bro_2008.pdf
10. Jaszczak RJ, Murphy PH, Huard D, et al. Radionuclide emission computed tomography of the head with 99mCc and a scintillation camera. *J Nucl Med*. 1977;18(4) ():373–380.
11. Gottschalk SC, Salem D, Lim CB, et al. SPECT resolution and uniformity improvements by noncircular orbit. *J Nucl Med*. 1983;24(9):822–828.
12. Gambhir SS, Berman DS, Ziffer J, et al. A novel high-sensitivity rapid-acquisition single-photon cardiac imaging camera. *J Nucl Med*. 2009;50(4):635–643.
13. Esteves FP, Raggi P, Folks RD, et al. Novel solid-state-detector dedicated cardiac camera for fast myocardial perfusion imaging: multicenter comparison with standard dual detector cameras. *J Nucl Cardiol*. 2009;16:927–934.
14. Garcia EV. Cardiac dedicated ultrafast spect cameras: new designs and clinical implications, *J Nucl Med*. 2011;52(2): 210–221.
15. Darambara DG. Solid state detectors in nuclear medicine. *Q J Nucl Med*. 2002;46:3–7.
16. Slomka PJ, Patton JA, Berman DS, et al. Advances in technical aspects of myocardial perfusion SPECT imaging. *J Nucl Cardiol*. 2009;16(2):255–276.
17. D-SPECT User Manual, version MAN0001 Rev. C
18. Sharir T, Pinskiy M, Pardes A, et al, Comparison of the diagnostic accuracies of very low stress-dose with standard-dose myocardial perfusion imaging: Automated quantification of one-day, stress-first SPECT using a CZT camera. *J Nucl Cardiol*. 2016;23(1):11–20.
19. Funk T, Kirch DL, Koss JE, et al. A novel approach to multi-pinhole SPECT for myocardial perfusion imaging. *J Nucl Med*. 2006;47(4):595–602.
20. Garcia EV, Tsukerman L, Keidar Z. A new solid state ultra fast cardiac multidetector SPECT system [abstract]. *J Nucl Cardiol*. 2008;15(suppl):S3.
21. Duvall L, Slomka PJ, Gerlach JR, et al. High-efficiency SPECT MPI: Comparison of automated quantification, visual interpretation, and coronary angiography. *J Nucl Cardiol*. 2013;20(5);763–773.
22. Ficaro EA, Fessler JA, Shreve PD, et al. Simultaneous transmission/emission myocardial perfusion tomography: diagnostic accuracy of attenuation corrected Tc-99m sestamibi single-photon emission computed tomography. *Circulation*. 1996;93:463–473.
23. Cullom SJ, Case JA, Bateman TM. Attenuation correction of cardiac SPECT: clinical and developmental challenges. *J Nucl Med*. 2000;41:860–862.
24. Corbett JR, Ficaro EP. Clinical review of attenuation-corrected cardiac SPECT. *J Nucl Cardiol*. 1999;6:54–68.
25. Perisinakis K, Theocharopoulos N, Karkavitsas N, Damilakis Patient effective radiation dose and associated risk from transmission scans using 153Gd line sources in cardiac SPECT studies. *J Health Phys*. 2002;83(1):66–74.
26. Bocher M, Balan A, Krausz Y, et al. Gamma camera mounted anatomical x-ray tomography: Technology, system characteristics and first images. *Eur J Nucl Med*. 2000;27:619–627.
27. Celler A, Dixon KL, Chang Z, et al. Problems created in attenuation-corrected SPECT images by artifacts in attenuation maps: a simulation study. *J Nucl Med*. 2005;46(2):335–343.
28. Dorbala S. Standard myocardial perfusion and cardiac FDG PET protocols and associated patient radiation doses. http://www.imagewisely.org/~/media/ImageWisely%20Files/NucMed/Standard%20Myocardial%20Perfusion.pdf. Accessed May 10, 2016.
29. McQuaid SJ, Hutton BF. Sources of attenuation-correction artefacts in cardiac PET/CT and SPECT/CT. *Eur J Nucl Med Mol Imaging*. 2008;35(6):1117–1123.
30. Goetze S, Brown TL, Lavely WC, et al. Attenuation correction in myocardial perfusion SPECT/CT: effects of misregistration and value of reregistration. *J Nucl Med*. 2007;48(7):1090–1095.
31. Chang S, Nabi F, Xu J, et al. The coronary artery calcium score and stress myocardial perfusion imaging provide independent and complementary prediction of cardiac risk. *J Am Coll Cardiol*. 2009;54(20):1872–1882.
32. Santana CA, Garcia EV, Faber TL, et al. Diagnostic performance of fusion of myocardial perfusion imaging (MPI) and computed tomography coronary angiography. *J Nucl Cardiol*. 2009;16:201–211.
33. Kadrmas DJ, Frey EC, Karimi SS, et al. Fast implementations of reconstruction-based scatter compensation in fully 3D SPECT image reconstruction. *Phys Med Biol*. 1998;43(4):857–873.
34. Borges-Neto S, Pagnanelli RA, Shaw LK, et al. Clinical results of a novel wide beam reconstruction method for shortening scan time of Tc-99m cardiac SPECT perfusion studies. *J Nucl Cardiol*. 2007;14(4):555–565.
35. Venero CV, Heller GV, Bateman TM, et al. A multicenter evaluation of a new post-processing method with depth-dependent collimator resolution applied to full-time and half-time acquisitions without and with simultaneously acquired attenuation correction. *J Nucl Cardiol*. 2009;16(5):714–725.
36. Radon J. Über die Bestimmung von Funktionen durch ihre Integralwerte längs gewisser Mannigfaltigkeiten", Berichte über die Verhandlungen der Königlich-Sächsischen Akademie der Wissenschaften zu Leipzig, Mathematisch-Physische Klasse [Reports on the proceedings of the Royal Saxonian

37. Shepp LA, Vardi Y. Maximum likelihood reconstruction for emission tomography. *IEEE Trans Med Imaging.* 1982;MI-1(2):113–122.
38. Hudson HM, Larkin RS. Accelerated image reconstruction using ordered subsets of projection data. *IEEE Trans Med Imaging.* 1994;13:601–609.
39. DiFilippo FP, Brunken RC. Do implanted pacemaker leads and ICD leads cause metal-related artifact in cardiac PET/CT? *J Nucl Med.* 2005;46(3):436–443.
40. Hsu BL, Case JA, Moser KW, et al. Reconstruction of rapidly acquired Germanium-68 transmission scans for cardiac PET attenuation correction. *J Nucl Cardiol.* 2007;14:706–714.
41. Muehllehner G. Effect of resolution improvement on required count density in ECT imaging: A computer simulation. *Phys Med Biol.* 1985;30(2):163–173.
42. Hutton BF. Cardiac single-photon emission tomography: Is attenuation correction enough? *Eur J Nucl Med.* 1997;24(7):713–715.
43. Heller EN, DeMan P, Liu YH, et al. Extracardiac activity complicates quantitative cardiac SPECT imaging using a simultaneous transmission–emission approach. *J Nucl Med.* 1997;38(12):1882–1890.
44. Rivero A, Santana C, Folks RD, et al. Attenuation correction reveals gender-related differences in the normal values of transient ischemic dilation index in rest–exercise stress sestamibi myocardial perfusion imaging. *J Nucl Cardiol.* 2006;13(3):338–344.
45. Ogawa K, Harata Y, Ichihara T, et al. A practical method for position-dependent Compton-scatter correction in single photon emission CT. *IEEE Trans Med Imaging.* 1991;MI-10(3):408–412.
46. Bowsher JE, Floyd CE Jr. Treatment of Compton scattering in maximum-likelihood, expectation-maximization reconstructions of SPECT images. *J Nucl Med.* 1991;32(6):1291–1293.
47. Brownwell GL, Sweet WH. Localization of brain tumors with positron emitters. *Nucleonics.* 1953;11:40–45.
48. Brownell GL, Burnham CA, Hoop B Jr, et al. Quantitative dynamic studies using short-lived radioisotopes and positron detection. In: *Proceedings of the Symposium on Dynamic Studies with Radioisotopes in Medicine.* Rotterdam. August 31–September 4, 1970. International Atomic Energy Agency, Vienna, 1971. pp. 161–172.
49. Schelbert HR, Phelps ME, Hoffman EJ, et al. Regional myocardial perfusion assessed with N-13 labeled ammonia and positron emission computerized axial tomography. *Am J Cardiol.* 1979;43:209–218.
50. Schelbert HR, Phelps ME, Huang SC, et al. N-13 ammonia as an indicator of myocardial blood flow. *Circulation.* 1981;63:1259–1272.
51. Gould KL. Clinical cardiac PET using generator-produced Rb-82: a review. *Cardiovasc Intervent Radiol.* 1989;12(5):245–251.
52. Goldstein R, Mullani N, Wong W, et al. Positron imaging of myocardial infarction with rubidium-82. *J Nucl Med.* 1986;27:1824–1829.
53. Bracco diagnostics. [Package Insert] CardioGen-82 Rubidium Rb 82 Generator, Bracco Diagnostics (NJ, USA) revised 04/2013. http://imaging.bracco.com/sites/braccoimaging.com/files/technica_sheet_pdf/Cardiogen%20Full%20Prescribing%20Information.pdf. Accessed June 30, 2016.
54. RUBY-FILL (rubidium Rb 82 generator) package insert, reference ID 3993017, September 2016, Jubilant DRAXIMAGE Inc. Kirkland, Quebec, Canada.
55. Tillisch J, Brunken R, Marshall R, et al. Reversibility of cardiac wall-motion abnormalities predicted by positron tomography. *N Engl J Med.* 1986;314:884–888.
56. Allman KC, Shaw LJ, Hachamovitch R, et al. Myocardial viability testing and impact of revascularization on prognosis in patients with coronary artery disease and left ventricular dysfunction: a meta-analysis. *J Am Coll Cardiol.* 2002;39:1151–1158.
57. Camici P, Ferrannini E, Opie LH. Myocardial metabolism in ischemic heart disease: basic principles and application to imaging by positron emission tomography. *Progr Cardiovasc Dis.* 1989;32:217–238.
58. Yamagishi H, Shirai N, Takagi M, et al. Identification of cardiac sarcoidosis with ^{13}N-NH$_3$/^{18}F-FDG PET. *J Nucl Med.* 2003;44:1030–1036.
59. Shoup TM, Elmaleh DR, Bohab AA, et al. Evaluation of trans-9-^{18}F-fluoro-3,4-Methyleneheptadecanoic acid as a PET tracer for myocardial fatty acid imaging. *J Nucl Med.* 2005;46(2):297–304.
60. Yu M, Bozek J, Kagan M, et al. Cardiac retention of PET neuronal imaging agent LMI1195 in different species: impact of norepinephrine uptake-1 and -2 transporters. *Nucl Med Biol.* 2013;40(5):682–688.
61. Lee S, Lee E, Choi H, et al. 11C-Pittsburgh B PET Imaging in Cardiac Amyloidosis. *J Am Coll Cardiol Imaging.* 2015; 8(1):50–59.
62. Glenn Wells R, deKemp RA, Beanlands RS. Positron emission tomography instrumentation. In: Heller GV, Mann A, Hendel RC, eds. *Nuclear Cardiology, Technical Applications.* New York: McGraw-Hill; 2008.
63. Esteves FP, Nye JA, Khan A. Prompt-gamma compensation in Rb-82 myocardial perfusion 3D PET/CT. *J Nucl Cardiol.* 2010;17(2):247–253.
64. Visvikis D, Griffiths D, Costa DC, et al. Clinical evaluation of 2D versus 3D whole-body PET image quality using a dedicated BGO PET scanner. *Eur J Nucl Med Mol Imaging.* 2005;32(9):1050–1056.
65. Cherry SR, Dahlborn M, Hoffman EJ. 3D PET using a conventional multislice tomography without septa. *J Comput Assist Tomogr.* 1991;15(4):655–668.
66. Dilsizian V, Bacharach SL, Beanlands RS, et al. ASNC imaging guidelines for nuclear cardiology procedures: PET myocardial perfusion and metabolism clinical imaging. *J Nucl Cardiol.* 2016;23(5):1187–1226. http://www.asnc.org/Files/Guidelines%20and%20Quality/PET%20GuidelineASNC%20SNMMI2016.pdf. Accessed June 13, 2017.
67. Loghin C, Sdringola S, Gould KL. Common artifacts in PET myocardial perfusion images due to attenuation-emission misregistration: Clinical significance, causes, and solutions. *J Nucl Med.* 2004;45(6):1029–1039.
68. Goerres GW, Kamel E, Heidelberg TN, et al. PET-CT image co-registration in the thorax: influence of respiration. *Eur J Nucl Med Mol Imaging.* 2002;29:351–360.

69. Alessio AM, Kohlmyer S, Branch K, et al. Cine CT for attenuation correction in cardiac PET/CT. *J Nucl Med.* 2007;48(5):794–801.
70. O'Daniel JC, Stevens DM, Cody DD. Reducing radiation exposure from survey CT scans. *Am J Roentgenol.* 2005;185(2):509–515.
71. Dorbala S, Di Carli MF, Delbeke D, et al. SNMMI/ASNC/SCCT Guideline for cardiac SPECT/CT and PET/CT 1.0. *J Nucl Med.* 2013:54(8);1485–1507.
72. Gould L, Pan T-S, Laghin C, et al. Frequent diagnostic errors in cardiac PET/CT due to misregistration of CT attenuation and emission PET images: A definite analysis of causes, consequences and corrections *J Nucl Med.* 2007;48(7):1112–1121.
73. Martinez-Moller A, Souvatzoglou M, Navab N, et al. Artifacts from misaligned CT in cardiac perfusion PET/CT studies: Frequency, effects, and potential solutions. *J Nucl Med.* 2007; 48:188–193.
74. Bentourkia M, Msaki P, Cadorette J, et al. Nonstationary scatter subtraction-restoration in high-resolution PET. *J Nucl Med.* 1996;37(12):2040–2046.
75. Levin CS, Dahlbom M, Hoffman EJ. A Monte Carlo correction for the effect of Compton scattering in 3-D PET brain imaging. *IEEE Trans Nucl Sci.* 1995;42: 1181–1188.
76. Watson CC, Newport D, Casey ME, et al. Evaluation of simulation-based scatter correction for 3-D PET cardiac imaging. *IEEE Trans Nucl Sci.* 1997;44:90–97.
77. Ollinger JM. Model-based scatter correction for fully 3D PET. *Phys Med Biol.* 1996;41:153–117.
78. Attix FH. Chapter 7. Gamma- and X-ray interactions in matter. *Introduction to Radiological Physics and Radiation Dosimetry.* New York: John Wiley & Sons; 1986.
79. Casey ME, Hoffman EJ. Quantitation in Positron Emission Computed Tomography: A technique to reduce noise in accidental coincidence measurements and coincidence efficiency calibration. *J Comput Assist Tomogr.* 1986;10:845–850.
80. Henzlova MJ, Cerqueria MD, Mahmarian JJ, et al. Stress protocols and tracers. *J Nucl Cardiol.* 2006. 13(6):e80–e90.
81. Hutchins GD, Schwaiger M, Rosenspire KC, et al. Noninvasive quantification of regional blood flow in the human heart using N-13 ammonia and dynamic positron emission tomographic imaging. *J Am Col Cardiol.* 1990;5:1032–1042.
82. Yoshida K, Mullani N, Gould KL. Coronary flow and flow reserve by PET simplified for clinical applications using rubidium-82 or nitrogen-13-ammonia. *J Nucl Med.* 1996;37(10):1701–1712.
83. Lortie M, Beanlands RS, Yoshinaga K, et al. Quantification of myocardial blood flow with 82Rb dynamic PET imaging. *Eur J Nucl Med Mol Imaging.* 2007;34(11):1765–1774.
84. Case JA, Van Vickle S, Courter SA, et al. A rapid protocol for measuring perfusion, gating and absolute blood flow using dedicated frame-mode 3D PET scanner. *J Nucl Cardiol.* 2014;21;768 (Abstract).
85. Defrise M, Kinahan PE, Townsend DW, et al. Exact and approximate rebinning algorithms for 3D-PET data. *IEEE Trans. Med Imaging.* 1997;16(2) 145–158.
86. Vandenberghe S, Mikhaylova E, D'Hoe E, et al. Recent developments in time-of-flight PET. *EJNMMI Physics.* 2016;3:3.

Quality Control in SPECT and PET Imaging

CHAPTER 5

Sue Miller, Frank DiGregorio, and Sunil Selvin

INTRODUCTION

Quality control (QC) of single-photon emission computed tomography (SPECT) and positron emission tomography (PET) nuclear cardiology procedures is a multiple-step process that begins before the patient enters the laboratory, continues during the acquisition, and after the patient leaves the laboratory. SPECT QC and PET QC require the close attention of all personnel and physicians that are involved with the laboratory. Requirements for imaging systems QC are based on Nuclear Regulatory Commission (NRC) requirements, agreement state requirements, accepted imaging guidelines, and the Intersocietal Accreditation Commission Nuclear/PET (IAC Nuclear/PET), and American College of Radiology (ACR) Accreditation standards.[1-8] The terminology used, requirements, and frequency may vary slightly between the standards, the model of scanners, and the original equipment manufacturers (OEM) recommendations. However, the basic premise of why it is necessary is the same in all situations: to ensure adequate camera performance, identify any potential sources of error or artifact within an acquisition, and ultimately provide the patient and referring physician with the best quality information possible. If QC procedures are not followed, it may lead to an equivocal or falsely interpreted study, which may result in increased downstream costs as well as poor outcomes. This chapter will review the routine QC procedures performed by the nuclear medicine technologist before, during, and after the acquisition of a nuclear cardiology study. Additional QC procedures and calibrations that are performed by camera service engineers or medical physicist will not be discussed.

QUALITY CONTROL BEFORE THE ACQUISITION

There are several required and recommended equipment QC procedures that should be performed on each imaging system.[2,5-31] The frequency of the procedures may vary among equipment manufacturers; however, all are important to ensure proper system performance (Tables 5-1 and 5-2). These tasks consist of daily, weekly, monthly, and quarterly system testing.

Table 5-1

Recommended Frequency for Gamma Camera Quality Control Procedures

Test	Frequency
Energy peaking	Daily
Uniformity	Daily
Sensitivity	Daily or weekly
Resolution and linearity	Weekly
Center of rotation	Weekly or monthly
SPECT phantom evaluation	Annually

Table 5-2 Recommended Frequency for PET Camera Quality Control Procedures	
Test	Frequency
Blank scan	Daily
Singles (PMT gain or Bucket setup)	Weekly
Coincidence timing	Weekly (or daily)
Normalization (Bucket scan)	Monthly (or per OEM recommendation)
Well counters	Quarterly

Single-Photon Emission Computed Tomography Systems

Daily

Energy Peaking

Energy peaking (photopeak analysis) should be performed daily to verify that the camera is counting photons using the correct energy.[2,3,9-11] Each imaging system should be checked before use to ensure that the camera peaking electronics are functioning properly, that the energy window has not drifted, and that the energy spectrum is in appropriate shape.

During the procedure, the pulse height analyzer's energy window should be manually or automatically placed over the correct photopeak energy. It is recommended that no greater than a 20% energy window be used in order to obtain the most accurate peak energy.[2,9-11] If the test is performed intrinsically, a point source should be placed at least 1.5 m away from the surface of the camera detector. If performed extrinsically, a sheet source should be used. In either case, the source should be enough to flood the entire field of view (FOV).

Verifying the photopeak daily will help prevent artifacts that may occur due to inappropriate photons entering the acquisition and degrading image quality. An off-centered photopeak may also result in poor count statistics, which will result in a poor-quality image.[2-4,9-11] If dual-isotope procedures are being performed, on some older imaging systems it may be necessary to perform this procedure between each acquisition of thallium-201 (Tl-201) and technetium-99m (Tc-99m) isotopes. It is also necessary to repeat this procedure whenever the camera is powered down for any reason during the day.

Daily Uniformity Flood

A daily uniformity flood should be performed to analyze system performance and to ensure the sensitivity response of the system is uniform across the detector surface.[2-15] This is performed by exposure of the detector surface to a radioactive source. The recommended method is to perform this procedure *intrinsically* using a Tc-99m point source of approximately 100 to 500 µCi in ≤0.5 mL of volume. The point source should be placed in the center and at a distance of approximately five useful fields of view (UFOV) away from the detector surface. An acquisition should be performed for approximately 2 to 5 million counts using a 20% energy window.[2,9,11,15] This may also be performed extrinsically using a 57-cobalt sheet source. This method is performed frequently on dual-head camera systems because the acquisition can be performed on both detectors at the same time. It is important to remember, however, that during the uniformity analysis of *extrinsic* floods, the outer 10% to 20% of the FOV should not be considered due to possible edge packing.[2,9,11,15]

After the acquisition of the flood field uniformity, the image should be evaluated visually, and a computerized analysis should be performed to measure the performance of the system. Central FOV and UFOV parameters should be <5% based on standards; <3% is preferred. This analysis should be performed following manufacturers' protocols and will be specific to each imaging system. If nonuniformities are detected, the system should not be used until service is performed. Severe artifacts, such as malfunctioning photomultiplier tubes, will be easily detected (Fig. 5-1). Smaller abnormalities may be more difficult to detect, however. These small, undetected nonuniformities may produce artifacts within patient acquisitions and result in a misinterpretation of the study.[2,9-15] It should be noted that the daily uniformity flood is not the same as the high count extrinsic uniformity flood that is completed on a monthly or per OEM recommendations to correct for detector and collimator nonuniformities.[2,5-8]

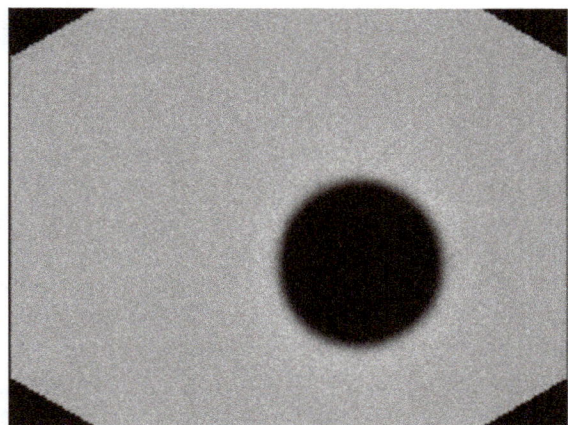

FIGURE 5-1 Illustration of a uniformity flood that had a cluster of photomultiplier tubes not functioning.

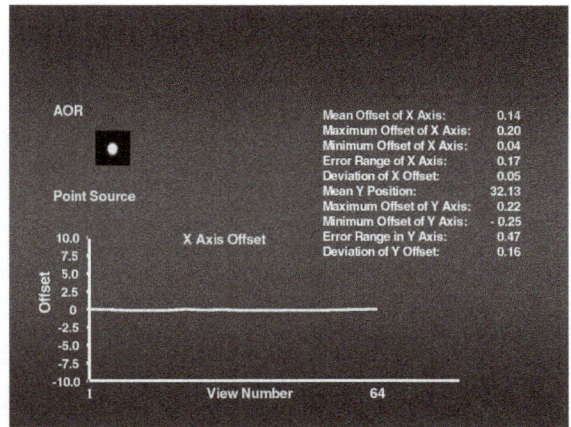

FIGURE 5-3 Example of a COR analysis. Mean × offset should be <0.5, and evaluation of the graph should be performed for any deviation as well.

Weekly or Monthly

Center of Rotation

A center of rotation (COR) evaluation may be performed weekly or monthly (depending on the manufacturer) in order to ensure and maintain the detector's electronic matrix alignment.[2,5-15] This is the x-axis position of the actual axis of rotation as seen by the image matrix.[2] If a COR error occurs, it may produce what has been characterized as a "doughnut"-shaped or "tuning fork" artifact (Fig. 5-2).[2] This artifact may appear similar to that caused by patient motion on the perfusion acquisition, but occurs on every patient study. This error becomes more pronounced if the deviation widens, particularly >2 pixels in a 64 × 64 matrix. Smaller deviations may not produce an artifact but could result in decreased spatial resolution and image contrast.[2,9,11,15]

Several manufacturers have recommended camera-specific protocols to follow when performing COR procedures. Most recommend using a 500 to 750 µCi point source placed off center in the FOV at approximately 4 to 8 in away from the detector surface.[2,9,11,15] The procedure is then performed using similar parameters as a standard SPECT acquisition. An analysis of this acquisition should be performed, and for any misalignment of >0.5 pixels of the x-axis, the COR should be recalibrated (Fig. 5-3).

System Resolution and Linearity Test

System spatial resolution and linearity evaluation should be performed weekly. This procedure is to document spatial resolution over time, as well as to evaluate the detector's ability to produce straight lines.[2,9-11,15] This should be performed *intrinsically* using a radioactive point source and a test phantom. This evaluation should not be performed extrinsically because the patterns of the lead bars in the phantom and the lead septa of the collimator may interfere with one another causing artifacts.

There are several bar phantoms available commercially that may be used for this test. The most commonly used are the parallel-line-equal-spaced (PLES), orthogonal hole, and four-quadrant phantoms.[2,5-15] The four-quadrant phantom has four sections of differing thickness lead bars that are equally spaced. If this type of phantom is used routinely, it should be placed over the detector surface so that each differing size lead bar is in a different position from the previously performed test (rotated 90 degrees from the previously placed position). This will allow the most tightly spaced bars of the phantom to appear over the

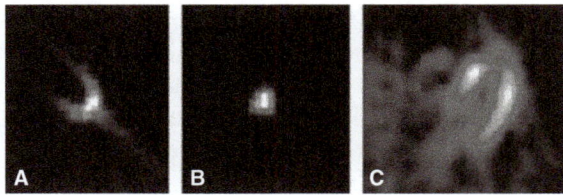

FIGURE 5-2 **A:** Tuning fork artifact. **B:** Normal COR image. **C:** Apical artifact as a result of COR deviation.

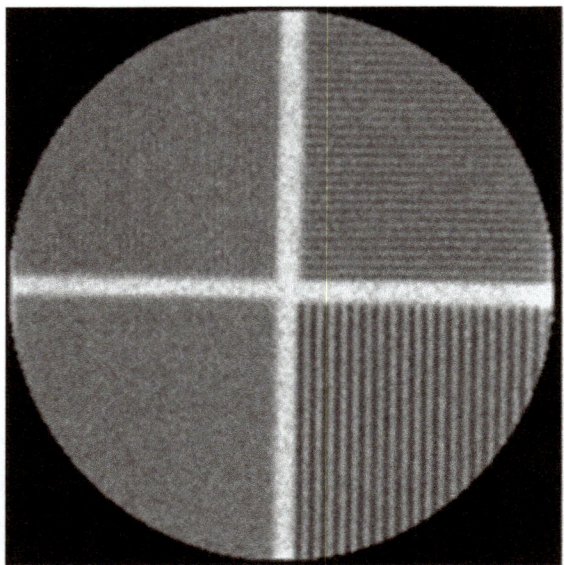

FIGURE 5-4 Example of four-quadrant bar phantom.

entire surface of the detector every fifth acquisition. This will provide the most thorough evaluation of the entire detector surface over time.[2,9,11,15]

Acquisition parameters for the resolution and linearity test should be similar to those used to perform a daily uniformity flood. On completion, the image should be evaluated visually to assess the straightness of the lines produced by the bar phantom and for how well each different-size lead bar is visualized (Fig. 5-4). The test should be stored in an electronic format for comparison of system resolution over time. As a decrease in resolution appears (loss of visualization of individual bars), preventive maintenance should be performed on the system. Manufacturers may supply software to evaluate linearity and resolution that should be used when available.

Annually

SPECT Phantom Study

The Intersocietal Accreditation Commission Nuclear/PET and ACR recommend that SPECT phantoms be performed annually.[5,6] This allows the evaluation of an imaging system's performance and limitations by providing a comparative means to judge previous performance with the most recent phantom acquisition.[2,9-11,15] Commercially available multipurpose Plexiglas and water-filled SPECT phantoms have attenuation and scattering properties similar to those of tissue, thus simulating clinical conditions in a three-dimensional (3D) view. This provides a realistic comparison of system performance similar to that in the clinical setting. Therefore, acquisition parameters used should be similar to those of standard SPECT.

▶ Solid-State SPECT Systems

Several manufacturers have recently brought solid-state imaging systems to market, such as the D-SPECT (Spectrum Dynamics Medical, Inc.).[18–21,23,24] Daily QC procedures are performed with either a Co-57 rod or phantom. Depending on the manufacturer, the camera software performs a pass/fail test for: energy resolution, energy peaking, detector registration, regional/global detector homogeneity, scan sensitivity, FOV, and faulty pixels.[18–21,23] If the daily QC fails, the camera service engineer should be contacted for repair.

▶ Positron Emission Tomography Systems

Daily

Blank Scan

A blank scan is performed daily prior to any patient testing to analyze system performance and stability.[5–8,16,18,24–26] The daily blank scan is the equivalent of the daily uniformity scan for SPECT and allows for detection of any sudden change in system performance such as a module malfunction.

Once a blank scan is acquired, it is processed using standard OEM reconstruction parameters and defaults, then displayed as a two-dimensional (2D) sinogram in gray scale. The blank scan is inspected visually (Fig. 5-5) and quantitatively (Fig. 5-6), if available on the system, for variations in image quality. Hot or cold streaks in the sinogram (Fig. 5-5) are an indication of a detector or block malfunction and identify blocks or modules (buckets) which are more (or less) sensitive than the respective system average.[16,18,24,26] It is also important to evaluate the results of the blank scan over time, looking for trends in system performance.[25] If blank scan quality is poor, corrective action is required. Updates to the PMT gain calibrations, coincidence timing calibration (CTC) or normalization files, and a repeat blank scan may be necessary.[16,18,24,26]

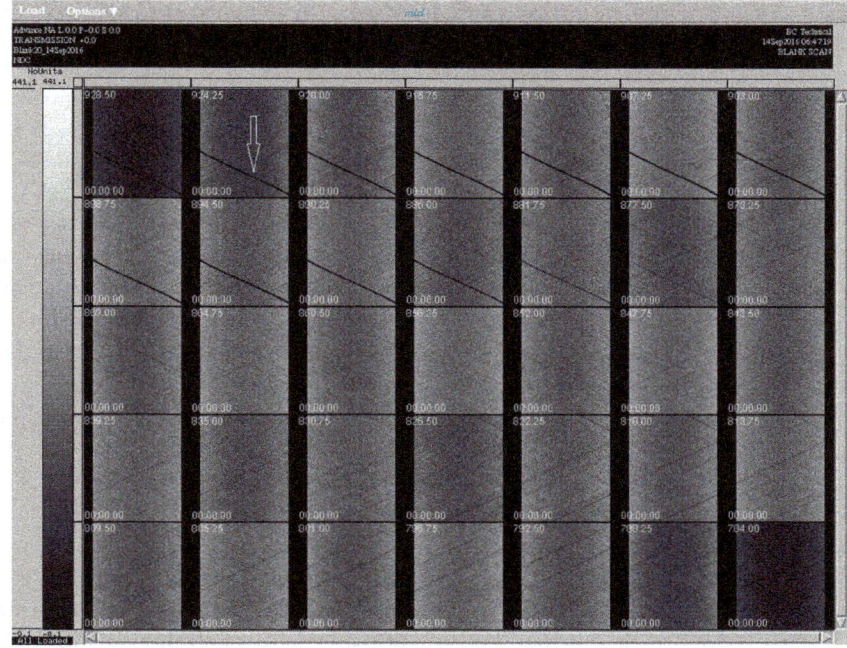

FIGURE 5-5 Example of Blank scan with cold streaks indicating detector or block malfunction.

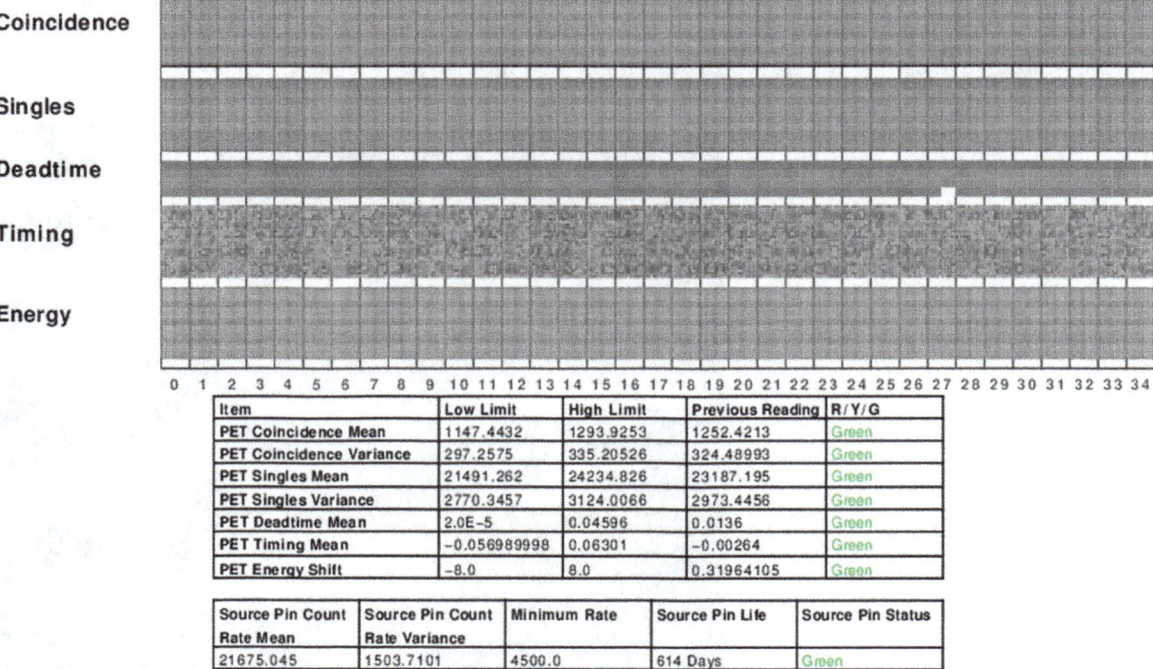

FIGURE 5-6 Example of Daily QC results page from GE PET/CT scanner.

If the blank scan fails after this step, then a service call should be placed and the system should be removed from service until repaired. If blank scan is acceptable, it is saved and set as the daily transmission reference scan for corrections when using Ge-68 or Cs-137 sources for attenuation correction.

Weekly

Singles Update Gain/Bucket Setup

Singles update gain or Bucket setup test is performed on a weekly basis, or as recommended by the manufacturer, using the Ge-68 rod sources.[2,25,27,30,31] The purpose of this calibration is to balance the gain characteristics of the photo multiplier tubes in each block. Singles or Bucket setup will compensate for photo multiplier tube drift caused by time and environmental changes.

Coincidence Timing Scan

The Coincidence Timing Calibration (CTC) scan is performed, at minimum, on a weekly basis, but may be performed daily.[2,25,27,31] The CTC scan is completed using Ge-68 rod sources to evaluate the constancy of the timing resolution. The duration of the scan is very short, typically 2 minutes. The calculation of the scan data compensates for differences in event detection hardware and adjusts for timing delays, ensuring events from all blocks are time stamped equally. This scan can be manufacturer and scanner model specific.

Monthly/Quarterly

Normalization

A normalization correction is routinely performed monthly or quarterly depending on the scanner's manufacturer.[16,18,24–27,30,31] It should also be acquired after a failed daily blank scan or scanner service. The normalization scan is used to correct for variations in the sensitivity of the blocks or buckets and adjustments in the efficiency in each line of response (LOR) in the sinogram.[16,18,24,26,30,31] A poor normalization scan will result in horizontal streaks through the image (Fig. 5-7).

A normalization correction is performed using radioactive rod (pin) sources or a solid phantom source; most commonly used is germanium-68 (Ge-68) source. Normalizations are performed in both the 2D and 3D mode, if available on the scanner.[2,24,26,30,31] Normalization scans may be performed by the technologist or the service provider. It is preferable to run the normalization scan overnight as the duration of the scan may range from 30 minutes to 12–18 hours, depending on the system type and age of the source. As the source decays, the normalization data should be monitored to ensure acceptable count statistics

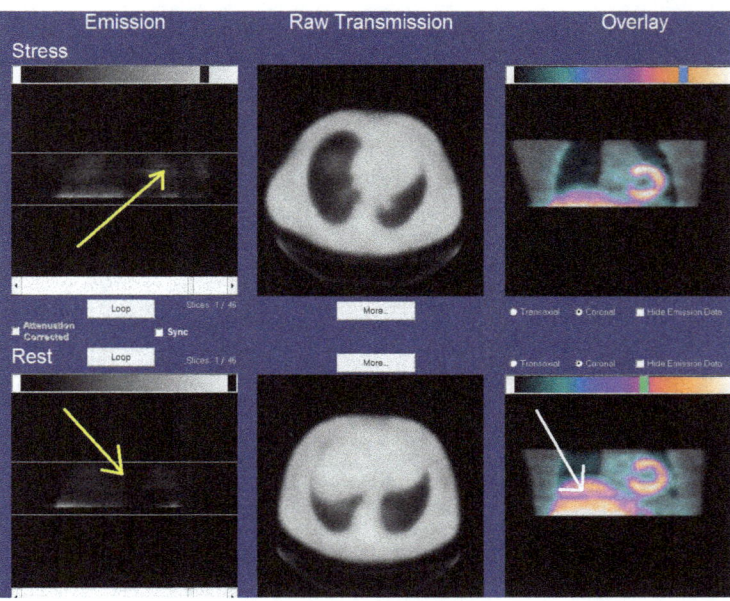

FIGURE 5-7 Example of PET scan with streaking artifact due to poor normalization.

and quality transmission maps are obtained. Sources should be routinely replaced based on manufacturer's recommendations, typically every 12 to 18 months depending on the system in use.

Once complete, the normalization scan is reconstructed and set as a new default based on OEM guidelines. A new blank scan must also be completed and applied each time a new normalization correction is completed.[16,18,24,26] Some systems have a pass or fail message upon completion of the scan. If the scan fails, the camera service engineer should be contacted for evaluation and repair.

Well Counter

Well counter correction (WCC) is an image pixel cross calibration to the dose calibrator. WCC uses a water-filled phantom and a known quantity of radioisotope to correlate the measured numerical value in each image pixel to a specific activity measured in physical units.[31] The 3D WCC also removes any axial sensitivity variation between images. Depending on the manufacturer, it is recommended that the 2D and 3D well counter acquisitions and corrections be updated quarterly to maintain good match of sensitivity. WCC can be performed by technologists, but are usually performed by service engineers during the quarterly preventative maintenance services.

▶ SPECT and PET Attenuation Correction

Attenuation correction for PET myocardial perfusion imaging (MPI), and more recently available for SPECT, requires additional QC procedures to be performed.[2,5–7,12–18,24,25,27] Currently the two available methods are either sealed source (gadolinium-153, cesium-137, or Ge-68) or computed tomography (CT).[2,12–18,24,25] When performing acquisitions with attenuation correction, it is important to understand the requirements and limitations of the specific hardware/software being used. It is also necessary to follow the manufacturer's recommendations for acquisition parameters and QC requirement to assure optimal image quality and system performance. In order to achieve a high-quality image study using attenuation correction, it is important to produce an optimal attenuation map to be applied to the images. This requires additional daily QC procedures.

Gadolinium-153 Sealed Sources for SPECT Systems

When performing SPECT attenuation correction with gadolinium-153 sealed sources, in order to produce an appropriate attenuation map, it is necessary to acquire a reference scan daily and ensure that the energy window is peaked accordingly.[2,12–18,28] The reference scan allows for the independent measure of the source with no attenuating media (table, patient, etc.). Since the source strength is stable, this can be performed once daily and applied to all patients. It is necessary to view this reference scan and evaluate for appropriate source strength. Based on the manufacturer's recommendations, if the reference scan does not have an adequate amount of counts, an inappropriate transmission scan will be acquired and may result in an under correction of the images. Therefore, if the reference scan produces an inadequate amount of counts, then the sources should not be used. Attenuation correction sources should be replaced based on the manufacturer's recommendations, typically every 12 to 18 months.

Germanium-68 Sealed Sources for Dedicated PET Systems

When performing PET attenuation correction with Ge-68 sealed sources, it is necessary to acquire a blank scan daily in order to produce an appropriate attenuation map.[16,18,24,25–27] The blank scan allows for the independent measure of the source with no attenuating media (table, patient, etc.). Since the source strength is stable, this can be performed once daily and applied to all patients. It is necessary to view this transmission scan and evaluate for appropriate source strength. Based on the manufacturer's recommendations, the transmission scan time may be adjusted between 20 and 30 minutes, based on the source counts. If the transmission scan does not have an adequate amount of counts, an inappropriate transmission scan will be acquired and may result in an under correction of the images. Sources should be replaced based on the manufacturer's recommendations, typically every 12 to 18 months.

CT-Based Attenuation Correction

With SPECT or PET/CT-based attenuation correction, it is important to ensure that the CT unit is in good working order and that the daily QC procedures are performed on the CT portion of the scanner in addition to the SPECT or PET QC procedures.[2,16,18,24–29] CT scanner QC is completed using a water-filled phantom and is often automatically performed by the system. Daily CT QC starts with x-ray tube warm up and air calibration and then typically includes accuracy of the CT number of water, evaluating uniformity, and image noise. Monthly or quarterly QC procedures may include laser alignment, slice thickness, spatial resolution, linearity, as well as low- and high-contrast resolution. Each manufacturer has specific requirements so it is recommended that you refer to your OEM manual and guidelines.[5–7] Similar to sealed source attenuation correction, it is necessary to have a reference scan to apply attenuation correction. This is acquired as a scout image on every patient prior to the start of the acquisition. If the CT unit is not functioning properly, this will result in a poor-quality scout and could adversely affect the corrected images.

With CT-based attenuation correction, additional testing must be completed to ensure proper alignment or registration of the CT and PET image sets. The PET and CT images are not performed simultaneously as the gantry bed position is different as a result of the two separate scanners. Electronic shift or "bed sag" can also be a factor in misregistration, and therefore, it is important to assess PET to CT registrations on an ongoing basis (Fig. 5-8).[25,32,33] Depending on your system, this is typically performed with a phantom or jig with multiple point sources and acquired in several bed positions. If "bed sag" is of concern, then it may be helpful to place a weight on the scanner bed for testing. Transaxial slices of the fused images are reviewed. It is recommended that any software registration errors after correction be under 1 mm.[25]

QUALITY CONTROL DURING THE ACQUISITION

The previous section focused on QC procedures related to the imaging system that should be performed prior to the image acquisition. There are also several QC techniques that should be performed during the acquisition to help achieve an optimal and interpretable study.[9,25,27,34]

In order to optimize image quality, it is necessary to ensure patient comfort, utilize appropriate imaging protocols, perform appropriate camera setup and acquisition parameters, and recognize potential sources of internal and external attenuation and artifacts. Artifacts and errors that occur during an

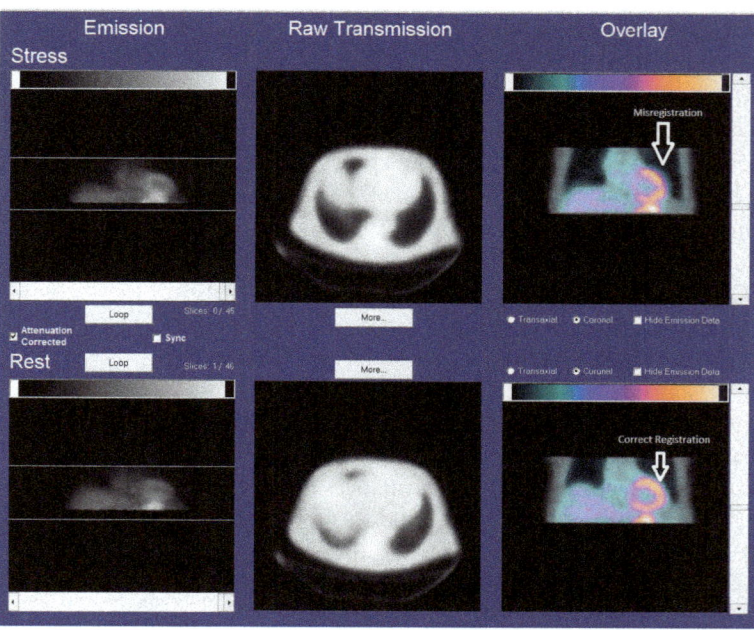

FIGURE 5-8 Example of dedicated PET scan before and after misregistration correction.

Table 5-3
Potential Sources of Artifacts Associated with Image Acquisition

Acquisition Setup	Patient-Related Artifacts
Collimation	Soft tissue attenuation
Radius	Extracardiac activity
Positioning	Motion
Number of projections	Irregular R–R interval with gated SPECT

acquisition may be the result of inappropriate camera setup or may be patient related (Table 5-3). Understanding potential sources of artifact and using proper imaging techniques may reduce potential errors due to artifact and increase overall test specificity.[9]

Protocols and Acquisition Setup

Single-Photon Emission Computed Tomography Systems

There are four commonly used SPECT imaging protocols for stress MPI.[11,17,35] These include 1- and 2-day Tc-99m–labeled isotope protocols, dual-isotope (Tl-201 rest/Tc-99m–labeled stress) protocol, and Tl-201 stress/delay protocol (see Chapter 9 SPECT Protocols). The protocol of choice for each laboratory should be based on the patient population being studied (inpatient vs. outpatient), the logistical considerations of the laboratory, the availability of personnel, including physician, nurse, and technologist, and finally availability of the radiopharmaceutical. It is important to maintain consistency with a chosen protocol. This will provide better recognition of abnormalities/artifacts based on deviation from standards and maintain high image quality.

There are several aspects that should be considered when performing acquisition setup. These include collimation, scan radius, number of projections, counts per projection, matrix size, and patient positioning.[9–11,17,34,36–42] When positioning the patient, it is necessary to center the heart in the FOV and reproduce this position for both the rest and stress. The scan radius should be as close to the patient as possible. If it is too large, excessive blurring may occur, resulting in contrast loss, resolution loss, and spatial distortion.[9,11,34,36–38] The number of projections and time per projection are also very important.[9,11,17,34,36–38]

Positron Emission Tomography Systems

There are two commonly used PET imaging protocols for stress MPI.[25,27] These include rubidium-82 (Rb-82) and ammonia (N-13) protocol (see Chapter 10 PET MPI Protocols). The protocol of choice for each laboratory should be based on the patient population being studied (inpatient vs. outpatient), the logistical considerations of the laboratory, the availability of personnel, including physician, nurse, and technologist, and finally availability of the radiopharmaceutical. It is important to maintain consistency with a chosen protocol. This will provide better recognition of abnormalities/artifacts based on deviation from standards and maintain high image quality.

There are several aspects that should be considered when performing PET acquisition setup. These include image mode (static, gated, or dynamic), total counts, matrix size, and patient positioning.[25,27] When positioning the patient, it is necessary to center the heart in the FOV and reproduce this position for both the rest and stress. The timing of the prescan delay before the start of the acquisition following an injection of Rb-82 and N-13 also very important to allow for blood pool clearance.[25,43] When using Rb-82 as a radiopharmaceutical, timing is a critical factor in quality due to the short half-life of Rubidium and the fast pace of the protocol. For 2D Rb-82 protocols, it is important to also understand the time activity profile of the Rb-82 generator over its life cycle. Each week technologists will need to adjust the dose activity and volumes to ensure you infuse the most optimal bolus dose. Infusing the same dose throughout the life of the generator can potentially cause decreased count statistics which can lead to artifacts or poor-quality images. In addition to understanding the Rb-82 generator's characteristics, the technologist will need to adjust the prescan delay based on each individual patient's cardiac function to acquire optimal images. The recommended prescan delay post Rb-82 infusion for patients with normal ventricular function, or a left ventricular ejection fraction (LVEF) greater than 50%, is 70 to 90 seconds. For patients that have reduced ventricular function or an LVEF from 30% to 50%, the recommended prescan delay post Rb-82 infusion is 90 to 110 seconds. For patients with poor function or an LVEF less than 30%, the recommended prescan delay post Rb-82 infusion is 110 to 130 seconds.[25]

In order to acquire high-quality image sets for both SPECT and PET, the studies must contain the appropriate count density. Perfusion defects may be created simply due to poor count statistics. To ensure each is optimal, it is necessary to customize the acquisition parameters to the protocol being performed and the imaging system being used. Manufacturers' system recommendations and various published imaging guidelines and standards may be used as a reliable reference.[5–7,17,25,35] The use of national standards, such as the American Society of Nuclear Cardiology, is very important for laboratory accreditation.[25]

▶ Potential Sources of Error during the Acquisition

An important reason to continue QC techniques during the acquisition is to help reduce artifacts and errors that may occur.[2,9,12,17,32,33,44,45] These artifacts can be camera related, as discussed in a previous section; however, they are more commonly related to the patient. The most common causes of artifacts include soft tissue attenuation, extracardiac activity, patient motion, and an irregular heart rate (R–R interval) with gated SPECT.

Soft Tissue Attenuation

Soft tissue attenuation is a common source of artifact on myocardial perfusion studies[9,12,17] unless attenuation correction is available. Dedicated PET, PET/CT and select SPECT systems have attenuation correction capability. For Cardiac PET, ASNC and SNMMI recommend imaging should only be performed with attenuation correction.[25] If attenuation correction is not available, the most common soft tissue attenuation artifact that appears is usually a result of breast tissue or the diaphragm (Fig. 5-9). These artifacts generally appear as an apparent localized decrease in count density on an acquired SPECT image. The location, size, and severity of the artifact produced are dependent on the attenuation in relation to the myocardium.[43] The severity is also dependent on the

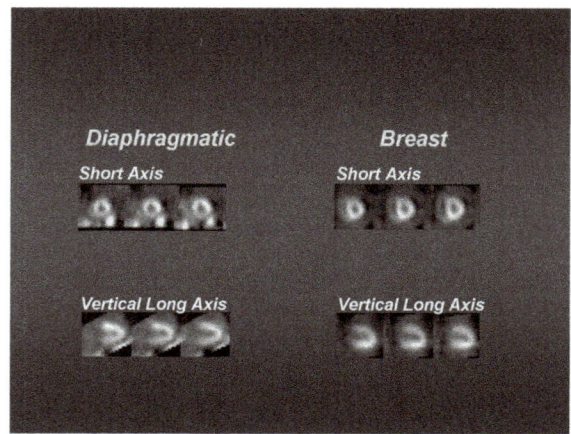

FIGURE 5-9 Example of diaphragm and breast attenuation. Diaphragm results in an area of decreased activity in the inferior wall and breast attenuation has an area of decreased activity in the anterior wall.

energy of the photon being acquired. For example, attenuation artifact occurs more frequently in SPECT MPI with the use of Tl-201 due to the lower (78 keV) energy in comparison to Tc-99m (140 keV).[44] Generally, attenuation artifacts are fixed; however, if there is a variation in the artifact location between stress and rest, it may appear reversible (Fig. 5-10).[44] If not recognized as such, these artifacts may result in a false positive interpretation.

To assist in the prevention of these artifacts, it is necessary to use an appropriate imaging protocol and maintain consistency. It is also helpful to image women with the bra off, as this helps position the breast tissue most uniformly between the detector and the myocardium.[9,44] In order to help avoid artifacts resulting from the diaphragm, stress imaging with Tc-99m–labeled agents should be performed after the patient's heart rate has returned to baseline (15–20 minutes post-stress injection). PET MPI protocols, with higher (511 keV) energy isotopes, may also be considered as an alternative to SPECT MPI when the potential for attenuation artifacts exists.

Other attenuation artifacts may be caused by external sources on the patient. Most common are pendants or necklaces, breast prostheses, metal components of pacemakers and implantable cardioverter defibrillators, or electrocardiogram (ECG) leads left on the patient. To prevent these artifacts, the patient should be asked to remove any metals or other attenuating sources if possible, and the chest area should

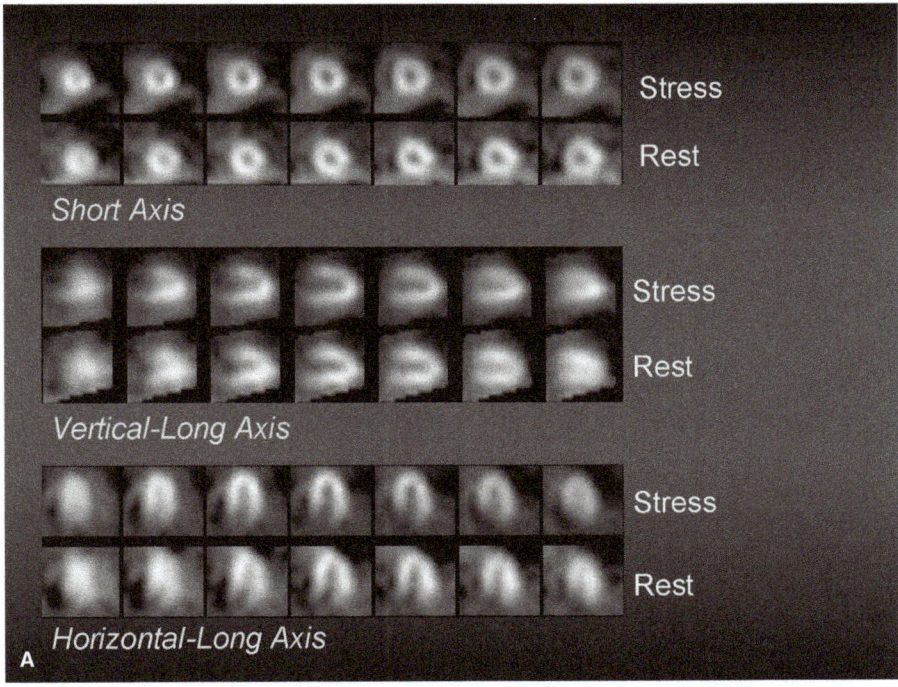

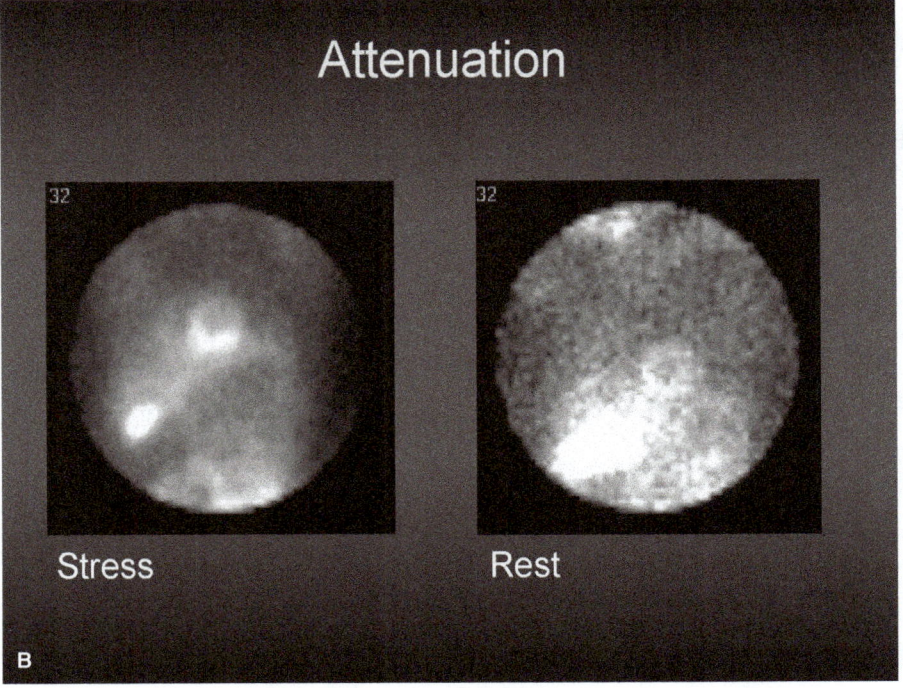

FIGURE 5-10 A: Stress images demonstrate a decrease in photon activity in the anterior wall that complete reverses at rest. **B:** Planar images demonstrate breast shadowing on stress not visualized at rest. This is most likely the cause of the reversible defect.

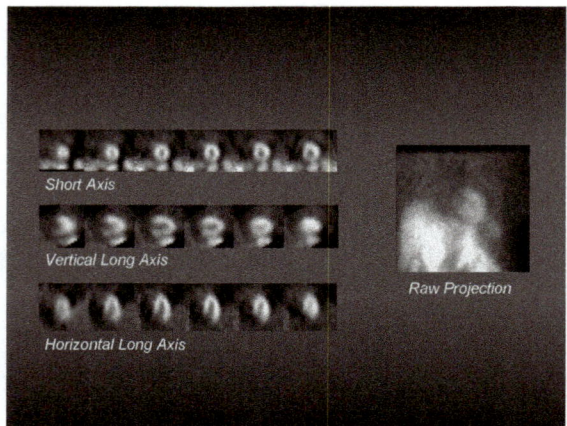

FIGURE 5-11 Increased liver activity creates a decrease of activity in the inferior wall.

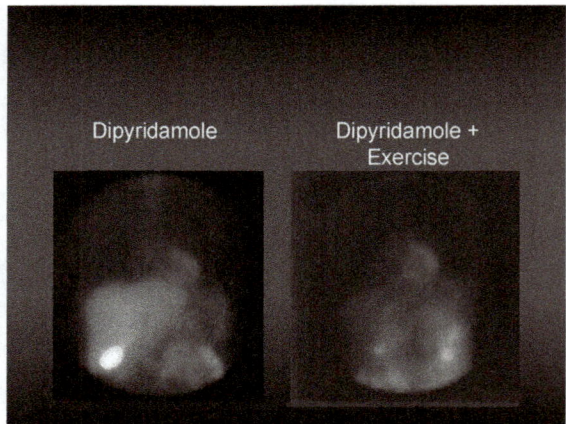

FIGURE 5-12 Example of patient pharmacologic stress image with and without supplemental exercise. Both images performed at 30 minutes. Image with supplemental exercise has less liver activity.

be visually inspected for these sources before beginning the acquisition.

Extracardiac Activity

Extracardiac activity may also affect both SPECT and PET MPI.[12,17,35,44,45] Such sources may be due to increased liver, blood pool, or bowel activity (Fig. 5-11). These artifacts are more common with the Tc-99m–labeled imaging agents, but can be a factor in all MPI imaging techniques. In SPECT, extracardiac activity may result in inferior wall defects, as it may create the appearance of more counts on the anterior wall due to a ramp artifact.[44] Artifacts may occur during back filter projection and polar plot generation. This can appear as fixed or reversible, depending on activity at both stress and rest.

To assist in prevention or reduction of these artifacts, it is necessary to allow for adequate clearance. When using Tc-99m–labeled SPECT imaging agents after injection at rest and/or pharmacologic stress, it is helpful to encourage some type of exercise with pharmacologic stress whenever possible to help stimulate liver clearance (Fig. 5-12). When using Rb-82 and N-13 PET imaging agents, it is important to choose the optimal post-injection delay prior to acquisition to ensure adequate blood pool clearance.[25,46] This is especially important when using Rb-82 due to its short half-life. With Rb-82, approximately 80% of the infused isotope counts are acquired in the first 3 minutes of the acquisition and within 5 minutes, 95% of the counts will have been attained.[25] Counts from excessive blood pooling can cause scatter into myocardial activity resulting in image degradation or may influence the size or severity of defects.

In the case of CT attenuation, streaking or "hot spot" artifacts can occur in images due to beam hardening with bone and overcorrection with metal objects such as the metal components of pacemakers and implantable cardioverter defibrillators.[25,46]

Patient Motion

Patient motion is another common cause of artifacts on myocardial perfusion studies.[2,9,12,17,25,45,47–52] Motion may occur in the horizontal or vertical axis or occasionally both. When this occurs during SPECT MPI, misalignment of data during back filter projection produces defects that generally occur in the anterior and posterior walls (Fig. 5-13).[2,9,12,17,45,48–52]

When performed with attenuation correction, patient motion can occur either within a single transmission or emission dataset or both since the studies are acquired in two separate datasets. When the patient motion occurs during the emission scan, artifacts may appear as blurred image contours or two opposing artifacts, 180 degrees apart.[25,27] When the patient motion occurs between the transmission and emission scans, misregistration artifacts may appear. In order to reduce motion artifact, it is important to always explain the procedure thoroughly and make the patient as comfortable as possible. The use of

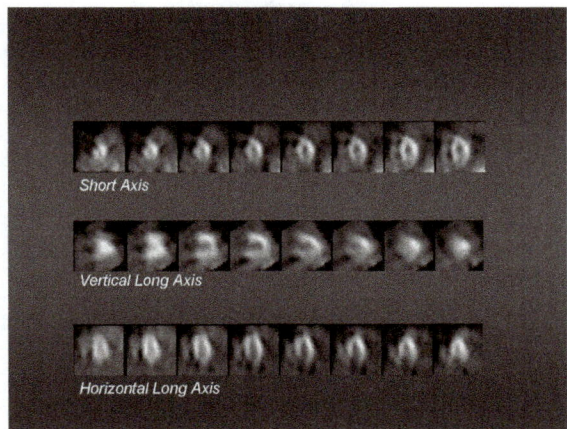

FIGURE 5-13 Motion artifact appears in the anterior and inferior walls of the myocardium.

pillows, blankets, and knee supports can be helpful. The inability of a patient to place the arms above the head comfortably may cause patient motion. In this group of patients, it may be helpful to image the patient with the arms at the side.[53] It is important to minimize the time under the camera by adopting the most efficient protocols and technologies (i.e., dual- or triple-head cameras). For patients receiving CT attenuation studies, respiratory averaging or shallow free breathing methods may be considered to reduce respiratory motion artifacts.[25,29,32] CT registration artifacts can be more significant if acquired at full or end inspiration.[25,29,32]

The SPECT raw cine projection data should always be reviewed before the patient is excused from the laboratory. As standard SPECT cameras acquire datasets over multiple projections by the rotating detector(s) around the patient, patient motion can easily be identified by a shift between sequential projections while reviewing the cine. If subtle motion is detected, it may be appropriate to apply motion correction software in order to correct the artifact.[2,9] If the scan motion is too severe, the acquisition should be repeated.

Unlike SPECT rotating detectors, PET scanners have nonmoving detectors that acquire all the patient datasets simultaneously which can make identification of motion artifacts more difficult.[18] For PET and PET/CT users, the axial images should be evaluated before proceeding to the next imaging sequence or excusing the patient from the laboratory. Currently, there is no motion correction software available to correct motion in PET MPI. For this reason, technologists must be vigilant when monitoring patients during the acquisition to reduce any patient motion. For dedicated PET and PET/CT users, a second transmission or CT attenuation scan preformed after gated stress emission images have been acquired may help correct for patient motion between rest and stress positions.[25,27,33] If available, attenuation correction software applications may be utilized to correct the misregistration when there is misalignment of transmission and emission scan due to subtle patient motion between the scans. If the software is not available or if the scan motion is too severe, the acquisition should be repeated as soon as the generator reaches equilibrium.

Irregular R–R Interval

When performing gated SPECT and PET MPI, the acquisition is triggered from the R–R interval of the three-lead ECG.[11,12,17,41,42,44,45,48-57] An irregular R–R interval (heart rate) may be a potential source of artifact on these acquisitions. If a patient has an arrhythmia, such as atrial fibrillation or atrial or ventricular premature beats, this may result in a lack of counts in each of the temporal frames that make up the projections during image acquisition. This is due to the variability in timing of each R–R interval causing misrepresentation of end diastole (ED) and end systole (ES) in the cardiac cycle. This in turn may cause perfusion artifacts as well as an underestimation of the LVEF.[11,12,54-57] While some systems have the capability to prevent this problem during the acquisition, others do not. It is important to understand the limitations of the imaging system being used. The length and number of rejected beats should be monitored. In some instances, gated imaging should not be performed on patients with an irregular heart rate in order to preserve image quality. This is especially important in Rb-82 PET protocols due to the short half-life in which repeating a scan would require an additional isotope administration. For this reason, when preforming a rest- and stress-gated protocol with Rb-82, the resting-gated scan should always be processed and evaluated for any gating issues prior to the start of stress-gated imaging.

Gated PET MPI studies are obtained using a similar gating device and acquired in 8 or 16 bins per

R–R interval.[25] Like SPECT, it is important to understand the limitations of your scanner and to monitor the R–R interval before and during acquisition. Atrial fibrillation, premature ventricular contractions (PVCs), and other abnormal rhythms should be noted before the start of acquisition. A non-gated or a list mode study should be considered for patients with gating difficulties. During the acquisition, the gate must be monitored for accepted and rejected beats. Any gating irregularities should be reported to the interpreting physician as an abnormal gate can lead to highly inaccurate gated information.[25]

QUALITY CONTROL AFTER THE ACQUISITION

QC should continue even after the patient has been discharged from the laboratory. There are steps that should be taken during processing, display, and interpretation of myocardial perfusion studies to ensure optimal image results and outcomes.

Processing

Processing of a myocardial perfusion study consists of three distinct steps.[9,10,12,24,25,58] Attention should be given to each step in order to prevent artifacts or errors that may result in a misinterpreted study. Before processing is started, the SPECT raw cine projection data should be evaluated. If any potential problems are visualized, repeating the acquisition should be considered. For PET and PET/CT users, the axial images should be evaluated before proceeding to the next imaging sequence.

The first step in processing is reconstruction. This involves selecting the upper and lower limits of the projection data that will be used to generate the perfusion slices. When selecting the upper and lower limits, care must be taken to ensure the limits are symmetrical, truncation of the myocardium is not occurring, and the limits are reproducible between the stress and rest images. If reconstruction limits are improperly selected, this may produce partial volume effects, difficulties in display scaling, and truncation of the myocardium. This may result in a loss of clinical accuracy.[10,12,14,17,58]

Choosing and applying the appropriate filtering parameters is the next step in processing. Filtering of the data optimizes the signal-to-noise ratio in the tomographic reconstructions, removes inherent reconstruction artifacts, and provides image enhancement.[10,12,14,58–62] Considerable care and attention should be given to this step of processing because overfiltering may mask a lesion or defect and underfiltering may create a lesion or defect. Filtering parameters should be chosen for each specific imaging system that allows for the most appropriate image enhancement and quality. These filtering parameters should then be consistent for each image set. For those patients who have low count statistics (i.e., obese patients and infiltrated dose), the acquisition should be performed for a longer time per projection or injected with a higher dose, rather than processed with different filters to increase image quality. Inappropriate filtering of the data may alter the interpretation and reduce clinical sensitivity.[9,14,58–62]

Reorientation of the transverse image is the last step in processing. This step determines the final creation of the slices, which includes the short, horizontal, and vertical long axes. The reorientation must reflect the accurate long axis of the left ventricle and should be consistent between the stress and rest images. Inappropriate reorientation may create or mask defects, cause geometric distortion of the myocardium, and prevent accurate slice matching during display.[9,14,58,63,64]

With sealed source attenuation, it is important to evaluate the attenuation map for truncation. The two patterns that may occur are critical and noncritical truncation.

Critical truncation is categorized as truncation occurring on the left and noncritical truncation occurs on the right (Fig. 5-14). If truncation occurs, then caution should be taken when interpreting the attenuation-corrected images.

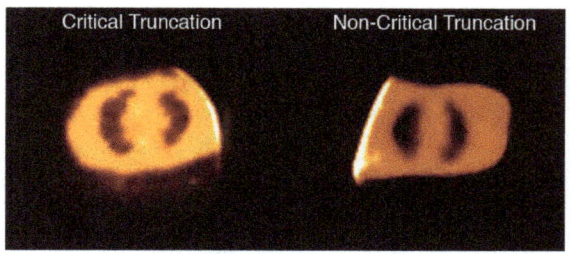

FIGURE 5-14 Example of an adequate and poor count density attenuation map.

Display and Interpretation

The last two components in the processing of MPIs are display and interpretation. QC techniques should be applied to these aspects of imaging as well to complete the process of providing the best quality information possible.

When displaying myocardial perfusion images, the software used should provide review of short, horizontal, and vertical long-axis slices and include at least eight slices per row.[5,17,64] The software should also allow one to review the gated SPECT and PET images, as well as the raw cine projection data in SPECT studies. This will provide improved efficiency for the interpreter by not having to change between applications to perform a thorough evaluation of the data. The images should be displayed in a linear or monochrome scale (gray or thermal) because some color scales are incremental and may cause a false positive interpretation. There are several commercially available software programs that incorporate all of these aspects for display.

Interpretation is one of the most important components of a myocardial perfusion study, as it is what allows the referring physician to make clinical decisions on the basis of the results. Referring physicians are looking for a result they can use, in particular a normal or abnormal finding. Equivocal results are not generally helpful, but should be used in cases of poor image quality or protocol violations rendering the study suboptimal for interpretation. MPI is best interpreted in a clinical context. Therefore, the interpreter should use all data available, including perfusion images, gated images for wall motion and ejection fraction, stress test findings, and clinical history in order to make a more informed decision.[17,65] However, it is important that the interpretation as normal or abnormal is based on the images, not the clinical or stress data. It is therefore recommended that images be reviewed blinded, and integration of clinical data be performed after a decision is made for the study.

The sequence of interpretation should be review of the SPECT raw cine projection first.[17,65] For PET and PET/CT users, the axial images should be reviewed first. This allows visualization of any potential sources that may cause artifacts, on the processed data. It is very important that the interpreting physician is aware and can recognize these artifacts, as they may result in a misinterpretation of the data as discussed earlier in the chapter. Next, the perfusion data should be reviewed for any defects, fixed or reversible. If quantitation is available, it should then be reviewed for comparison. For practices in which there is only one interpreter, quantitation may be a good second reader. Finally, the gated data should be reviewed to assess wall motion and LVEF. The review of the gated data may also help resolve questions of true scar due to myocardial infarction (MI) versus artifact with fixed perfusion abnormalities.[54,65,66]

CONCLUSION

QC is a very important component of nuclear cardiology laboratory procedures. It is a process that is continual and requires attention from both the technologist and the physician. It begins before the patients enter the laboratory and continues after they are discharged. In order to achieve optimal image quality, it is important to have a thorough QC program in place within the laboratory. The explanations and procedures provided are just a few of the several components that make up such a program. For a more thorough understanding, it may be helpful to refer to the references provided, as well as several others that are currently available. This process and understanding will result in better referring physician, as well as patient satisfaction, and ultimately result in better patient outcomes.

REFERENCES

1. National Committee on Radiation Protection. *Safe Handling of Radioactive Materials. Recommendation of NCRP, Report 30*. Washington, DC: National Bureau of Standards Handbook 92; 1964.
2. Nichols KJ, Bacharach SL, Bergmann SR, et al. Instrumentation quality assurance and performance. ASNC imaging guidelines for nuclear cardiology procedures. *J Nucl Cardiol*. 2007;14:e61–e78.
3. National Electrical Manufacturer's Association. *Performance Measurements of Gamma Cameras. Standards Publication No. NU1-2012*. Rosslyn, VA: National Electrical Manufacturer's Association; 2012.
4. National Electrical Manufacturer's Association. *Performance Measurements of Positron Emission Tomography. Standards Publication No. NU2-2012*. Rosslyn, VA: National Electrical Manufacturer's Association; 2012.

5. The Intersocietal Accreditation Commission. The IAC Standards and Guidelines for Nuclear/PET Accreditation. http://www.intersocietal.org/nuclear/standards/IACNuclearPETStandards2012.pdf
6. American College of Radiology. *Nuclear Medicine Accreditation Program Requirements.* Reston, VA; 2017. http://www.acraccreditation.org/~/media/ACRAccreditation/Documents/NucMed-PET/Nuclear-Medicine-Requirements.pdf?la=en
7. American College of Radiology. *PET Accreditation Program Requirements.* Reston, VA; 2017. http://www.acraccreditation.org/~/media/ACRAccreditation/Documents/NucMed-PET/PETRequirements.pdf?la=en
8. American College of Radiology (ACR) and the Society of Pediatric Radiology (SPR). ACR-SPR Technical Standard for Diagnostic Procedures using Radiopharmaceuticals; 2016. https://www.acr.org/~/media/5E5C2C7CFD7C45959FC2BDD6E10AC315.pdf
9. Nichols KJ, Galt, JR. Quality control for SPECT imaging. In: DePuey EG, Garcia EV, Berman DA, eds. *Cardiac SPECT Imaging.* 2nd ed. Philadelphia, PA: Lippincott Williams and Wilkins; 2001.
10. Kritzman J. SPECT instrumentation. In: Heller GV, Mann A, Hendel RC, eds. *Nuclear Cardiology Technical Applications.* New York: The McGraw-Hill Companies; 2009.
11. Mann A. Protocols and acquisition parameters for SPECT myocardial perfusion imaging. In: Heller GV, Mann A, Hendel RC, eds. *Nuclear Cardiology Technical Applications.* New York: The McGraw-Hill Companies; 2009.
12. Cullom SJ. Artifacts and quality control for myocardial perfusion SPECT including attenuation correction. In: Heller GV, Mann A, Hendel RC, eds. *Nuclear Cardiology Technical Applications.* New York: The McGraw-Hill Companies; 2009.
13. Early PJ, Sodee DB. Quality assurance. In: *Principles and Practice of Nuclear Medicine.* St. Louis, MO: CV Mosby; 1985.
14. Cullom SJ. Principles of cardiac SPECT imaging. In: DePuey EG, Garcia EV, Berman DA, eds. *Cardiac SPECT Imaging.* 2nd ed. Philadelphia, PA: Lippincott Williams and Wilkins; 2001.
15. Baron JM, Choraguai P. Myocardial single-photon emission computed topography quality assurance. *J Nucl Cardiol.* 1996;3:157–166.
16. Zanzonico P. Routine quality control of clinical nuclear medicine instrumentation: A brief review*. *J Nucl Med.* 2008;49:1114–1131.
17. Holly TA, Abbott BG, Al-Mallah M, et al. Single photon-emission computed tomography. In: *ASNC Imaging Guidelines for Nuclear Cardiology Procedures.* Bethesda, MD: American Society of Nuclear Cardiology; 2010. http://www.asnc.org/files/SPECT%202010.pdf
18. Case JA, Bateman TA. Taking the perfect nuclear image: Quality control, acquisition, and processing techniques for cardiac SPECT, PET, and hybrid imaging. *J Nucl Cardiol.* 2013;20:891–907.
19. Esteves FP, Raggi P, Folks RD, et al. Novel solid-state detector dedicated cardiac camera for fast myocardial perfusion imaging: Multicenter comparison with standard dual detector cameras. *J Nucl Card.* 2009;16:927–934.
20. Garcia EV, Faber TL, Esteves FP. Cardiac dedicated ultrafast SPECT cameras: New designs and clinical implications. *J Nucl Med.* 2011;52:210–217. http://jnm.snmjournals.org/content/52/2/210.full.pdf
21. Slomka PJ, Patton JA, Berman DS, et al. Advances in technical aspects of myocardial perfusion SPECT imaging *J Nucl Cardiol.* 2009;16:255–276.
22. International Atomic Energy Agency (IAEA). *Human Health Series no 6. Quality Assurance for SPECT Systems.* Vienna, Austria: IAEA; 2009. http://www-pub.iaea.org/MTCD/Publications/PDF/Pub1394_web.pdf
23. Spectrum Dynamics Medical, Inc., D-SPECT User Manual, version MAN00003 Rev. G.1. Spectrum Dynamics Medical, Inc.; September 2011.
24. Society of Nuclear Medicine and Molecular Imaging–Technologist Section. *SNMMI-TS: Myocardial Perfusion Imaging 2016: Quality, Safety, and Dose Optimization.* Reston, VA: Society of Nuclear Medicine and Molecular Imaging–Technologist Section; 2016.
25. Dilsizian V, Bacharach SL, Beanlands RS, et al. ASNC imaging guidelines/SNMMI procedure standard for positron emission tomography (PET) nuclear cardiology procedures. *J Nucl Med.* 2016;23(5):1187–1226.
26. International Atomic Energy Agency (IAEA). *Human Health Series no 1.Quality Assurance for PET and PET/CT Systems.* Vienna, Austria: IAEA; 2009. http://www-pub.iaea.org/MTCD/Publications/PDF/Pub1393_web.pdf
27. Dorbala S, Di Carli1 MF, Delbeke D, et al. SNMMI/ASNC/SCCT guideline for cardiac SPECT/CT and PET/CT 1.0*. society of nuclear medicine and molecular imaging. *J Nucl Med.* 2013;54:1485–1507. http://jnm.snmjournals.org/content/54/8/1485.full.pdf
28. Hendel RC, Corbett JR, Cullom SJ, at al. The value and practice of attenuation correction for myocardial perfusion spect imaging: A joint position statement from the American society of nuclear cardiology and the society of nuclear medicine. *J Nucl Cardiol.* 2002;9:135–143. http://jnm.snmjournals.org/content/43/2/273.full.pdf
29. Slomka PJ, Le Meunier L, Hayes SW, et al. Comparison of myocardial perfusion 82Rb PET performed with CT- and transmission CT-based attenuation correction. *J Nucl Med.* 2008;49:1992–1998. http://jnm.snmjournals.org/content/49/12/1992.full.pdf
30. CPS Innovations. *Siemens ECAT Accel PET software version 7.2.2 Operating Instructions Rev.* A July 2002 (User Manual). Knoxville, TN: CPS Innovations; 2002.
31. General Electric Medical Systems Company. PET Advance Operator Manual, Direction 2280383-100, Rev. 4. General Electric Medical Systems Company; August 2002.
32. Gould LK, Pan T, Loghin C, et al. Frequent diagnostic errors in cardiac PET/CT due to misregistration of CT attenuation and emission PET images: A definitive analysis of causes, consequences, and corrections. *J Nucl Med.* 2007;48:1112–1121. http://jnm.snmjournals.org/content/48/7/1112.full.pdf
33. Loghin C, Sdringola S, Gould LK. Common artifacts in pet myocardial perfusion images due to attenuation–emission misregistration: Clinical significance, causes, and solutions. *J Nucl Med* 2004;45:1029–1039. http://jnm.snmjournals.org/content/54/1/50.full.pdf
34. Galt JR, Garcia EV. Advances in instrumentation for cardiac SPECT. In: DePuey EG, Garcia EV, Berman DA, eds. *Cardiac SPECT Imaging.* 2nd ed. Philadelphia, PA: Lippincott Williams and Wilkins; 2001.

35. Henzlova MJ, Duvall WL, Einstein AJ, et al. Stress, protocols and tracers. In: *ASNC Imaging Guidelines for Nuclear Cardiology Procedures*. Bethesda, MD: American Society of Nuclear Cardiology; 2016. http://www.asnc.org/files/Guidelines%20 and%20Quality/ASNC%20SPECT%20ProtocolsTracers%20 Guidelines2016.pdf
36. Breszk JA, Hawman EG. Evaluation of SPECT angular sampling effects: Continuous vs. step and shoot. *J Nucl Med*. 1987;28:1308–1314.
37. Maniawski PJ, Morgan HT, Whackers FJ. Orbit-related variation in spatial resolution as a source of artifactual defects in thallium-201 SPECT. *J Nucl Med*. 1991;32(5):871–875.
38. Garcia EV, Cooke CD, Van Train KF, et al. Technical aspects of myocardial SPECT imaging with technetium-99m sestamibi. *Am J Cardiol*. 1990;66(13):23E.
39. Go RT, MacIntyre WJ, Houser TS, et al. Clinical evaluation of 360° and 180° data sampling techniques for transaxial SPECT thallium-201 myocardial perfusion imaging. *J Nucl Med*. 1985;26:695–706.
40. Hoffman EJ. 180° compared with 360° sampling in SPECT. *J Nucl Med*. 1982;23:745–746.
41. Maublant JC, Peycelon P, Kwiatkowski F, et al. Comparison between 180° and 360° data collection in technetium-99m MIBI SPECT of the myocardium. *J Nucl Med*. 1989;30: 295–300.
42. Eisner RL, Nowak DJ, Pettigrew R, et al. Fundamentals of 180° reconstruction in SPECT imaging. *J Nucl Med*. 1986;27:1717–1728.
43. Di Carli1 MF, Dorbala S, Jolene Meserve J, et al. Clinical Myocardial Perfusion PET/CT*. *J Nucl Med*. 2007;48:783–793.
44. DePuey EG. How to detect and avoid myocardial perfusion SPECT artifacts. *J Nucl Med*. 1994;35:699–702.
45. DePuey EG, Garcia EV. Optimal specificity of thallium-201 SPECT through recognition of imaging artifacts. *J Nucl Med*. 1989;30:441–449.
46. DiFilippo FP, Brunken RC. Do Implanted Pacemaker Leads and ICD Leads Cause Metal-Related Artifact in Cardiac PET/CT?. *J Nucl Med* 2005;46:436–443.
47. Martinez-Moller A, Souvatzoglou M, Navab N, et al. Artifacts from misaligned CT in cardiac perfusion PET/CT studies: Frequency, effects, and potential solutions. *J Nucl Med*. 2007; 48:188–193.
48. Friedman J, Berman DS, Van Train K, et al. Patient motion in thallium-201 myocardial SPECT imaging: An easily identified frequent source of artifactual defect. *Clin Nucl Med*. 1988;13:321–324.
49. Cooper JA, Neumann PH, McCandless BK. Effect of patient motion on tomographic myocardial perfusion imaging. *J Nucl Med*. 1992;33:1566–1571.
50. Eisner RL. Sensitivity of SPECT thallium-201 myocardial perfusion imaging to patient motion. *J Nucl Med*. 1992;33: 1571–1573.
51. Geckle WJ, Frank TL, Links JM, et al. Correction for patient motion and organ movement in SPECT: Application to exercise thallium-201 cardiac imaging. *J Nucl Med*. 1988;28:441–450.
52. Cooper JA, Neumann PH. Visual detection of patient motion during tomographic myocardial perfusion imaging. *Radiology*. 1992;185:283.
53. Toma DM, White MP, Mann A, et al. Influence of arm positioning upon rest/stress Tc-99m sestamibi tomographic imaging. *J Nucl Cardiol*. 1999;6:163–168.
54. White MP, Mann A, Saari MA. Gated SPECT imaging 101. *J Nucl Cardiol*. 1998;5:523–526.
55. Cullom SJ, Case JA, Bateman TM. Electrocardiographically gated myocardial perfusion SPECT: Technical principles and quality control considerations. *J Nucl Cardiol*. 1998;5:418–425.
56. Nichols K, Dorbala S, DePuey EG, et al. Influence of arrhythmias on gated SPECT myocardial perfusion and function quantification. *J Nucl Med*. 1999;40:924–934.
57. Arrighi JA. ECG-gated SPECT imaging. In: Heller GV, Mann A, Hendel RC, eds. *Nuclear Cardiology Technical Applications*. New York: The McGraw-Hill Companies; 2009.
58. Folks RD. Myocardial SPECT processing. In: Heller GV, Mann A, Hendel RC, eds. *Nuclear Cardiology Technical Applications*. New York: The McGraw-Hill Companies; 2009.
59. Galt JR, Hise LH, Garcia EV, et al. Filtering in frequency space. *J Nucl Med Technol*. 1986;14:152–162.
60. Zubal GW, Wisniewski G. Understanding Fourier space and filter selection. *J Nucl Cardiol*. 1997;4(3):234–243.
61. King MA, Schwiger RB, Doherty PW, et al. Two-dimensional filtering of SPECT images using Metz and Wiener filters. *J Nucl Med*. 1984;25:1234–1240.
62. Boulfelfel D, Rangayyan RM, Hahn LJ, et al. Prereconstruction restoration of myocardial single photon emission computed tomography images. *IEEE Trans Med Imaging*. 1992;11(3):336–341.
63. Borello JA, Clinthorne NH, Rogers WE, et al. Oblique-angle tomography. A restructuring algorithm for transaxial tomographic data. *J Nucl Med*. 1981;22:471–473.
64. The Cardiovascular Imaging Committee. Standardization of cardiac tomographic imaging. *J Am Coll Cardiol*. 1992;20:255–256.
65. Tilkemeier PL, Cooke CD, Grossman GB, et al. Standardized reporting of radionuclide myocardial perfusion and function. In: *ASNC Imaging Guidelines for Nuclear Cardiology Procedures*. Bethesda, MD: American Society of Nuclear Cardiology; 2009. http://www.asnc.org/files/Radionuclide%20MP%20&%20 Function.pdf.
66. DePuey EG, Rozanski A. Using gated technetium-99msestamibi SPECT to characterize fixed myocardial defects as infarct or artifact. *J Nucl Med*. 1995;36:952–955.

Quality Performance in Nuclear Cardiology: A Global Perspective

CHAPTER 6

Peter L. Tilkemeier

INTRODUCTION

Analyzing and reporting quality processes are an integral component of today's world, regardless of the area of application, be it medical, manufacturing, customer service, or other areas. In order to allow an exploration of quality in nuclear cardiology, this chapter will provide definitions of quality today and examine five common cycles that have been used to promote quality improvement, each with their own unique characteristics that make them particularly well suited for specific applications. Utilization of quality-driven processes and their impact on cost and value will also be addressed. In this context, the importance of quality and its integration into global accreditation and certification processes, including the similarities and differences among the various bodies providing accreditation will be discussed. Clinical application of quality improvement methodologies regarding patient and test selection, performance, interpretation, reporting, and the development of a quality improvement program for each of these areas will be the next area of focus. Finally, the chapter will provide information regarding reporting of quality performance initiatives and the use of registries and benchmarks in clinical nuclear cardiology today.

QUALITY DEFINITIONS

▶ Components of Quality

Quality in nuclear cardiology today has much broader implications than just producing high-quality images.

With the advent of appropriate use criteria, the availability of multiple imaging modalities and protocols, multiple settings in which nuclear cardiology imaging can be delivered, interpretation of nuclear cardiology tests by multiple specialties, pay-for-performance initiatives including accreditation and certification and the regulatory requirements for reporting, "quality" has become a much larger topic in everything we do in nuclear cardiology.[1] This chapter will address the many facets of quality today.

The current definition of quality can vary greatly depending upon the perspective of an individual or organization. It is clearly a perception that is supported by data depending upon the metrics utilized. Quality can range from the daily quality control testing performed to insure optimal camera performance to the ability of a nuclear cardiology study to reduce downstream healthcare expense. Given this broad range of quality in current practice it is important to understand some basic definitions. The traditional quality assurance activities that have been used in nuclear cardiology have focused on insuring high-quality imaging. These have been focused around quality control and quality assurance whose definitions imply maintaining performance of a process, for example, image acquisition, over a period of time and within specified parameters. The performance of this type of testing is addressed in Chapter 6 of this book. A well-functioning nuclear cardiology laboratory today has an established protocol for maintenance and assurance of quality control. More recently, quality improvement has become a focus of processes within the nuclear cardiology laboratory, in large part to maintain accreditation. Quality improvement initiatives were initially focused on process-driven measures of performance, such as report turnaround times or availability of the next appointment. More recently quality improvement has expanded to more outcome-driven measures such as radiation reduction, correlation with downstream testing results, and patient/physician satisfaction surveys.

It is no longer adequate to just insure the quality of the images. Quality improvement in nuclear cardiology must include all aspects of the complex nuclear cardiology imaging process from order entry and test selection to reporting and impact on future testing and patient outcomes including functional status, quality of life, and reductions in morbidity and mortality. In order for any quality improvement program to be successful, the program must be iterative continuously striving to improve on prior performance through a cyclical assessment. Cyclical models of quality improvement will be addressed next.

Quality Improvement Cycles

Five quality improvement cycles that have had their greatest success and healthcare applications include the FOCUS-PDCA model, LEAN, Six-Sigma, FMEA, and the Milestones models. Selection of one of these tools as a mechanism to assist with improving quality will depend on the type of project, the team members involved, and the need for one time versus continued quality improvement. As a laboratory looks to improve processes, selection of the best cycle will facilitate the greatest potential for change in the least amount of time with greatest cost efficiency. The cycles have their unique features which will be independently examined and are summarized in Table 6-1.

FOCUS-PDCA

FOCUS-PDCA is designed to maximize the performance of pre-existing processes. This includes: Finding a process that is in need of improvement, Organizing a team of knowledgeable stakeholder's regarding the process crossing various levels of the organization, Clarifying current processes and the changes needed to achieve improvement, Understanding the potential for variability by measuring performance and whether or not the process is currently under control or not and Selecting actions that are necessary to improve the process. After this initial assessment has been performed a traditional plan-do-check-act quality improvement project can be undertaken. The planning phase of this model includes projections of what leadership believes will

Table 6-1

Models for Quality Improvement Cycles

Quality Cycle	Project Scope	Project Size	Special Features
FOCUS-PDCA	Maximize performance of pre-existing processes	Small to large	Developed by Hospital Corporation of America; variation of PDCA
LEAN	Reduction of inefficiencies and waste adversely affecting performance	Usually large and multi-step serial processes	Numerous tools developed to facilitate. Need trained staff to facilitate improvement process
Six-Sigma	Reduce variation in currently functioning processes	Usually large and complex projects involving numerous teams	Reduces variability in process resulting in reduced waste and inventory and improved throughput
FMEA	Predict future product failures due to prior failures; usually applied to new designs and processes	Usually utilized in multi-step cross departmental processes	Analysis based on severity, likelihood of occurrence and ability to detect future failure
Milestones	Assessment of process most likely to succeed	Small to large	Serial process requiring completion of a step before proceeding to next step

Adapted with permission from Tilkemeier PL, Hendel RC, Heller GV, et al. *Quality Evaluation in Non-Invasive Cardiovascular Imaging*. Switzerland: Springer; 2016.

happen as a result of the improvement project. The "doing" phase is comprised of four major components including educating and training staff, developing a plan that allows implementation on a small scale before broader implementation, documenting any problems or unexpected observations and adjust as necessary, and developing the tools that will be utilized to analyze the data. The third phase, check, assesses the effectiveness of the intervention with regard to the goals outlined in the earlier planning phase. The final phase, act, is the broad scale implementation of the change within the organization. It is intended that this cycle back to the first step in the process to understand if further process improvement is necessary.[2,3]

LEAN

The LEAN model is specifically focused on reducing insufficiency in a repetitive process such as unnecessary human movement, waiting for supplies, doing more than necessary to meet requirements, poor-quality work resulting in rework, inventory not matching need, unnecessary movement of resources, delivery of services that are unwanted by the customer, and finally overproduction. To focus on these areas of inefficiency the lean process includes six steps including problem definition from the customer's perspective, examination of current work procedures and processes, team-based identification of improvement opportunities, identifying root causes of the problem, define a new process to address root causes, and design of an implementation plan including measures to determine success and the timeline to achieve them.[2]

Six-Sigma

Six-Sigma is a tool that is widely used in healthcare today and is primarily focused on reducing performance variability. The most successful Six-Sigma projects would result in a defect rate of less than 4 per 1 million opportunities. The Six-Sigma process emphasizes variation control, results oriented activities, and the use of data to drive the process. It can be highly impactful and can also have significant limitations in healthcare applications due to patient care variability that cannot be accounted for in a process control model.[2,4]

FMEA

The Failure Mode Effect Analysis is a tool that has been used to predict future failure based on past failures and has been traditionally used for evaluation of newly designed clinical processes. The tool focuses on those steps that have the greatest risk for failure and identifying and mitigating them prior to their occurrence. This has unique significance in the healthcare industry given the high rate of change we are currently experiencing and the significant potential impact of change with negative patient outcomes.[4]

Milestones

Given the many opportunities for improvement in quality in healthcare, the Milestones model has particular applicable ability because it focuses on evaluating processes and Majors which have the greatest opportunity for improvement. The seven steps are as follows: Involving measurement and performance in the daily activities of the organization, identifying the typical categories of concepts to be measured, identifying specific measures for improvement, development of operational definitions of specific measures, developing a robust plan for data collection plan and data gathering, data analysis and, finally, actual data collection necessary for the organization to develop plans for implementation. This is an extremely data-driven model which depending upon the organization and its culture and infrastructure has a greater potential for success.[5]

The importance of cycles in quality improvement should be evident from the five models examined. As we implement change to improve processes and outcomes in the nuclear cardiology laboratory, it is important to continuously monitor the impact of those changes on the real outcome. Many times changes in one area result in unintended consequences in other portions of the process that may have greater adverse impact on the outcome than the original improvement was designed to address. As a new process stabilizes and the outcome is consistent, given the critical nature of patient care, it is important to move from an improvement to a monitoring program to insure that changes elsewhere in the complex nuclear cardiology imaging cycle have not affected a process with an established outcome.

Quality: Cost and Value

Nuclear cardiology has been on the leading edge of the cost and value discussion as it regards overall quality of cardiovascular care. As a result, there have been numerous studies evaluating the clinical value relative to the cost of care delivery of a nuclear cardiology study as noted in a recent information statement from the American Society of Nuclear Cardiology.[6] Quality plays an important role in this discussion because a poor-quality study has no value and only cost. It is therefore essential that we strive to perform only the highest-quality studies. A useful quality indicator in all laboratories could be that a poor-quality study is of such importance that a root cause analysis be performed to understand how to prevent this in the future. This should result in the lowest number possible poor-quality studies being performed.

Having controlled the number of poor-quality studies, emphasis can then be placed on the cost of performing the test. Opportunities to understand the cost of each component of a study and evaluate mechanisms for reducing the cost are essential. Analysis of cost reduction opportunities can result in the need to improve infrastructure in such a way that new lower cost methodologies can be implemented, such as cameras with more highly sensitive detectors allowing faster imaging time and reduced use of radiopharmaceuticals. A major area of cost savings is the utilization of appropriate use criteria, an inappropriately performed study is the most expensive from a population health-based perspective, increasing the total cost of care with the potential to increase cost and risk to the patient by adding further downstream testing that is likely to have minimal clinical impact.

The value of a test is dependent upon its ability to impact clinical outcomes, future testing, and future therapy. A test may have a high cost but be of greater value due to its ability to influence morbidity, mortality, and cost of future therapy in a positive manner, such as positron emission tomography. In order for a test to have high value, it must have significant clinical impact to change or affirm a therapeutic course, at a reasonable cost. The value of testing will be dependent on a number of factors including the quality and cost of the test itself, the quality and cost of downstream diagnostic testing resulting from the nuclear cardiology test, the cost of a therapeutic intervention and its impact on morbidity and mortality. Many of these will be local factors dependent upon the expertise and infrastructure available at the clinical site. The END multicenter study group demonstrated this through the observation that stable chest pain patients who underwent a more aggressive diagnostic strategy of cardiac catheterization first had higher initial costs, increased interventional procedures and great follow-up cost over a composite 3-year follow-up period.[7]

ACCREDITATION AND CERTIFICATION

Accreditation of laboratories and certification of physician qualifications are important measures of quality in our nuclear cardiology laboratories today. This is true no matter where you are practicing nuclear cardiology worldwide. The methodologies for accreditation and certification do vary based upon your geographic location, especially outside of the United States. Accreditation and/or certification can be governmentally mandated and regulated or performed in the private sector. In the United States, accreditation is mandated for payment of nuclear cardiology studies performed on patients covered by Medicare in the outpatient setting and this accreditation is done by an approved but nongovernmental organization. In Europe, accreditation of laboratories and certification of physicians are government-regulated processes. Table 6-2 shows the comparison between the United States and European systems. The available pathways will be examined in further detail.

Accreditation in the United States

There are presently four organizations qualified to provide accreditation of advanced imaging services including nuclear cardiology in the United States. These include the American College of Radiology, the Inter-societal Accreditation Commission (IAC), RadSite, and The Joint Commission. Although there are minor variations in the requirements for each of their programs, they are all based on a multi-faceted assessment of the nuclear cardiology imaging laboratory including policies and procedures, image quality, reporting, and an ongoing quality improvement program. Examples of quality improvement projects for nuclear cardiology and templates to assist in their implementation are available from the IAC website at

Table 6-2
Characteristics of Accreditation Compared between European and United States Based Methodologies

Characteristic	European	United States
Mechanism of accreditation	Societal	Independent
Mandated for payment	No	Yes (CT, CMR, Nuclear medicine, PET)
Modalities available		
Echocardiography	Yes	Yes—IAC
Nuclear medicine/PET	Yes	Yes—ACR, IAC, RadSite, TJC
CMR	No	Yes—ACR, IAC, RadSite, TJC
CT	No	Yes—ACR, IAC, RadSite, TJC
Noninvasive vascular	No	Yes—IAC
Government regulation	Local and national regulations	Indirectly through MIPPA

PET, positron emission tomography; CMR, cardiac magnetic resonance; CT, computed tomography; IAC, Inter-societal Accreditation Commission; ACR, American College of Radiology; TJC, The Joint Commission; MIPPA, Medicare Improvements for Patients and Providers Act.
Reproduced with permission from Tilkemeier PL, Hendel RC, Heller GV, et al. *Quality Evaluation in Non-Invasive Cardiovascular Imaging.* Switzerland: Springer; 2016.

http://www.intersocietal.org/nuclear/seekings/sample_qualitycontrol.htm. The methodology for assessing each of these varies among the organizations including direct review by the accrediting body, random audit of current process, and reporting of self-study activities. The programs are based on standards developed by each of the organizations based on societal guidelines for performance of nuclear cardiology studies.[8–11]

Physician certification is now performed through the Alliance for Physician Certification and Advancement™ as a result of the merger of the former Certification Board of Nuclear Cardiology into this organization. There has been no change in the process of physician certification as a result of this merger. The physician certification pathway will continue to support nuclear regulatory commission authorized user status as well as maintenance of certification activities for other board certification.

International Accreditation

From an international perspective, programs specific to the accreditation and performance of nuclear cardiology laboratories and physicians exist in the United Kingdom, Europe, and are in development in Japan. Each of these are evolving current standards or developing new standards to assure that high-quality high-value nuclear cardiology studies are available to patients and referring physicians. This has included using centers of excellence, documentation of training experience, the development of syllabi outlining the core curriculum for performance of high-quality studies and founding of new societies to oversee the process as required. Specifically, the European approach is overseen by the European Association of Cardiovascular Imaging in concert with the European Society of Cardiology and is somewhat less prescriptive with regard to its standards than its counterpart organizations in the United States. There is greater emphasis on outcome than on process. The United Kingdom model is in the middle ground between these two with slightly more detailed guidelines for accreditation. The Japanese are in the early development phases of accreditation criteria and guideline development for the practice of nuclear cardiology in Japan.[12–14]

EVALUATION OF TESTING PROCEDURES

Patient Selection

Quality improvement activities can focus on many aspects of selection for myocardial perfusion imaging testing. This can include correct patient selection for the test and followed by selection of the best test for the patient who has been referred to answer the clinical question. In order to assure correct patient selection for the test, there have been multi-societal documents developed addressing appropriate use criteria for testing based either on the type of test to be performed or more recently on the clinical condition that is to be assessed.[15] The latter are more focused on multimodality imaging and selecting the appropriate test for the diagnosis. The American College of Cardiology Foundation has developed and revised the definitions for the appropriate use criteria. The current definitions are as follows: Appropriate—An appropriate option for management of patients in this population due to benefits generally outweighing risks; effective option for individual care plans although not always necessary, depending on physician judgment and patient-specific preferences (i.e., procedure is generally acceptable and is generally reasonable for the indication); May be Appropriate—At times, an appropriate option for management of patients in this population due to variable evidence or agreement regarding the benefits/risks ratio, potential benefit based on practice experience in the absence of evidence, and/or variability in the population; effectiveness for individual care must be determined by a patient's physician in consultation with the patient based on additional clinical variables and judgment along with patient preferences (i.e., procedure may be acceptable and may be reasonable for the indication); and Rarely Appropriate Care—Rarely an appropriate option for management of patients in this population due to the lack of a clear benefit/risk advantage; rarely an effective option for individual care plans; exceptions should have documentation of the clinical reasons for proceeding with this care option (i.e., procedure is not generally acceptable and is not generally reasonable for the indication).[16] An important opportunity in the quality assessment of the laboratory is the implementation of appropriate use criteria to determine that the clinical condition warrants the study.[17] Understanding that "rarely appropriate" studies do need to occur, it is important to note their incidence as well as patterns of referrals for patients with such indications. This can be the basis for a quality improvement project regarding physicians referring patients to the laboratory.[18] The American Society of Nuclear Cardiology patient-centered imaging preferred practice statement can be a helpful reference when addressing appropriate patient selection for testing.[19]

Once the patient has been deemed appropriate for either PET or SPECT imaging, the next area for potential evaluation for quality improvement would be appropriate testing protocol selection, such as one day, two day, pharmacologic with exercise, or stress only imaging for example. Quality improvement projects as part of the accreditation process could be performed evaluating potential mechanisms to improve patient test selection. In addition, it is important to note that the results of myocardial perfusion imaging studies are an important decision point in the algorithm to proceed to further invasive diagnostic imaging.[20] Examination of downstream testing can provide an opportunity for the laboratory as a quality improvement project that is related to outcome. Such a project may evaluate the referral pattern to coronary angiography and the results of the angiogram relative to the risk of future cardiac events as determined by the myocardial perfusion imaging study, such as whether the nuclear study was normal, low, or high risk. Again, complete agreement is probably not obtainable; however, correlation based on the risk of the study results should be meaningful.

Examination of Testing Performance

Once the appropriate patient and testing protocol have been determined, the performance of the test in a way that will result in a high-quality, accurate, and highly reliable manner is the next important step in the quality chain. The performance of high-quality imaging includes quality control, quality assurance, and quality improvement. Basic quality control is necessary to insure the equipment is performing according to manufacturer's standards necessary to produce high-quality images. Examples of quality control include daily flood field images, center of rotation, and other quality control measures as required by the manufacturer. Quality assurance activities are required to insure that standardized processes continue to function at the level for which they are expected to on a daily basis. Examples of quality assurance activities may include accurate image processing by the technologist, optimal stress test performance, implementation of methodology to minimize radiation exposure to the staff and patients, and evaluation of appointment availability to meet the needs of the referring physician and patient.[21,22] Quality improvement activities would be based on those processes which are not meeting expected quality standards or have not stabilized to the point of ongoing monitoring as part of quality assurance. Utilization of quality improvement cycles described earlier in this chapter and appropriate to the clinical setting could be implemented as a mechanism to improve and insure ongoing control of quality performance.

▶ Interpretation Evaluation

The next step in the myocardial perfusion imaging quality chain is the evaluation of interpretation of the image. As with all of the other steps the interpretation has many components. The image interpretation plays an important role in the quality assurance and improvement process because it requires an assessment of the patient selection, protocol selection, test performance, and data processing that all contribute to high-quality images for interpretation. The first step in interpretation examination is to assure the previous steps have been taken. Interpretation of the study should include all of the elements noted in the associated societal guidelines for the study being performed. Quality assurance and improvement projects evaluating study interpretation could include interobserver and intraobserver variability in image interpretation through comparison of independent interpretation of the images by two observers or by the same observer temporarily dissociated. Review of studies with discrepancies can be an important learning and quality improvement activity. Other quality improvement activities related to image interpretation can be correlation with further studies such as catheterizations performed as well as interventions and "outcomes" from the myocardial perfusion imaging study. These types of studies can be facilitated by participation in multiple registries that track these data. Substantial lack of correlation could be related to multiple factors in the complex myocardial perfusion imaging chain and should trigger an examination of the potential source of error.

▶ Reporting Evaluation

The report of a myocardial perfusion imaging study is the next to last step in the process. The true final interpretation is by the referring physician or healthcare provider who receives the report and his/her perception of the information that was included in the report. It is therefore of utmost importance that the report accurately conveys the results of the study in a meaningful way to the healthcare provider such that the results can be incorporated into the care plan for the patient. If the report does not answer the clinical question or allow the referring physician to act on the information contained in it, the report can have the impact equal to a technically poor-quality study. We know from prior studies that the nuclear cardiology report is a significant potential area for improvement.[23] Insuring that the report contains all of the required components is an essential component of any lab quality program. Furthermore, it is important that the report utilize "plain English" to describe the findings in a way that is meaningful to the referring physician. The report should not utilize phrases specific only to cardiology or nuclear cardiology trained physicians' "dictionaries" and in a large majority of cases state clearly whether the findings are normal or abnormal.[24] The findings may also carry some assessment of patient risk and whether this risk has been lowered or raised by the test results. The American Society of Nuclear Cardiology has an established guideline for nuclear cardiology reporting.[25] This guideline is currently under revision with an update due in early 2017.

Multiple potential quality assurance and improvement projects can be centered on myocardial perfusion imaging reports. This can include comparison of results when the report is read by a physician not familiar with the patient, audits to insure the report contains all of the required elements utilizing standardized reporting guidelines, ability of the report to meet the requirements for Registry submission and whether or not the report reads timeliness and critical result guidelines. The report truly is the final product from a very complex process with multiple opportunities for poor quality to adversely affect patient care.

▶ Developing a Quality Improvement Program

If quality is to be improved, given the complexity of the myocardial perfusion imaging process, it takes a "large" number of engaged individuals. The team will need to include individuals from every aspect of the process including referring physicians, information technology staff, business planning, marketing, development, nursing, technologists, and nuclear cardiologists. Potentially, the most important member of the team would be a patient advocate. All of the individuals must be engaged in the common purpose of improving the process to prevent sabotage. In order to be successful, the team must work through three phases of the quality improvement process including: (1) discovery—during which they identify an opportunity, the needs to attain the opportunity, the appropriate team members and baseline data; (2) analysis—including data analysis, insuring that the baseline processes in control, identifying opportunities for change and identifying appropriate comparative data; and (3) action—composed of developing a plan for change, implementing those changes, analyzing the effectiveness of the change, developing a monitoring plan and most importantly celebrating the accomplishment. Potential mechanisms for identifying areas of improvement include comparisons to national benchmarks, patient, staff and physician surveys, patient safety reporting, direct observation, peer-review, and internal analyses. Once all of these analytics have been performed, it is necessary for the team to generate potential solutions utilizing such stools as brainstorming, surveys, root cause analysis, accreditation and certification feedback, and national bench marking. Probably the most important part and the most frequently overlooked is the implementation of tools to monitor results and insure that improvements are maintained over time. If nuclear cardiology is to survive into the future implementation of strong quality improvement plans and engaged dedicated quality improvement teams will be necessary.

REPORTING QUALITY AND USE OF BENCHMARKS

▶ Continuous Quality Improvement

As has been emphasized throughout this chapter, quality improvement should be a continuous process. Some quality majors will need to be continuously improved while others can move into a quality assurance on monitoring mode once the improvement appears to be stable. Quality improvement is clearly a cyclical process that requires dedicated time and individuals as well as infrastructure and resources from the organization to insure the greatest impact on our patients. As we move forward into new payment models in the United States and with the existing impact of quality on payment in other parts of the world, quality will play an ever-increasing role in the performance of myocardial perfusion imaging studies.

▶ Utilization of Benchmarks

Benchmarks play an important role today and will in the future regarding quality reporting and improvement. The use of public reporting and comparison to benchmarks will be an integral part of quality improvement moving forward. Utilizing these two mechanisms will result in transparency of program quality to payors, referring physicians, and patients. It is important to realize the limitations of both public reporting and bench marking. One of the most important aspects of using benchmarks is to understand the source of the data that was used to derive the information. When choosing a benchmark to compare to, it is important to understand how the data were reported; the demographic information of the benchmark, such as was it derived from practice sites or large health systems; and the mechanism of data reporting whether it was self-reported, harvested from electronic health records, or claims based. It is also important to realize the impact of public reporting because facilities may choose to avoid high-risk cases when data cannot be adjusted for risk and the impact this can have on the program as well as patient care.

Utilization of immediate benchmark feedback has been of use in numerous clinical settings such that through the electronic health record a caregiver can be reminded when their performance is not aligned with benchmark or guideline-derived care models. Furthermore, the use of behavioral theory and the potential of the Hawthorne effect (knowing you are being observed) can make the use of benchmark data very impactful on changing behavior. In summary, benchmarks will become much more prominent in our everyday clinical care and it will be important to realize how they have been developed to insure their maximal impact.

Registries

Participation in imaging registries will have an important impact on informing all of us regarding the daily practice of myocardial perfusion imaging. Registries allow us to gather and evaluate data outside of the clinical trial setting which can vary significantly from the day-to-day practice of nuclear cardiology. Moving forward, data gathered from registries will help inform the development of guidelines, quality improvement activities, changes in payment models, and healthcare policy. The integration of data from our laboratories in registries will allow us to perform retrospective randomized controlled trials on large populations of patients without the expense of a randomized controlled trial. For example, is there a difference in additional downstream testing for patients of a similar body habitus with similar imaging results, depending on whether there initial perfusion study was performed with a low dose stress only protocol or a two day protocol? Answering this type of question from a registry will be significantly more cost-effective and allow more timely answers to important clinical questions that will continue to prove the value of myocardial perfusion imaging. The ability to combine information from different registries such as myocardial perfusion imaging and cardiac catheterization will allow us to understand the complex clinical interaction between these two tests and their impact on future therapies and patient outcomes. Participation in patient registries will become the norm for everything we do and will need to be integrated into our daily workflows to be most successful.[26–28]

SUMMARY

Quality performance is a requirement for successful myocardial perfusion imaging globally. There are many methodologies to assist with continuous quality improvement utilizing quality cycles and data from numerous sources to insure that the complex process of myocardial perfusion imaging results and the highest quality in greatest improvement in outcomes for patients. In addition, as we improve quality, the value of nuclear cardiology in the future will be better defined. Through the use of quality improvement tools in all aspects of nuclear cardiology starting with patient selection and ending with a high-quality report, we will insure the future role for myocardial perfusion imaging. If nuclear cardiology is to remain successful, quality will need to be integrated into all of the daily procedures and transparency regarding our outcomes will be required for success.

REFERENCES

1. Depuey EG. Journal of Nuclear Cardiology News Update "Why Quality Counts". *J Nucl Cardiol.* 2014;21:1041.
2. Spath PL. *Introduction to Healthcare Quality Management.* 2nd ed. Chicago, IL: Health Administration Press; 2013. Chapter 5, Continuous improvement; 111–130.
3. McLauglin CP, Kaluzny AD. *Continuous Quality Improvement in Healthcare: Theory, Implementation, and Applications.* 2nd ed. Gaithersburg, MD: Aspen Publishers; 1999. Chapter 1, Defining quality improvement: past, present, and future; 3–33.
4. Warren K. Quality improvement: The foundation, processes, tools, and knowledge transfer techniques. In: Ransom ER, Joshi MS, Nash DB, Ransom SB, eds. *The Healthcare Quality Book: Vision, Strategy, and Tools.* 2nd ed. Chicago, IL: Health Administration Press; 2008.
5. Lloyd RC. Milestones in the quality measurement journey. In: Ransom ER, Joshi MS, Nash DB, Ransom SB, eds. *The Healthcare Quality Book: Vision, Strategy, and Tools.* 2nd ed. Chicago, IL: Health Administration Press; 2008.
6. DesPrez RD, Shaw LJ, Gillespie RL, et al. Cost-effectiveness of myocardial perfusion imaging: A summary of the currently available literature. *J Nucl Cardiol.* 2005;12:750–759.
7. Shaw LJ, Hachamovitch R, Berman DS, et al. The economic consequences of available diagnostic and prognostic strategies for the evaluation of stable angina patients: An observational assessment of the value of precatheterization ischemia. Economics of Non-invasive Diagnosis (END) Multicenter Study Group. *J Am Coll Cardiol.* 1999;33(3):661–669.
8. Jarvinen H, Wilcox P. Clinical audit and practice accreditation. In: Lau L, Ng K, eds. *Radiological Safety and Quality: Paradigms in Leadership and Innovation.* Netherlands: Springer; 2014.
9. Heller G, Katanick S, Sloper T, et al. Accreditation for cardiovascular imaging: Setting quality standards for patient care. *JACC Cardiovasc Imaging.* 2008;1(3):390–397.
10. 2014 Ambulatory care accreditation overview: a snapshot of the accreditation process. Oak Brook, IL: Joint Commission Resources; 2014 [cited October 14, 2016]. http://www.jointcommission.org/assets/1/6/2014_AHC_Overview_Guide.pdf
11. RadSite Accreditation Standards http://www.radsitequality.com/products-and-services. Accessed November 10, 2016.
12. Gimelli A, Neglia D, Schindler T, et al. Nuclear cardiology core syllabus of the European association of cardiovascular imaging (EACVI). *Eur Heart J Cardiovasc Imaging.* 2015;16(4):349–350.
13. Underwood SR. NICE in the United Kingdom: A milestone for nuclear cardiology. *J Nucl Cardiol.* 2004;11:660–663.
14. Yoshinaga K, Tamaki N. Current status of nuclear cardiology in Japan: Ongoing efforts to improve clinical standards and to establish evidence. *J Nucl Cardiol.* 2015;22:690–699.
15. Arrighi JA. Nuclear cardiology: Call to action. *J Nucl Cardiol.* 2013;20:315–316.

16. Hendel RC, Patel MR, Allen JM, et al. Appropriate Use of Cardiovascular Technology 2013 ACCF Appropriate Use Criteria Methodology Update: A Report of the American College of Cardiology Foundation Appropriate Use Criteria Task Force. *J Am Coll Cardiol.* 2013;61(12):1305-1317.
17. Wolk MJ, Bailey SR, Doherty JU, et al. ACCF/AHA/ASE/ASNC/HFSA/HRS/SCAI/SCCT/SCMR/STS 2013 multimodality appropriate use criteria for the detection and risk assessment of stable ischemic heart disease. *J Am Coll Cardiol.* 2014;63(4):380-406.
18. Johnson TV, Rose GA, Fenner DJ, et al. Improving appropriate use of echocardiography and single-photon emission computed tomographic myocardial perfusion imaging: a continuous quality improvement initiative. *J Am Soc of Echocardiogr.* 2014;27(7):749-757.
19. DePuey EG, Mahmarian JJ, Miller TD, et al. ASNC Preferred Practice Statement: Patient centered imaging. *J Nucl Cardiol.* 2012; 19:185-215.
20. Patel MR, Bailey SR, Bonow RO, et al. ACCF/SCAI/AATS/AHA/ASE/ASNC/HFSA/HRS/SCCM/SCCT/SCMR/STS 2012 appropriate use criteria for diagnostic catheterization. *JACC.* 2012;59(22):1995-2027.
21. Nichols KJ, Bacharach SL, Bergmann SR, et al. Instrumentation quality assurance and performance. *J Nucl Cardiol.* 2006;13:e25-e41.
22. Case JA, Bateman TM. Taking the perfect nuclear image: Quality control, acquisition, and processing techniques for cardiac SPECT, PET, and hybrid imaging. *J Nucl Cardiol.* 2013;20:891-907.
23. Tilkemeier PL, Serber ER, Farrell MB. The nuclear cardiology report: Problems, predictors, and improvement. A report from the ICANL database. *J Nucl Cardiol.* 2011;18:858-868.
24. Wackers F. The art of communicating: The nuclear cardiology report. *J Nucl Cardiol.* 2011;18:833-835.
25. Tilkemeier PL, Cooke CD, Grossman GB, et al. Standardized reporting of radionuclide myocardial perfusion and function. *J Nucl Cardiol.* 2009;16(4):650.
26. Williams KA, McKinley AP. How the ASNC Image guide registry will guide healthcare policy. *J Nucl Cardiol.* 2013;20: 948-950.
27. DePuey EG. Facing the current challenges in nuclear cardiology. *J Nucl Cardiol.* 2014;21:222-224.
28. Mahmarian JJ, Nuclear cardiology—taking the high road. *J Nucl Cardiol.* 2012;19:392-403.

Radiation Reduction Strategies in Myocardial Perfusion Imaging

CHAPTER 7

Michael C. Desiderio and Gary V. Heller

INTRODUCTION

Patient radiation exposure during medical procedures is a growing concern among health care providers, professional organizations as well as the general public. Medical radiation (of all subtypes) has increased by over 700% since 1980. Because of its value in diagnosis and prognosis in patients with known or suspected obstructive coronary disease, radionuclide myocardial perfusion imaging use has also increased over the last 25 years. Nuclear imaging accounts for approximately 25% of medical radiation. Cardiac imaging represents ~50% of all nuclear imaging procedures but is responsible for nearly 85% of all nuclear radiation doses.[1-4]

Optimizing radiation exposure for patients is of considerable importance for patient safety and should be taken into account when ordering tests. For the nuclear cardiologist, this impacts choices in testing protocols, equipment, and even tracers. Radiation-reduction strategies should also take into account the value of the testing procedure and should not be performed at the expense of image quality, and thus the value of the examination itself. This chapter will present concepts of the consequences of radiation exposure, methods of measuring radiation exposure in medical imaging and in particular, nuclear cardiology, describe current radiation exposure in common cardiovascular single-photon emission computed tomography (SPECT) and positron emission tomography (PET) myocardial perfusion imaging (MPI) procedures, and discuss methods of reducing radiation exposure through instrumentation changes, protocol changes, and tracer choice.

▶ Radiation Exposure: The Data

The exact consequences of radiation exposure are uncertain. The deterministic effects of direct radiation to an organ system, such as epidermal reactions, are well studied. However, understanding the consequences of radiation exposure to an individual is more obscure and difficult to assess. These stochastic effects of radiation exposure acquired during medical imaging are indeed difficult to apply to an individual's lifetime risk of developing cancers. This is in part due to variations in radiation types, exposure rates and quantities, and tissue susceptibilities as well as timing of procedures. In addition, malignancy generated by radiation exposure is often indistinguishable from those occurring from other causes.[2] Data estimated from the coronary computed tomography (CT) literature suggest that a 10-mSv radiation exposure increases lifetime risk of developing a fatal malignancy by 0.0005%.[4] This represents a small, but measureable increase in lifetime risk, but is difficult to quantify when considering an individual patient. For perspective, Table 7-1 illustrates comparative risks of death from both radiation sources and other causes.[4]

Evaluating lifetime risk due to radiation exposure, one must consider age and life expectancy at time of exposure. Certainly, as demonstrated in Figure 7-1, augmenting a patient's lifetime malignancy risk is weighed more heavily at younger decades when many

Table 7-1

Estimated Risk of Fatal Malignancy or Death Resulting from Radiation Exposure and the Lifetime Odds of Dying as the Result of Selected Activities of Everyday Life

Exposure	Estimated Risk of Fatal Malignancy or Lifetime Odds of Dying (per 1000 Individuals)
Effective radiation dose	
1 mSv (calcium score/lung screen)	0.05
10 mSv (coronary CTA/abdomen CT, invasive coronary angiography, radionuclide myocardial perfusion study)	0.5
50 mSv (yearly radiation worker allowance)	2.5
100 mSv (definition of low exposure)	5
Natural fatal cancer	212
Passive smoking	
Low exposure	4
High exposure, married to a smoker	10
Radon in home	
US average	3
High exposure (1–3%)	21
Arsenic in drinking water	
2.5 µg/L (US estimated average)	1
50 µg/L (acceptable limit before 2006)	13
Motor vehicle accident	11.9
Pedestrian accident	1.6
Drowning	0.9
Bicycling	0.2
Lightning strike	0.013

CTA indicates CT angiogram.
National Safety Council estimates are based on data from National Center for Health Statistics and US Census Bureau. Deaths are classified on the basis of the Tenth Revision of the World Health Organization's *International Classification of Diseases*. Lifetime odds are approximated by dividing the 1-year odds by the life expectancy of a person born in 2005 (77.8 years).
Reproduced with permission from Gerber TC, Carr JJ, Arai AE, et al. Ionizing radiation in cardiac imaging: A science advisory from the American Heart Association Committee on Cardiac Imaging of the Council on Clinical Cardiology and Committee on Cardiovascular Imaging and Intervention of the Council on Cardiovascular Radiology and Intervention. *Circulation*. 2009;119(7):1056–1065.

tissues are more rapidly replicating than when older and cell lines tend to be more senescent. Gender differences exist as well, and should also be acknowledged when considering testing in nuclear cardiology.[4-6]

▶ Measurement of Radiation Exposure in Nuclear Cardiology and Current Status

Measures of radiation and subsequent exposure are complex and more thoroughly discussed elsewhere (see Chapters 3 and 4). Typically, the Sievert unit (or milliSievert) is the most commonly used stochastic variable to compare radiation exposure levels from different sources. A Sievert (Sv), or milliSievert (mSv), is a unit which estimates the biological effect that 1 joule of radiation energy has on 1 kilogram of body tissue. Background radiation (from sources such as radon) produces exposure on the order of 3 mSv/year. The estimated radiation exposure from a typical rest/stress SPECT MPI is approximately 12 to 15 mSv

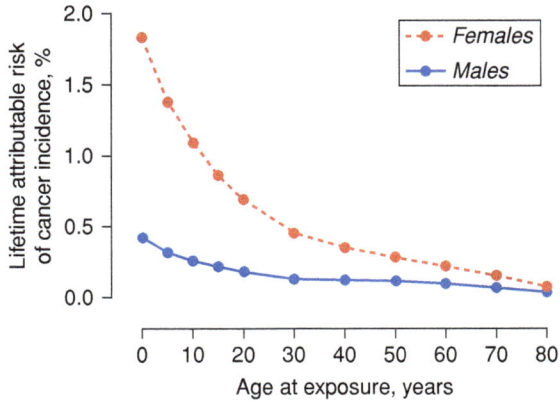

FIGURE 7-1 Lifetime attributable risk estimated of all-cancer incidence as a function of age and gender based on estimated effective exposure of 18 mSv. (Reproduced with permission from Hill KD, Einstein AJ: New approaches to reduce radiation exposure. *Trends Cardiovasc Med.* 2016;26(1):55–65.)

of radiation. This classifies nuclear cardiac imaging as a high-dose procedure by regulatory bodies.[1,2,4]

Table 7-2 represents the recommended radiotracer doses and estimated radiation exposure from recently published American Society of Nuclear Cardiology (ASNC) Guidelines.[3] The number of radiopharmaceuticals that are available, combined with a variety of the protocols, create a heterogeneous potential of exposure to US patients undergoing cardiac nuclear testing.

Radiation exposure has been a concern for professional societies for several years. As a result, ASNC published an "Information Statement" in 2010 intended to address radiation exposure.[1] The recommended reduction in nuclear cardiac imaging was to utilize less than 9 mSv per patient in at least 50% of nuclear cardiology studies. The writing committee also recommended methods of reducing radiation to an individual patient, illustrated in Figure 7-2, such as the use of technetium-based tracers rather than thallium-201, stress-only imaging and cardiac PET over SPECT, if available.

Despite the published statements, it is unclear whether these recommendations resonated within the community. A recent study using the Intersocietal Accreditation Commission (IAC) database examined compliance with these recommendations 2 years after the information statement publication.[5] Utilizing accreditation data submitted from 1047 laboratories in the United States, only 1% of laboratories were adhering to the <9 mSv standard (see Fig. 7-3). Furthermore, 10% of laboratories were still using thallium as their primary imaging agent although

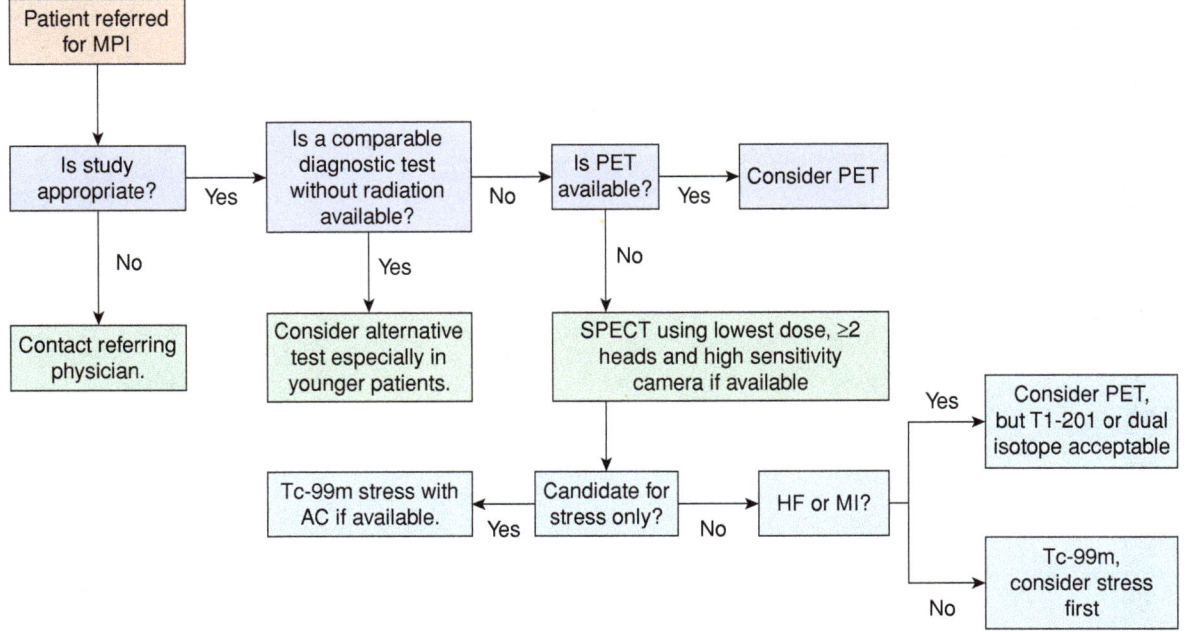

FIGURE 7-2 Recommended means of reducing radiation exposure in patients. (Reproduced with permission from Cerqueira MD, Allman KC, Ficaro EP, et al. Recommendations for reducing radiation exposure in myocardial perfusion imaging. *J Nucl Cardiol.* 2010;17(4):709–718.)

Table 7-2
Current SPECT Myocardial Perfusion Imaging Protocols and Estimated Radiation Exposure

	First Injection				Second Injection				Total Dose (mSv)	Total Dose if Stress Only (mSv)
	Given at	Activity (mCi)	Activity (MBq)	Dose (mSv)	Given at	Activity (mCi)	Activity (MBq)	Dose (mSv)		
Tc-99m protocols										
Tc-99m one-day stress first/stress only	Stress	8–12	296–444	2.0–3.0	Rest	24–36	888–1332	7.0–10.5	9.0–13.5	2.0–3.0
Tc-99m one-day rest/stress	Rest	8–12	296–444	2.3–3.5	Stress	24–36	888–1332	6.1–9.1	8.4–12.6	n/a
Tc-99m two-day stress/rest	Stress	8–12	296–444	2.0–3.0	Rest	8–12	888–1332	2.3–3.5	4.3–6.5	2.0–3.0
Tc-99m two-day stress/rest—large patient	Stress	18–30	666–1110	4.5–7.6	Rest	18–30	666–1110	5.2–8.7	9.8–16.3	4.5–7.6
Tc-99m two-day rest/stress	Rest	8–12	296–444	2.3–3.5	Stress	8–12	296–444	2.0–3.0	4.3–6.5	n/a
Tc-99m two-day rest/stress large patient	Rest	18–30	666–1110	5.2–8.7	Stress	18–30	666–1110	4.5–7.6	9.8–16.3	n/a
Tl-201 protocols										
Tl-201 stress/redistribution rest	Stress	2.5–3.5	92.5–129.5	10.9–15.3	n/a	n/a	n/a	n/a	10.9–15.3	10.9–15.3
Tl-201 stress/redistribution rest/reinjection	Stress	2.5–3.5	92.5–129.5	10.9–15.3	Rest	1–2	37–74	4.4–8.8	15.3–24.1	n/a
Tl-201 rest/redistribution	Rest	2.5–3.5	92.5–129.5	10.9–15.3	n/a	n/a	n/a	n/a	10.9–15.3	n/a
Dual-isotope Tl-201 rest/Tc-99m stress	Rest	2.5–3.5	92.5–129.5	10.9–15.3	Stress	8–12	296–444	2.0–3.0	13.0–18.3	n/a
Dual-isotope Tl-201 rest/Tc-99m stress—large patient	Rest	3.0–3.5	111–129.5	13.1–15.3	Stress	18–30	666–1110	4.5–7.6	17.7–22.9	n/a
I-123 protocol										
MIBG	Rest	10	370	4.6	n/a	n/a	n/a	n/a	4.6	n/a
Newer technology reduced-dose protocols										
Tc-99m one-day stress first/stress only	Stress	4–6	148–222	1.0–1.5	Rest	12–18	444–666	3.5–5.2	4.5–6.7	1.0–1.5
Tc-99m one-day rest/stress	Rest	4–6	148–222	1.2–1.7	Stress	12–18	444–666	3.0–4.5	4.2–6.3	n/a
Tc-99m two-day stress/rest	Stress	4–6	148–222	1.0–1.5	Rest	4–6	148–222	1.2–1.7	2.2–3.3	1.0–1.5
Tc-99m two-day stress/rest—large patient	Stress	9–15	333–555	2.3–3.8	Rest	9–15	333–555	2.6–4.4	4.9–8.1	2.3–3.8
Tc-99m two-day rest/stress	Rest	4–6	148–222	1.2–1.7	Stress	4–6	148–222	1.0–1.5	2.2–3.3	n/a
Tc-99m two-day rest/stress—large patient	Rest	9–15	333–555	2.6–4.4	Stress	9–15	333–555	2.3–3.8	4.9–8.1	n/a

Data from Henzlova MJ, Duvall WL: The future of SPECT MPI: Time and dose reduction. *J Nucl Cardiol*. 2011;18(4):580–587.

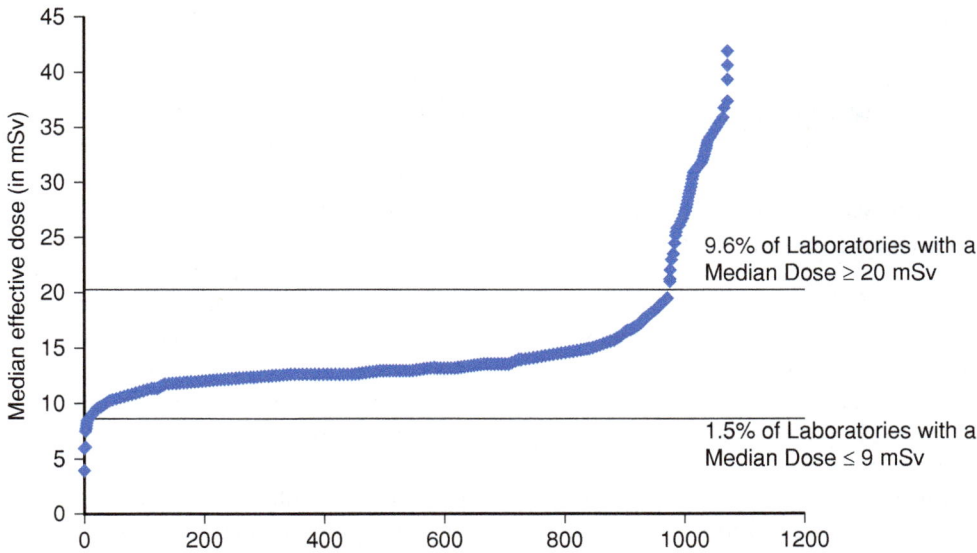

FIGURE 7-3 Cumulative radiation dose in IAC-accredited US sites in 2012 for cardiac PET and SPECT. The cumulative plot of myocardial perfusion imaging effective doses demonstrates that only 1.5% of laboratories reported a median dose of ≤9 mSv while 9.6% of laboratories reported a median dose of >20 mSv. Most laboratories reported a median effective dose between 10.1 and 20.0 mSv. (Reproduced with permission from Jerome SD, Tilkemeier PL, Farrell MB, et al. Nationwide laboratory adherence to myocardial perfusion imaging radiation dose reduction practices. A report from the Intersocietal Accreditation Commission Data Repository. *JACC Cardiovasc Imaging.* 2015;8(10):1170–1176.)

strongly discouraged by the information statement, and less than 1% of sites had incorporated stress-only imaging into their protocols to reduce radiation exposure. These findings suggest that other means may be necessary to gain accepted reductions of radiation from nuclear cardiology testing procedures.

Methods to Reduce Radiation Exposure: Patient Testing

Cardiac testing, whether it be for diagnostic or prognostic purposes, is based on risk–benefit analysis. The decision to pursue testing is based on pretest probabilities and estimated benefit from attaining the subsequent diagnosis. The practice of contemporary medicine offers a variety of imaging modalities. Not infrequently, patients undergo multiple testing procedures (for multiple indications) which incur some radiation exposure. For this reason there has been considerable attention paid to which patients would be most likely, and by default, least likely, to benefit from nuclear cardiac imaging for further investigation of obstructive coronary disease. The ASNC/ACC guidelines are important clinical recommendations meant to increase diagnostic yield and reduce patient risk.[1] A review of appropriate-use criteria is discussed elsewhere (see Chapter 13). Recent data from Doukky et al. suggest patients who undergo cardiac nuclear studies for "rarely appropriate" indications have significantly fewer abnormal studies, indicating less value.[6] In conclusion, appropriate utilization of nuclear cardiac imaging is the first step toward reducing excessive radiation exposure to the individual patient and the population as a whole.

Reducing Radiation Exposure: Imaging Protocols

Various radiopharmaceutical choices and protocols exist for SPECT MPI, utilizing blood flow differential (see Table 7-2). The most widely utilized tracers, those that are technetium (Tc-99m) based, typically require rest and poststress images in order to sufficiently diagnose and risk stratify patients. Tc-99m protocols are preferred over Tl-201 (thallium) or dual-isotope (Tl-201 rest/Tc-99m stress) protocols due to the increased radiation of Tl-201 (>25 mSv). Despite this, IAC data demonstrates that over 1.5

million dual-isotope MPI studies are performed each year in the United States.[5] Thus, an immediate means of reducing radiation exposure would be to eliminate thallium as a primary imaging tracer in all laboratories, as currently recommended.[1,7,8]

▶ Stress-Only or Stress-First Imaging to Reduce Patient Radiation

In more than 95% of laboratories in the United States, a patient undergoes the rest study first, followed by stress. Despite this common protocol, it has been recently estimated that perhaps only 8% to 15% of studies are found to be positive for ischemia or infarction.[9] Thus in the overwhelming majority of studies, rest imaging is of no clinical value. It has been proposed for several years that performing the stress first, and rest only when necessary would be a reasonable means of increasing laboratory efficiency and reducing patient radiation. The "stress-only" or "stress-first" protocols which utilize poststress MPI have been advocated by European centers since 2005[10–12] as well as editorials and recommendations from ASNC.[1,3] In the United States, studies by Chang, Duvall, Heller, and others have demonstrated the utility of stress-only imaging.[3,7,10–12] Stress-only protocols have been shown to confer similar mortality to similar patients who underwent rest/poststress protocols.[11]

An important consideration of stress-only imaging is the administered dose. In older camera systems, a low dose of 8 to 15 mCi of Tc-99m may yield an image that is difficult to interpret due to poor image quality and attenuation artifact. Thus, this protocol may require a high-dose stress study but still avoids the rest images in most circumstances. Comparison of cumulative radiation exposure of various tissues during stress-only, standard rest–stress, and dual-isotope protocols are demonstrated in Figure 7-4. Even without high-sensitivity equipment, utilizing stress-only protocols and standard radiopharmaceutical dosing provides decreased radiation exposure that can comply with ASNC recommendations. This reduction is even greater when low-dose stress-only protocols are utilizing appropriate camera systems. The susceptibility to artifact is a significant obstacle to providing high-specificity stress-only images. Significant reduction (by 35–85%) in the need for rest images is seen when attenuation correction (AC) is applied to image processing.[13] In a study by Mathur et al., using stress only with AC in a chest pain center environment, only 8% required a rest study, and at least half of these patients had evidence of scar.[14] In conclusion, modification of stress protocols to perform stress before ordering rest imaging represents an attainable method to reduce radiation exposure to patients unlikely to benefit from a rest study.

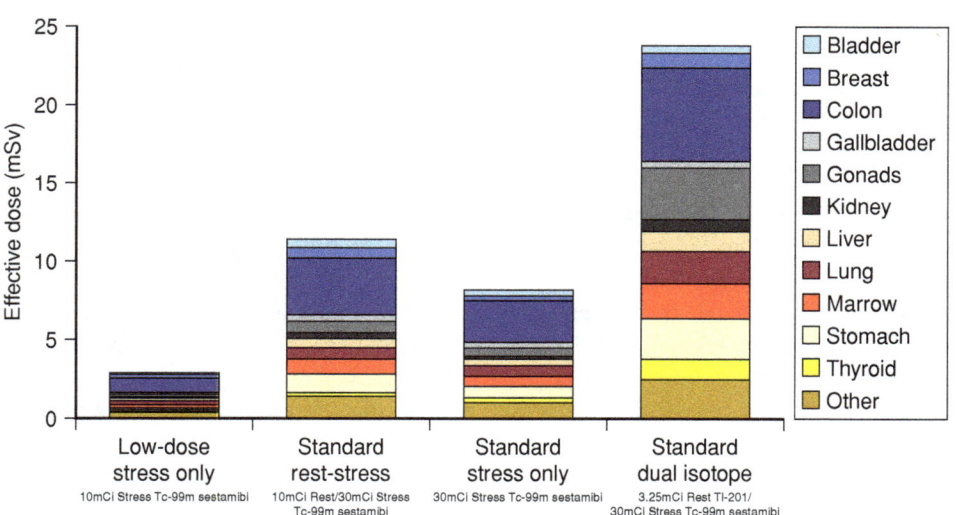

FIGURE 7-4 Radiation exposure of various tissues during stress-only, standard rest-stress, and dual-isotope protocols. (Reproduced with permission from Henzlova MJ, Duvall WL: The future of SPECT MPI: Time and dose reduction. *J Nucl Cardiol.* 2011;18(4):580–587.)

Image Processing and Software for Existing Systems

The generation of high-quality images from SPECT MPI data is paramount to ensuring diagnostic accuracy and utility of testing. To successfully reduce imaging doses as recommended by Cerqueira et al.[1] either new cameras with different technologies (see next section) or software solutions are required. Using software to enhance images can be used to either reduce image acquisition times or use lower doses with standard acquisition times, or sometimes both. For example, improvements to standard methods for image reconstruction (filtered back projection) such as iterative reconstruction (ordered subset expectation maximization or OSEM) can suppress background noise and improve count statistics. Compared with filtered back projection, iterative reconstruction algorithms require 50% to 75% less counts to produce similar images.[1,15,16] Proprietary software algorithms from the large medical technology companies (UltraSPECT Inc., GE Healthcare, Siemens, Philips) can be purchased to augment resolution of images without additional radiation. Wide-beam reconstruction (WBR) is one such algorithm that compensates for the complicated beam angles and spread of counts when reconstructing the image, and can be applied to standard camera systems with standard collimators. This technology provides the ability to reduce radiation exposure on the order of 50% to 75% without impacting image quality.[17] Algorithms by Philips (Astonish) combine multiple levels of processing by utilizing OSEM, noise-reduction algorithms, collimator design, scatter modeling, and AC to produce high-quality images during half-time acquisition. Which software system is applicable to a given camera is dependent upon the age of the camera, the type (manufacturer), and available computer system. Generally, the manufacturer solutions (GE, Philips, Siemens) are limited to newer systems and only for the given company producing the software. WBC (UltraSPECT) and ImagenSPECT (CVIT, Kansas City, MO) technologies are available and use existing cameras from multiple vendors.[14,16]

Impact of Technology: Hardware and Cameras

In the vast majority of US SPECT laboratories, standard Anger cameras are used. The design for these cameras was developed over 40 years ago and has changed little since conception. These cameras utilize collimators to physically resolve signals prior to processing. Standard collimators for general purpose studies attempt to balance count sensitivity with spatial resolution on the order of 9 to 10 mm. High-sensitivity collimator designs produce images with spatial resolutions of 8 to 8.5 mm; however, this is at the expense of doubling the radiation dose.[1,3,16] Clinically, 1.0-mm resolution differences in image resolution do not warrant doubling the radiation exposure to patients. However, specialized collimator designs can lead to decreased radiation dose. Custom cardiac design collimators have been designed that focus on increasing spatial resolution and sensitivity for counts from the cardiac region. These collimators are designed to be utilized within a certain camera system and require accompanying reconstruction algorithms.[1]

In contrast to sodium iodide (NaI) cameras, new solid detectors have been developed which utilize cadmium zinc telluride (CZT) arrays. These new camera arrays demonstrate better sensitivities in the range of 2.2 to 4.7 kcps compared to 0.5 to 0.7 kcps of standard Anger NaI cameras. Detailed descriptions of SPECT camera systems are discussed in Chapter 4. Data suggest that higher-count sensitivity of CZT cameras can produce images of comparable diagnostic quality with 15% to 30% of amount of standard radiation dose at the same scan duration.[1,18] Table 7-2 demonstrates the substantial reduction in radiation exposure that is possible with "new-technology" camera systems. Again, application of new camera systems to additional radiation-reduction techniques such as stress-only imaging (last column) significantly reduces radiation exposure when compared to standard Tc-99m stress/rest protocols utilizing standard anger cameras.

The development of these high-efficiency cameras and their incorporation into imaging systems have provided high-quality images to be constructed at a fraction of the standard isotope dose. Examples of combination software/hardware systems include the Cardius-3 XPO camera system produced by Digirad, Inc. (Poway, California, USA). This system utilizes triple-head geometry of indirect, solid-state (CsI[Tl]) detectors which are allowed to vary source distance to produce images with spatial resolution of 8.95 mm. This is, in part, accomplished through OSEM methods for reconstruction (discussed previously). Recent studies have also demonstrated that

Table 7-3

Estimated PET Radiation Exposure for Stress/Rest and Viability

Agent	Injected Dose (mCi)	Estimated Total Body Radiation Exposure (mSv)
^{82}Rubidium (2D)[1]	30–60 (rest/stress protocol)	2.7–5.4
^{82}Rubidium (3D)[1]	15–30 (rest/stress protocol)	1.4–2.7
N-13 Ammonia[2]	10–20 (rest/stress protocol)	2.0–4.0
F-18 FDG[2]	10 (viability study)	7.0

Data from Hunter CR, Hill J, Ziadi MC, et al. Biodistribution and radiation dosimetry of (82)Rb at rest and during peak pharmacological stress in patients referred for myocardial perfusion imaging. *Eur J Nucl Med Mol Imaging*. 2015;42:1032–1042; Hays MT, Watson EE, Thomas SR, et al. MIRD dose estimate report no. 19: Radiation absorbed dose estimates from (18)F-FDG. *J Nucl Med*. 2002;43:210–214.

total patient radiation exposure can be reduced to 4 to 9 mSv with very high-quality images.[13]

Cardiovascular PET Radiation Exposure

This review, thus far, has been confined to SPECT radiation exposure. Recently, cardiovascular PET has been entering the clinical arena for myocardial perfusion imaging as well as other applications such as myocardial viability and infection/inflammation imaging. The value of cardiovascular PET as well as instrumentation is described in Chapters 3, 4 and 10.

Cardiovascular PET utilizes three primary tracers for imaging, rubidium and ammonia for perfusion imaging as 18-fluorodeoxyglucose (F-18 FDG) for viability, infection, and inflammation imaging. The radiation exposure for each of these is represented in Table 7-3. PET systems typically employ line source (utilizing gadolinium) or CT sources for AC. It is noteworthy that AC requires the use of additional radiation. This radiation exposure is generally quite small, usually less than 1 mSv.[19,20]

The two FDA-approved PET tracers for myocardial perfusion imaging are rubidium (Rb-82) and ammonia (NH$_3$). Due to the short half-life of these tracers (76 seconds and 9.8 minutes, respectively), the radiopharmaceuticals can be administered at higher doses than SPECT but result in overall lower radiation exposure. The most commonly used PET perfusion tracer is Rb-82. Several studies have examined the human radiation exposure with this tracer.[19–21] In normal subjects undergoing pharmacologic stress with Rb-82, Senthamizhchelvan et al. determined that 20 mCi results in 0.9-mSv exposure.[22] Given that a rest and stress dose is 30 to 60 mCi, the total radiation exposure is estimated to be 2.7 to 5.4 mSv per patient, well below ASNC recommendations and current SPECT procedures. Hunter et al. carefully calculated radiation exposure to patients undergoing Rb-82 at the University of Ottawa and found the average to be 2.4 mSv.[20] Other advances in cardiac PET imaging include 3D imaging which utilizes the high-sensitivity PET cameras to quickly image low-dose activity without loss of diagnostic sensitivity.[19–22] With 3D imaging, the patient exposure would be half that of 2D imaging (1.8–3.5 mSv).[23]

Another albeit, less commonly utilized tracer is ^{13}N-ammonia. ^{13}N-Ammonia demonstrates a more linear response to blood flow compared not only to SPECT tracers but ^{82}Rb as well. Subsequent studies have confirmed the accuracy of ^{82}Rb with ^{13}N-ammonia in the detection of coronary artery disease with low radiation exposure levels of approximately 4 mSv per study utilizing a 20-mCi dose.[5] With 3D imaging, the radiation exposure is lower (2–3 mSv).

For nonperfusion PET imaging, the myocardium can be imaged directly with F-18-FDG. FDG viability protocols are discussed in Chapter 21. Data suggest radiation exposure levels of approximately 7 mSv per study for viability assessment using the standard 15-mCi dose.[24] In addition, FDG imaging has emerging clinical utility in identifying inflammation and infection in conditions such as sarcoidosis and endocarditis, respectively discussed in Chapter 24.[25]

RADIATION EXPOSURE AND REDUCTION: SUMMARY

Cardiac nuclear imaging is a popular and valuable tool in the practice of cardiology.

These noninvasive diagnostic procedures have high diagnostic accuracy when applied to the appropriate patient. Since these techniques use radioactive tracers, the risk of developing cancers due to radiation exposure is present but not fully understood. This risk has become a societal concern and has resulted in safe practice guidelines to mitigate risk. There is a wide variety of protocols, isotopes, and systems utilized in cardiac nuclear testing, each with varying degrees of radiation exposure. Clinicians must balance the risk and benefits in order to practice for safe and fiscally responsible medicine and then the utilization of techniques becomes critical to their appropriate application. Current ASNC recommendations for radiation exposure during cardiac nuclear imaging are below 9 mSv per study. Unfortunately, data have demonstrated that few nuclear laboratories are able to achieve these goals. The current ASNC goal is attainable through application of stress-only protocols, CZT camera, application of PET tracers, and other techniques noted in this chapter.

REFERENCES

1. Cerqueira MD, Allman KC, Ficaro EP, et al. Recommendations for reducing radiation exposure in myocardial perfusion imaging. *J Nucl Cardiol.* 2010;17:709–718.
2. Thompson RC, Cullom SJ. Issues regarding radiation dosage of cardiac nuclear and radiography procedures. *J Nucl Cardiol.* 2006;13:19–23.
3. Henzlova MJ, Duvall WL. The future of SPECT MPI: Time and dose reduction. *J Nucl Cardiol.* 2011;18:580–587.
4. Gerber TC, Carr JJ, Arai AE, et al. Ionizing radiation in cardiac imaging: A science advisory from the American Heart Association Committee on Cardiac Imaging of the Council on Clinical Cardiology and Committee on Cardiovascular Imaging and Intervention of the Council on Cardiovascular Radiology and Intervention. *Circulation.* 2009;119:1056–1065.
5. Jerome SD, Tilkemeier PL, Farrell MB, Shaw LJ. Nationwide laboratory adherence to myocardial perfusion imaging radiation dose reduction practices. A report from the Intersocietal Accreditation Commission Data Repository. *JACC Cardiovasc Imaging.* 2015;8:1170–1176.
6. Doukky R, Hayes K, Frogge N, et al. Impact of appropriate use on the prognostic value of single-photon emission computed tomography myocardial perfusion imaging. *Circulation.* 2013;128:1634–1643.
7. Hill KD, Einstein AJ. New approaches to reduce radiation exposure. *Trends Cardiovasc Med.* 2016;26:55–65.
8. Henzlova MJ, Duvall WL, Einstein AJ, Travin MI, Verberne HJ. ASNC imaging guidelines for SPECT nuclear cardiology procedures: Stress, protocols, and tracers. *J Nucl Cardiol.* 2016;23:606–639.
9. Rozanski A, Gransar H, Hayes SW, et al. Temporal trends in the frequency of inducible myocardial ischemia during cardiac stress testing: 1991 to 2009. *J Am Coll Cardiol.* 2013;61:1054–1065.
10. Gowd BM, Heller GV, Parker MW. Stress-only SPECT myocardial perfusion imaging: A review. *J Nucl Cardiol.* 2014;21:1200–1212.
11. Chang SM, Nabi F, Xu J, Raza U, Mahmarian JJ. Normal stress-only versus standard stress/rest myocardial perfusion imaging: Similar patient mortality with reduced radiation exposure. *J Am Coll Cardiol.* 2010;55:221–230.
12. Heller GV, Bateman TM, Johnson LL, et al. Clinical value of attenuation correction in stress-only Tc-99m sestamibi SPECT imaging. *J Nucl Cardiol.* 2004;11:273–281.
13. Ardestani A, Ahlberg AW, Katten DM, et al. Risk stratification using line source attenuation correction with rest-stress Tc-99m sestamibi SPECT myocardial perfusion imaging. *J Nucl Cardiol.* 2014;21:118–126.
14. Mathur S, Heller GV, Bateman TM, et al. Clinical value of stress-only Tc-99m SPECT imaging: Importance of attenuation correction. *J Nucl Cardiol.* 2013;20(1):27–37.
15. DePuey EG, Gadiraju R, Clark J, Thompson L, Anstett F, Shwartz SC. Ordered subset expectation maximization and wide beam reconstruction "half-time" gated myocardial perfusion SPECT functional imaging: A comparison to "full-time" filtered backprojection. *J Nucl Cardiol.* 2008;15:547–563.
16. Slomka PJ, Patton JA, Berman DS, Germano G. Advances in technical aspects of myocardial perfusion SPECT imaging. *J Nucl Cardiol.* 2009;16:255–276.
17. DePuey EG, Bommireddipalli S, Clark J, Leykekhman A, Thompson LB, Friedman M. A comparison of the image quality of full-time myocardial perfusion SPECT vs wide beam reconstruction half-time and half-dose SPECT. *J Nucl Cardiol.* 2011;18:273–280.
18. Duvall WL, Croft LB, Ginsberg ES, et al. Reduced isotope dose and imaging time with a high-efficiency CZT SPECT camera. *J Nucl Cardiol.* 2011;18:847–857.
19. Kaster T, Mylonas I, Renaud JM, Wells GA, Beanlands RS, deKemp RA. Accuracy of low-dose rubidium-82 myocardial perfusion imaging for detection of coronary artery disease using 3D PET and normal database interpretation. *J Nucl Cardiol.* 2012;19:1135–1145.
20. Hunter CR, Hill J, Ziadi MC, Beanlands RS, deKemp RA. Biodistribution and radiation dosimetry of (82)Rb at rest and during peak pharmacological stress in patients referred for myocardial perfusion imaging. *Eur J Nucl Med Mol Imaging.* 2015;42:1032–1042.
21. Nogueira SA, Dimenstein R, Cunha ML, Wagner J, Funari MB, Lederman HM. Low-dose radiation protocol using 3D mode in a BGO PET/CT. *Radiol Med.* 2015;120:251–255.
22. Senthamizhchelvan S, Bravo PE, Lodge MA, Merrill J, Bengel FM, Sgouros G. Radiation dosimetry of 82Rb in humans under pharmacologic stress. *J Nucl Med.* 2011;52:485–491.
23. Knesaurek K, Machac J, Krynyckyi BR, Almeida OD. Comparison of 2-dimensional and 3-dimensional 82-Rb myocardial perfusion PET imaging. *J Nucl Med.* 2003;44:1350–1356.
24. Hays MT, Watson EE, Thomas SR, Stabin M. MIRD dose estimate report no. 19: Radiation absorbed dose estimates from (18)F-FDG. *J Nucl Med.* 2002;43:210–214.
25. Blankstein R, Lundbye J, Heller G. Proceedings of the ASNC cardiac PET summit meeting, May 12, 2014, Baltimore, MD: 4. Novel applications of cardiovascular PET. *J Nucl Cardiol.* 2015;22:720–729.

SECTION 2

RADIONUCLIDE MYOCARDIAL PERFUSION IMAGING (MPI)

Exercise and Pharmacologic Stress Testing

CHAPTER 8

Robert C. Hendel and Archana Ramireddy

INTRODUCTION

Using radiopharmaceuticals to visualize the regional distribution of myocardial perfusion during rest and stress is a well-established modality for the evaluation of known or suspected coronary artery disease (CAD). In 1964, the first scintigraphic images of myocardial perfusion were acquired by Carrea et al.,[1] while Zaret et al. were the first to demonstrate exercise-induced myocardial ischemia using radioactive potassium in 1973.[2] Since then, the field of nuclear cardiology has grown dramatically, and numerous studies have validated the utility of both exercise and pharmacologic stress myocardial perfusion imaging (MPI) for risk assessment and the prediction of future cardiac events. With >8 million such studies being performed yearly in the United States alone, understanding the logistics of and options available for radionuclide stress testing is critical.[3]

EXERCISE STRESS TESTING

Whenever possible, exercise is the preferred modality for stress testing, because it allows for a physiologic assessment of functional capacity, hemodynamics, and symptoms. In addition, when compared to pharmacologic stress testing, exercise is associated with less extensive hepatic and gastrointestinal tracer uptake, which significantly improves image quality.[4,5]

MPI in conjunction with exercise stress testing enhances diagnostic sensitivity and specificity, particularly among patients with resting electrocardiographic (ECG) abnormalities that preclude the interpretation of ST-segment deviation. Similarly, MPI can differentiate true-positive from false-positive ST-segment depression (STD), which is helpful, because among patients referred for exercise ECG testing with a low to intermediate pretest probability of CAD, approximately 40% of those who develop STD will not have CAD.[6] When compared to ECG interpretation in isolation, MPI not only provides a more accurate assessment of the extent and severity of disease, but it can also localize ischemia to a particular vascular distribution. MPI is also useful when patients fail to achieve their target heart rate during exercise, because myocardial perfusion abnormalities in response to stress occur earlier than ECG changes.[7] Finally, when combined with exercise, MPI not only improves diagnostic capability, but is also predictive of short- and long-term cardiac events.[8] This important prognostic ability does not apply to ECG interpretation without concurrent use of the Duke treadmill score (Table 8-1) or

Table 8-1
Duke Treadmill Score
Exercise time (minutes) − (5 × maximum ST depression) − (4 × angina score), where angina score is none (0); present (1); reason for test termination (2).
Low risk: >5
Intermediate risk: −10 to +4
High risk: <−10

Data from Mark DB, Hlatky MA, Harrell FE, et al. Exercise treadmill score for predicting prognosis in coronary artery disease. *Ann Intern Med.* 1987;106(6):793–800.

Table 8-2
Indications for Exercise Stress Myocardial Perfusion Imaging

Indications	Class
1. Diagnosis of ischemic heart disease in patients with intermediate risk of CAD and/or risk stratification of patients with intermediate or high likelihood of CAD	
Identification of extent, severity, and location of ischemia	I
Assess functional significance of intermediate (25–75%) stenosis	I
Intermediate Duke treadmill score	I
Repeat testing when symptoms have changed	I
Repeat testing in 1–3 years in high-likelihood patients	IIb
Severe coronary calcification with uninterpretable ECG	IIb
Asymptomatic but with high-risk occupation	IIb
Screening of asymptomatic patients with a low likelihood of disease	III
2. Assessment of interventions and therapy in ischemic heart disease	
3–5 years after revascularization in high-risk asymptomatic patients	IIa
Repeat testing to evaluate therapeutic efficacy	IIb
Routine assessment of asymptomatic patients after PTCA or CABG	III
3. Prior to noncardiac surgery	
Low-risk surgery	III
Intermediate-risk surgery or vascular surgery and adequate functional capacity (>4 METS)	III
Intermediate-risk surgery or vascular surgery *and* risk factors with poor functional capacity (≤4 METS)	IIb

PTCA, percutaneous coronary intervention; CABG, coronary artery bypass grafting; ECG, electrocardiogram; Class I, usually appropriate and considered helpful; Class II, acceptable but usefulness less well established; Class IIa, weight in favor of usefulness; Class IIb, can be helpful but not well established; Class III, generally not appropriate.
Data from Klocke FJ, Baird MG, Lorell BH, et al. ACC/AHA/ASNC guidelines for the clinical use of cardiac radionuclide imaging—executive summary: A report of the American College of Cardiology/American Heart Association Task Force on Practice Guidelines (ACC/AHA/ASNC Committee to Revise the 1995 Guidelines for the Clinical Use of Cardiac Radionuclide Imaging). *J Am Coll Cardiol.* 2003;42(7):1318–1333; Fleisher LA, Beckman JA, Brown KA, et al. ACC/AHA 2007 guidelines on perioperative cardiovascular evaluation and care for noncardiac surgery. *J Am Coll Cardiol.* 2007;50;1707–1732.

Table 8-3
Indications for Noninvasive Stress Testing in Patients with Suspected Ischemic Heart Disease

Noninvasive Test	Class
1. Standard Exercise ECG	
Intermediate likelihood of ischemic heart disease, able to exercise, no prior coronary revascularization, and with interpretable resting ECG	I
Low likelihood of ischemic heart disease, able to exercise, no prior coronary revascularization, and with interpretable resting ECG	IIa
2. Pharmacologic Stress MPI or Echo	
Intermediate or high likelihood of ischemic heart disease and unable to exercise	I
Low likelihood of ischemic heart disease and unable to exercise	IIa
3. MPI or Echo with Exercise	
Previous coronary revascularization and able to exercise	I
Intermediate to high likelihood of ischemic heart disease, able to exercise, no prior coronary revascularization, and with interpretable resting ECG	IIa

ECG, electrocardiogram; MPI, myocardial perfusion imaging; CMR, cardiac magnetic resonance imaging; CCTA, cardiac/coronary computed tomography angiography; Class I, usually appropriate and considered helpful; Class IIa, weight in favor of usefulness.
Data from Fihn SD, Gardin JM, Abrams J, et al. 2012 ACCF/AHA/ACP/AATS/PCNA/SCAI/STS Guideline for the diagnosis and management of patients with stable ischemic heart disease: executive summary. *J Am Coll Cardiol.* 2012;60;2564–2603.

the presence of significant ischemic changes, such as ST-segment elevation (STE). Despite the clear advantages of MPI in conjunction with exercise testing, an important consideration should be made for patients who are able to achieve ≥10 METS on exercise stress testing. A recent study by Bourque et al.[9] showed that individuals who are at intermediate risk for CAD or those who have known CAD and are able to accomplish ≥10 METS have an excellent cardiovascular prognosis regardless of peak heart rate achieved, and thus the addition and utility of MPI in this population is questionable.

▶ Logistics and Procedures

The indications and contraindications for exercise MPI are listed in Tables 8-2, 8-3, and 8-4. Of note, the appropriate use of exercise and pharmacologic radionuclide imaging is specifically addressed in Chapter 13. Among patients who are capable of physical exercise, MPI is usually performed using one of the several standardized treadmill protocols. Individuals who are generally healthy should perform treadmill exercise using the Bruce protocol, which calls for 3-minute stages of gradually increasing speed and grade. Older individuals, or those with limited exercise capacity, can be evaluated with a modified Bruce protocol that incorporates two warm-up stages. Other protocols, such as the Naughton or Weber, use 1- or 2-minute stages with incremental 1-MET increases, and are appropriate for patients with significantly limited exercise tolerance. Cycle ergometers, while less expensive than treadmills, are infrequently used in the United States. They are unfamiliar to many patients, and often preclude maximum levels of exercise due to muscle fatigue. Regardless of the particular protocol or equipment, 6 to 12 minutes of continuous and progressive exercise produces maximal myocardial metabolic demand and is optimal for diagnostic and prognostic purposes.[6,10–12]

From a procedural standpoint, patients should be instructed not to eat, drink, or smoke for 8 hours prior to exercise testing, and to wear comfortable shoes and loose-fitting clothing. Antihypertensive and antianginal medications can limit the development of ischemia and blunt the physiologic heart rate response during exercise, resulting in a lower level of sensitivity for detecting CAD. Thus, whenever clinically feasible, these medications (beta blockers, calcium channel blockers, and long-acting nitrates) should be tapered and discontinued at least 12 hours prior to exercise testing,[5,13] especially if the study is being performed for diagnostic purposes.

After explaining the logistics of the test as well as the potential risks and benefits, informed consent is obtained, after which a brief history and physical examination should be conducted in order to elicit any medical issues that may limit or preclude exercise. An intravenous line is then placed for injection of the radiopharmaceutical agent. During exercise, the heart rate, blood pressure, and ECG should be

Table 8-4

Contraindications to Exercise Stress Testing

Absolute	Relative[a]
Acute MI (<2 days[b])	Left main coronary stenosis
High-risk unstable angina	Moderate valvular stenosis
Uncontrolled, symptomatic arrhythmias	Electrolyte abnormalities
Decompensated heart failure	High-grade AV block
Uncontrolled hypertension (BP >200/110)	Hypertrophic cardiomyopathy or outflow tract obstruction
Symptomatic severe aortic stenosis	Significant tachy- or bradyarrhythmias
Acute PE or pulmonary infarction	LBBB, pacemaker, or pre-excitation
Acute myocarditis or pericarditis	Mental or physical impairment
Acute aortic dissection	
Severe pulmonary hypertension	
Acute medical illness	

MI, myocardial infarction; PE; pulmonary embolism; BP, blood pressure.
[a]Relative contraindications can be suspended if the benefits of exercise stress testing outweigh the risks.
[b]<4 days per ASNC guidelines 2009.
Data from Gibbons RJ, Balady GJ, Bricker JT, et al. ACC/AHA 2002 guideline update for exercise testing: summary article. A report of the American College of Cardiology/American Heart Association Task Force on Practice Guidelines (Committee to Update the 1997 Exercise Testing Guidelines). J Am Coll Cardiol. 2002;40(8):1531–1540; Henzlova MJ, Duvall WL, Einstein AJ, et al. ASNC imaging guidelines for SPECT nuclear cardiology procedures: Stress, protocols, and tracers. J Nucl Cardiol. 2016;23(3):606–639.

recorded toward the end of each stage, along with symptoms should they occur. When the endpoint of exercise is reached, the radiopharmaceutical is injected rapidly and followed by a saline flush, and the patient is encouraged to continue exercising for at least 1 to 2 more minutes. Continuation of exercise is crucial because it allows for myocardial extraction of radiopharmaceutical during peak blood flow and maximum ischemic stress. If necessary, the speed and grade of the treadmill can be decreased to allow for continuation of exercise. Following completion of the test, monitoring should continue for at least 5 to 10 minutes or until any symptoms resolve. The indications for terminating exercise MPI, aside from patient fatigue, are listed in Table 8-5.

ECG Interpretation

Prior to stress testing, a standard 12-lead ECG should be recorded along with blood pressure and heart rate in both the supine and standing positions, since postural changes can elicit ST–T-wave abnormalities. Hyperventilation, which can also produce nonspecific ST-segment changes, is no longer recommended as a routine prior to stress testing.[14] If false-positive ST-segment changes due to hyperventilation are suspected, a hyperventilation ECG can always be obtained after the test is complete,[6] and then compared with the maximal ST-segment abnormalities observed during exercise.

Multiple ECG changes can occur as part of the normal physiologic response to exercise, including PR, QRS, and QT interval shortening, and J point, or junctional, depression with rapid, upsloping ST segments. In the presence of underlying ischemia, the ST segment classically becomes horizontal during exercise, a finding that may be associated with angina or become more pronounced with increasing workload (Fig. 8-1).ABnormal ECG findings during exercise include ≥1 mm of horizontal or downsloping STD, and 1.5 mm of upsloping STD, all measured 60 to 80 ms after the J point.[15-17] Of these criteria, downsloping STD is the strongest predictor of underlying CAD. Precordial STD, especially in lead V_5, is more reliable for detecting CAD in patients without prior myocardial infarction (MI) and normal resting ECGs than is STD in the inferior leads, which carries a high false-positive rate.

Table 8-5

Indications for Termination of Exercise Stress Testing

Absolute	Relative
Drop in SBP of ≥10 mm Hg from baseline despite increasing workload, when evidence of ischemia is present	Drop in SBP of ≥10 mm Hg from baseline despite increasing workload, without evidence of ischemia
Moderate–severe angina	Profound (>2 mm) ST-segment depression
Ataxia, dizziness, or near syncope Signs of poor perfusion (pallor, cyanosis)	Multifocal PVCs, triplets of PVCs, SVT, heart block, or bradyarrhythmias
Technical difficulties	Marked fatigue, shortness of breath, or claudication
Subject wishes to stop	New bundle branch block or IVCD that cannot be distinguished from ventricular tachycardia
ST-segment elevation without Q waves (except in leads V_1 and AVR)	Increasing chest pain
Sustained ventricular tachycardia or ventricular fibrillation	Hypertensive response (BP >250/115 mm Hg)

SBP, systolic blood pressure; PVC, premature ventricular complex; SVT, supraventricular tachycardia; IVCD, intraventricular conduction delay; BP, blood pressure.
Data from Gibbons RJ, Balady GJ, Bricker JT, et al. ACC/AHA 2002 guideline update for exercise testing: Summary article. A report of the American College of Cardiology/American Heart Association Task Force on Practice Guidelines (Committee to Update the 1997 Exercise Testing Guidelines). *J Am Coll Cardiol*. 2002;40(8):1531–1540; Henzlova MJ, Duvall WL, Einstein AJ, et al. ASNC imaging guidelines for SPECT nuclear cardiology procedures: Stress, protocols, and tracers. *J Nucl Cardiol*. 2016;23(3):606–639.

STD may first appear after exercise is complete or persist during recovery,[11,12] emphasizing the need for continuous monitoring throughout the procedure. STD that begins after the cessation of exercise is not more significant than STD that occurs during exercise,[18-20] but when ST changes during exercise are equivocal, downsloping STD during recovery indicates a significant ischemic burden, and portends a poor long-term prognosis.[21] In general, true

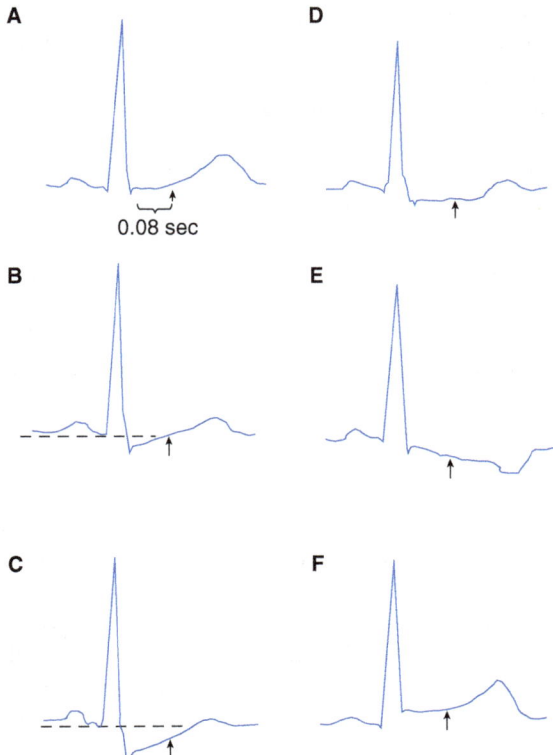

FIGURE 8-1 Potential ST-segment changes during exercise. **(A)** Normal. **(B)** Upsloping ST-segment depression that returns to baseline within 0.08 s (*arrow*). **(C)** Persistent upsloping ST-segment depression. **(D)** Horizontal ST-segment depression. **(E)** Downsloping ST-segment depression. **(F)** ST-segment elevation. (Reproduced with permission from Tavel ME. Stress testing in cardiac evaluation: Current concepts with emphasis on the ECG. *Chest* 2001;119(3):907–925.)

ischemic STD tends to coincide with the termination of exercise, and frequently persists or intensifies for at least 2 to 3 minutes during recovery. If STD does not occur until >2 or 3 minutes into recovery, or if it occurs near peak exertion and resolves rapidly in early recovery, a false-positive response is likely.[16–22]

Overall, the diagnostic accuracy of the exercise ECG in isolation is extremely variable, with an overall mean sensitivity and specificity of ~70%, based on meta-analyses of 147 consecutively published reports involving >20,000 patients who underwent both coronary angiography and exercise testing.[14] The sensitivity of exercise-induced ECG changes is higher in populations with a greater prevalence of disease, such as the elderly or those with multiple cardiac risk factors. Likewise, specificity is reduced when false-positive results are likely, as when resting ECG abnormalities or confounding clinical conditions are present.

The location of the exercise-induced STD (leads) does not reliably predict the location of coronary stenoses.[23] In contrast, the rare finding of exercise-induced STE without prior MI implies a high-grade coronary lesion,[23,24] and localizes myocardial ischemia quite accurately. Exercise-induced STE in the presence of a previous transmural MI is relatively common and of debatable significance. The mechanism is unclear, but has been ascribed to wall-motion abnormalities or residual viability in the infarcted area.[25–29]

Confounders of Stress ECG Interpretation

The clinical conditions associated with false-positive ST-segment responses to exercise are listed in Table 8-6. In addition to postural changes and hyperventilation, several additional factors deserve further comment. *Resting STD* of <1 mm in the absence of other abnormal findings is nonspecific, but it is also a relatively sensitive marker for significant CAD, and has been shown to be associated with adverse outcomes.[30–34] Thus, exercise-induced ST-segment changes can be reasonably well interpreted in this cohort,[14] with the potential exception of patients taking *digoxin* and those with *left ventricular*

Table 8-6

Confounders of Exercise ECG Interpretation

- Resting ST-segment depression of >1 mm. Low risk: >5
- Left bundle branch block
- Right bundle branch block (precludes interpretation of ST-segment changes in leads V_1–V_3)
- Left ventricular hypertrophy
- Digoxin
- Beta blockers or calcium channel blockers (inadequate heart rate response to exercise)
- Other medications (nitrates, antihypertensive agents, antiarrhythmic agents)
- Pre-excitation (e.g., Wolff–Parkinson–White syndrome)
- Ventricular-paced rhythm

Data from Gibbons RJ, Balady GJ, Bricker JT, et al. ACC/AHA 2002 guideline update for exercise testing: Summary article. A report of the American College of Cardiology/American Heart Association Task Force on Practice Guidelines (Committee to Update the 1997 Exercise Testing Guidelines). *J Am Coll Cardiol.* 2002;40(8):1531–1540.

hypertrophy (LVH). Digoxin produces abnormal ventricular repolarization and STD in response to exercise.[35-37] Similarly, the repolarization abnormalities associated with LVH decrease the specificity of any ECG changes during exercise. Thus, current consensus guidelines for stress testing recommend imaging modalities in combination with exercise among patients taking digoxin, or for those with LVH.[14]

Exercise-induced STD usually occurs in the presence of *left bundle branch block* (LBBB), and has no diagnostic significance or association with ischemia.[38] However, during exercise, both increased heart rate and augmented myocardial workload decrease septal blood flow in the setting of LBBB, which often results in falsely abnormal MPI. Therefore, vasodilator pharmacologic stress MPI is the preferred modality when baseline LBBB or a ventricular-paced rhythm is present. Exercise in the setting of *right bundle branch block* (RBBB) is associated with nonischemic anterior STD (in leads V_1–V_3) secondary to abnormal repolarization.[39] Nonetheless, ischemic changes can still be interpreted in the presence of RBBB using the left chest leads (V_5 and V_6) and inferior leads (II, III, and aVF) without reduced sensitivity, specificity, or predictive value. The induction of complete RBBB or LBBB during exercise is a nonspecific finding in isolation, but it may suggest myocardial ischemia if noted in conjunction with hemodynamic or clinical symptoms.[16]

▶ Additional Stress Testing Parameters

Aside from exercise-induced STD, other modalities may provide supplementary clinical and prognostic information during and after stress testing. Michaelides et al.[40] evaluated the utility of *right-sided precordial leads* during exercise testing in a group of 245 patients, and found that the sensitivity and specificity of the ECG to detect CAD were enhanced when compared to standard leads, yielding comparable results to those obtained with stress MPI. However, there was a high pretest prevalence of CAD in their patient population, and without confirmatory studies involving larger groups, the routine use of right-sided leads during stress testing is not currently recommended.[14]

The degree of ST-segment displacement relative to the maximum heart rate achieved during exercise, or *ST/HR index*, has also been suggested as a means to enhance the detection of CAD. This measurement can be derived manually or generated by computer, although its use among symptomatic patients has been limited.[41-46] Thus, the ST/HR index has not been validated for routine use during stress testing, but it may be helpful in certain situations, such as when there is equivocal STD associated with a high exercise heart rate.[14,47] Also of note, *computer processing* of exercise ECG data to calculate STD is part of most standard software programs, but a significant number of false-positive findings can result.[47] Computerized scores or measurements of ST-segment deviation, while useful, should always be preceded by and compared to the raw ECG data, and never used in isolation.

The increase in heart rate during exercise is a function of parasympathetic withdrawal and sympathetic activation, while heart rate recovery immediately after exercise is mediated by reactivation of the parasympathetic nervous system. *Chronotropic incompetence* during exercise in the absence of rate-limiting medications, although variably defined, generally signifies significant cardiac disease, and among patients with known or suspected CAD is independently associated with higher all-cause mortality.[48] *Heart rate recovery* after exercise can also provide prognostic information. In a study involving 2428 consecutive patients undergoing exercise MPI, Cole et al.[49] were the first to demonstrate that a delayed decrease in the heart rate during the first minute after exercise was an independent predictor of overall mortality regardless of workload, changes in heart rate during exercise, or perfusion defects. Their findings have been independently confirmed in several subsequent studies.[50-53] Adverse outcomes are also more frequent with persistently elevated *systolic blood pressure* after exercise[54] or an inability to adequately augment systolic blood pressure in response to exercise.

Finally, the *Duke treadmill score* (Table 8-1) is a valuable clinical tool that is used for diagnosis as well as risk assessment and prognosis. It was originally devised by Mark et al.[55] using clinical and ECG data from almost 3000 inpatients with known or suspected CAD who underwent exercise stress testing prior to coronary angiography. Briefly, the formula incorporates exercise time, ECG changes, and angina to calculate a score from −11 to +5 that has been shown to be a powerful predictor of mortality. It works equally well with men and women, and has subsequently been validated in outpatients, patients at other centers, and in those with resting nonspecific ST–T-wave changes.[55–58]

PHARMACOLOGIC STRESS TESTING

Even when MPI is combined with exercise stress testing, failure to attain an adequate heart rate response during exercise reduces the sensitivity of stress MPI for detecting CAD, diminishes the extent of defects seen on perfusion scintigraphy,[59–63] and can result in a substantial number (up to 25%) of false-negative results.[64–66] Many individuals referred for stress testing are elderly, and are unable to perform maximum exercise because of chronic obstructive pulmonary disease (COPD), physical deconditioning, musculoskeletal and peripheral vascular disease, previous stroke, extremity amputation, unfamiliarity with the treadmill, or simply poor motivation. Heart rate responsiveness is also frequently affected by the use of medications, particularly beta blockers. In addition, as noted above, complete LBBB or a ventricular paced rhythm can produce artifactual septal perfusion defects with exercise.

Pharmacologic stress testing is increasingly being utilized for stress perfusion imaging, and currently accounts for nearly 50% of all nuclear stress tests in the United States.[67] Pharmacologic stress MPI has been well validated when compared to exercise MPI in terms of diagnostic sensitivity, specificity, and risk stratification, and can safely be accomplished with vasodilating agents such as adenosine and dipyridamole, and recently with selective $A2_a$ adenosine agonists, such as regadenoson. Alternatively, catecholamines, such as dobutamine, may be used, primarily in the setting of contraindications to the use of vasodilators. In general, pharmacologic stress testing should be reserved for patients who are unable to exercise adequately or who possess contraindications for exercise; the indications for pharmacologic stress MPI are listed in Table 8-7. A listing of general and specific contraindications for pharmacologic testing is noted in Table 8-8.

▶ Vasodilators: Adenosine and Dipyridamole

Adenosine is a small, ubiquitous heterocyclic compound that is produced endogenously in myocardial smooth muscle and vascular endothelium, or derived

Table 8-7

Indications for Pharmacologic Vasodilator Stress Imaging

- Inability to perform adequate exercise
- Left bundle branch block
- Ventricular pacemaker
- Ventricular pre-excitation
- Concurrent use of medications that may blunt the heart rate response (calcium channel blockers, beta blockers)
- Evaluation of patients very early after acute myocardial infarction (≥3 days), or following ED presentation with presumptive ACS

Data from Henzlova MJ, Duvall WL, Einstein AJ, et al. ASNC imaging guidelines for SPECT nuclear cardiology procedures: Stress, protocols, and tracers. *J Nucl Cardiol.* 2016;23(3):606–639.

via the extracellular dephosphorylation of adenosine triphosphate (ATP) and adenosine diphosphate (ADP). It acts on four known receptor subtypes (A1, $A2_a$, $A2_b$, and A3). When adenosine binds to cardiac-specific $A2_a$ receptors, it triggers several reactions, including increased production of adenylate cyclase and intracellular cyclic adenosine monophosphate (cAMP), all of which ultimately lead to coronary vasodilatation. After activating its receptors, adenosine enters endothelial and red blood cells by a facilitated transport mechanism, where it is rapidly inactivated.

Table 8-8

Contraindications for Pharmacologic Stress Testing

- Asthma with on-going wheezing (not for dobutamine)
- Second- or third-degree AV block (adenosine, dipyridamole, regadenoson)
- Systolic BP <90
- Methylxanthine use (aminophylline, caffeine) (not for dobutamine)
- Recent use of dipyridamole (adenosine, regadenoson)
- Known hypersensitivity of stress agent
- Uncontrolled hypertension (BP >200/110)
- Recent ACS
- For dobutamine only: severe aortic stenosis, LV outflow obstruction, supraventricular tachycardias with uncontrolled rate, history of VT, aortic dissection or large aneurysm, receiving beta blockers

Data from Henzlova MJ, Duvall WL, Einstein AJ, et al. ASNC imaging guidelines for SPECT nuclear cardiology procedures: Stress, protocols, and tracers. *J Nucl Cardiol.* 2016;23(3):606–639.

Although commonly referred to as such, by definition pharmacologically induced coronary artery vasodilatation is not a "stress test," since it does not significantly increase the rate–pressure product. The vasodilatory effects of adenosine predominate; it produces little, if any, chronotropic or inotropic response.[68] When cardiac $A2_a$ adenosine receptors are activated in patients without CAD, resistance vessel blood flow is increased three to five times above baseline levels. In patients with CAD, the resistance vessels distal to a hemodynamically significant stenosis are usually maximally dilated in order to maintain normal resting flow and are consequently unaffected by adenosine. However, any adjacent myocardium that is supplied by relatively normal coronary arteries will experience a substantial increase in blood flow when exposed to adenosine. This flow disparity translates into relative hypoperfusion of the ischemic myocardium, which can then be detected by means of MPI (Fig. 8-2).

The preprocedure routine for dipyridamole or adenosine stress MPI is similar to that of exercise MPI. In addition to not eating or drinking for 2 hours before testing, patients should not take xanthine derivatives (e.g., aminophylline) or consume caffeine-containing products for 12 hours prior to testing,[4] because xanthines block adenosine receptors and can cause false-negative results.[69] Some data did suggest that small amounts of caffeine, such as those contained in a single cup of coffee, do not impact on the detection or extent of ischemia.[70,71] However, the most recent studies, including that from Reyes et al., did show a reduction of ischemic defects when patient had received caffeine before an adenosine study.[72] The attenuation of the hyperemic response to adenosine may be overcome by increasing the dose by 50% (210 mcg/kg/min).[72]

Neither dipyridamole nor adenosine should be administered if there is a history of asthma or bronchospasm. Other contraindications to vasodilatory pharmacologic stress testing include persistent hypotension (systolic blood pressure <90 mm Hg), unstable angina, or recent acute MI (<2 days), high-grade AV block without a permanent pacemaker, uncontrolled arrhythmias, and critical aortic stenosis.[4]

Dipyridamole blocks the cellular reuptake of adenosine. It is infused slowly over 4 minutes (0.142 mg/kg/min), at which point maximum vasodilatation is achieved, and the radiopharmaceutical is injected. Frequently, low-level exercise is performed after the infusion is complete in order to minimize side effects, which occur frequently and include headache, flushing, hypotension, nausea, dyspnea, jaw pain, various forms of AV block, and chest discomfort. These effects can often persist for hours because of the lengthy half-life of dipyridamole. Fortunately, major adverse events during dipyridamole stress MPI (death, MI, or stroke) are extremely rare (<0.001%), as has been demonstrated in >73,000 patients.[73] If necessary, the effects of dipyridamole can be reversed with intravenous aminophylline, a competitive adenosine receptor antagonist, although its administration should be delayed for at least 1 minute after the radioisotope injection so as not to compromise the perfusion images.

Adenosine is typically administered at a rate of 140 μg/kg/min over 6 minutes, although a protocol using four infusions has proven to be equally efficacious.[74-76] A 3-minute infusion should be avoided, however.[76] Peak vasodilatation after adenosine administration occurs earlier than with dipyridamole, usually within 1 to 2 minutes after the start of the infusion. When using a standard 6-minute protocol, the radiopharmaceutical is injected 3 minutes into the infusion (or at 2 minutes into a 4-minute infusion). Exogenous administration of adenosine results in side effects that are similar to those seen with dipyridamole, but they occur more frequently, particularly AV block. Cerqueira et al.[77] prospectively reported the incidence of adenosine-related side effects in a large, multicenter trial. More than 80% of 9256 patients experienced adverse effects, including flushing (37%), chest pain (35%), dyspnea (35%), headache (14%), and AV block (8%). However, in contrast to dipyridamole, adenosine has an extremely short half-life (seconds), and thus side effects usually resolve rapidly on termination of the infusion. Aminophylline may be used, but is rarely necessary. The safety profile of adenosine as a pharmacologic stress MPI agent has been proven through evaluation of >15,000 patients.[77,78]

▶ Synthetic Catecholamines: Dobutamine

Although adenosine and dipyridamole are the preferred agents for pharmacologic stress MPI, they are contraindicated in the presence of asthma or bronchospasm. In such cases, dobutamine can be

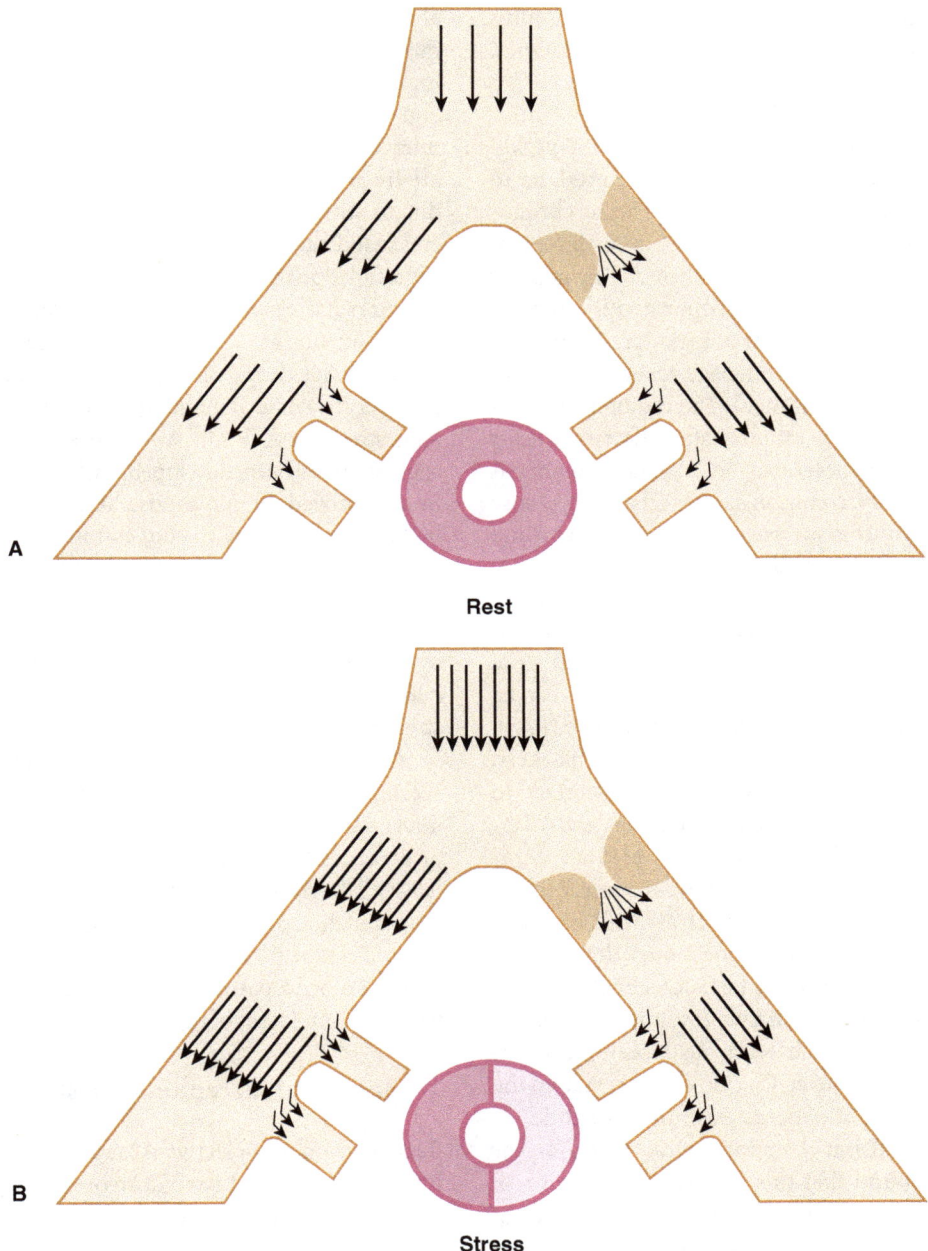

FIGURE 8-2 Schematic representation of rest and stress myocardial blood flow. **(A)** At rest, the presence of a non–flow-limiting stress does not alter regional perfusion and the representative image appears homogenous. **(B)** With vasodilation, coronary blood flow more than doubles. The presence of the stenosis and the limited flow reserve now limits regional perfusion and creates a "defect" on the resultant image.

substituted as a pharmacologic stressor. Dobutamine is a beta-adrenergic receptor agonist with a relatively short biologic half-life (2 minutes) that increases myocardial oxygen demand via positive chronotropic and inotropic effects. It also acts as a vasodilator by increasing blood flow in normal coronary arteries, thereby reducing perfusion pressure distal to significant coronary stenoses.[79-82]

Dobutamine is administered as a continuous infusion, beginning at 5 or 10 μg/kg/min for 3 minutes. It is then increased to 10 μg/kg/min for another 3 minutes, and subsequently increased every 3 minutes by 10 μg/kg up to a maximum dose of 50 μg/kg/min. If an adequate heart rate is not achieved, up to 1 mg of atropine can be given to augment the chronotropic response, which safely results in achievement of target heart rate in >90% of patients.[83] The goal for titration of the dobutamine infusion (with atropine) should be similar to the physiologic target for exercise, approximately 85% of the age-related maximum predicted heart rate (220-age). The radiopharmaceutical is injected 1 to 2 minutes after the target heart rate or maximum tolerable dose of dobutamine is reached. The most common side effects of high-dose dobutamine infusion are palpitations, chest pain, and hypertension. Occasionally, patients will experience a hypotensive response to dobutamine because of beta$_2$-adrenergic agonism. Less frequently, ventricular tachycardia (which is rarely sustained) or rapid atrial fibrillation can develop.[84] These adverse effects can be countered with cessation of the dobutamine infusion or by the administration of intravenous beta blockers.

Dobutamine is a safe and effective adjunct to SPECT MPI. The sensitivity, specificity, and diagnostic accuracy of dobutamine stress MPI are comparable to both adenosine and dipyridamole.[84,85] The prognostic value of dobutamine stress MPI has been questioned, because in the canine model, dobutamine attenuates the myocardial uptake of technetium-99m (Tc-99m) sestamibi, which may result in an underestimation of blood flow heterogeneity seen on perfusion images.[86,87] However, Calnon et al.[88] reviewed the clinical outcomes of patients who underwent dobutamine stress MPI at their institution over a 4-year period, and found that this cohort was at high risk for future cardiac events, especially the subgroup of patients with dobutamine-induced STD and abnormal SPECT imaging. Of note, failure to achieve the target heart rate (85% of maximum predicted heart rate) with dobutamine increases the annual cardiac event rate, irrespective of the clinical risk category.[89]

▶ Selective A2$_a$ Receptor Agonists

Adenosine and dipyridamole are well-established for use during pharmacologic MPI. However, as noted above, both agents have multiple side effects largely due to their nonselective activation of multiple adenosine receptors, which can result in patient discomfort and at times cause premature study termination. The intraventricular conduction delays and chest pain that are frequently noted during infusion of adenosine are due to stimulation of A1 receptors,[90,91] while peripheral vasodilatation, bronchoconstriction, and mast cell degranulation that leads to flushing are mediated by A2$_b$ receptors.[92,93] Since coronary vasodilatation is mediated by adenosine A2$_a$ receptors, selective A2$_a$ receptor agonists offer the advantage of eliminating unwanted side effects while remaining an effective pharmacologic stress agent. While several selective A2$_a$ receptor agonists have been developed, only regadenoson has been approved for clinical use. A second agent which had completed phase III studies, binadenoson, did not obtain FDA approval due to concerns of similar efficacy as adenosine, and the continued development of a third A2$_a$ agonist, apadenoson, has been placed on hold by the pharmaceutical company.[94-99] Regadenoson is currently the most commonly utilized pharmacologic stress agent compared to the other vasodilators.[3]

Clinical experience, to date, with all of the selective A2$_a$ agonists has demonstrated comparable diagnostic information with somewhat less hypotension, minimal or no effect on the AV node, and a reduction in side effects.[94,100] The potential of the A2$_a$ agonists to expand the population of patients undergoing vasodilator stress is based on the potential use of these agents in the setting of bronchospastic lung disease and those patients who were intolerant of dipyridamole or adenosine.

▶ Selective A2$_a$ Receptor Agonist: Regadenoson

Regadenoson is a selective A2$_a$ agonist that is administered as a standard fixed dose of 400 mcg by means of a bolus injection delivered over 10 seconds.[101-103] The radiopharmaceutical may be injected within 30 seconds of regadenoson, as hyperemia is rapidly achieved. No infusion pump or specialized tubing is required and regadenoson is available as prefilled, single-dose syringe, as no dose calibration is needed. A weight-adjusted dosage regime is not required due to the presence of a large A2$_a$ receptor reserve and the need for only a small fraction of receptors to be activated by regadenoson. The fixed dose of 400 mcg has been shown to be safe and is better tolerated than adenosine, irrespective of the age, gender, and body habitus of the patient.[103] Reduced renal clearance of regadenoson is present in the setting of renal impairment[104]; the clinical impact of this finding remains under investigation, but thus far does not appear to represent a serious concern.[105] Though prior studies have suggested that ingestion of one 8-oz cup of coffee prior to stress testing may not have significant effects on the utility of regadenoson MPI, a more recent study confirms the initial concerns about loss of maximal hyperemia if caffeine is present. Ingestion of 200 to 400 mg of caffeine prior to regadenoson can decrease the detection and magnitude of ischemia on SPECT MPI, and thus should be avoided for at least 12 hours prior to testing.[71,106]

Clinical trials in >1300 patients (ADVANCE MPI trials) demonstrate noninferiority in the level of agreement between regadenoson and adenosine compared with other patients undergoing two adenosine studies.[102] The extent of ischemia that was detected with regadenoson was similar to that noted with adenosine. Blood pressure changes were similar between regadenoson and adenosine, but a more robust increase in heart rate response was noted with regadenoson. Regadenoson caused less incidence of first- and second-degree AV block than noted with adenosine, although a single patient did have an isolated dropped beat, consistent with second-degree AV block. Side effects appear to be less with regadenoson, especially related to chest pain and flushing, although headache was more frequently observed. Severe and/or persistent adverse reactions should be reversed with 50 to 250 mg of aminophylline. Of note, there has been an increased incidence of seizures associated with regadenoson administration.[107]

There has been conflicting data in regards to the significance of vasodilator-induced ischemic changes seen on EKG in the setting of normal MPI and their prognostic implications.[108–111] In a smaller study with 396 patients, regadenoson and adenosine were compared in terms of their effects on EKG changes (STD or STE), symptoms of chest pain during stress testing, and their ability to reliably detect ischemia based on those criteria.[112] While symptoms of chest pain were more common with adenosine and EKG changes occurred infrequently in both groups (16% in the regadenoson group and 10% in the adenosine group), there was no significant correlation between either of these findings and true ischemia on MPI. Interestingly, women were more commonly found to have symptoms with adenosine injection, but there were no significant gender differences in the side effects associated with regadenoson administration. In contrast, other studies have shown that when these ischemic EKG changes occur, albeit infrequently, in postmenopausal women, there may be greater prognostic significance in regards to underlying cardiac disease and increased cardiovascular mortality.[110]

As selective $A2_a$ stimulation is present with regadenoson, there is potential to use this agent in patients with COPD and/or asthma. Several small studies[113–115] have confirmed this potential application, but further trials are needed to fully evaluate regadenoson radionuclide imaging in this context.

COMBINED EXERCISE AND PHARMACOLOGIC MPI

Combining exercise with pharmacologic stress testing is an attractive option, because it facilitates the assessment of ischemia while still permitting a determination of functional capacity among patients who might not achieve their target heart rate. In addition, concomitant exercise reduces the quantity and severity of adenosine-related side effects.[66,116–121] Furthermore, image quality is enhanced due to the redistribution of blood flow to the skeletal muscle and away from intra-abdominal organs and the lungs, thereby increasing heart:background (lung and liver) ratios and improving contrast.[116–120,122]

Exercise has been successfully combined with adenosine[116–119,123,124] and dipyridamole,[64,65] using several different protocols. Elliot et al.[116] compared a standard 6-minute adenosine infusion to limited treadmill exercise combined with 4-minute adenosine infusion, and showed a significant reduction in adverse effects as well as improved image quality with the combined protocol (Fig. 8-3). Casale et al.[64] studied 100 patients who received an infusion of dipyridamole combined with treadmill exercise to another 100 patients who received dipyridamole alone. They found that their experimental protocol was safe, resulted in fewer side effects, and yielded better quality perfusion images when compared with standard dipyridamole stress MPI. Stern et al.[65] evaluated dipyridamole infusion combined with different exercise modalities, and

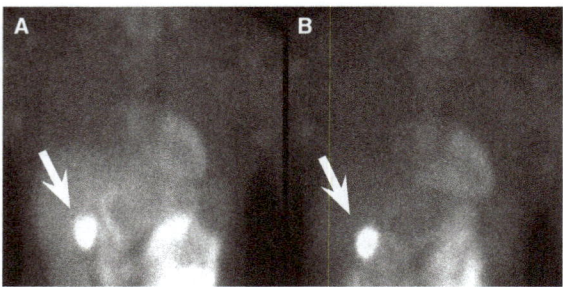

FIGURE 8-3 Myocardial perfusion imaging: adenosine versus adenosine + exercise. Panel **A** demonstrates similar intensity in the liver (*arrow*) as noted in the myocardium following an adenosine infusion. However, when exercise is combined with adenosine (panel **B**), much less hepatic activity (*arrow*) is present when compared with the myocardium.

concluded that low-level treadmill exercise in combination with dipyridamole was superior to either handgrip and dipyridamole or dipyridamole alone. Similarly, Ignaszewski et al.[66] reported that symptom-limited exercise in combination with dipyridamole was safe and well tolerated, even in elderly patients or those with known significant CAD.

Holly et al.[121] directly compared standard treadmill exercise to a protocol combining treadmill exercise with a 4-minute adenosine infusion in a group of patients who were thought to be incapable of reaching their target heart rate. The combined adenosine and exercise protocol was well tolerated, with no adverse effects noted as a result of the adenosine infusion. Combining vasodilation with exercise stress also permits an earlier acquisition of imaging data, thereby improving efficiency and allowing for the potential to detect myocardial stunning.[125] In addition, combined vasodilator and exercise stressor provides prognostic data in patients with known or suspected coronary disease.[126] Although limited data are presently available regarding the use of adjunctive exercise with $A2_a$ selective agonists, data from small studies with regadenoson demonstrate the feasibility and safety of such an approach.[127,128] The use of a fixed-dose, bolus stressor, such as regadenoson, may be ideally suited for this combined protocol, as the injection of regadenoson may be performed immediately (30 seconds) before tracer delivery, ensuring the performance of maximal exercise. In a recent study by Ross et al., 75 patients who were unable to reach their target heart rate during exercise alone were randomized to receiving either regadenoson at peak exercise or at rest after exercise, and it appeared that both protocols were well tolerated and resulted in similar imaging findings, thereby supporting the safety of combined peak exercise with regadenoson.[128] Notably, 62% of patients scheduled to undergo regadenoson stress testing were able to reach their target heart rate, therefore making the administration of the vasodilator unnecessary. Similar findings with regard to the safety of combined regadenoson-exercise and the lack of need for regadenoson have been shown in other studies.[129] The addition of isometric exercise with handgrip also appears to be effective in increasing heart rate response but important in reducing adverse effects with regadenoson and concomitantly improving image quality.[130]

In summary, the combination of exercise and pharmacologic MPI is recommended and accepted as a safe and well-tolerated diagnostic option when choosing a stress test, as it allows for improved image quality and minimizes or eliminates side effects. Patients with a tendency for hypotension or bradycardia should undergo a combined protocol as well as those who have sustained significant side effects or technical problems with prior vasodilator studies.[120] These combined protocols are applicable to a broad range of patients, including virtually all patients who are sufficiently ambulatory to enter an outpatient laboratory without assistance. In addition, when using regadenoson, patients who are able to reach their target response to exercise do not require the administration of the pharmacologic stress agent.

CONCLUSIONS

Stress testing in combination with SPECT MPI is a well-established procedure that has been in widespread clinical use for many years. The vast majority of stress testing is performed in order to evaluate either known or suspected CAD. If patients are capable of exercise and have a normal baseline ECG (including complete RBBB and/or <1 mm of resting STD), they should undergo standard exercise testing without concurrent imaging. If confounding conditions are present, SPECT MPI should be performed along with exercise.

Exercise stress testing with or without SPECT MPI is preferable to any form of pharmacologic stress testing, because it allows for an assessment of functional capacity and provides better quality perfusion images. However, if contraindications to exercise exist, pharmacologic stress with an infusion of adenosine, dipyridamole, regadenoson, or dobutamine can be substituted without diminishing the sensitivity, specificity, or predictive value of SPECT MPI. It is advised to withhold caffeine and other methylxanthines for at least 12 hours prior to vasodilator stress. The side effects of adenosine, dipyridamole, and regadenoson may be frequent, but are usually inconsequential, and can be easily managed with cessation of the infusion or administration of aminophylline in the case of dipyridamole or regadenoson.

Recent studies combining exercise with vasodilating agents appear to reduce or eliminate these medication-induced side effects while providing an assessment of functional capacity. As such, combined exercise and pharmacologic SPECT MPI may ultimately supplant pharmacologic stress alone among patients who are capable of submaximal exercise. Regadenoson, the only FDA-approved selective $A2_a$ receptor agonist, is now the most commonly used vasodilator. It appears to be hemodynamically superior and better tolerated than either adenosine or dipyridamole, while providing comparable imaging data and allows for flexibility during exercise stress, as it may be administered if a patient is unable to achieve an adequate level of exercise or alternatively may not be given when the exercise test is diagnostic.

REFERENCES

1. Carrea JR, Gleason G, Shaw J, et al. The direct diagnosis of myocardial infarction by photoscanning after administration of Cesium-131. *Am Heart J.* 1964;68:627–636.
2. Zaret BL, Strauss HW, Martin ND, et al. Noninvasive regional myocardial perfusion with radioactive potassium. Study of patients at rest, with exercise and during angina pectoris. *N Eng J Med.* 1973;288(16):809–812.
3. Zoghbi GJ, Iskandrian AE. Selective adenosine agonists and myocardial perfusion imaging. *J Nucl Cardiol.* 2012;19(1):126–141.
4. Henzlova MJ, Duvall WL, Einstein AJ, et al. ASNC imaging guidelines for SPECT nuclear cardiology procedures: Stress, protocols, and tracers. *J Nucl Cardiol.* 2016;23(3):606–639.
5. Klocke FJ, Baird MG, Lorell BH, et al. ACC/AHA/ASNC guidelines for the clinical use of cardiac radionuclide imaging—executive summary: A report of the American College of Cardiology/American Heart Association Task Force on Practice Guidelines (ACC/AHA/ASNC Committee to Revise the 1995 Guidelines for the Clinical Use of Cardiac Radionuclide Imaging). *J Am Coll Cardiol.* 2003;42(7):1318–1333.
6. Balady GJ, Morise AP. Exercise Testing. In: Mann DL, Zipes DP, Libby P, et al., eds. *Braunwald's Heart Disease: A Textbook of Cardiovascular Medicine.* 10th ed. Philadelphia, PA: WB Saunders; 2015:155–176.
7. Esquivel L, Pollock SG, Beller GA, et al. Effect of the degree of effort on the sensitivity of the exercise thallium-201 stress test in symptomatic coronary artery disease. *Am J Cardiol.* 1989;63(3):160–165.
8. Hachamovitch R, Berman DS, Kiat H, et al. Exercise myocardial perfusion SPECT in patients without known coronary artery disease: Incremental prognostic value and use in risk stratification. *Circulation.* 1996;93(5):905–914.
9. Bourque JM, Charlton GT, Holland BH, et al. Prognosis in patients achieving >/= 10 METS on exercise stress testing: Was SPECT imaging useful? *J Nucl Cardiol.* 2011;18(2):230–237.
10. Myers J, Froelicher VF. Optimizing the exercise test for pharmacological investigations. *Circulation.* 1990;82(5):1839–1846.
11. Ellestad MH, Mishkin FS, Selvester RH, et al. *Stress Testing: Principles and Practice.* 5th ed. New York, NY: Oxford University Press, Inc.; 2003.
12. Froelicher VF, Myers J. *Exercise and the Heart.* 5th ed. Philadelphia, PA: WB Saunders; 2006.
13. Barbour MM, Garber CE, Agarwal KC, et al. Effect of dipyridamole therapy on myocardial ischemia in patients with stable angina pectoris receiving concurrent anti-ischemic therapy. *Am J Cardiol.* 1992;69(5):449–452.
14. Gibbons RJ, Balady GJ, Bricker JT, et al. ACC/AHA 2002 guideline update for exercise testing: Summary article. A report of the American College of Cardiology/American Heart Association Task Force on Practice Guidelines (Committee to Update the 1997 Exercise Testing Guidelines). *J Am Coll Cardiol.* 2002;40(8):1531–1540.
15. Stuart RJ, Ellestad MH. Upsloping S-T segments in exercise stress testing. Six year follow-up study of 438 patients and correlation with 248 angiograms. *Am J Cardiol.* 1976;37(1):19–22.
16. Tavel ME. Stress testing in cardiac evaluation: Current concepts with emphasis on the ECG. *Chest.* 2001;119(3):907–925.
17. Eagle KA, Guyton RA, Davidoff R, et al. ACC/AHA Guidelines for Coronary Artery Bypass Graft Surgery: A Report of the American College of Cardiology/American Heart Association Task Force on Practice Guidelines (Committee to Revise the 1991 Guidelines for Coronary Artery Bypass Graft Surgery). American College of Cardiology/American Heart Association. *J Am Coll Cardiol.* 1999;34(4):1262–1347.
18. Rywik TM, Zink RC, Gittings NS, et al. Independent prognostic significance of ischemic ST-segment response limited to recovery from treadmill exercise in asymptomatic subjects. *Circulation.* 1998;97(21):2117–2122.
19. Karnegis JN, Matts J, Tuna N, et al. Comparison of exercise-positive with recovery-positive treadmill graded exercise tests. *Am J Cardiol.* 1987;60(7):544–547.
20. Savage MP, Squires LS, Hopkins JT, et al. Usefulness of ST-segment depression as a sign of coronary artery disease when confined to the postexercise recovery period. *Am J Cardiol.* 1987;60(16):1405–1406.

21. Rodriguez M, Moussa I, Froning J, et al. Improved exercise test accuracy using discriminant function analysis and "recovery ST slope". *J Electrocardiol.* 1993;26(3):207–218.
22. Barlow JB. The "false positive" exercise electrocardiogram: Value of time course patterns in assessment of depressed ST segments and inverted T waves. *Am Heart J.* 1985;110(6):1328–1336.
23. Kang X, Berman DS, Lewin HC, et al. Comparative localization of myocardial ischemia by exercise electrocardiography and myocardial perfusion SPECT. *J Nucl Cardiol.* 2000;7(2):140–145.
24. Gallik DM, Mahmarian JJ, Verani MS. Therapeutic significance of exercise-induced ST-segment elevation in patients without previous myocardial infarction. *Am J Cardiol.* 1993;72(1):1–7.
25. Manvi KN, Ellestad MH. Elevated ST segments with exercise in ventricular aneurysm. *J Electrocardiol.* 1972;5(4):317–323.
26. Haines DE, Beller GA, Watson DD, et al. Exercise-induced ST segment elevation 2 weeks after uncomplicated myocardial infarction: Contributing factors and prognostic significance. *J Am Coll Cardiol.* 1987;9(5):996–1003.
27. Margonato A, Ballarotto C, Bonetti F, et al. Assessment of residual tissue viability by exercise testing in recent myocardial infarction: Comparison of the electrocardiogram and myocardial perfusion scintigraphy. *J Am Coll Cardiol.* 1992;19(5):948–952.
28. Margonato A, Chierchia SL, Xuereb RG, et al. Specificity and sensitivity of exercise-induced ST segment elevation for detection of residual viability: Comparison with fluorodeoxyglucose and positron emission tomography. *J Am Coll Cardiol.* 1995;25(5):1032–1038.
29. Lombardo A, Loperfido F, Pennestri F, et al. Significance of transient ST-T segment changes during dobutamine testing in Q wave myocardial infarction. *J Am Coll Cardiol.* 1996;27(3):599–605.
30. Blackburn H. Canadian Colloquium on Computer-Assisted Interpretation of Electrocardiograms. VI. Importance of the electrocardiogram in populations outside the hospital. *Can Med Assoc J.* 1973;108(10):1262–1265.
31. Cullen K, Stenhouse NS, Wearne KL, et al. Electrocardiograms and 13 year cardiovascular mortality in Busselton study. *Br Heart J.* 1982;47(3):209–212.
32. Aronow WS. Correlation of ischemic ST-segment depression on the resting electrocardiogram with new cardiac events in 1,106 patients over 62 years of age. *Am J Cardiol.* 1989;64(3):232–233.
33. Califf RM, Mark DB, Harrell FE, Jr., et al. Importance of clinical measures of ischemia in the prognosis of patients with documented coronary artery disease. *J Am Coll Cardiol.* 1988;11(1):20–26.
34. Harris PJ, Harrell FE, Lee KL, et al. Survival in medically treated coronary artery disease. *Circulation.* 1979;60(6):1259–1269.
35. Sketch MH, Mooss AN, Butler ML, et al. Digoxin-induced positive exercise tests: Their clinical and prognostic significance. *Am J Cardiol.* 1981;48(4):655–659.
36. LeWinter MM, Crawford MH, O'Rourke RA, et al. The effects of oral propranolol, digoxin and combination therapy on the resting and exercise electrocardiogram. *Am H J.* 1977;93(2):202–209.
37. Sundqvist K, Atterhög JH, Jogestrand T. Effect of digoxin on the electrocardiogram at rest and during exercise in healthy subjects. *Am J Cardiol.* 1986;57(8):661–665.
38. Whinnery JE, Froelicher VF, Stewart AJ, et al. The electrocardiographic response to maximal treadmill exercise of asymptomatic men with left bundle branch block. *Am Heart J.* 1977;94(3):316–324.
39. Whinnery JE, Froelicher VF, Longo MR, et al. The electrocardiographic response to maximal treadmill exercise of asymptomatic men with right bundle branch block. *Chest.* 1977;71(3):335–340.
40. Michaelides AP, Psomadaki ZD, Dilaveris PE, et al. Improved detection of coronary artery disease by exercise electrocardiography with the use of right precordial leads. *N Engl J Med.* 1999;340(5):340–345.
41. Okin PM, Roman MJ, Schwartz JE, et al. Relation of exercise-induced myocardial ischemia to cardiac and carotid structure. *Hypertension.* 1997;30(6):1382–1388.
42. Fletcher GF, Flipse TR, Kligfield P, et al. Current status of ECG stress testing. *Curr Probl Cardiol.* 1998;23(7):353–423.
43. Morise AP. Accuracy of heart rate-adjusted ST segments in populations with and without posttest referral bias. *Am Heart J.* 1997;134(4):647–655.
44. Okin PM, Kligfield P. Heart rate adjustment of ST segment depression and performance of the exercise electrocardiogram: A critical evaluation. *J Am Coll Cardiol.* 1995;25(7):1726–1735.
45. Viik J, Lehtinen R, Malmivuo J. Detection of coronary artery disease using maximum value of ST/HR hysteresis over different number of leads. *J Electrocardiol.* 1999;32 Suppl:70–75.
46. Froelicher VF, Lehmann KG, Thomas R, et al. The electrocardiographic exercise test in a population with reduced workup bias: Diagnostic performance, computerized interpretation, and multivariable prediction. Veterans Affairs Cooperative Study in Health Services #016 (QUEXTA) Study Group. Quantitative Exercise Testing and Angiography. *Ann Intern Med.* 1998;128(12 Pt 1):965–974.
47. Milliken JA, Abdollah H, Burggraf GW. False-positive treadmill exercise tests due to computer signal averaging. *Am J Cardiol.* 1990;65(13):946–948.
48. Lauer MS, Francis GS, Okin PM, et al. Impaired chronotropic response to exercise stress testing as a predictor of mortality. *JAMA.* 1999;281(6):524–529.
49. Cole CR, Blackstone EH, Pashkow FJ, et al. Heart-rate recovery immediately after exercise as a predictor of mortality. *N Engl J Med.* 1999;341(18):1351–1357.
50. Cole CR, Foody JM, Blackstone EH, et al. Heart rate recovery after submaximal exercise testing as a predictor of mortality in a cardiovascularly healthy cohort. *Ann Intern Med.* 2000;132(7):552–555.
51. Diaz LA, Brunken RC, Blackstone EH, Snader CE, Lauer MS. Independent contribution of myocardial perfusion defects to exercise capacity and heart rate recovery for prediction of all-cause mortality in patients with known or suspected coronary heart disease. *J Am Coll Cardiol.* 2001;37(6):1558–1564.
52. Watanabe J, Thamilarasan M, Blackstone EH, et al. Heart rate recovery immediately after treadmill exercise and left ventricular systolic dysfunction as predictors of mortality: The case of stress echocardiography. *Circulation.* 2001;104(16):1911–1916.

53. Nishime EO, Cole CR, Blackstone EH, et al. Heart rate recovery and treadmill exercise score as predictors of mortality in patients referred for exercise ECG. *JAMA.* 2000;284(11):1392–1398.
54. Shetler K, Marcus R, Froelicher VF, et al. Heart rate recovery: Validation and methodologic issues. *J Am Coll Cardiol.* 2001;38(7):1980–1987.
55. Mark DB, Hlatky MA, Harrell FE, et al. Exercise treadmill score for predicting prognosis in coronary artery disease. *Ann Intern Med.* 1987;106(6):793–800.
56. Kwok JM, Miller TD, Christian TF, et al. Prognostic value of a treadmill exercise score in symptomatic patients with nonspecific ST-T abnormalities on resting ECG. *JAMA.* 1999;282(11):1047–1053.
57. Mark DB, Shaw L, Harrell FE, et al. Prognostic value of a treadmill exercise score in outpatients with suspected coronary artery disease. *N Engl J Med.* 1991;325(12):849–853.
58. Bruce RA, DeRouen TA, Hossack KF. Pilot study examining the motivational effects of maximal exercise testing to modify risk factors and health habits. *Cardiology.* 1980;66(2):111–119.
59. Iskandrian AS, Heo J, Askenase A, et al. Dipyridamole cardiac imaging. *Am Heart J.* 1988;115(2):432–443.
60. Brown KA. Prognostic value of thallium-201 myocardial perfusion imaging. A diagnostic tool comes of age. *Circulation.* 1991;83(2):363–381.
61. Brown KA, Rowen M. Impact of antianginal medications, peak heart rate and stress level on the prognostic value of a normal exercise myocardial perfusion imaging study. *J Nucl Med.* 1993;34(9):1467–1471.
62. Iskandrian AS, Heo J, Kong B, et al. Effect of exercise level on the ability of thallium-201 tomographic imaging in detecting coronary artery disease: Analysis of 461 patients. *J Am Coll Cardiol.* 1989;14(6):1477–1486.
63. Heller GV, Ahmed I, Tilkemeier PL, et al. Influence of exercise intensity on the presence, distribution, and size of thallium-201 defects. *Am Heart J.* 1992;123(4 Pt 1):909–916.
64. Casale PN, Guiney TE, Strauss HW, et al. Simultaneous low level treadmill exercise and intravenous dipyridamole stress thallium imaging. *Am J Cardiol.* 1988;62(10 Pt 1):799–802.
65. Stern S, Greenberg ID, Corne RA. Quantification of walking exercise required for improvement of dipyridamole thallium-201 image quality. *J Nucl Med.* 1992;33(12):2061–2066.
66. Ignaszewski AP, McCormick LX, Heslip PG, et al. Safety and clinical utility of combined intravenous dipyridamole/symptom-limited exercise stress test with thallium-201 imaging in patients with known or suspected coronary artery disease. *J Nucl Med.* 1993;34(12):2053–2061.
67. Lam F. Medtech 360 Report: Diagnostic Imaging Systems -U.S.-2015-Market Analysis. *Decision Resources Group Reports website.* 2014. https://decisionresourcesgroup.com/report/6392-medtech-diagnostic-imaging-systems-us-2015-market/. Accessed August 8, 2016.
68. Verani MS. Stress approaches: Techniques. In: Pohost GM, O'Rourke RA, Shah PM, eds. *Imaging in Cardiovascular Medicine.* Philadelphia, PA: Lippincott Williams & Wilkins; 2000:155.
69. Bottcher M, Czernin J, Sun KT, et al. Effect of caffeine on myocardial blood flow at rest and during pharmacological vasodilation. *J Nucl Med.* 1995;36(11):2016–2021.
70. Zoghbi GJ, Htay T, Aqel R, et al. Effect of caffeine on ischemia detection by adenosine single-photon emission computed tomography perfusion imaging. *J Am Coll Cardiol.* 2006;47(11):2296–2302.
71. Gaemperli O, Schepis T, Koepfli P, et al. Interaction of caffeine with regadenoson-induced hyperemic myocardial blood flow as measured by positron emission tomography: A randomized, double-blind, placebo-controlled crossover trial. *J Am Coll Cardiol.* 2008;51(3):328–329.
72. Reyes E, Loong CY, Harbinson M, et al. High-dose adenosine overcomes the attenuation of myocardial perfusion reserve caused by caffeine. *J Am Coll Cardiol.* 2008;52(24):2008–2016.
73. Lette J, Tatum JL, Fraser S, et al. Safety of dipyridamole testing in 73,806 patients: The Multicenter Dipyridamole Safety Study. *J Nucl Cardiol.* 1995;2(1):3–17.
74. Treuth MG, Reyes GA, He ZX, et al. Tolerance and diagnostic accuracy of an abbreviated adenosine infusion for myocardial scintigraphy: A randomized, prospective study. *J Nucl Cardiol.* 2001;8(5):548–554.
75. O'Keefe JH, Jr., Bateman TM, Handlin LR, et al. Four- versus 6-minute infusion protocol for adenosine thallium-201 single photon emission computed tomography imaging. *Am Heart J.* 1995;129(3):482–487.
76. Bokhari S, Ficaro EP, McCallister BD, Jr. Adenosine stress protocols for myocardial perfusion imaging. *J Nucl Cardiol.* 2007;14(3):415–416.
77. Cerqueira MD, Verani MS, Schwaiger M, et al. Safety profile of adenosine stress perfusion imaging: Results from the Adenoscan Multicenter Trial Registry. *J Am Coll Cardiol.* 1994;23(2):384–389.
78. Abreu A, Mahmarian JJ, Nishimura S, et al. Tolerance and safety of pharmacologic coronary vasodilation with adenosine in association with thallium-201 scintigraphy in patients with suspected coronary artery disease. *J Am Coll Cardiol.* 1991;18(3):730–735.
79. Coma-Canella I. Dobutamine stress test to diagnose the presence and severity of coronary artery lesions in angina. *Eur Heart J.* 1991;12(11):1198–1204.
80. Mazeika PK, Nadazdin A, Oakley CM. Dobutamine stress echocardiography for detection and assessment of coronary artery disease. *J Am Coll Cardiol.* 1992;19(6):1203–1211.
81. Previtali M, Lanzarini L, Ferrario M, et al. Dobutamine versus dipyridamole echocardiography in coronary artery disease. *Circulation.* 1991;83(5 Suppl):III27–31.
82. Martin TW, Seaworth JF, Johns JP, et al. Comparison of adenosine, dipyridamole, and dobutamine in stress echocardiography. *Ann Int Med.* 1992;116(3):190–196.
83. Elhendy A, Valkema R, van Domburg RT, et al. Safety of dobutamine-atropine stress myocardial perfusion scintigraphy. *J Nucl Med.* 1998;39(10):1662–1666.
84. Hays JT, Mahmarian JJ, Cochran AJ, et al. Dobutamine thallium-201 tomography for evaluating patients with suspected coronary artery disease unable to undergo exercise or vasodilator pharmacologic stress testing. *J Am Coll Cardiol.* 1993;21(7):1583–1590.
85. Geleijnse ML, Elhendy A, Fioretti PM, Roelandt JR. Dobutamine stress myocardial perfusion imaging. *J Am Coll Cardiol.* 2000;36(7):2017–2027.
86. Calnon DA, Glover DK, Beller GA, et al. Effects of dobutamine stress on myocardial blood flow, 99mTc sestamibi uptake, and systolic wall thickening in the presence of

coronary artery stenoses: Implications for dobutamine stress testing. *Circulation*. 1997;96(7):2353–2360.
87. Wu JC, Yun JJ, Heller EN, et al. Limitations of dobutamine for enhancing flow heterogeneity in the presence of single coronary stenosis: Implications for technetium-99m-sestamibi imaging. *J Nucl Med*. 1998;39(3):417–425.
88. Calnon DA, McGrath PD, Doss AL, et al. Prognostic value of dobutamine stress technetium-99m-sestamibi single-photon emission computed tomography myocardial perfusion imaging: Stratification of a high-risk population. *J Am Coll Cardiol*. 2001;38(5):1511–1517.
89. Navare SM, Katten D, Johnson LL, et al. Risk stratification with electrocardiographic-gated dobutamine stress technetium-99m sestamibi single-photon emission tomographic imaging: Value of heart rate response and assessment of left ventricular function. *J Am Coll Cardiol*. 2006;47(4):781–788.
90. Bertolet BD, Belardinelli L, Franco EA, et al. Selective attenuation by N-0861 (N6-endonorboran-2-yl-9-methyladenine) of cardiac A1 adenosine receptor-mediated effects in humans. *Circulation*. 1996;93(10):1871–1876.
91. Gaspardone A, Crea F, Tomai F, et al. Muscular and cardiac adenosine-induced pain is mediated by A1 receptors. *J Am Coll Cardiol*. 1995;25(1):251–257.
92. Linden J, Thai T, Figler H, et al. Characterization of human A(2B) adenosine receptors: Radioligand binding, western blotting, and coupling to G(q) in human embryonic kidney 293 cells and HMC-1 mast cells. *Mol Pharmacol*. 1999;56(4):705–713.
93. Auchampach JA, Jin X, Wan TC, et al. Canine mast cell adenosine receptors: Cloning and expression of the A3 receptor and evidence that degranulation is mediated by the A2B receptor. *Mol Pharmacol*. 1997;52(5):846–860.
94. Cerqueira MD. Advances in pharmacologic agents in imaging: New A2A receptor agonists. *Curr Cardiol Repor*. 2006;8(2):119–122.
95. Glover DK, Ruiz M, Yang JY, et al. Pharmacological stress thallium scintigraphy with 2-cyclohexylmethylidenehydrazinoadenosine (WRC-0470). A novel, short-acting adenosine A2A receptor agonist. *Circulation*. 1996;94(7):1726–1732.
96. He ZX, Cwajg E, Hwang W, et al. Myocardial blood flow and myocardial uptake of (201)Tl and (99m)Tc-sestamibi during coronary vasodilation induced by CGS-21680, a selective adenosine A(2A) receptor agonist. *Circulation*. 2000;102(4):438–444.
97. Glover DK, Ruiz M, Takehana K, et al. Pharmacological stress myocardial perfusion imaging with the potent and selective A(2A) adenosine receptor agonists ATL193 and ATL146e administered by either intravenous infusion or bolus injection. *Circulation*. 2001;104(10):1181–1187.
98. Udelson JE, Heller GV, Wackers FJ, et al. Randomized, controlled dose-ranging study of the selective adenosine A2A receptor agonist binodenoson for pharmacological stress as an adjunct to myocardial perfusion imaging. *Circulation*. 2004;109(4):457–464.
99. Hendel RC, Taillefer R, Crane PD, et al. Preliminary experience with BMSO68645, a selective A2a adenosine agonist, for pharmacologic stress myocardial perfusion Imaging. *Circulation*. 2005;112(suppl 2):474.
100. Murray JJ, Weiler JM, Schwartz LB, et al. Safety of binodenoson, a selective adenosine A2A receptor agonist vasodilator pharmacological stress agent, in healthy subjects with mild intermittent asthma. *Circ Cardiovasc Imaging*. 2009;2(6):492–498.
101. Trochu J-N, Zhao G, Post H, et al. Selective A2A adenosine receptor agonist as a coronary vasodilator in conscious dogs: Potential for use in myocardial perfusion imaging. *J Cardiovasc Pharmacol*. 2003;41(1):132–139.
102. Iskandrian AE, Bateman TM, Belardinelli L, et al. Adenosine versus regadenoson comparative evaluation in myocardial perfusion imaging: Results of the ADVANCE phase 3 multicenter international trial. *J Nucl Cardiol*. 2007;14(5):645–658.
103. Cerqueira MD, Nguyen P, Staehr P, et al. Effects of age, gender, obesity, and diabetes on the efficacy and safety of the selective A2A agonist regadenoson versus adenosine in myocardial perfusion imaging integrated ADVANCE-MPI trial results. *JACC Cardiovasc Imaging*. 2008;1(3):307–316.
104. Gordi T, Blackburn B, Lieu H. Regadenoson pharmacokinetics and tolerability in subjects with impaired renal function. *J Clin Pharmacol*. 2007;47(7):825–833.
105. Laighold S, Druz R. Initial clinical experience with a selective A2A receptor agonist, regadenoson, in a patient with end-stage renal disease on hemodialysis. *J Nucl Cardiol*. 2009;16(3):478–480.
106. Tejani FH, Thompson RC, Kristy R, et al. Effect of caffeine on SPECT myocardial perfusion imaging during regadenoson pharmacologic stress: A prospective, randomized, multicenter study. *Int J Cardiovasc Imaging*. 2014;30(5):979–989.
107. Agarwal V, DePuey EG. Regadenoson and seizures: A real clinical concern. *J Nucl Cardiol*. 2014;21(5):869–870.
108. Hage FG, Dubovsky EV, Heo J, et al. Outcome of patients with adenosine-induced ST-segment depression but with normal perfusion on tomographic imaging. *Am J Cardiol*. 2006;98(8):1009–1011.
109. Klodas E, Miller TD, Christian TF, et al. Prognostic significance of ischemic electrocardiographic changes during vasodilator stress testing in patients with normal SPECT images. *J Nucl Cardiol*. 2003;10(1):4–8.
110. Uthamalingam S, Gurm GS, Ahmado I, et al. Outcome of patients with regadenoson-induced ST-segment depression but normal perfusion on single-photon emission computed tomography. *Angiology*. 2013;64(1):46–48.
111. Shaw LJ, Mieres JH, Hendel RH, et al. Comparative effectiveness of exercise electrocardiography with or without myocardial perfusion single photon emission computed tomography in women with suspected coronary artery disease: Results from the What Is the Optimal Method for Ischemia Evaluation in Women (WOMEN) trial. *Circulation*. 2011;124(11):1239–1249.
112. Zahid M, Kapila A, Eagan CE, et al. Prevalence and significance of electrocardiographic changes and side effect profile of regadenoson compared with adenosine during myocardial perfusion imaging. *J Cardiovasc Dis Res*. 2013;4(1):7–10.
113. Leaker BR, O'Connor B, Hansel TT, et al. Safety of regadenoson, an adenosine A2A receptor agonist for myocardial perfusion imaging, in mild asthma and moderate asthma patients: A randomized, double-blind, placebo-controlled trial. *J Nucl Cardiol*. 2008;15(3):329–336.
114. Thomas GS, Tammelin BR, Schiffman GL, et al. Safety of regadenoson, a selective adenosine A2A agonist, in patients

with chronic obstructive pulmonary disease: A randomized, double-blind, placebo-controlled trial (RegCOPD trial). *J Nucl Cardiol.* 2008;15(3):319-328.
115. Prenner BM, Bukofzer S, Behm S, et al. A randomized, double-blind, placebo-controlled study assessing the safety and tolerability of regadenoson in subjects with asthma or chronic obstructive pulmonary disease. *J Nucl Cardiol.* 2012;19(4):681-692.
116. Elliott MD, Holly TA, Leonard SM, et al. Impact of an abbreviated adenosine protocol incorporating adjunctive treadmill exercise on adverse effects and image quality in patients undergoing stress myocardial perfusion imaging. *J Nucl Cardiol.* 2000;7(6):584-589.
117. Thomas GS, Prill NV, Majmundar H, et al. Treadmill exercise during adenosine infusion is safe, results in fewer adverse reactions, and improves myocardial perfusion image quality. *J Nucl Cardiol.* 2000;7(5):439-446.
118. Muller-Suur R, Eriksson SV, Strandberg LE, et al. Comparison of adenosine and exercise stress test for quantitative perfusion imaging in patients on beta-blocker therapy. *Cardiology.* 2001;95(2):112-118.
119. Pennell DJ, Mavrogeni SI, Forbat SM, et al. Adenosine combined with dynamic exercise for myocardial perfusion imaging. *J Am Coll Cardiol.* 1995;25(6):1300-1309.
120. Elhendy AA, Gregory SA, Holly TA, et al. ASNC Announcement. *J Nucl Cardiol.* 2009;16(1):163-163.
121. Holly TA, Satran A, Bromet DS, et al. The impact of adjunctive adenosine infusion during exercise myocardial perfusion imaging: Results of the Both Exercise and Adenosine Stress Test (BEAST) trial. *J Nucl Cardiol.* 2003;10(3):291-296.
122. Vitola JV, Brambatti JC, Caligaris F, et al. Exercise supplementation to dipyridamole prevents hypotension, improves electrocardiogram sensitivity, and increases heart-to-liver activity ratio on Tc-99m sestamibi imaging. *J Nucl Cardiol.* 2001;8(6):652-659.
123. Jamil G, Ahlberg AW, Elliott MD, et al. Impact of limited treadmill exercise on adenosine Tc-99m sestamibi single-photon emission computed tomographic myocardial perfusion imaging in coronary artery disease. *Am J Cardiol.* 1999;84(4):400-403.
124. Samady H, Wackers FJ, Joska TM, et al. Pharmacologic stress perfusion imaging with adenosine: Role of simultaneous low-level treadmill exercise. *J Nucl Cardiol.* 2002;9(2):188-196.
125. Vitola J, Ludwig V, Cunha Pereira Neto C. Exercise and dipyridamole combined myocardial scintigraphy allows early evaluation of perfusion and function. *J Nucl Cardiol.* 2003;10(1):87.
126. Ahlberg AW, Baghdasarian SB, Athar H, et al. Symptom-limited exercise combined with dipyridamole stress: Prognostic value in assessment of known or suspected coronary artery disease by use of gated SPECT imaging. *J Nucl Cardiol.* 2008;15(1):42-56.
127. Thomas GS, Thompson RC, Miyamoto MI, et al. The RegEx trial: A randomized, double-blind, placebo- and active-controlled pilot study combining regadenoson, a selective A(2A) adenosine agonist, with low-level exercise, in patients undergoing myocardial perfusion imaging. *J Nucl Cardiol.* 2009;16(1):63-72.
128. Ross MI, Wu E, Wilkins JT, et al. Safety and feasibility of adjunctive regadenoson injection at peak exercise during exercise myocardial perfusion imaging: The Both Exercise and Regadenoson Stress Test (BERST) trial. *J Nucl Cardiol.* 2013;20(2):197-204.
129. Parker MW, Morales DC, Slim HB, et al. A strategy of symptom-limited exercise with regadenoson-as-needed for stress myocardial perfusion imaging: A randomized controlled trial. *J Nucl Cardiol.* 2013;20(2):185-196.
130. Janvier L, Pinaquy J, Douard H, et al. A useful and easy to develop combined stress test for myocardial perfusion imaging: Regadenoson and isometric exercise, preliminary results. *J Nucl Cardiol.* 2015.

SPECT Myocardial Perfusion Imaging Protocols

CHAPTER 9

Milena J. Henzlova

INTRODUCTION

Single photon-emission computerized tomographic (SPECT) myocardial perfusion imaging (MPI) remains the dominant noninvasive functional imaging perfusion method for the diagnosis as well as prognosis of epicardial coronary artery disease (CAD). The advent and advances of other methods used for similar purposes (cardiac positron emission tomography [PET], stress echocardiography, coronary computerized tomography [CTA], and magnetic resonance imaging [MRI]) have all contributed to recent re-examination of traditional MPI protocols to optimize its use.[1] This task was facilitated by introduction of high-efficiency cadmium zinc telluride (CZT) nuclear cameras and innovative software. With changes in society and concern of radiation exposure, emphasis has shifted from "one size fits all" to patient-centered imaging with individualized approach to each patient's unique constellation of reasons and urgency of testing, comorbidities, age, body habitus, physical ability, and results of previous tests and procedures.[2] In-depth knowledge of the advantages and disadvantages of available radionuclide tracers and stressors by those who perform stress testing and imaging is paramount. Patient participation in decision making becomes desirable, as well.

With an acknowledgment of possibly harmful effects of low radiation doses used at times frequently over an extended period of time due to the chronic nature of CAD, attention has shifted to dose reduction[3] and potentially mandatory tracking of all received radiation doses.[4]

In view of competing noninvasive imaging modalities, cost effectiveness has also been addressed. The length of "traditional" MPI is almost ½ a day, which poorly compares to on average 1 hour to completion and diagnosis using CTA, stress echo, or PET. Many of the newer imaging protocols therefore address the need for increased throughput and improved productivity of a Nuclear Cardiology Laboratory. This chapter will describe protocols for SPECT MPI for the two primary imaging agents, thallium-201 and technetium-based products.

SPECT PROCEDURES

The primary indication for a SPECT MPI study is the assessment of the relative distribution of coronary flow in patients with suspected or known CAD. Since this distribution of coronary flow both at rest and stress is equal in all segments of the left ventricle, the presence of perfusion defects suggests intraluminal coronary obstruction, and if worse at stress than rest, ischemia. An increase in coronary flow is needed for the detection of significant coronary artery stenosis (>50% of luminal narrowing) since rest flow distribution is even unless prior infarction is part of the history. Coronary flow can be increased most physiologically with physical effort (treadmill exercise), or in patients who are unable to exercise adequately, using coronary vasodilators (adenosine, dipyridamole, and regadenoson) or dobutamine (for a more complete description, see Chapter 8).

Evaluation of left ventricular size and function became possible with the development of gating algorithms used in conjunction with MPI. The combination of perfusion and function data improved both the diagnostic and the prognostic value of SPECT studies. ECG-gated SPECT imaging is a powerful tool for evaluating fixed attenuation artifact. Ventricular function assessment and interpretation is described in Chapter 11.

The availability of more than one perfusion tracer and different modes of stress provides a multitude of imaging protocols. Ideally, the imaging protocol should be tailored for the individual patient, taking into account the patient's age, gender, size, physical ability, various comorbidities, and particularly the clinical question to be answered. Laboratory logistics, test urgency, and cost effectiveness also dictate imaging sequences. Knowledge of tracer and stressor characteristics is critical for the right choice and best results.

▶ Thallium-201 Tracer Protocols

Tl-201 (clinically used since the 1970s) is a monovalent cation, analogous to potassium, with a physical half-life of 73.1 hours. Decay is by electron capture to Hg-201, with principal emission of 68- to 80-keV x-rays. First-pass extraction is high (approximately 85%). The tracer is actively transported to the myocyte as well as to other organs and washed out (redistributed) beginning 10 to 15 minutes after an IV injection. The relationship between flow and uptake is almost linear at physiologic flows and even during vasodilator-induced hyperemia. Recommended Tl-201 dose, injected at peak stress is 2.5 to 3.5 mCi. Lower Tl-201 doses are recommended with use of high-efficiency cameras (as low as 1 mCi). The standard effective radiation dose for Tl-201 is approximately 4.4 mSv per 1 mCi of Tl-201, or 10.9 to 15.3 mSv per patient. For a more detailed description, refer to Chapter 3.

▶ Tl-201 Imaging Protocols

Tl-201 is injected approximately 1 minute prior to termination of the exercise or at peak effect of a coronary vasodilator. SPECT imaging must begin within 10 to 15 minutes (Fig. 9-1). The delay is needed for poststress monitoring, patient positioning in the camera, and avoidance of "upward creep," which is caused by cranial motion of the diaphragm due to hyperventilation during stress. Delay in imaging beyond this time may lead to missed ischemia as redistribution begins within 10 to 15 minutes. Tl-201 is by design "stress-first" imaging. Stress images should be reviewed, and, if there are no perfusion defects, rest imaging is unnecessary. The purpose of rest imaging is to ascertain reversibility (redistribution) of perfusion defects seen on stress images. The mechanism of Tl-201 "redistribution" is for the most part due to differential washout from the myocardium. In segments with high initial tracer uptake, that is, in segments supplied by nonobstructed coronary flow and with functional myocytes, washout rate is high. At the time of initial equilibrium (shortly after peak stress tracer injection), intravascular tracer concentration is negligible. In segments supplied by an obstructed epicardial coronary artery, coronary flow is limited and initial tracer uptake is decreased; the intracellular:intravascular tracer gradient is lower and washout rate is slower. After 3 to 4 hours of injection, a second SPECT imaging is obtained (rest scan). If there are no abnormalities, the study is considered normal. If a stress defect appears less prominent or absent on rest, the defect is considered due to ischemia and is consistent with viable but hypoperfused myocardium. If no stress defect reversibility is seen on rest images, the defect is assumed to be scar, possibly due to prior myocardial infarction. If there is concern for missed ischemia, additional imaging can be done either with additional delay (up to 24 hours) or after 1-mCi Tl-201 reinjection. (See strategies as outlined by ASNC guidelines in Fig. 9-1.)

Apart from using Tl-201 for diagnostic or prognostic purposes, Tl-201 is also indicated for detection of myocardial "viability" (Fig. 9-2). The testing should be limited to patients with resting LVEF ≤35% and who are also candidates for myocardial revascularization (surgical or percutaneous). In this case, a rest injection is performed and imaging at 15 to 20 minutes and 3 to 4 hours later. The presence of viability is judged by 50% or greater uptake in the region or vascular territory under consideration (left anterior descending, right or circumflex arteries). If

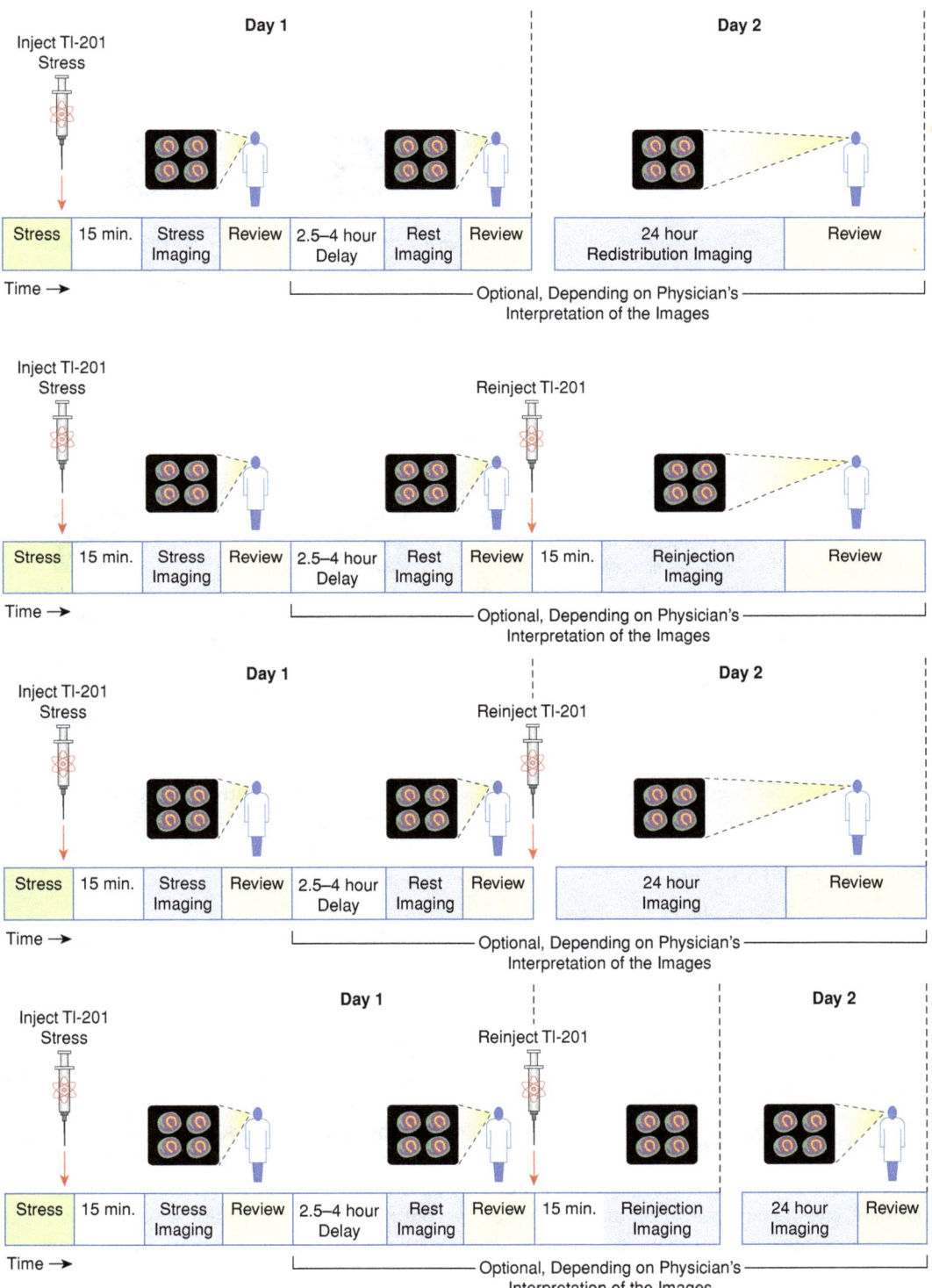

FIGURE 9-1 Thallium-201 protocols from the ASNC imaging guidelines for SPECT. (Reproduced with permission from Henzlova MJ, Duvall WL, Einstein AJ, et al. ASNC imaging guidelines for SPECT nuclear cardiology procedures: Stress, protocols, and tracers. *J Nucl Cardiol.* 2016;23(3):606–639.)

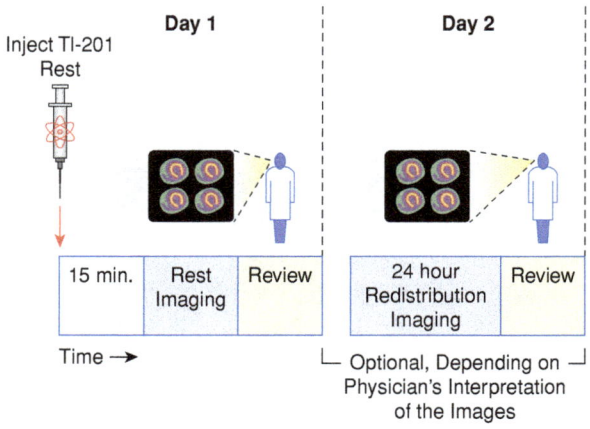

FIGURE 9-2 Thallium-201 viability protocols from ASNC imaging guidelines for SPECT. The primary protocol is rest (15 minutes) followed by 3- to 4-hour delayed imaging. A secondary protocol is delay imaging 24 hours later. (Reproduced with permission from Henzlova MJ, Duvall WL, Einstein AJ, et al. ASNC imaging guidelines for SPECT nuclear cardiology procedures: Stress, protocols, and tracers. *J Nucl Cardiol.* 2016;23(3):606–639.)

viability is not demonstrated on 3- to 4-hour imaging, a 24-hour image can be obtained (Fig. 9-2).

Advantages of Tl-201 Imaging

1. Extensive experience, evidence-based data.
2. No need for delay after stress injection, possible "stress-only" protocol.
3. Good flow-uptake linearity, high first-pass extraction.
4. Absence of liver uptake.
5. Assessment of myocardial viability.

Disadvantages of Tl-201 Imaging

1. Low photon energy (68–80 keV) leads to more prominent soft tissue attenuation artifacts. Also, gated images may be count poor, requiring at times extended imaging time.
2. The long half-life of Tl-201 limits the dosage that can be safely administered to a patient (2.5–4 mCi). This affects the image quality and interpretive certainty due to relatively low counts, making accurate diagnosis more difficult.
3. High radiation dose (>15 mSv) compared to other available tracers.

Technetium-Based SPECT Protocols

Two Tc-99m–based perfusion tracers, Tc-99m-sestamibi (Cardiolite) and Tc-99m-tetrofosmin (Myoview™), are available for clinical use in the United States. Tc-99m agents are lipid soluble, cationic, with a physical half-life of 6 hours, and decay with the emission of 140-keV photons. The first-pass extraction of sestamibi and tetrofosmin is lower (45–50%) compared to Tl-201; therefore, stress needs to continue for at least 1 minute (preferably 2 minutes) after peak stress injection. The tracers are excreted via the hepatobiliary system to the gastrointestinal tract. Tetrofosmin's GI clearance is slightly faster than that of sestamibi. Considerable gut and liver uptake is frequently seen with exercise and pharmacologic stress, although liver activity is more prominent with pharmacologic stress.

Myocardial uptake of Tc-99m-sestamibi and Tc-99m-tetrofosmin is almost linear with increased coronary flow at moderate increases in physiologic coronary flows (such as moderate exercise), but not so with high flows (200–300% increase over rest) at the peak of the vasodilator effect (roll-off phenomenon) or at high exercise level, which could affect sensitivity, and ability to identify multivessel ischemia. The tracers enter the myocytes by passive distribution and are retained in the mitochondria, with negligible tracer redistribution. Therefore, two injections are required: a rest and a separate stress dose. Imaging is usually begun 30 to 45 minutes after the rest injection while poststress injection imaging time is shorter after exercise (15–30 minutes) and longer after coronary vasodilation (45–60 minutes). The reason for delay is subdiaphragmatic tracer uptake, which interferes with image interpretation and lessens over time, and generally is considered worse during pharmacologic stress. Different recommendations have been proposed to reduce these effects, but none have been uniformly successful or accepted. However, it is commonly understood that some level of exercise in conjunction with pharmacologic stress reduces liver uptake.

ECG gating for ventricular function should be done with all Tc-99m studies, when possible. Gating should be performed during both the rest and poststress acquisitions. If using a 1-day rest/stress protocol, the quality of the high-dose images is superior due to higher count rate than at rest, but still can be used for comparative purposes, especially wall motion abnormalities. Since imaging is done early after stress (15–45 minutes), the calculated left ventricular ejection fraction (LVEF) and ventricular volumes do not represent true resting values, but rather "early poststress EF/LV volumes" and should be reported as such. In patients with extensive ischemia, these obtained values can reflect transient stunning; underestimation of the true rest LVEF is possible and has consequences for therapeutic decisions (e.g., AICD implantation and ACE inhibitor initiation). For a more detailed description, refer to Chapter 11.

Knowledge of Tc-99m–based agent's characteristics provides considerable flexibility of imaging protocols. The test can be completed in 1 or 2 days and the study protocol can be tailored to individual patient needs with stress–rest, rest–stress, or stress-only sequences.

Given the 6-hour physical half-life of Tc-99m, a 24-hour separation between the two injections is optimal to minimize background radioactivity for the second set of images. In clinical practice, however, having patients undergo imaging on 2 separate days may be inconvenient or impractical. In addition, it is more efficacious to have all the information from both studies available on the same day. However, both 2- and 1-day protocols for rest and stress imaging have been developed (Fig. 9-3).

For 2-day protocols, the Tc-99m–labeled agent is injected at peak stress (20–30 mCi) and imaged within 15 to 45 minutes. This is followed at least 24 hours (approximately 4 half-lives) later by a second injection at rest and a second set of images. A 2-day protocol is often needed in patients with a high BMI (>30), since low-dose rest images, as used in 1-day protocols, are more likely nondiagnostic due to poor image quality. Alternatively, the order of the injections for a 2-day test can be reversed, with the stress study being performed first and rest injection at least 24 hours later, using high tracer dose (20–30 mCi) for both injections.

The more common protocol is that in which both the rest and stress are performed on the same day.[5] It is estimated that this protocol is used 90% of the time. In general, the rest is performed first, followed by the stress portion. In order to offset the residual activity of the first injection, it has been determined that the rest: stress tracer dose should be 1:3. The suggested[1] rest dose is 8 to 12 mCi and stress dose is 24 to 36 mCi. A rest–stress sequence is preferable when using a 1-day protocol because the rest image performed initially represents a "true" rest study. This is not necessarily the case with the stress–rest sequence due to cross-talk from the stress study present in the rest images. If the stress–rest sequence is used, a longer time interval or a higher rest dose is needed. In addition, the first study is of lesser quality due to the lower dose and using standard equipment in most laboratories it is preferable that this be the rest study. For newer cameras such as with CZT detectors or OSEM processing, the image quality of a low-dose stress may be acceptable and the sequence preferable if considering a "stress-only" or "stress-first"

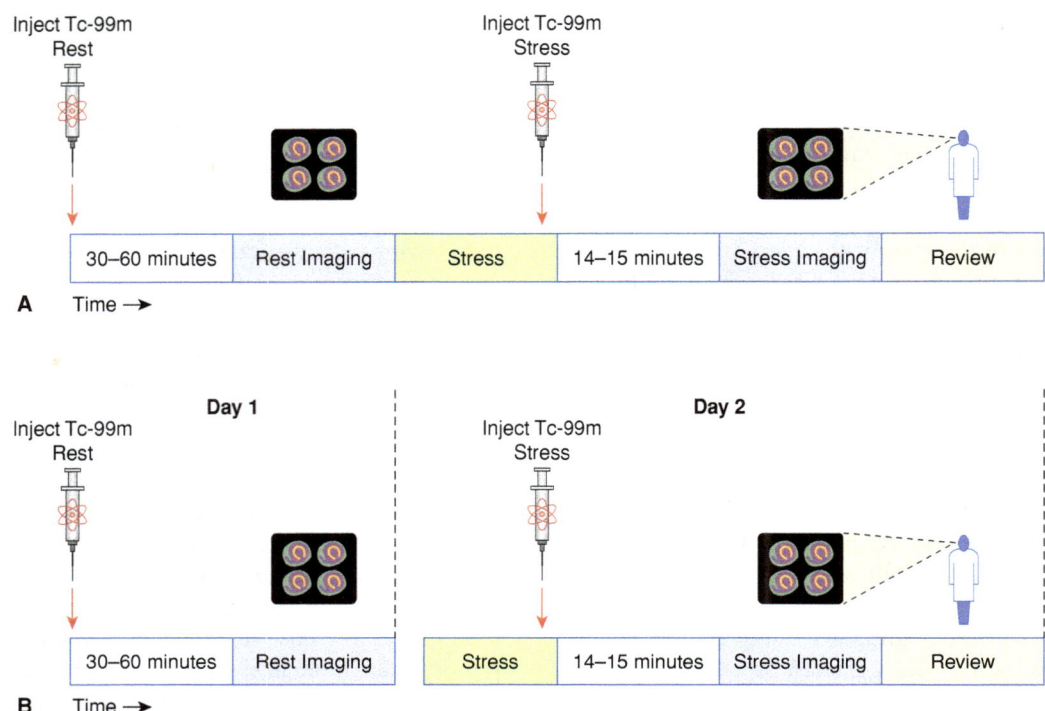

FIGURE 9-3 One- and 2-day technetium-99 protocols from ASNC guidelines for SPECT. The 1-day rest/stress protocol is in Panel **A** and 2-day protocol is in Panel **B**. (Reproduced with permission from Henzlova MJ, Duvall WL, Einstein AJ, et al. ASNC imaging guidelines for SPECT nuclear cardiology procedures: Stress, protocols, and tracers. *J Nucl Cardiol.* 2016;23(3):606–639.)

protocol. As many new protocols are being suggested it is advised to follow the current literature.

Rest–stress and stress–rest protocols for Tc-99m-sestamibi SPECT imaging have been compared and demonstrated that the former sequence provides better image contrast and an increased ability to detect reversibility of perfusion defects. The 1-day stress–rest protocol offers advantages that must be taken into consideration: it allows for the elimination of the rest study if the stress study is found to be normal similar to a planned 2-day study (see section on stress-only imaging).

The estimated radiation dose to a 70-kg adult using ICRP 60 calculation is 15.7 mSv for a 2-day high-dose study, 11.3 mSv for a 1-day rest–stress study, and 7.9 mSv for a stress-only study.[6]

Tc-99m–labeled agents, compared to Tl-201, allow more flexibility and more "tailoring" of the test sequences to patient needs. Other advantages include a higher photon flux (higher injected dose) and higher photon energy (140 keV), which result in better image quality and clarity. Images are of higher quality, attenuation artifacts are slightly less prominent, and gated images are also of higher quality than thallium-201. The disadvantages in relation to Tl-201 include considerably more gut and liver uptake and less linearity of blood flow, potentially reducing diagnostic accuracy.

Advantages of Tc-99m Agents

1. Flexibility of imaging protocols.
2. Higher image quality, reduced soft tissue attenuation compared to Tl-201.
3. Well-documented accuracy and risk stratification data.
4. Lower radiation exposure compared to Tl-201.

Disadvantages of Tc-99m Agents

1. Nonlinearity of flow and uptake may affect detection of moderate coronary lesions and multivessel ischemia.

2. Considerable gut and liver uptake resulting in reduced specificity.
3. Modest diagnostic accuracy.

Dual-Isotope Imaging

A dual-radionuclide imaging protocol was introduced, validated, and popularized in the early 1990s.[7] This protocol consists of an injection of 3.0 to 3.5 mCi of Tl-201 at rest, imaging and of 25 to 30 mCi of Tc-99m-sestamibi at peak stress (Fig. 9-4).[7] SPECT imaging begins 10 to 15 minutes after the initial injection of Tl-201 at rest. Immediately following Tl-201 imaging, the patient performs the stress part of the test (exercise or pharmacologic). At peak stress, a dose of 25 to 30 mCi of Tc-99m-sestamibi or Tc-99m-tetrofosmin is injected. Imaging starts 15 to 45 minutes later depending upon whether exercise or pharmacologic stress (generally 15 minutes after exercise stress, 45 minutes after pharmacologic stress). The separate acquisition dual-radionuclide imaging procedure can be completed in approximately 2 to 3 hours.

The dual-radionuclide imaging protocol is shorter than a 1-day Tc-99m-sestamibi/tetrofosmin protocol. Although imaging time does not change, time is saved since Tl-201 rest images are acquired shortly after the tracer injection as there is minimal liver or gut uptake. Sequential imaging is performed without contribution of the rest counts to the stress image (as is the case of low-dose–high-dose Tc-99m imaging). However, this protocol also presents some

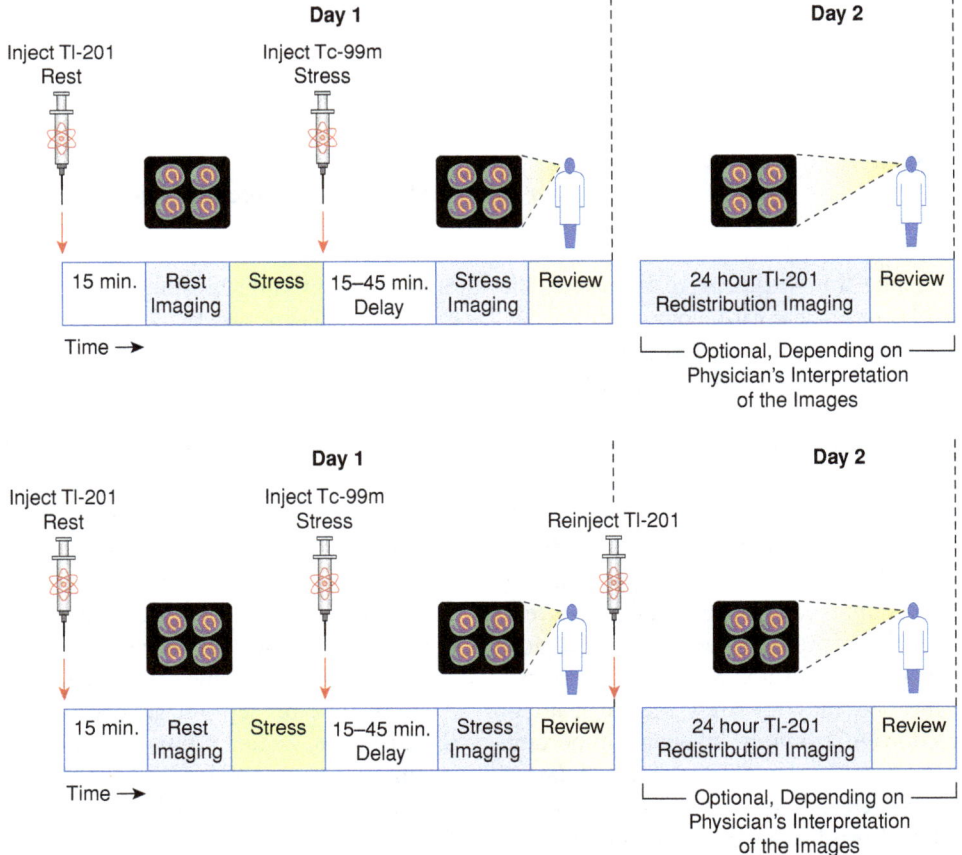

FIGURE 9-4 Dual-isotope protocols from ASNC guidelines for SPECT. Thallium-201 is used as the rest tracer followed by Tc-99m technetium as the stress tracer (either sestamibi or tetrofosmin). (Reproduced with permission from Henzlova MJ, Duvall WL, Einstein AJ, et al. ASNC imaging guidelines for SPECT nuclear cardiology procedures: Stress, protocols, and tracers. *J Nucl Cardiol.* 2016;23(3):606–639.)

disadvantages. The physical characteristics of the two radionuclides involved are quite different, resulting in a different count density. This may affect the evaluation of the degree of defect reversibility, especially in patients with prior myocardial infarction and an abnormal Tl-201 rest study. Furthermore, the quality of the rest Tl-201 studies is sometimes suboptimal. Visual interpretation of transient ischemic cavity dilation (TID) is difficult to assess due to inherent differences in thallium and technetium images.

A major concern and disadvantage is the radiation exposure of this protocol. The estimated radiation dose of a dual-isotope study could be very high: >20 mSv. Thus, as with the Tl-201 only study, routine use of this protocol is not recommended by national societies and guidelines.[1,8] It may be justified in the evaluation of patients with severe congestive heart failure, when viability detection is of importance for therapeutic decisions (revascularization, medical therapy, or cardiac transplantation).

▶ Stress-Only or Stress-First Imaging to Reduce Patient Radiation

The most common stress protocol is that of rest imaging first, followed by stress MPI, as previously described. Despite this, it has been estimated that only 8% to 10% of nuclear cardiology studies demonstrate ischemia.[9] Thus, in a majority of studies, a rest study is of no clinical value, particularly when the stress study is completely normal. It has been proposed for several years that performing the stress first, and rest only when necessary would be a reasonable means of reducing patient radiation. The "stress-only" or "stress-first" protocols have been recommended by ASNC for several years.[10,11] Using this approach, the number of rest studies can be substantially reduced, thus shortening the protocol for the patient and reducing radiation exposure. Since decisions are made with only one study, the stress, the use of attenuation correction (AC) or prone imaging is important in reducing the number of unnecessary rest studies.[10]

An important consideration of stress-only imaging is the administered stress dose. In older camera systems, a low stress dose of 8 to 15 mCi of Tc-99m may yield an image that is difficult to interpret due to poor image quality and attenuation artifact. Thus, with these systems, this protocol may require a high-dose stress study (25–30 mCi), but will still avoid the rest radiation exposure in most circumstances. The radiation reduction is even greater when low-dose stress only (8–15 mCi) protocols are utilized with appropriate and newer camera systems (see below). Significant reduction (35–85%) in the need for rest images is seen when AC is applied to image processing.[10] In a study by Mathur et al. using stress only with AC in a chest pain center environment, only 8% required a rest study, and at least ½ of these patients had evidence of scar.[11]

The optimal candidates for stress-only imaging are patients with no known history of CAD and secondarily those with CAD but no history of myocardial infarction or bypass surgery. In addition, patient with CAD who had a recent stress MPI study for comparison could also be considered candidates. Less optimal candidates are those with prior MI, CABG, or ventricular dysfunction. Ideally an interpreting physician should be available to decide on whether a rest study is indicated in order to complete the study in an efficacious manner.

▶ Use of Newer Technologies

There have been many recent advancements in camera technology and software which impact protocols and radiation exposure.[12]

Solid state cameras employ the use of different detector technology from the more common Anger cameras. Solid-state cameras use CZT or cesium-iodide (CsI) semiconductor detectors. CZT cameras are also called high-efficiency cameras,[1,12] and hold the potential to dramatically decrease tracer doses and reduce imaging times. Laboratory efficiency is improved particularly for high-volume laboratories, thus potentially offsetting higher purchase prices of these new cameras. The downside of a CZT camera includes lack of efficient motion detection and AC, presence of new imaging artifacts unique to these systems, limited utility for morbidly obese and immobile patients and lack of versatility compared to traditional NaI cameras (only cardiac imaging is feasible). A more complete discussion of this technology is in Chapter 4.

Novel processing software is offered for most newly purchased traditional SPECT cameras; most <10 years old NaI Anger cameras can be retrofitted. Proprietary variation of resolution recovery/noise reduction is implemented into iterative reconstruction software. Software is offered by Philips (Astonish™), Siemens (Flash 3D), GE Healthcare (Evolution), Digirad (Nspeed); wide beam reconstruction (WBR) is offered by a third-party vendor (Ultra SPECT), as well as ImagenSPECT from Cardiovascular Imaging Technologies (CVIT). Each of the algorithms has been clinically validated and will allow ½ dose and/or ½ time acquisition.

CONCLUSIONS

This chapter has described the current protocols for SPECT MPI with Tl-201 and Tc-99m. Careful attention is given to the time required for each protocol as well as radiation exposure. Stress-only or stress-first imaging should be considered for selected patients as a means of reducing radiation exposure and improving laboratory efficiency. Newer camera technologies and software innovations offer the potential of radiation dose reduction as well as more time-efficient protocols.

REFERENCES

1. Henzlova MJ, Duvall WL, Einstein AJ, et al. ASNC imaging guidelines for SPECT nuclear cardiology procedures: Stress, protocols, and tracers. *J Nucl Cardiol.* 2016;23:606–639.
2. DePuey EG, Mahmarian JJ, Miller TD, et al. Patient centered imaging. *J Nucl Cardiol.* 2012;19:185–215.
3. Jerome SD, Tilkemeier PL, Farrell MB, et al. Nationwide Laboratory adherence to myocardial perfusion imaging radiation dose reduction practices. A report from Intersocietal Accreditation Commission Data Repository. *JACC Cardiovascular Imaging.* 2015;8:1170–1176.
4. Neumann RD, Bluemke DA. Tracking radiation exposure from diagnostic imaging devices at the NIH. *J Am Coll Radiol.* 2010;7:87–89.
5. Taillefer R, Gagnon A, Laflamme L, et al. Same day injections of Tc-99m methoxy isobutyl isonitrile (hexamibi) for myocardial tomographic imaging: Comparison between rest–stress and stress–rest injection sequences. *Eur J Nucl Med.* 1989;15:113–117.
6. Mattsson S, Johansson L, Leide Svegborn S, et al.; International Commission on Radiological Protection. Radiation dose to patients from radiopharmaceuticals: A compendium of current information related to frequently used substances. ICRP Publication 128. *Ann ICRP.* 2015;44(2S):7–321.
7. Berman DS, Kiat H, Friedman JD, et al. Separate acquisition rest thallium-201/stress technetium-99m sestamibi dual-isotope myocardial perfusion single-photon emission computed tomography: A clinical validation study. *J Am Coll Cardiol.* 1993;22:1455–1464.
8. Cerqueira M, Allman K, Ficaro E, et al. Recommendations for reducing radiation exposure in myocardial perfusion imaging. *J Nucl Cardiol.* 2010;17:709–718.
9. Rozanski A, Gransar H, Hayes S, et al. Temporal trends in the frequency of inducible myocardial ischemia during cardiac stress testing: 1991–2009. *J Am Coll Cardiol.* 2013;61:1054–1065.
10. Gowd BM, Heller GV, Parker MW. Stress-only SPECT myocardial perfusion imaging: A review. *Nucl Cardiol.* 2014;21:1200–1212.
11. Mathur S, Heller G, Bateman T, et al. Clinical value of stress-only Tc-99m SPECT Imaging: Importance of attenuation correction. *J Nucl Cardiol.* 2013;20:27–37.
12. Slomka PJ, Dey D, Duvall WL, et al. Advances in nuclear cardiac instrumentation with a view towards reduced radiation exposure. *Curr Cardiol Rep.* 2012;14:208–216.

Cardiovascular Positron Emission Tomography

CHAPTER 10

Justin B. Lundbye and Gary V. Heller

INTRODUCTION

Cardiac positron emission tomography (PET) myocardial perfusion imaging is an outstanding tool for diagnosis and risk stratification of patients with known or suspected coronary artery disease with many important differences compared to SPECT imaging. Its clinical use in assessing patients for CAD as well as other nonperfusion indications is expanding rapidly. Cardiac PET offers excellent diagnostic accuracy and image quality, low radiation exposure as well as a noninvasive means of measuring myocardial blood flow reserve. Cardiovascular PET is becoming an important tool for nuclear cardiologists to consider not only for perfusion imaging, but also for a growing number of other cardiovascular conditions such as myocardial viability, infection, and inflammation. Its role in nuclear cardiology has expanded with the increased and continuous availability of PET radiopharmaceuticals and PET camera systems (see Chapters 3 and 4 on radiopharmaceuticals and instrumentation). This chapter will review the principles of cardiovascular PET, data on diagnostic accuracy, image quality, radiation exposure, indications, and addition of myocardial blood flow (MBF) for myocardial perfusion imaging (MPI), as well as exciting new nonperfusion applications.

PRINCIPLES OF CARDIAC PET

PET imaging provides superior temporal and spatial resolution of radioactive atoms as they decay. A PET radioactive tracer, which has been engineered to be taken up in to the organ of interest, is injected into the patient. After it reaches the target organ, the radioactive agent begins to decay and emits a positron (Fig. 10-1). This positron then collides with a nearby electron. The resulting collision causes annihilation of both an electron and a positron, creating a high-energy discharge of 1.02 MeV.

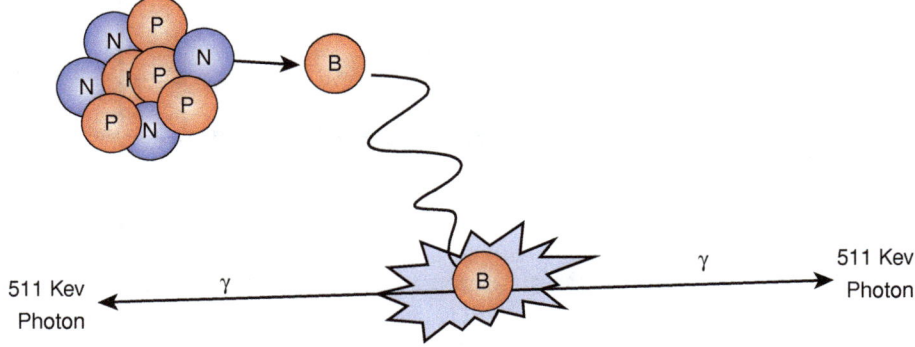

FIGURE 10-1 Annihilation event during PET imaging.

This energy is split into two gamma rays of 511-keV energy, which are emitted 180 degrees from each other. For image collection, multiple detectors encircle the patient; absorption from both emissions simultaneously occurs, and events that are not 180% are eliminated. The distance to the annihilation event impacts ultimate image quality. The processing of these simultaneous events forms the basis of PET imaging.[1]

CARDIAC PET INSTRUMENTATION

Cardiac PET instrumentation is discussed in detail in Chapter 4. A PET camera appearance is similar to a computed axial tomography (CT) system. However, in the gantry of the PET camera are multiple detectors placed circularly around the patient (Fig. 10-2). These detectors are grouped into cassettes filled with a specified number of crystals (4,000–24,000). Data from the crystals are then transmitted to photomultiplier tubes similar to Single Photon Emission Computed Tomography (SPECT) imaging. In contrast to SPECT acquisition which requires multiple acquisitions from the same crystals rotating spatially around the patient, PET data acquisition occurs simultaneously surrounding the patient. Most scanners are full-ring design but some have partial-ring detectors with a rapidly rotating gantry.[2] An attenuation correction scan with either PET radionuclide line source or computed tomography (CT) is an integral part of the acquisition and is applied to each study.

RADIOACTIVE ISOTOPES USED FOR CARDIAC PET MYOCARDIAL IMAGING

While there are several myocardial tracers available for PET imaging, only three are presently used for clinical imaging: rubidium-82 (Rb-82), N-13 ammonia (N-13), and fluorine-18 (^{18}F) fluorodeoxyglucose (FDG). For complete review of PET isotopes, see Chapter 3.

▶ Rubidium-82

Rubidium (Rb)-82 is a potassium analog radiopharmaceutical that is produced with commercially available generators which can be stored on site. It is produced by the decay of strontium-82 (^{82}Sr) which has a half-life of 25.5 days. Rb-82 has a half-life of 75 seconds. The extraction fraction of Rb-82 is estimated to be 65% to 75%, substantially higher than SPECT technetium agents.

The use of Rb-82 is provided by an on-site generator and delivery system, which can be stored conveniently in the camera room. The generator is replaced every 4 to 6 weeks and supplied at a fixed cost, independent of the number of studies performed. Because of the cost involved with the generator, consideration for PET use in a facility should include adequate patient volumes. When in use, the generator is replenished quickly, within 10 minutes via ^{82}Sr to Rb-82 decay. This permits minimal downtime between stress and rest imaging, allowing efficient utilization of the generator. The protocol for

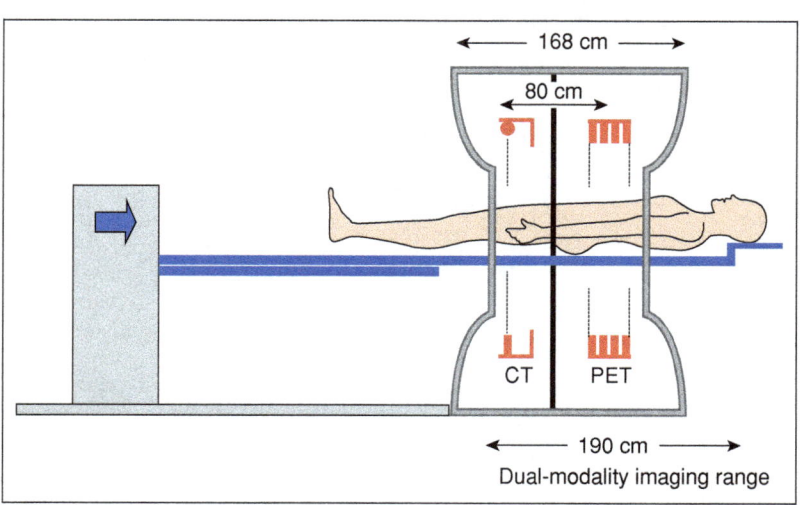

FIGURE 10-2 PET-CT camera. CT instrumentation is in the front of the camera, PET in the back. (Reproduced with permission from Townsend DW. Dual-modality imaging: Combining anatomy and function. *J Nucl Med.* 2008;49(6):938–955.)

stress imaging requires the use of a pharmacologic stress agent because of the short half-life of Rb-82.

Advantages of Rb-82 include the ability to have rapid acquisition times for rest and stress imaging and continuous availability. Another advantage was studied by Parkash et al.[3] They used Rb-82 with PET/CT imaging and were able to detect smaller perfusion abnormalities and more accurate detecting multivessel disease. This suggests that PET may be able to detect multivessel disease more accurately than with SPECT-imaging techniques.[4]

There are also disadvantages to Rb-82 imaging. Due to the half-life of ^{82}Sr, the same generator is used for 4 to 6 weeks, but with reduced activity during the last weeks, which can impact image quality, with cameras using 2D acquisition. This limitation, however, can be overcome by 3D imaging.[5] The short half-life of rubidium limits its clinical use to pharmacologic stress and not exercise.

N-13 Ammonia

N-13 has been used as a cardiac tracer for over 20 years. Implementation requires the presence of an on-site cyclotron as it has a half-life of 9.96 minutes. N-13 has an extraction fraction of up to 80%. The overall trapping of N-13 is dependent on a properly functioning metabolism and trapping may be decreased in myocytes that are ischemic.[6,7] Advantages of N-13 ammonia include the high tomographic counts and a clear blood-to-myocardial delineation. Because of the longer half-life, exercise is possible, in contrast to rubidium. Limitations include the finding that even in normal subjects, the retention of N-13 in the lateral wall is 10% less than other segments creating false-positive results.[8] Prominent liver activity in some studies can complicate interpretation of the inferior wall.[9] Finally, the necessity for on-site or close proximity cyclotron availability due to short half-life limits its practical use. This has severely limited its use, with perhaps 15 to 20 laboratories using this agent according to recent data. This may change with the availability of a small cyclotron designed for ammonia production only that is much more manageable and can be placed onsite.

Fluorine-18 Fluorodeoxyglucose

FDG is fluorine-labeled with 2-deoxyglucose. It is cyclotron produced and decays into O-18 oxygen. When it decays, its positron range is very short (0.5 mm). This fact, combined with its half-life of 109.8 minutes, allows it to provide images with the highest spatial resolution of any of the commonly used radionuclides.

FDG is a glucose analog and is brought into the myocardium via diffusion across glucose-specific transporters that are located on the myocytes. Once in the cell, it is transformed into FDG-6-P. There are low levels of glucose-6-phosphatase to reverse this step; there the FDG-6-P is essentially trapped in the myocardial cell. The use of F-18-FDG is further elaborated on the viability discussion later in the chapter as well as Chapter 21. Active research is underway to validate F-18 Flurpiridaz, a blood flow agent for the detection of CAD.

BENEFITS OF CARDIAC PET MYOCARDIAL PERFUSION IMAGING

The increasing clinical use of cardiac PET MPI is due to several features that clinicians find important for their laboratories as well as patient care. This section will outline demonstrated advantages including imaging quality, diagnostic accuracy, radiation exposure, assessment of MBF, and conclude with a section on which patients are either recommended or preferred for PET MPI.[10]

Excellent Image Quality

Myocardial PET perfusion imaging utilizes high-energy level radiopharmaceutical tracers, with short half-lives. This translates into relatively higher doses being administered (but with lower radiation exposure) and better acquisition characteristics. The result is high myocardial counts, high spatial and contrast resolution, and high signal-to-noise ratio. Improved PET image quality was demonstrated by Yoshinaga et al., in which patients with equivocal SPECT studies were referred for cardiac PET imaging.[11] In a very high percentage of patients, the PET study resulted in good to excellent image quality. Using a comparison of similar but matched patients undergoing SPECT or PET, Bateman et al. also reported a significant improvement in image quality with PET over SPECT, with fewer equivocal reports.[12]

The routine use of attenuation correction plus higher-energy levels of PET tracers substantially reduces attenuation artifacts in images, reducing the potential for false-positive studies for interpretation.

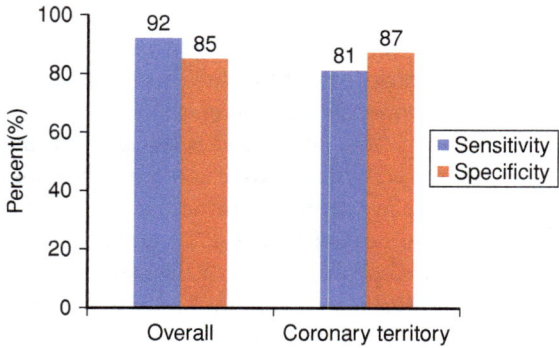

FIGURE 10-3 Meta-analysis of diagnostic accuracy literature for cardiac PET perfusion imaging. (Data from Nandalur KR, Dwamena BA, Choudhri AF, et al. Diagnostic performance of positron emission tomography in the detection of coronary artery disease: A meta-analysis. *Acad Radiol.* 2008;15:444–451.)

patients. Thus, while obese patients or patients with prior equivocal SPECT studies are excellent candidates for PET imaging, the high accuracy among all patients suggests even broader application.[10] In addition, the incidence of gut activity affecting interpretation was significantly and substantially reduced with PET in relation to pharmacologic SPECT.[12]

▶ Diagnostic Accuracy with Cardiac PET Perfusion

The literature suggests that PET has high sensitivity and specificity. A meta-analysis of Nandalur et al. demonstrated high diagnostic accuracy from the available PET literature in over 1400 patients (Fig. 10-3).[13] Two subsequent and larger studies have confirmed these findings, including a systematic review by Mc Ardle et al. which demonstrated that the sensitivity and specificity utilizing Rb-82 was 90% and 88%, respectively.[14] A separate meta-analysis of 11,862 patients by Parker et al., PET MPI, also demonstrated a higher diagnostic accuracy for coronary artery disease than SPECT MPI (Figs. 10-4 and 10-5).[15] Both of these studies also compared PET to

This may be particularly useful in obese patients however, in a study by Bateman et al. the specificity of PET was significantly higher in comparison to SPECT, regardless of body habitus.[12] Similarly, patients who had equivocal SPECT studies were found to have diagnostically useful PET studies in 98% of the referred

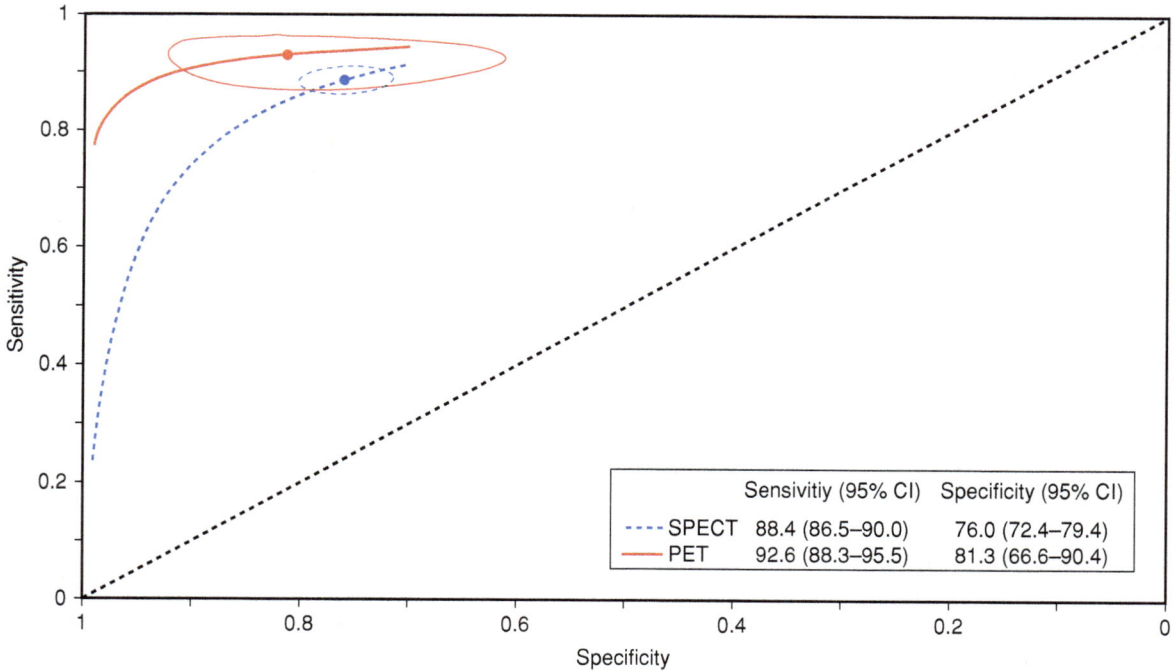

FIGURE 10-4 Meta-analysis of the diagnostic accuracy of PET perfusion. (Data from Parker MW, Iskandar A, Limone B, et al. Diagnostic accuracy of cardiac positron emission tomography versus single photon emission computed tomography for coronary artery disease: A bivariate meta-analysis. *Circ Cardiovasc Imaging.* 2012;5:700–707.)

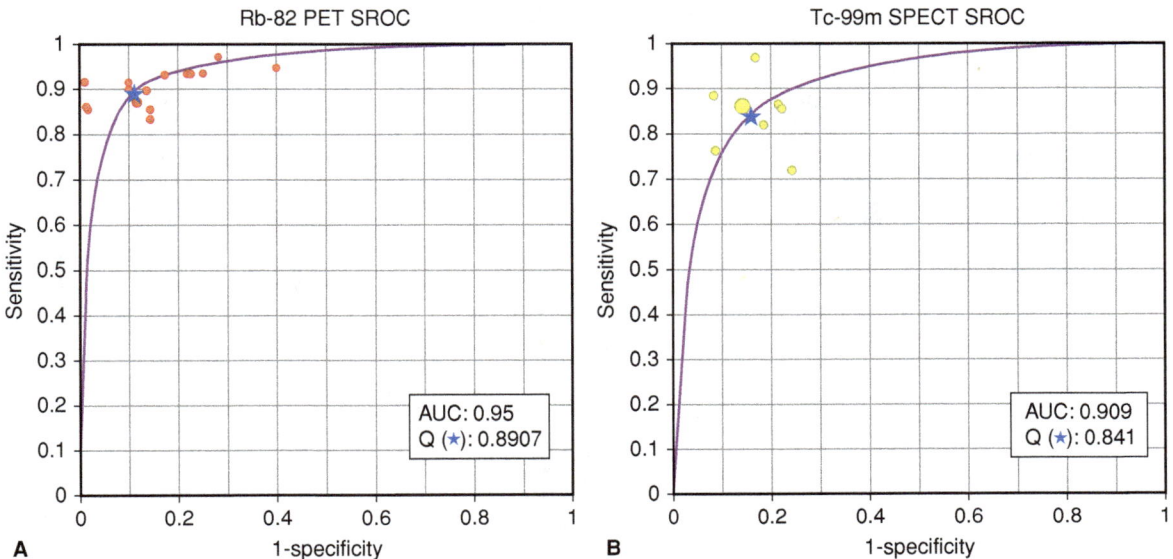

FIGURE 10-5 A systematic review and meta-analysis of PET perfusion. Panel A: PET and Panel B: SPECT. (Data from Mc Ardle BA, Dowsley TF, deKemp RA, et al. Does rubidium-82 PET have superior accuracy to SPECT perfusion imaging for the diagnosis of obstructive coronary disease? A systematic review and meta-analysis. *J Am Coll Cardiol.* 2012;60:1828–1837.)

SPECT literature and found significantly higher diagnostic accuracy for PET. Many of these reported studies in these two analyses used dedicated PET cameras with line source attenuation correction. A study by Sampson et al. also confirmed high diagnostic accuracy with the PET/CT instrumentation.[16]

A direct clinical comparison of SPECT to PET in similar patients was performed by Bateman et al.[12] Over 120 age-, body habitus-, and risk factor-matched patients underwent SPECT or PET imaging and cardiac catheterization. Significantly improved diagnostic accuracy was identified in patients undergoing PET perfusion imaging. Importantly, the ability to identify multivessel ischemia with PET was also significantly higher (74% vs. 41%) than with SPECT perfusion imaging, confirming the findings of Parkash.[3] In sub-study analysis, diagnostic accuracy held regardless of body mass index or gender (Fig. 10-6).

RADIATION EXPOSURE WITH CARDIAC PET IMAGING

Minimizing radiation exposure is an important consideration when ordering a diagnostic test. Efforts have been made on a national level to encourage the lowest radiation exposure possible in patients undergoing diagnostic testing with either CT or nuclear imaging, without sacrificing on image quality and diagnostic accuracy. With these concerns, the American Society of Nuclear Cardiology (ASNC) published an information statement in 2010 recommending radiation exposure for a patient study to be less than 9 mSv.[17] However, a report by Jerome et al. subsequent to this recommendation, found that <1% of SPECT studies met these criteria and the mean radiation exposure was 14.6 mSv, far exceeding doses recommended.[18] In contrast, radiation exposure for cardiac PET studies is substantially less than ASNC recommendations. For example, in a study by Senthamizhchelvan et al., radiation exposure from an Rb-82 PET study was calculated to be 9 mSv/20 mCi, translating to 3 to 6 mSv per patient depending on instrumentation.[19] These findings were confirmed by Hunter et al. in a single-center study in which the PET radiation exposure was calculated to be as low as 1 to 3 mSv.[20] On a national basis, a recent study by Lundbye et al.[21] confirmed that radiation exposure to patients using either Rb-82 or NH_3 ammonia was an average of 3.59 mSv in 122 laboratories undergoing accreditation evaluation by the Intersocietal Accreditation Commission (Fig. 10-7). These data support

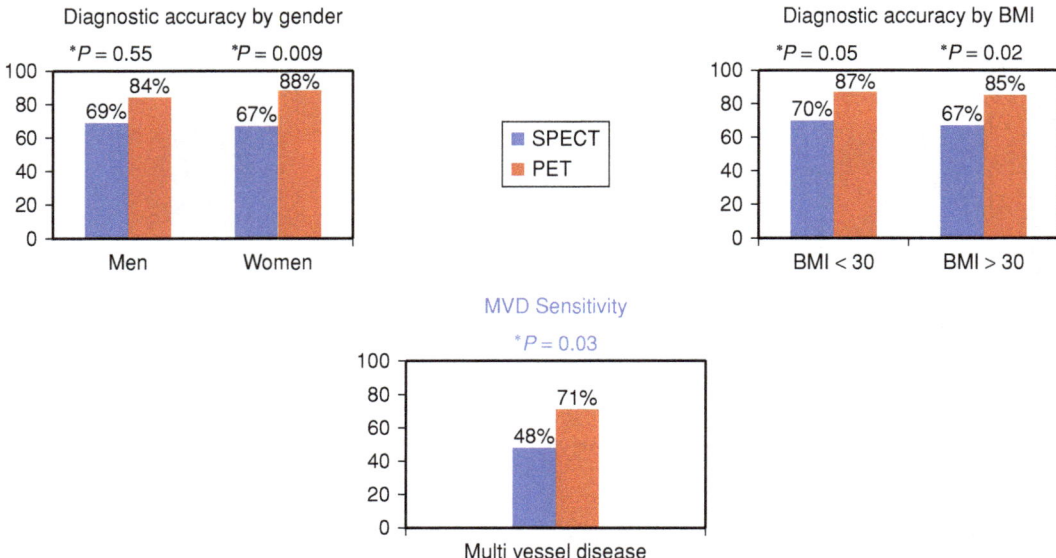

FIGURE 10-6 Cardiac diagnostic accuracy comparing SPECT with PET. (Data from Bateman TM, Heller GV, McGhie AI, et al. Diagnostic accuracy of rest/stress ECG-gated Rb-82 myocardial perfusion PET: Comparison with ECG-gated Tc-99m sestamibi SPECT. *J Nucl Cardiol.* 2006;13(1):24–33.)

the ASNC information statement recommendation of using cardiac PET for radiation reduction in patients undergoing nuclear cardiology studies when available.[17,22] In summary, cardiac PET perfusion imaging radiation exposure to patients is low and generally consistent with annual background levels (3–4 mSv), substantially lower than current SPECT practices and is lower than ASNC recommendations.

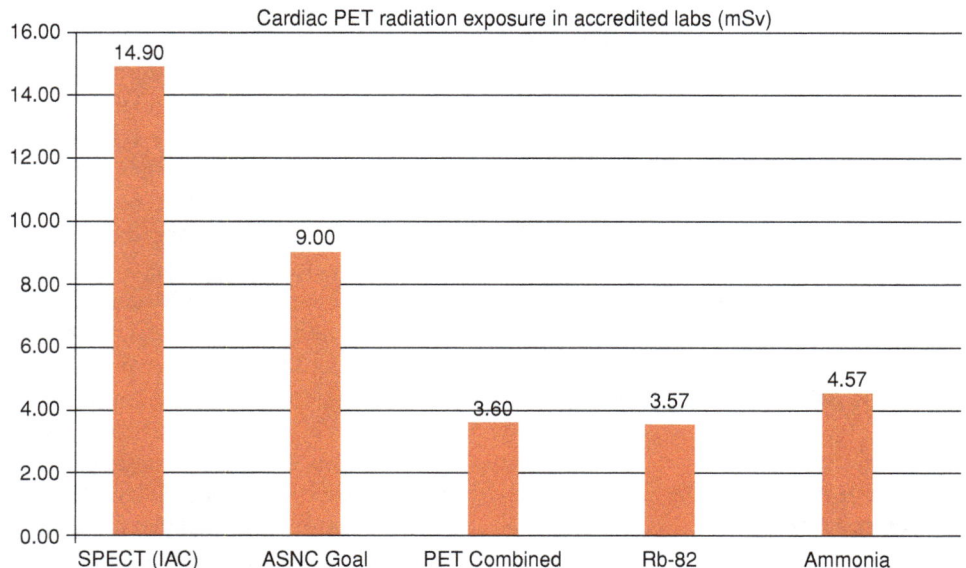

FIGURE 10-7 Cardiac PET compared to SPECT and ASNC recommendations. (Reproduced with permission from Abstracts of Original Contributions ASNC2016 The 21st Annual Scientific Session of the American Society of Nuclear Cardiology: September 22-25, 2016 Boca Raton, FL. *J Nucl Cardiol.* 2016;23(4):899–937.)

Risk Stratification with Cardiac PET Perfusion Imaging

Risk stratification with SPECT imaging has become a very important aspect of the success of this modality. There now is growing evidence supporting the substantial prognostic value of cardiac PET. Several small and limited studies demonstrated the concept that the size and severity of the PET perfusion study predicts subsequent cardiac events. The largest study to date was that of Dorbala et al. published in 2013 (Fig. 10-8).[23] This multicenter study of over 7000 patients, evaluated outcomes in patients undergoing pharmacologic stress Rb-82 PET imaging. In a 2- to 3-year follow-up evaluation, the ability of the rubidium PET study to characterize patients into low, intermediate, and high risk for either cardiac death or all-cause mortality was demonstrated (Panels A, B). Two important aspects of that study emerged. First, the patients in the moderate- to high-risk category had a much higher event rate than similar SPECT studies, most likely due to the ability of the imaging procedure

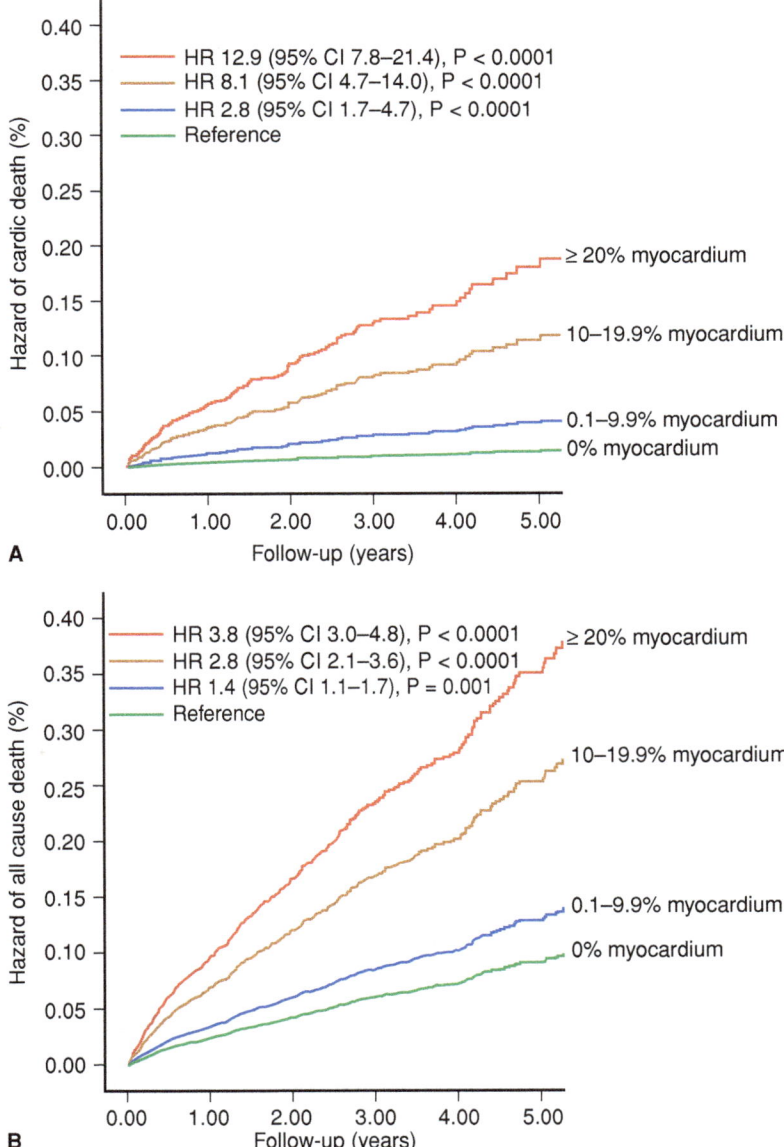

FIGURE 10-8 Prognostic value of positron emission tomography (PET) myocardial perfusion imaging (MPI) and the improved classification of risk. Panel A: cardiac death and Panel B: all cause death. (Reproduced with permission from Dorbala S, Di Carli MF, Beanlands RS, et al. Prognostic value of stress myocardial perfusion positron emission tomography: results from a multicenter observational registry. *J Am Coll Cardiol.* 2013;61(2):176-184.)

to more accurately identify multivessel CAD. Second, those in the lower-risk group had annualized event rates of less than 1%. This finding is in contrast to a pharmacologic SPECT study in which the risk of events is higher, 1% to 2%.[24] This is a reassuring finding for patients undergoing pharmacologic stress imaging with PET.

In a subset of patients separated by gender, similar risk stratification was demonstrated for both male and female patients.[23] These data are particularly important in an era in which women undergo evaluation at an earlier stage than previously and are expected to have a longer longevity than men, placing radiation exposure reduction of considerable importance.

Rb-82 left ventricular ejection fraction reserve (peak stress minus rest ejection fraction) provides incremental prognostic value to clinical data, rest left ventricular ejection fraction, and myocardial perfusion data including the identification of multivessel disease.[25-27] In a study by Lertsburapa et al. in 1600 patients, the relationship between all-cause mortality, perfusion-summed stress score, and ejection fraction was evaluated. The results indicate that the highest-risk patients were those with a high-summed stress score and a low ejection fraction (Fig. 10-9),[28] as also noted with SPECT.

CLINICAL VALUE OF MYOCARDIAL BLOOD FLOW ASSESSMENT

An important and unique capability of cardiac PET perfusion imaging is the ability to measur myocardial blood flow (MBF). Typically, both PET and SPECT evaluate differences in regional uptake between rest and stress to identify patterns consistent with coronary stenosis. While this approach has been very useful, and this chapter has emphasized the important advantages of PET MPI, there are still limitations. The presence of normal perfusion does not exclude "balanced" ischemia ever with PET the abnormality present may underestimate the extent of CAD, and with pharmacologic stress one does not know whether the stress agent is successful at increasing blood flow. Currently, PET is unique as a noninvasive tool in its documented ability to measure regional and global MBF. MBF is commonly provided as a relationship between rest and stress

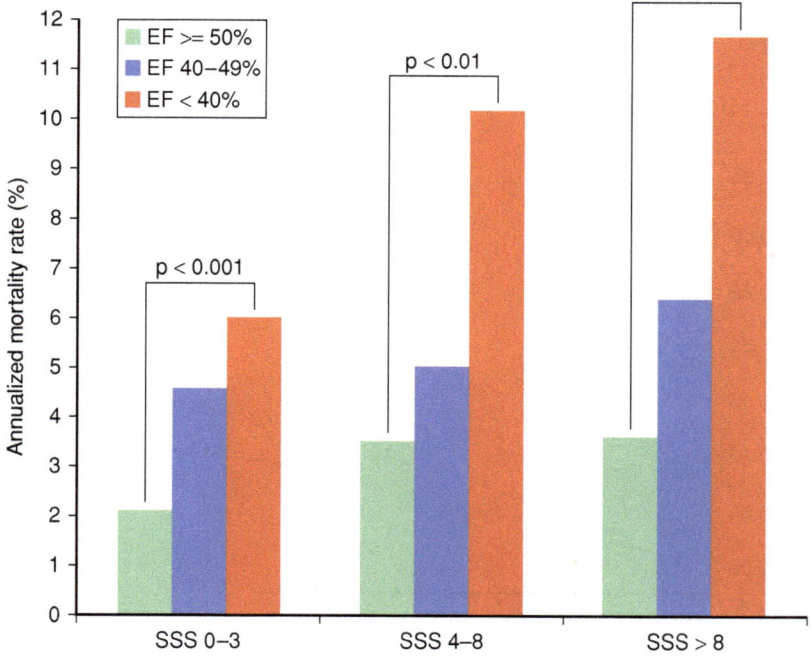

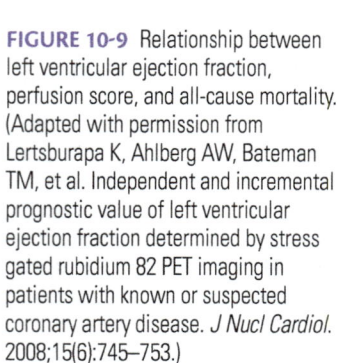

FIGURE 10-9 Relationship between left ventricular ejection fraction, perfusion score, and all-cause mortality. (Adapted with permission from Lertsburapa K, Ahlberg AW, Bateman TM, et al. Independent and incremental prognostic value of left ventricular ejection fraction determined by stress gated rubidium 82 PET imaging in patients with known or suspected coronary artery disease. *J Nucl Cardiol.* 2008;15(6):745–753.)

conditions as MBF reserve, although proper use of blood flow should include examination of both the rest and stress data. There are several commercially available software tools for measuring MBF with both Rb-82 and N-13 ammonia which have been extensively validated. Data collection generally occurs within the first 2 minutes after injection of tracer, thus not extending the acquisition time.

The evaluation of MBF has now moved into the clinical arena adding both diagnostic and prognostic value to the perfusion imaging data. An important notion is that abnormal MBF can occur in the presence of normal or abnormal perfusion, and if abnormal in the presence of a single localized stenosis, multiple stenosis, diffuse epicardial disease, endothelial inflammation, isolated microvascular dysfunction, or combinations of all. Irrespective of perfusion abnormality, MBF offers incrementally significant improvements in diagnosis of hemodynamically significant CAD.

The clinical significance of the addition of MBF to perfusion data with cardiac PET is well established. The information of normal MBF in addition to normal PET perfusion substantially reduces the likelihood of obstructive CAD (several studies indicate 99% negative predictive value) and future cardiac events (see Fig. 10-10). Abnormal MBF can reflect other cardiac conditions such as endothelial dysfunction, diffuse microvascular disease and assess the efficacy of the stress agent.[29] Prognostic data from several sources suggest worse cardiac outcomes occur in patients with perfusion abnormalities and a severe reduction of MBF and myocardial flow reserve. Thus, the addition of MBF to PET perfusion imaging has added another dimension to the study that contributes considerably to the clinical information and subsequent decisions following a study. Any laboratory now performing or entering into the PET perfusion arena should strongly consider the value of MBF.

Multiple publications have demonstrated the prognostic value of MBF. Normal MBF values are associated with low coronary risk, compared to abnormal values which predict higher cardiac risk. These measurements additionally predict the presence and extent of perfusion defects and outcomes. Studies have demonstrated the prognostic value of flow measurements beyond information from the relative perfusion images in consecutive patient populations, in diabetics, in patients with renal failure, and in patients following heart transplants.[30-33] Thus, a patient with a single-vessel PET perfusion pattern but with markedly low myocardial blood flow reserve (difference between rest and stress) indicates more severe disease, and also high-grade stenosis that may require intervention. Another important scenario is that of lack of augmentation of blood flow in the presence of normal perfusion. This indicates that the pharmacologic stress agent has failed, perhaps due to caffeine ingestion or some other factor.

The prognostic value of MBF has been demonstrated by several studies, including a recent publication by Murthy et al. (Fig. 10-11).[34] The cumulative incidence of cardiac mortality was calculated by tertiles of MBFR, demonstrating a significant relationship between lowest to highest flow in cardiac mortality.

The incorporation of MBF into clinical reports is now occurring and referring physicians/health care providers are finding benefit. However, unlike perfusion reports in which national standards have been established for several years, there is no national consensus on when and what to report. Recently, guidance was provided by a publication of Bateman et al.[29] They recommend three general categories as follows:

1. Clearly normal-flow augmentation. If the study is well above the normal MBF for a particular software program, this finding indicates adequate pharmacologic stress and the risk of a major coronary event is very low.
2. Abnormally low-flow augmentation. This should raise concern for possible significant CAD in an otherwise normal perfusion study, and places the patient in a higher-risk category.
3. No-flow augmentation. This circumstance is either due to a technical error in the study or pharmaceutical failure due to antagonists such as caffeine. This is particularly important in a study in which normal perfusion is identified.

In summary, assessment of MBF during a cardiac PET perfusion study has been found to add considerable diagnostic and prognostic information. It should be strongly encouraged in clinical PET laboratories.

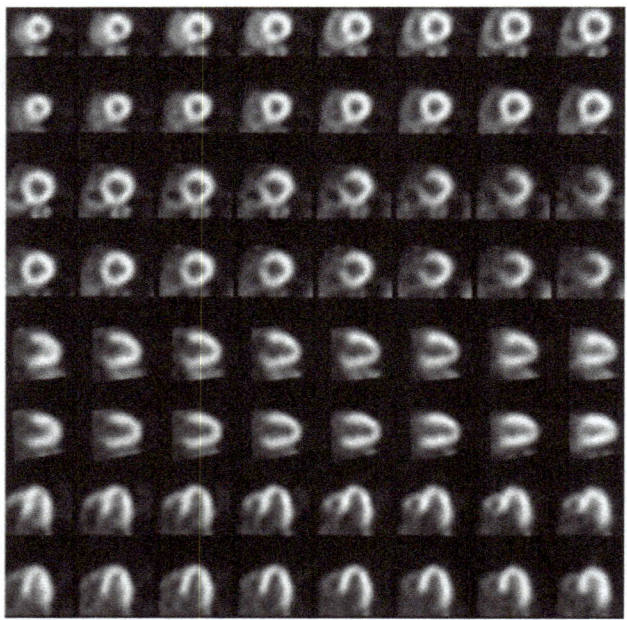
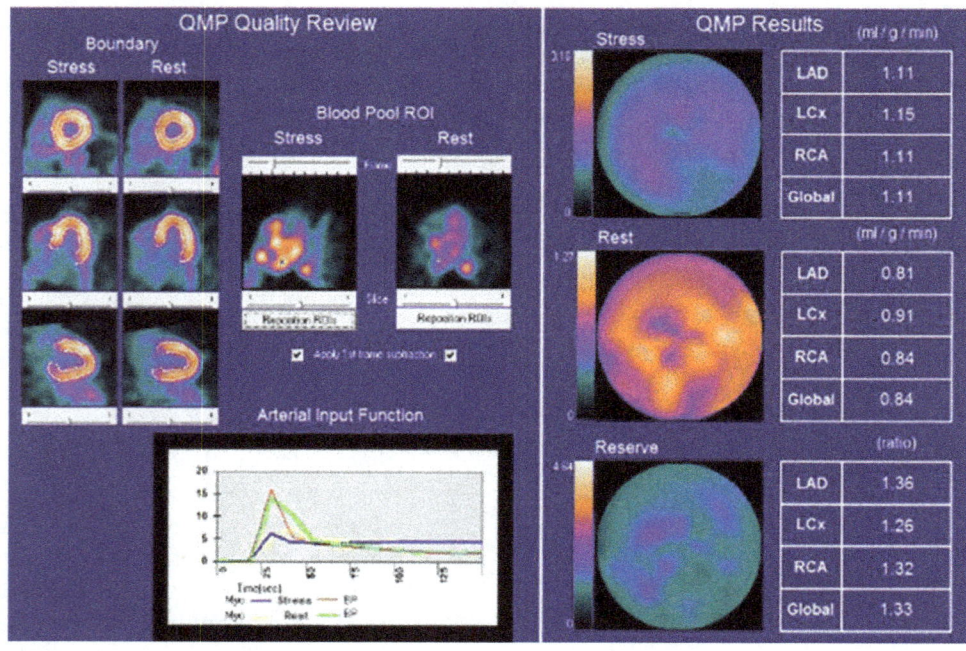

FIGURE 10-10 Example of severe diffuse CAD with normal relative uptake PET **(A)** images but severely reduced peak stress MBF and stress/rest MBFR, **(B)** globally and for all three coronary distributions. (Reproduced with permission from Bateman TM, Lance Gould K, Di Carli MF. Proceedings of the Cardiac PET Summit, 12 May 2014, Baltimore, MD: 3: Quantitation of myocardial blood flow. *J Nucl Cardiol*. 2015;22(3):571–578.)

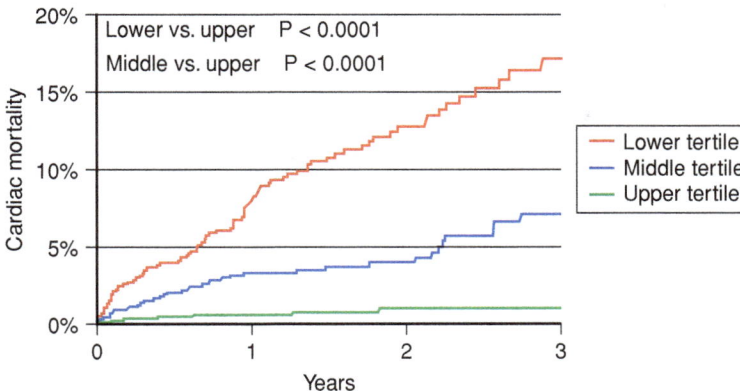

FIGURE 10-11 Cardiac mortality. Cumulative incidence of cardiac mortality for tertiles of MBFR. (Data from Murthy VL, Naya M, Foster CR, et al. Association between coronary vascular dysfunction and cardiac mortality in patients with and without diabetes mellitus. *Circulation.* 2012;126(15):1858–1868.)

ACQUISITION PROTOCOLS FOR CARDIAC PET

Cardiac PET perfusion imaging can be performed using several available radiotracers; the most common cardiac PET perfusion agent is Rb-82. There are over 200 laboratories using this tracer in the United States. N-13 ammonia is also being used clinically, but is far less prevalent (estimated 20 laboratories in the United States).

Cardiac PET perfusion imaging with rubidium is performed using pharmacologic stress because of the very short half-life of 75 seconds. This can be performed using vasodilator stress (regadenoson and dipyridamole) or inotropic stress (dobutamine). In general, adenosine is not recommended due to excessive patient motion during the acquisition. The protocol for cardiac PET perfusion imaging using the radiotracer Rb-82 is substantially faster than a SPECT protocol. A rest/stress protocol for SPECT imaging, regardless of radiopharmaceutical, requires at least 2.5 to as much as 4 hours for completion. In contrast, cardiac PET perfusion imaging protocols require 25 to 30 minutes for PET/CT camera (Fig. 10-12) and 35 to 40 minutes for a "dedicated" line source PET camera protocol (Fig. 10-13). The acquisition time for Rb-82 at both rest and stress is approximately 5 minutes. The strontium generator can produce a second dose of rubidium within 10 minutes of injection, thus the second dose is available when the stress protocol is completed. Because of the short protocol, it is recommended that the patient stay under the camera during the stress pharmaceutical injection. If MBF is being collected, most recommend the first 2 minutes after injection of both the rest and stress dose, thus not prolonging the procedure.

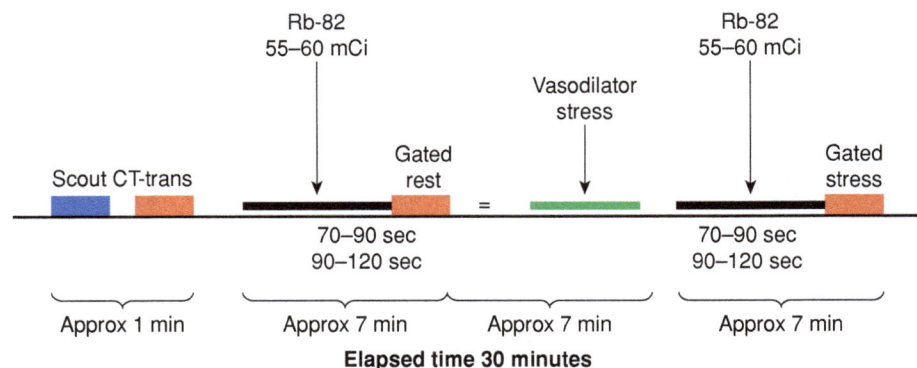

FIGURE 10-12 Cardiac PET protocol with CT attenuation correction.

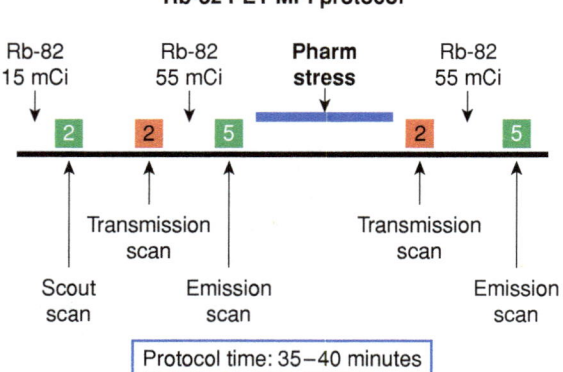

FIGURE 10-13 Cardiac PET protocol with line-source attenuation correction.

PATIENT SELECTION FOR CARDIAC PET PERFUSION

Cardiac PET perfusion studies offer high diagnostic accuracy and image quality, short protocols, low radiation exposure, and now additional information from MBF data. Thus, this test provides considerable value to the patient, which generally supersedes current SPECT procedures. Recently, a Joint Position Statement[10] was published by the ASNC and the Society of Nuclear Medicine and Molecular Imaging (SNMMI) that addressed the choices between PET and SPECT (Table 10-1). These professional societies stated that PET was the "preferred test" for patients recommended for pharmacologic stress imaging in both patients with suspected or known coronary artery disease that met proper indications. The societies also extended their position on PET as a "recommended test" for several patient conditions beyond pharmacologic stress alone, as noted in Table 10-1. These conditions include challenging body habitus, a previous inconclusive test, "high-risk" patients in whom a diagnostic error test would result in other downstream testing, younger patients in whom radiation exposure is of considerable concern, and those patients in which MBF data would be clinically important. These patient groups are independent of exercise status. This document elucidates the current patients in which cardiac PET would be most useful. If longer-acting agents for PET perfusion such as F-18 based tracers (2-hour half-life) are developed, this may be extended.

Nonperfusion Indications for Cardiovascular PET

Within the last several years, indications for cardiovascular PET imaging beyond myocardial perfusion imaging have increased considerably. Many of these indications are addressed in more detail on subsequent chapters (Chapters 21 and 24). Currently, many of these indications utilize 2-[18F]-fluoro-2-deoxy-d-glucose (FDG). FDG is a glucose analog used extensively for oncology studies in identifying presence, severity, location, and treatment success of a wide range of tumors. This glucose agent is now

Table 10-1

Preferred and Recommended Patient Type for Cardiac PET

	Preferred	Recommended
Unable to complete an ETT	√	
Prior poor quality stress imaging		√
Anticipated significant attenuation artifact		√
High-risk patients in whom diagnostic errors carry even greater clinical implications		√
Anticipated repeated radiation exposure to minimize exposure		√
Patients in whom myocardial blood flow quantification is identified by clinicians to be a needed adjunct to the image findings		√

Data from Bateman TM, Dilsizian V, Beanlands RS, et al. American Society of Nuclear Cardiology and Society of Nuclear Medicine and Molecular Imaging Joint Position Statement on the Clinical Indications for Myocardial Perfusion PET. *J Nucl Cardiol.* 2016;23(5):1227–1231.

being used in a variety of cardiovascular conditions described below.

CARDIAC PET FOR MYOCARDIAL VIABILITY

Congestive heart failure is one of the most common cardiac reasons for admission to a hospital in the United States. This disease affects close to 6 million people with an incidence that approaches 10 per 1000 people who are older than age 65 years.[26] Heart failure is associated with a very high morbidity and mortality. Any improvement in left ventricular function would be beneficial to such patients. Cardiac revascularization is extremely beneficial in those patients who demonstrate myocardial viability and potentially detrimental to those patients who do not.

The identification of heart failure patients who would benefit from revascularization can be aided by conducting viability studies. It is known that under normal conditions the cardiac myocytes preferentially undergo fatty acid metabolism for energy. In contrast, myocytes that are under stress or that are damaged change to glucose metabolism for their energy source. As FDG is a glucose analog, this shift allows the use of FDG-labeled isotopes to test for myocardial viability. The FDG uptake can be enhanced by glucose loading a patient prior to the administration. This increase in serum glucose causes a reflexive increase in insulin levels that then causes a decrease in fatty acid metabolism. This results in an imaging mismatch between perfusion and metabolic imaging, resulting in an increase in glucose uptake into the myocytes. Myocardial viability assessment using PET procedures is fully discussed in Chapter 21.

CARDIAC SARCOID AND INFECTION IDENTIFICATION

Sarcoidosis is a multi-organ disease with no known etiology. It can affect many organ systems including the lymph nodes, skin, eyes, and the nervous, musculoskeletal, renal, and endocrine systems, and importantly the heart.[35] Patients inflicted with this systemic disease carry a good prognosis overall. In sharp contrast, however, patients with cardiac sarcoid involvement carry a considerably higher morbidity and mortality.

Cardiac sarcoidosis can affect any part of the heart, including both the left and right ventricles. The clinical severity depends on the location of the sarcoid granuloma, the degree of infiltration, and the amount of inflammation. The most clinically significant manifestations are heart failure and fatal and nonfatal arrhythmias, which account for the high incidence of death in these patients. The presenting signs and symptoms warranting evaluation are varied and may also include heart block, chest pain, pleural effusions, dyspnea, and new onset of heart failure. Arrhythmias range from asymptomatic conduction abnormalities to fatal ventricular tachycardia or fibrillation.

The diagnosis of cardiac sarcoid remains a difficult one to make, short of biopsy. The use of FDG has become a novel way to identify active cardiac sarcoid occurrence. The images obtained provide the clinician with evidence of location and severity of infiltration. A recent review demonstrates the value of this identification both for diagnosis as well as measuring treatment success versus failure.[36] For a full discussion of this procedure and its clinical value, see Chapter 24.

Cardiac sarcoid imaging takes advantage of the ability of FDG to identify in-glucose activity in inflammation conditions. More recently, this agent has been extended to identify infectious processes within the cardiovascular system, such as prosthetic valves, implanted devices or pockets, and graft infections.[37] There are emerging data on various vasculitis conditions as well, although this should be considered preliminary. Finally, the evaluation of coronary plaque is also becoming possible with the use of F-18 sodium fluoride (NaF). These conditions and applications are also discussed in Chapter 24.

CONCLUSIONS

A growing body of literature supports the value of cardiac PET perfusion imaging in clinical practice. Advantages include high diagnostic accuracy, excellent image quality with minimal attenuation artifact, rapid protocols, and low radiation exposure. This chapter presented the supporting clinical data, procedures, and radiopharmaceuticals available for cardiac

PET studies; recent recommendations from ASNC/SNMMI support cardiac PET as the "preferred" imaging study in all patients undergoing pharmacologic stress. Optimal patients also include those with equivocal SPECT studies, obese patients, those with a high suspicion for coronary artery disease, and patients with known coronary artery disease. Emerging non-perfusion indications for cardiovascular PET including viability assessment, inflammation, and infection imaging have expanded the role of this modality.

REFERENCES

1. Early PJ, Sodee DB. *Principles and Practice of Nuclear Medicine*. 2nd ed. St. Louis, MO: Mosby; 1995.
2. DiCarli MF. *Cardiac PET and PET/CT Imaging*. New York: Springer; 2007.
3. Parkash R, deKemp RA, Ruddy TD, et al. Potential utility of rubidium 82 PET quantification in patients with 3-vessel coronary artery disease. *J Nucl Cardiol*. 2004;11:440–449.
4. Di Carli MF, Murthy VL. Cardiac PET/CT for the evaluation of known or suspected coronary artery disease. *Radiographics*. 2011;31:1239–1254.
5. Renaud JM, Yip K, Guimond J, et al. Characterization of 3-dimensional PET systems for accurate quantification of myocardial blood flow. *J Nucl Med*. 2017;58:103–109.
6. Bergmann SR, Hack S, Tewson T, Welch MJ, Sobel BE. The dependence of accumulation of 13NH3 by myocardium on metabolic factors and its implications for quantitative assessment of perfusion. *Circulation*. 1980;61:34–43.
7. Muzik O, Beanlands RS, Hutchins GD, Mangner TJ, Nguyen N, Schwaiger M. Validation of nitrogen-13-ammonia tracer kinetic model for quantification of myocardial blood flow using PET. *J Nucl Med*. 1993;34:83–91.
8. Beanlands RS, Muzik O, Hutchins GD, et al. Heterogeneity of regional nitrogen 13-labeled ammonia tracer distribution in the normal human heart: comparison with rubidium 82 and copper 62-labeled PTSM. *J Nucl Cardiol*. 1994;1:225–235.
9. Vitola JV, Delbeke D. *Nuclear Cardiology and Correlative Imaging: A Teaching File*. New York: Springer; 2004.
10. Bateman TM, Dilsizian V, Beanlands RS, DePuey EG, Heller GV, Wolinsky DA. American Society of Nuclear Cardiology and Society of Nuclear Medicine and Molecular Imaging Joint Position Statement on the Clinical Indications for Myocardial Perfusion PET. *J Nucl Cardiol*. 2016;23(5):1227–1231.
11. Yoshinaga K, Chow BJ, Williams K, et al. What is the prognostic value of myocardial perfusion imaging using rubidium-82 positron emission tomography? *J Am Coll Cardiol*. 2006;48:1029–1039.
12. Bateman TM, Heller GV, McGhie AI, et al. Diagnostic accuracy of rest/stress ECG-gated Rb-82 myocardial perfusion PET: comparison with ECG-gated Tc-99m sestamibi SPECT. *J Nucl Cardiol*. 2006;13:24–33.
13. Nandalur KR, Dwamena BA, Choudhri AF, Nandalur SR, Reddy P, Carlos RC. Diagnostic performance of positron emission tomography in the detection of coronary artery disease: a meta-analysis. *Acad Radiol*. 2008;15:444–451.
14. Mc Ardle BA, Dowsley TF, deKemp RA, Wells GA, Beanlands RS. Does rubidium-82 PET have superior accuracy to SPECT perfusion imaging for the diagnosis of obstructive coronary disease? A systematic review and meta-analysis. *J Am Coll Cardiol*. 2012;60:1828–1837.
15. Parker MW, Iskandar A, Limone B, et al. Diagnostic accuracy of cardiac positron emission tomography versus single photon emission computed tomography for coronary artery disease: a bivariate meta-analysis. *Circ Cardiovasc Imaging*. 2012;5:700–707.
16. Sampson UK, Dorbala S, Limaye A, Kwong R, Di Carli MF. Diagnostic accuracy of rubidium-82 myocardial perfusion imaging with hybrid positron emission tomography/computed tomography in the detection of coronary artery disease. *J Am Coll Cardiol*. 2007;49:1052–1058.
17. Cerqueira MD, Allman KC, Ficaro EP, et al. Recommendations for reducing radiation exposure in myocardial perfusion imaging. *J Nucl Cardiol*. 2010;17:709–718.
18. Jerome SD, Tilkemeier PL, Farrell MB, Shaw LJ. Nationwide laboratory adherence to myocardial perfusion imaging radiation dose reduction practices: A report from the Intersocietal Accreditation Commission Data Repository. *JACC Cardiovasc Imaging*. 2015;8:1170–1176.
19. Senthamizhchelvan S, Bravo PE, Esaias C, et al. Human biodistribution and radiation dosimetry of 82Rb. *J Nucl Med*. 2010;51:1592–1599.
20. Hunter CR, Hill J, Ziadi MC, Beanlands RS, deKemp RA. Biodistribution and radiation dosimetry of (82)Rb at rest and during peak pharmacological stress in patients referred for myocardial perfusion imaging. *Eur J Nucl Med Mol Imaging*. 2015;42:1032–1042.
21. Lundbye J, Desiderio MC, Farrell MB, et al. Abstracts of Original Contributions ASNC2016 The 21st Annual Scientific Session of the American Society of Nuclear Cardiology: September 22–25, 2016 Boca Raton, FL. *J Nucl Cardiol*. 2016;23:899–937.
22. Cerqueira MD, Batista JF, Prvulovich L, et al. Journal of Nuclear Cardiology News Update. *J Nucl Cardiol*. 1997;4:344–346.
23. Dorbala S, Di Carli MF, Beanlands RS, et al. Prognostic value of stress myocardial perfusion positron emission tomography: results from a multicenter observational registry. *J Am Coll Cardiol*. 2013;61:176–184.
24. Navare SM, Mather JF, Shaw LJ, Fowler MS, Heller GV. Comparison of risk stratification with pharmacologic and exercise stress myocardial perfusion imaging: a meta-analysis. *J Nucl Cardiol*. 2004;11:551–561.
25. Dorbala S, Vangala D, Sampson U, Limaye A, Kwong R, Di Carli MF. Value of vasodilator left ventricular ejection fraction reserve in evaluating the magnitude of myocardium at risk and the extent of angiographic coronary artery disease: a 82Rb PET/CT study. *J Nucl Med*. 2007;48:349–358.
26. Marwick TH, Shan K, Patel S, Go RT, Lauer MS. Incremental value of rubidium-82 positron emission tomography for prognostic assessment of known or suspected coronary artery disease. *Am J Cardiol*. 1997;80:865–870.

27. Dorbala S, Hachamovitch R, Curillova Z, et al. Incremental prognostic value of gated Rb-82 positron emission tomography myocardial perfusion imaging over clinical variables and rest LVEF. *JACC Cardiovasc Imaging*. 2009;2:846–854.
28. Lertsburapa K, Ahlberg AW, Bateman TM, et al. Independent and incremental prognostic value of left ventricular ejection fraction determined by stress gated rubidium 82 PET imaging in patients with known or suspected coronary artery disease. *J Nucl Cardiol*. 2008;15:745–753.
29. Bateman TM, Gould LK, Di Carli MF. Proceedings of the Cardiac PET Summit, 12 May 2014, Baltimore, MD: 3: Quantitation of myocardial blood flow. *J Nucl Cardiol*. 2015;22:571–578.
30. Shah NR, Charytan DM, Murthy VL, et al. Prognostic value of coronary flow reserve in patients with dialysis-dependent ESRD. *J Am Soc Nephrol*. 2016;27:1823–1829.
31. Fukushima K, Javadi MS, Higuchi T, et al. Impaired global myocardial flow dynamics despite normal left ventricular function and regional perfusion in chronic kidney disease: a quantitative analysis of clinical 82Rb PET/CT studies. *J Nucl Med*. 2012;53:887–893.
32. Mc Ardle BA, Davies RA, Chen L, et al. Prognostic value of rubidium-82 positron emission tomography in patients after heart transplant. *Circ Cardiovasc Imaging*. 2014;7:930–937.
33. Murthy VL, Naya M, Foster CR, et al. Association between coronary vascular dysfunction and cardiac mortality in patients with and without diabetes mellitus. *Circulation*. 2012;126:1858–1868.
34. Murthy VL, Naya M, Foster CR, et al. Improved cardiac risk assessment with noninvasive measures of coronary flow reserve. *Circulation*. 2011;124:2215–2224.
35. Judson MA. The diagnosis of sarcoidosis. *Clin Chest Med*. 2008;29:415–427, viii.
36. Blankstein R, Lundbye J, Heller G. Proceedings of the ASNC cardiac PET summit meeting, May 12, 2014, Baltimore MD: 4. Novel applications of cardiovascular PET. *J Nucl Cardiol*. 2015;22:720–729.
37. Blankstein R, Miller EJ. Quantifying FDG uptake to diagnose cardiac device infections: When and how should we do it? *J Nucl Cardiol*. 2016;23:1467–1469.

ECG-Gated SPECT Imaging for Assessment of Ventricular Function and Dyssynchrony

CHAPTER 11

Prem Soman and Saurabh Malhotra

INTRODUCTION

The introduction of electrocardiographic (ECG)-gated myocardial single-photon emission computed tomography (SPECT) in the 1990s expanded the application of myocardial perfusion imaging to routinely include the assessment of LV systolic function.[1] The development and use of this technique occurred when technetium-based imaging agents were placed into clinical use as these tracers provided much higher counts, and therefore image quality for measuring function. This was a critical development in the evolution of myocardial perfusion imaging. Currently, the majority of myocardial perfusion studies performed in the United States use gated SPECT technology and Tc-99m tracers. A more recent development has been the evaluation of ventricular dyssynchrony by SPECT, providing further data beyond myocardial perfusion. This chapter will discuss both aspects of ventricular assessment.

PRINCIPLES OF ECG-GATED SPECT IMAGING

▶ Technical Considerations

Hardware Requirements

Gated SPECT images can be acquired using single- or multiple-detector cameras. More recently, dual-headed cameras in the 90-degree configuration have been preferred, as images can be acquired in half the time required using a single-headed system without sacrificing image quality. The majority of gated SPECT imaging is performed with high-resolution parallel hole collimators for Tc-99m studies, while all-purpose collimators are used for thallium-201 (Tl-201) studies. A 180-degree imaging arc (45-degree right anterior oblique to 45-degree left posterior oblique projections) with a circular orbit is most commonly used, although noncircular (body contour) orbits can also be used. The most common detector rotation mode is the "continuous step and shoot" acquisition method, in which the detector records events when stationary at each projection, and then rotates (moves) to the next projection. A "continuous" acquisition mode is also available. The standard image matrix size for gated and nongated SPECT imaging is 64 × 64 pixels, with pixel sizes of 5 to 7 mm. This size offers adequate image resolution for interpretation and quantitation of both Tl-201 and Tc-99m tomograms. Contemporary computers possess adequate processing speed and internal hard disk space to process and store large amounts of scintigraphic data. Acquisition computers are usually separate from processing computers to allow for efficient laboratory operations. In addition, unsophisticated, relatively inexpensive, three-lead gating devices are provided by manufacturers to supply the trigger to the acquisition computer.[2]

Gated SPECT Acquisition and Processing

In an ECG-gated acquisition, a three-lead ECG provides the R-wave trigger to the acquisition computer, with two successive R-wave peaks on the ECG

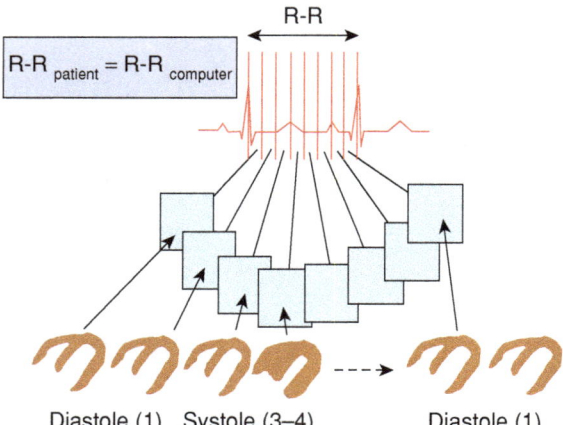

FIGURE 11-1 Principle of ECG-gated SPECT acquisition. Separate temporal frames corresponding to different phases of the cardiac cycle are acquired for each angular projection. Perfusion images are obtained from summation of the individual frames. (Reproduced with permission from Cullom SJ, Case JA, Bateman TM: Electrocardiographically gated myocardial perfusion SPECT: Technical principles and quality control considerations. *J Nucl Cardiol.* 1998;5(4):418–425.)

defining a cardiac cycle. Counts from each phase of the cardiac cycle are binned to a corresponding temporal "frame" within the computer. Perfusion projection images are obtained from summation of the individual frames (Fig. 11-1).[1] There is a trade-off between the temporal resolution of gated Tc-99m-sestamibi images and the count density of the individual frames. Gating of myocardial perfusion is usually performed at 8 or 16 frames per R–R interval per projection to maintain the count density using a single-headed camera, although 32 frames per cycle are also possible. With dual-headed cameras, 16 frames per cycle (rather than 8 frames) are preferred as the ejection fraction (EF) results are more in line with other imaging modalities. With a multiheaded SPECT system, more frames can be acquired with no increase in acquisition time, as these systems can obtain higher count density images.

Most manufacturers provide one of two modes of gated SPECT acquisition—"fixed" or "variable"—to define the R–R interval. In fixed acquisition mode, the R–R interval is estimated by the acquisition computer prior to the study, based on previously observed 10 to 20 heartbeats, and remains fixed throughout the study. In the variable acquisition mode, the heart rate is continuously monitored throughout the study and the acquisition computer alters the duration of temporal frames as needed to bin counts equally into the prespecified intervals (8 or 16) per each previously detected R–R interval. In both of these modes "fixed" and "variable," the data cannot be reformatted after acquisition is complete. An alternative to this is the list mode, a technique increasingly used in contemporary radionuclide studies.[3] This technique allows counts to be reformatted into temporal frames after acquisition is complete. The computer records the spatial coordinates of each detected count as well as the timing marker that identifies at what time the count was detected. After acquisition, gated SPECT frames are generated by selecting the mean R–R interval and the beat rejection criteria followed by appropriate binning of the data. The advantage of the list mode is its flexibility, and thus potentially avoids the gating artifacts seen in the fixed- and the variable-mode acquisitions. A disadvantage, however, is that it requires storage of massive amounts of data, and therefore was rarely used in clinical practice until recently, when high-capacity computers became ubiquitous.[2]

Variations in heart rate due to a variety of factors (sinus arrhythmia, other arrhythmias, patient anxiety or motion, poor ECG lead contact, etc.) can result in temporal "blurring," that is, mixing of counts from adjacent frames. To limit acquired data to those heartbeats that are representative of the patient's average heartbeat and to minimize temporal blurring, a beat rejection window is set by specifying the acceptable deviation of R–R interval from the expected value. A 20% (±10) window has historically been applied, although in patients with highly variable heart rates, up to a 100% (±50) acceptance window can be set. Some camera manufacturers provide an extra frame in which counts from all rejected beats are accumulated. The counts within the extra frame can be added to the nongated data after the acquisition is complete in order to generate a summed SPECT dataset for interpretation of the static perfusion images. On most commercial systems, a premature ventricular contraction (PVC) mode may be set that programs the computer to skip one or more cardiac beats before the R–R gating is reestablished. This is done to avoid mixing counts from the two successive cardiac cycles.[2]

As can be inferred from the above discussion, the detection of an adequate R-wave signal is essential to the successful collection of image data synchronized to heart rate. In patients with severe arrhythmias, the triggering mechanism is incapable of properly identifying the R wave and EF fluctuations, artifactual perfusion abnormalities, and wall thickening discordance may occur.[3] Thus, in this situation, a nongated SPECT study may be preferred.

A variety of single- and 2-day protocols may be used in conjunction with gated SPECT. As long as counts are adequate, either Tl-201 or Tc-99m perfusion tracers may be used. Either or both the acquisitions composing the stress/rest or rest/stress protocol can be gated, although the most commonly utilized is the high-dose technetium stress study because of its superior count density. Although the common practice is to gate only the poststress image, a study by Johnson et al.[4] reported that in 36% of patients with reversible perfusion defects, the poststress left ventricular ejection fraction (LVEF) was >5% lower than at rest. This implies that global and regional LV functions obtained from poststress–gated acquisitions are not representative of basal LV function in patients with stress-induced ischemia, and that perhaps both rest and stress images should be gated routinely, as long as count density is adequate. It is currently recommended that both rest and stress ECG gating be performed. In general, resting function is of lesser quality due to lower counts and information is not reported unless changes occur between the post stress and rest images.

The ECG-gated SPECT procedure results in the derivation of a time–*volume* curve, based on the volume of the left ventricle derived by endocardial definition at each of the 8 or 16 bins (frames) within one cardiac cycle. This is in contrast to the time–*activity* curve derived from radionuclide ventriculography (RVG), a technique that calculates EF from the difference in LV cavity counts between end-systole and end-diastole, rather than from LV volumes determined by endocardial definition. This technique is reviewed in Chapter 22.

▶ Procedure for Interpretation of ECG-Gated SPECT Imaging

To maximize the value of functional ECG-gated SPECT data, a systematic approach to interpretation is essential. Ventricular function should be interpreted only in the context of the perfusion data, as the latter

Table 11-1

Sequence of Interpretation of ECG-Gated SPECT Function

1. Observation of unprocessed (raw) data
2. Evaluation of individual perfusion slices
3. Application of quantitative perfusion software
4. Evaluation of individual slices for ventricular function
5. Quantitation of left ventricular ejection fraction
6. Evaluation of three-dimensional–gated images
7. Evaluation of right ventricular function

has potential to influence the results and, the two sets of information are complementary. The sequence of interpretation is listed in Table 11-1, and should begin with the evaluation of rotation images followed by perfusion data and finally ventricular function. The final step is integration of clinical information.

Evaluation of Unprocessed (Raw) Data

The interpretation of gated SPECT begins with evaluation of the rotating unprocessed data for overall image quality and any information that might impact function. This includes potential soft tissue attenuation from breast or diaphragm, and interference from extra cardiac liver or gut activity. Inspection of raw data provides assessment of the technical quality of gated SPECT acquisition. In general, images with poor counts should be interpreted with caution as they could be associated with artifacts. Periodic flashing of the display results from gating errors, occurring as a result of wide variation in the cardiac cycle during the acquisition leading to variation in counts between images. Wide variability of R–R interval can also cause a radial blurring artifact in the gated tomographic images. This may limit the definition of end-systolic frame, affecting LVEF and end-systolic volume (ESV) measurements. The presence of gating errors can be further confirmed by graphs displaying accepted counts as a function of the projection number. If there are no gating errors, all projection curves should superimpose nearly perfectly.

Evaluation of Myocardial Perfusion Data

Tomographic slices of the myocardium should be displayed according to the standardized model recommended by the American Society of Nuclear

Cardiology,[5] and interpreted prior to assessment of ventricular function. Using this model, the myocardium is divided into 17 segments based on three short-axis slices (the apical, mid-ventricular, and basal) and a mid-ventricular vertical long-axis slice. The presence of a defect and the degree of reversibility (differences between stress and rest) should also be noted. Quantitative confirmation of the visual observations of the perfusion data should generally be made. Fixed and reversible perfusion deficits should be carefully evaluated for regional function as described in the next section.

Evaluation of Ventricular Function

Assessment of wall motion should be performed for both the left and the right ventricle. Assessment should include both global left and right ventricular function, and regional function for the left ventricle. The latter is critically important in the presence of a perfusion abnormality. It is generally recommended that ventricular function be interpreted using at least three short-axis slices and one horizontal and vertical long-axis slice at a magnification sufficient to easily assess regional changes. The short-axis slices selected should be similar to those used for perfusion interpretation to enable meaningful comparison.

Assessment of Global Ventricular Function

The interpreter should first estimate the global LVEF by visual interpretation, and then confirm with the quantitative software. Confirmation of quantitated LVEF should include examining the contours, as gut and liver activity might be mistakenly included. It is important for the reader to know the lower limit of normal for a given software quantitation package, since the absolute number varies by imaging modality as well as among software and hardware vendors. Global function can be categorized as normal (EF >50%), mild (EF 40–50%), moderate (EF 30–40%), or severe (EF <30%).

Evaluation of Regional Ventricular Function

Parameters of regional ventricular function assessed by gated SPECT include segmental myocardial wall motion and myocardial thickening. Segmental wall motion analysis consists of observing both epicardial and endocardial surfaces. Wall motion in one region should be compared to adjacent regions (i.e., inferior compared with anterior). In general, wall motion is best observed using monochrome display scales (thermal, gray, etc.), while wall thickening is best observed using color scale (e.g., isocontour). Assessment of both wall motion and wall thickening contributes to overall evaluation of ventricular function. A visual semi-quantitative assessment of regional wall motion and thickening can be performed using the same 17-segment model used for perfusion assessment. For assessing wall motion, a six-point (0, normal; 1, mild hypokinesis; 2, moderate hypokinesis; 3, severe hypokinesis; 4, akinesis; and 5, dyskinesis) scoring system is used.[5] This includes estimation and quantification of LVEF and quantification of LV volumes. Completely automated algorithms, both count based and geometry based, are available.

Right ventricular (RV) size and global functions should also be noted, and important clinical data points. Reports should reflect the best estimation of RV size and function.

While 8- and 16-bin gating are routinely performed for data acquisition, ASNC guidelines recommend the latter. Recent data demonstrate that a larger number of gating bins results in higher fidelity of the time–volume curve, a fact that has practical implications. First, a 16-bin study routinely results in a higher EF value (by approximately 4–5 EF units) compared to 8-bin gating,[6] which is more in line with other modalities. In our institution the EF threshold for normality is 45% and 50%, for 8-bin and 16-bin gating, respectively. Second, it is generally accepted that at least 32-bin gating is required for optimal assessment of LV diastolic function, an approach that is generally impractical during SPECT acquisition due to the long acquisition time required.[7]

The assessment of LV systolic function by gated SPECT has undergone an extensive validation.[8] However, the 50% threshold for normality of EF was derived from RVG.[9,10] It is well established that the absolute EF numbers are not interchangeable between modalities, and that the threshold for normality should really be modality specific.[11] Nevertheless, the 50% threshold is applied across modalities for convenience, and the intermodality variability in absolute EF has been ignored even in the design of landmark clinical trials which have recruited patients based on an absolute EF value. For example, in the Multicenter Automatic Defibrillator Implantation (MADIT) trials the inclusion criteria of EF <35% could be determined by "angiography, radionuclide scanning, or echocardiography."[12] Furthermore, this intermodality variability is exaggerated in patients with LV systolic dysfunction.[13]

The clinically important attributes of biological measurements are accuracy and precision (reproducibility and repeatability). In the case of EF measurements, the absence of a truth standard makes accuracy difficult to determine. However, measurements of precision are particularly important for serial assessment, and is a strength of radionuclide-based approaches which are largely automated and rely less on operator input. Reproducibility refers to the serial processing of an acquired dataset by the same or different individual, and reflects the effects of operator input on the technique. Repeatability refers to variability in serial acquisition of the data and its subsequent processing. High reproducibility is therefore an inherent requirement for high repeatability. In the context of LVEF, when serial studies are performed in close temporal proximity (e.g., within minutes of each other), technical variability is measured, whereas studies performed days apart reflect both technical and biological variability.[14] It is important to use the same processing software processing protocol for EF determination as there is considerable variability among vendors.

In general, EF determination by gated SPECT requires less operator input than RVG, unless completely automatic border detection options are chosen for the processing of the latter. However, several factors affect EF determination by SPECT. Equipment and processing software have profound influences and should be kept constant for serial imaging.[15] Patient position, tracer dose, interval between tracer injection and imaging, image reorientation angle, and the presence of large perfusion defects can affect EF determination, often surreptitiously.[16-19] The tracer dose and time to imaging affect the target to background ratio and thus, delineation LV borders and segmentation. Available data suggest that the repeatability coefficients (obtained by Bland Altman plotting) for RVG and gated SPECT for serial LVEF assessment are comparable, and in the range of 6% to 8% (EF units).[14,20] LVEF changes on serial imaging beyond this range generally reflect a true difference. It must be noted that the contractile reserve of a normal LV is much higher (50–85%) than that of a dysfunctional ventricle. Thus biological variability is higher in the normal LV.[21]

As the left ventricle becomes dysfunctional and dilated, count statistics in the LV cavity improve, in contrast to the thinned out LV myocardium. Myocardial count statistics are further compromised by large perfusion defects. Thus, RVG may have some inherent advantages over SPECT myocardial perfusion imaging in the assessment of the dysfunctional left ventricle.

Clinical Uses of Gated SPECT Imaging

There are numerous clinical applications of the gated functional data (Table 11-2). The additive value of functional data to nongated perfusion data has been consistently shown in prior studies.

Differentiating Attenuation Artifacts from Scar

A useful clinical application of gated SPECT imaging is in adjudicating fixed perfusion defects which could be either scar or soft tissue attenuation. The basic assumption using ECG-gated SPECT imaging for this purpose is that a fixed perfusion abnormality associated with CAD should represent either prior myocardial infarction (MI) or stunned myocardium, both of which are associated with wall motion abnormalities. In contrast, if wall motion in the same area as the fixed perfusion abnormality is normal, this should represent attenuation artifact. Thus, a fixed perfusion abnormality with normal wall motion should be considered normal. This interpretation would therefore reduce the number of "false-positive" studies and

Table 11-2

Clinical Use of Ventricular Function Using ECG-Gated SPECT Imaging

1. Identification of attenuation artifact
2. Enhanced detection of coronary artery disease
3. Prognosis and risk stratification
4. To determine etiology of LV systolic dysfunction
5. Assessment of myocardial viability
6. Evaluation of right ventricular function

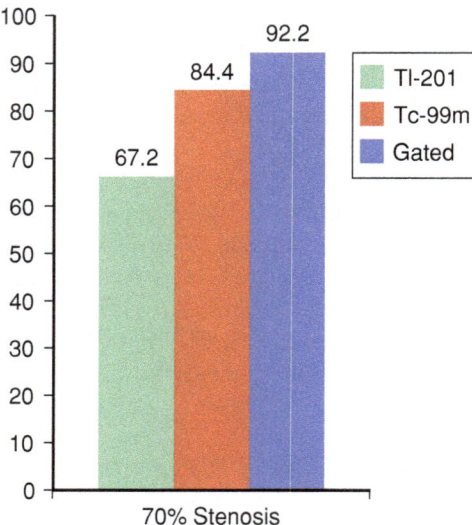

FIGURE 11-2 Specificity of Tl-201, Tc-99m-sestamibi perfusion, and gated SPECT studies for both patients without CAD and the group of normal volunteers. (Data from Taillefer R, DePuey EG, Udelson JE, et al. Comparative diagnostic accuracy of Tl-201 and Tc-99m-sestamibi SPECT imaging (perfusion and ECG-gated SPECT) in detecting coronary artery disease in women. *J Am Coll Cardiol.* 1997;29:69–77.)

improve specificity. Several studies have been published,[22,23] demonstrating improved specificity using this assumption (Fig. 11-2).

By incorporating regional wall motion data in the interpretation of perfusion imaging, DePuey and Rozanski[22] demonstrated that false-positive perfusion studies could be reduced from 14% to 3%. In patients with low likelihood of CAD, the normalcy rate increased from 74% to 93%. In patients with a high likelihood for CAD, the trend was also toward a higher number of unequivocally abnormal interpretations. In women, where the false-positive rate of stress ECGs is relatively high and breast attenuation artifact common, ECG gating was shown to further enhance the diagnostic specificity of Tc-99m perfusion imaging from 84% to 94%.[23] Subsequently, Smanio et al.[24] demonstrated that the addition of gated SPECT for the assessment of regional systolic function reduces the degree of uncertainty in the interpretation of Tc-99m-sestamibi perfusion studies. The numbers of "borderline normal" or "borderline abnormal" interpretations were significantly reduced (Fig. 11-3).

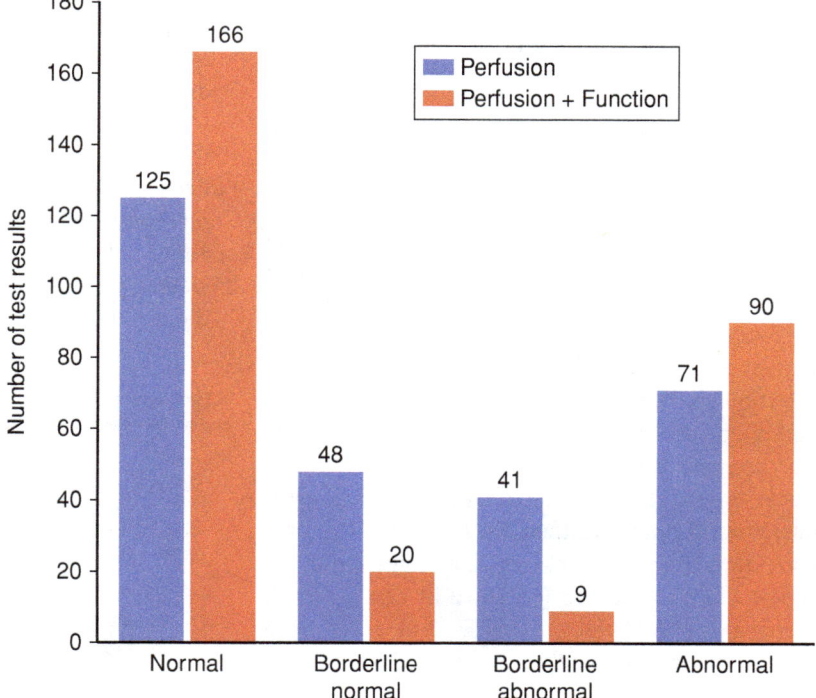

FIGURE 11-3 Changes in test interpretations after interpretation of perfusion and function images (*hatched bars*) compared with stress and rest perfusion images alone (*solid bars*) for all 285 patients in the study referred for evaluation for coronary artery disease (CAD). (Reproduced with permission from Smanio PE, Watson DD, Segalla DL, et al. Value of gating of technetium-99m-sestamibi single-photon emission computed tomographic imaging. *J Am Coll Cardiol.* 1997;30(7):1687–1692.)

Gated SPECT imaging is limited in distinguishing attenuation artifact in those patients with reversible perfusion abnormalities or those with either stress-only imaging or acute rest myocardial perfusion in the emergency department (ED) with no reference image. In any of these circumstances, if wall motion is normal, one cannot exclude the presence of ischemia as an etiology of the perfusion abnormality. Since ventricular function is assessed 30 to 60 minutes later, any wall motion abnormality created by ischemia would, for the most part, have resolved by the time of imaging. In both ED and stress-only imaging, a reference image must be obtained for comparison. Reversible perfusion abnormalities must be considered abnormal despite normal wall motion.

Enhanced Detection of Coronary Artery Disease

In addition to improving diagnostic specificity, the capability to obtain functional information through gating may also enhance the detection of CAD, particularly multivessel disease. While proven in various studies that SPECT MPI reliably detects CAD, the question of underestimating ischemia in the case of multivessel disease or left main disease because of balanced global hypoperfusion comes into question. Several reports have estimated that only 13% to 50% of patients with three-vessel CAD or left main disease actually have perfusion abnormalities in multiple territories, thus potentially leading clinicians to underestimate risk.[25–27] Several studies have demonstrated the incremental value of utilizing both functional and perfusion data in detecting multivessel disease or high-grade stenoses over perfusion data alone. Sharir et al.[28] examined a population of 99 patients who underwent dual-isotope resting Tl-201/exercise-gated Tc-99m-sestamibi SPECT with normal resting perfusion. Multivariate regression analysis suggested that both extensive perfusion abnormalities and the presence of wall motion abnormalities in multiple territories were independent predictors of severe multivessel CAD, but that the addition of wall motion variables to perfusion data resulted in a significant increase in accuracy for predicting severe proximal left anterior descending (LAD) as well as multivessel CAD. For perfusion alone, sensitivity was 49%, while combined perfusion and wall motion abnormality yielded a sensitivity of 82%.

Furthermore, the use of rest and stress LVEF may assist in the detection of multivessel coronary disease, as demonstrated in a study by Yamagishi et al.[29] wherein the combination of perfusion data and worsening of the LVEF significantly increased sensitivity in detecting multivessel CAD over Tl-201 perfusion defects or rest LVEF and postexercise LVEF alone (43.3% vs. 26.9%, 25.4%, and 25.4%, respectively). Another study sought to correlate degree of angiographic stenosis with the presence of regional wall motion abnormalities (RWMAs) on exercise stress/rest-gated technetium-99m SPECT studies.[30] Reversible RWMAs were found to be highly specific for angiographic stenoses >70%, both overall and for specific vascular territories (94–100%). Furthermore, when patients were stratified according to severity of angiographic stenoses (50–79% and 80–99%), the presence of reversible RWMA distinguished a higher angiographic severity with positive predictive values between 77% and 88% for specific vascular territories.

Prognosis and Risk Stratification

As is the case with perfusion imaging in general, gated SPECT imaging has also found an important role in the risk assessment of patients with known or suspected CAD. This is not surprising, given the well-recognized prognostic role of LV function with regard to long-term survival, as has been shown using a variety of techniques for LV functional assessment. Among a large series of 1690 consecutive patients who underwent dual-isotope–gated SPECT imaging, those patients in whom EFs were <45% were associated with reduced survival, irrespective of the perfusion defect size or severity.[31] In addition, those patients with normal ESV of <70 mL or an EF of >45% had a very low cardiac mortality rate, despite severe perfusion abnormalities (Fig. 11-4). This group also examined the relative value of perfusion and function in the risk stratification in 2686 patients into low-, intermediate-, and high-risk categories for cardiac death and MI.[32] LVEF was most predictive of death, and the amount of ischemia (summed difference score on perfusion imaging) was the best predictor of nonfatal MI. Functional information was found to be of incremental value in the prediction of cardiac death beyond the perfusion imaging parameters. The presence of ischemia did not influence

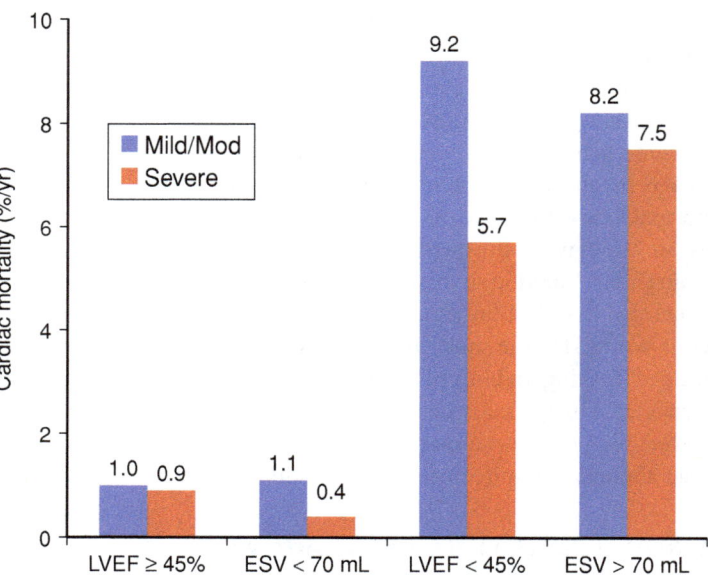

FIGURE 11-4 Annual cardiac death rates stratified by LV volume and ejection fraction. Patients with an LVEF of >45% or ESV <70 mL have a low mortality rate regardless of severity of perfusion defects. Similar findings are noted for patients with a low ejection fraction (<45%). (Data from Yamagishi H, Shirai N, Yoshiyama M, et al. Incremental value of left ventricular ejection fraction for detection of multivessel coronary artery disease in exercise (201)Tl gated myocardial perfusion imaging. *J Nucl Med.* 2002;43:131–139.)

prognosis in patients with LVEF <30%, due to the already high mortality rate.

LV function has long been a key determinant for survival following an acute MI. Recently, a study of 128 postinfarct survivors confirmed the value of gated SPECT imaging for risk stratification in post-MI patients, as an LVEF of <40% with this method was found to increase the risk of subsequent cardiac event by almost threefold.[33] The presence of a fixed or reversible defect had no independent predictive value in this study, although the latter finding may be a result of the censoring of high-risk patients who underwent early revascularization.

Differentiation of Etiology of Dilated Cardiomyopathy

The role of radionuclide image in heart failure is described in Chapter 22. An important step in the evaluation of new-onset heart failure is the distinction between LV systolic dysfunction due to CAD and other etiologies. In this regard, the addition of regional function data to perfusion data may be of benefit,[34] particularly the presence of regional dysfunction in coronary vascular territories, which is more consistent with ischemic cardiomyopathy etiology. Table 11-3 lists findings suggestive of ischemic and nonischemic etiologies for LV systolic dysfunction.

Assessment of Left Ventricular Dyssynchrony

Dyssynchrony refers to a temporal dispersion in the activation and contraction of the normally coordinated ventricle. Since, minor differences in the amplitude and timing of LV contraction exist in normally functioning hearts,[35] pathophysiologic dyssynchrony needs to be defined using threshold rarely encountered in the normal population. Thus, LV dyssynchrony is not an all-or-none phenomenon, but represents a continuum of severity. LV dyssynchrony is identified clinically by the presence of a bundle

Table 11-3

SPECT Patterns in Ischemic and Nonischemic Cardiomyopathies

Condition	Pattern on Perfusion Scan
Ischemic Cardiomyopathy	
Myocardial perfusion	Large fixed or reversible defect
Myocardial function	Regional dysfunction in coronary vascular territories
Nonischemic Cardiomyopathy	
Myocardial perfusion	Normal or mild (usually fixed) perfusion abnormalities
Myocardial function	Global dysfunction, RV dysfunction

branch block on ECG (electrical dyssynchrony), which is an indicator of interventricular conduction delay and hence interventricular dyssynchrony.[36] The presence of a wide (>150 ms) left bundle branch block (LBBB) is currently considered the strongest predictor of improvement in LV function after cardiac resynchronization therapy (CRT) among patients with drug-refractory heart failure and severely reduced LVEF.[37] Dyssynchrony can also be intraventricular (within the LV), and characterized by global or regional intraventricular variations in myocardial contractility. Studies have shown intraventricular dyssynchrony to be more strongly associated with poor cardiac performance and adverse events, than interventricular dyssynchrony.[38] The mechanisms of LV dyssynchrony are poorly understood, but thought to be dependent on a complex interplay of numerous factors including severity of LV systolic dysfunction, electrical abnormalities (QRS width and pattern), and LV scar burden. In general, the prevalence of mechanical dyssynchrony increases with worsening systolic dysfunction and increasing QRS duration. Among patients with severely reduced LV systolic function, dyssynchrony has been reported in up to 75% of the patients.[39] Among all patients with systolic heart failure, the reported prevalence of mechanical dyssynchrony measured by echocardiography varies from 27% in patients with narrow QRS (<120 ms) to 89% in those with QRS duration >150 ms.[35,40] Traditionally, intraventricular mechanical dyssynchrony has been measured using echocardiographic techniques (m-mode and tissue Doppler imaging) that have poor inter- and intraobserver reproducibility.[41] Contemporaneous echo approaches utilizing speckle tracking and real-time 3D echocardiography have better repeatability,[42] but have not proven effective in predicting response to CRT.[42] The reason for this dissociation between the presence of mechanical dyssynchrony and response to CRT is unclear, but is most likely related to the complexity of the CRT response, which is influenced by many other factors including location and extent of myocardial scar, location of the latest contracting myocardial segment and its relation with the LV lead of the biventricular pacemaker.

Radionuclide-based synchrony measurement utilizes phase analysis of regional or global time activity curves to determine timing of regional contraction, and can be performed using RVG or tomographic techniques (SPECT or PET). Since the vast majority of current cardiac radionuclide studies are gated SPECT, this approach has accrued the most supporting data, and will be focus of this review. The poor spatial resolution of SPECT makes it subject to partial-volume effects, resulting in a relatively linear relationship between myocardial thickening and myocardial count density in any segment of the myocardium.[43] This can be visually appreciated on gated SPECT images where the myocardium is brighter in systole. Thus the count activity curve of a myocardial sample (voxel) during a cardiac cycle essentially represents a myocardial thickening curve, albeit with poor temporal fidelity because of the 8- or 16-bin gating that is generally used for myocardial SPECT. Fourier transformation of the count-activity curve of the myocardium in phase analysis improves the temporal resolution of the gated SPECT images and also generates a continuous thickening curve that delineates the timing of contraction of a myocardial sample (Fig. 11-5).[44,45]

In addition, the timing (phase) of the peak contraction of a myocardial sample is also identified (referred to as "onset of mechanical contraction") and

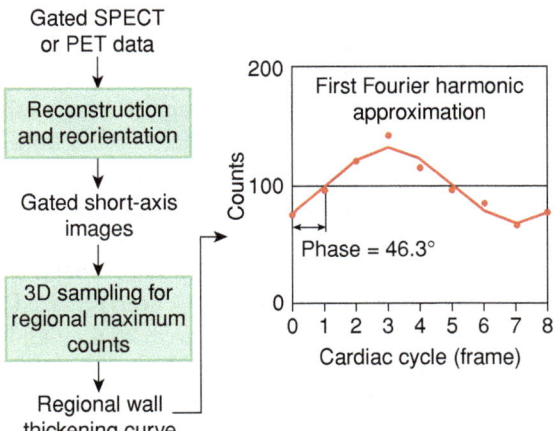

FIGURE 11-5 First-harmonic Fourier analysis of regional myocardial thickening. The points in the plot represent counts from one myocardial voxel at each frame of the cardiac cycle. The curve represents the Fourier transform of the individual points. The horizontal line represents the average count intensity of the voxel over one cardiac cycle. The point at which the upslope of the curve intersects the horizontal line represents the onset of mechanical contraction (OMC) of this particular myocardial voxel. In this way, the phase of OMC of each myocardial voxel can be determined.

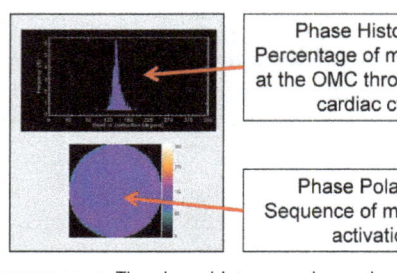

FIGURE 11-6 The phase histogram shows the percentage of myocardium contracting (y-axis) at each point in the cardiac cycle (x-axis). The phase polar map is a bull's-eye representation of the LV, showing the sequence of mechanical activation, using a color-coded scheme. This is an example of synchronous LV contraction with a narrow and highly peaked histogram and a uniform color on the phase polar map.

can be compared to that of other myocardial samples. Data on thickening and the onset of mechanical contraction are collected for over 600 myocardial samples during a standard myocardial perfusion–gated SPECT acquisition, and allows for the comparison of the timing of thickening among the various samples. This information can be displayed as a phase histogram or a phase polar map (Fig. 11-6).

Interpretation of Dyssynchrony

Gated SPECT phase analysis parameters that have been validated to represent LV dyssynchrony are the histogram bandwidth (HBW): the range (in degrees) during which 95% of the myocardial samples initiate contraction, and the phase standard deviation (PSD): the standard deviation (in degrees) of the timing of contraction from all the myocardial samples, and entropy. Using Emory Cardiac Toolbox® (ECTb), gender-specific cut-offs have been reported, by which a PSD value of >24.4 degrees in men and >22.2 degrees in women or an HBW value of >62.2 degrees in men and >49.8 degrees in women identifies presence of dyssynchrony.[46] Phase analysis–derived PSD and HBW value of gated SPECT data has been known to have shown excellent reproducibility[47] in single-center studies, due to the automated generation of these parameters with minimal operator input. However, repeatability has not been testing in a multi-center setting. In general, PSD and HBW are considered to represent a measure of global LV dyssynchrony. The assessment of regional V dyssynchrony can be derived by partitioning of the global phase data in accordance with the standard 17-segment LV model.[48] The segmental mean phase value provides an assessment of regional differences in LV contraction, from which the segmental location of the site of latest activation (SOLA) can be determined.[48] It is important to note that assessment of dyssynchrony from gated SPECT is software dependent, in a fashion similar to the known variations in measurement of LV volume and EF.[49] It is known that, Quantitative-Gated SPECT® (QGS) excludes myocardial regions with the lowest 5% of phase amplitude in the derivation of the HBW, and therefore is expected to produce values of HBW that are systematically different from those obtained from ECTb.[46,50] Given these computational differences between software, it is important to use software specific cut-offs when evaluating dyssynchrony, and to utilize the same software to process-gated SPECT data when serial changes in LV dyssynchrony is to be determined. Despite the low temporal resolution, when compared to ERNA, the wider availability and the ability to simultaneously obtain comprehensive information on perfusion, function, and dyssynchrony (both global and regional) from a standard acquisition, makes gated SPECT a very attractive tool for dyssynchrony assessment.

Clinical Application of Dyssynchrony

The natural application of LV dyssynchrony assessment would be in guiding CRT in patients with medically refractory heart failure and severely reduced EF, where approximately two-thirds of patients selected based on clinical criteria (NYHA class II-IV, EF <35% and QRS >120 ms) will show improvement in symptomatic and or LV function. Thus, there is interest in using imaging approaches to improve patient selection and response rates. However, more recent iterations of selection criteria afford a class I indication only to patients with QRS >150 ms with LBBB pattern, where the response rates is >80%. Gated SPECT and ERNA studies have shown that presence of LV dyssynchrony and its severity prior to CRT determines LV reverse remodeling and symptomatic benefit following CRT.[51-55] While threshold values of abnormal dyssynchrony have been associated with CRT response in small, single-center studies, specific cut-off values of HBW or PSD, hitherto considered in

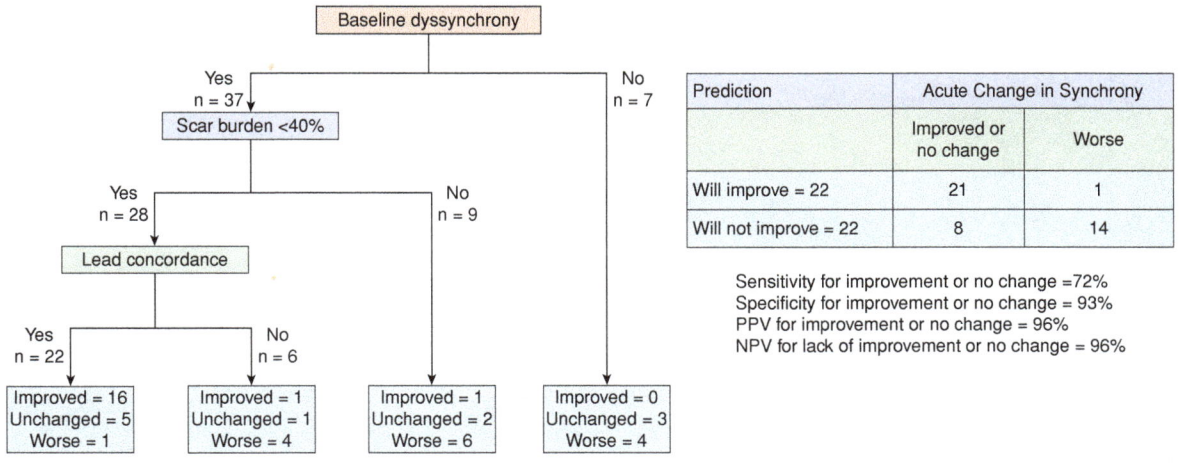

FIGURE 11-7 Algorithm for predicting acute change in synchrony following CRT.

isolation, have not been useful in improving patient selection for CRT. Recent studies have suggested an important role of myocardial scar burden in predicting CRT response,[56-58] and also a relationship between SOLA with the position of the LV lead of a biventricular pacemaker.[59-61] Gated SPECT is an established technique to imaging MI or scar, and its ability to identify SOLA by regional phase analysis to guide LV lead position has been recently reported.[62] Identification of regional phase on gated SPECT in a population with HF, low EF has demonstrated the SOLA to be always located in the lateral wall among those with LBBB,[63] but only in 50% of patients with non–LBBB wide QRS. This finding may partly explain the high response rate to CRT in patients with LBBB, and suggests a role of image guidance in the placement of

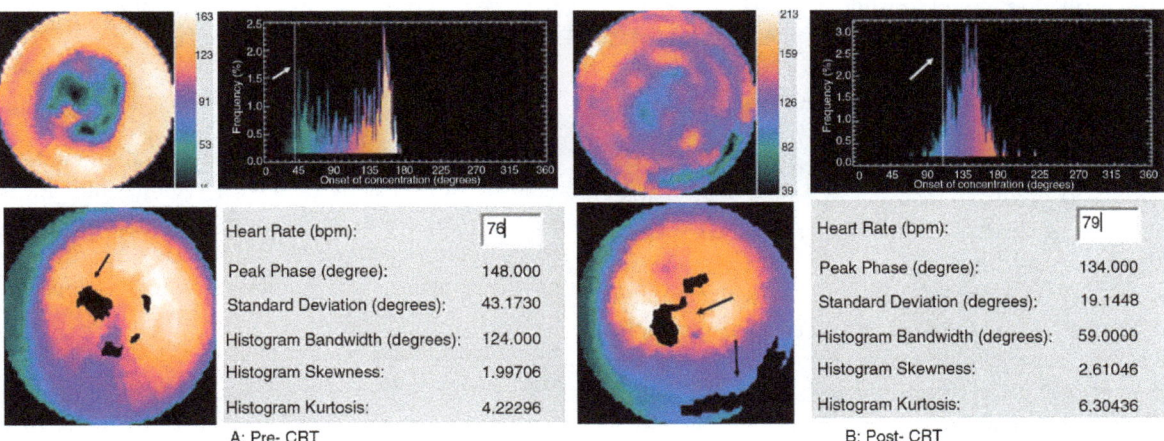

FIGURE 11-8 Example of serial assessment of dyssynchrony before (**A**, left panel) and immediately after (**B**, right panel) CRT. The top panel shows a phase polar map (left) and a phase histogram (right). The left image in the bottom panel shows the site of initial contraction of the LV as a blackout area(s) on a perfusion polar map, corresponding to the position of the cursor on the histogram (*arrows*). The bottom panel also shows the quantitative results of dyssynchrony assessment. This patient has a right ventricular pacemaker at baseline. The pre-CRT image shows a heterogeneous phase polar map, with the onset of contraction at the LV apex. The histogram and quantitative indices indicate the presence of LV dyssynchrony. Following CRT, the phase polar map is more homogenous, and LV contraction is initiated almost simultaneously at the apex and posterolateral wall, as would be expected with biventricular pacing. The histogram and quantitative measure indicate significant improvement in LV synchrony. In this patient, LV ejection fraction improved from 34% pre-CRT to 44% post-CRT.

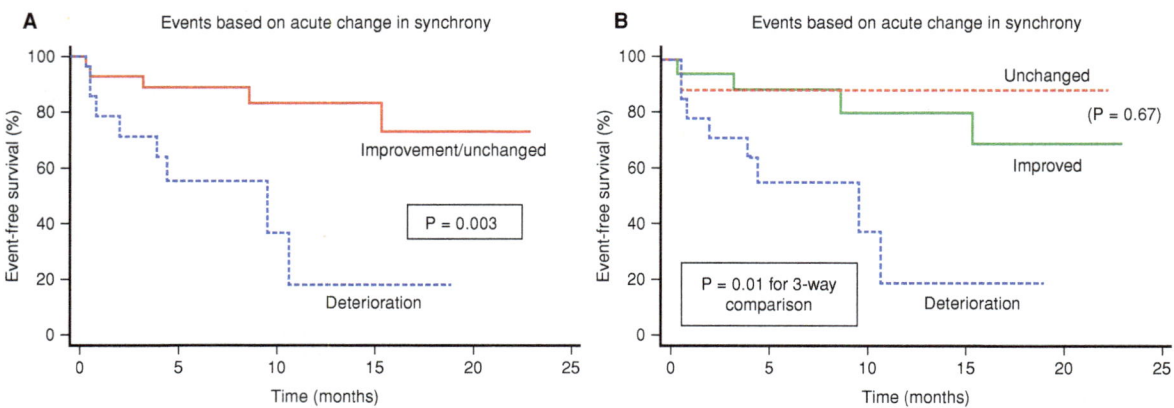

FIGURE 11-9 Kaplan–Meier event-free survival analysis based on acute response of left ventricular (LV) synchrony to cardiac resynchronization therapy (CRT). **(A)** Patients with an acute deterioration in LV synchrony after CRT had worse event-free survival compared with patients who had an acute improvement or no change (hazard ratio, 4.6 [1.3 to 16.0]). **(B)** Patients with no acute change in synchrony were similar in prognosis to patients who improved synchrony acutely after CRT (hazard ratio, 0.62 [0.09 to 4.4]).

the LV lead in patients with non–LBBB QRS patterns. Indeed, single-center studies do suggest improved outcome when the LV lead is targeted to a viable myocardial segment with delayed activation.[64–66]

The combined value of dyssynchrony, myocardial scar and LV lead concordance with SOLA, in predicting CRT response was evaluated in a prospective study of 44 HF patients undergoing CRT implantation.[64] The presence of baseline dyssynchrony and its change immediately following resynchronization was studied on gated SPECT with a novel "single-injection protocol." A prespecified algorithm comprising of (a) presence of baseline dyssynchrony, (b) scar burden of <40%, and (c) LV lead concordance with SOLA (Fig. 11-7), predicted acute improvement or no change in LV dyssynchrony with 93% specificity and 96% positive predictive value, with a 96% negative predictive value (NPV) for acute deterioration in dyssynchrony.

Figure 11-8 shows a representative example. Patients experiencing acute improvement or no change in LV dyssynchrony with CRT had lower composite outcome of death, heart failure hospitalization, and ventricular arrhythmia compared to those in whom dyssynchrony acutely deteriorated (Fig. 11-9), thus providing some mechanical insight into CRT response mechanisms.

Most patients with drug refractory, symptomatic HF, severe LV systolic dysfunction and a wide (>150 ms) LBBB QRS morphology will benefit from CRT if they do not have extensive scar. In these patients, the imaging of the severity and pattern of LV dyssynchrony is unlikely to offer additive value, but imaging to exclude extensive scar has direct relevance to CRT outcome. In patients with a narrow QRS complex, CRT has been shown to be detrimental even in the presence of echo evidence of LV dyssynchrony.[42] In patients with non–LBBB types of conduction abnormalities, the potential role of imaging dyssynchrony remains to be determined.

SUMMARY

The introduction of ECG gating and the resultant ability of SPECT to determine LV regional and global function has been an important addition to the scope of radionuclide MPI. LV function information provides critical information that has established diagnostic and prognostic value. In addition, it has expanded the application of MPI to other evolving areas such as LV dyssynchrony assessment.

REFERENCES

1. Cullom SJ, Case JA, Bateman TM. Electrocardiographically gated myocardial perfusion SPECT: Technical principles and quality control considerations. *J Nucl Cardiol*. 1998;5:418–425.
2. Germano G NK, Cullom SJ. Cardiac SPECT Imaging. In: DePuey EG GE, Berman DS, eds. *Gated Perfusion SPECT: Technical Considerations*. 2nd ed. Philadelphia, PA: Lippincott Williams & Wilkins; 2001:103.

3. Nichols K, Dorbala S, DePuey EG, et al. Influence of arrhythmias on gated SPECT myocardial perfusion and function quantification. *J Nucl Med.* 1999;40:924–934.
4. Johnson LL, Verdesca SA, Aude WY, et al. Postischemic stunning can affect left ventricular ejection fraction and regional wall motion on post-stress gated sestamibi tomograms. *J Am Coll Cardiol.* 1997;30:1641–1648.
5. Cerqueira MD, Weissman NJ, Dilsizian V, et al. Standardized myocardial segmentation and nomenclature for tomographic imaging of the heart. A statement for healthcare professionals from the Cardiac Imaging Committee of the Council on Clinical Cardiology of the American Heart Association. *J Nucl Cardiol.* 2002;9:240–245.
6. Manrique A, Koning R, Cribier A, et al. Effect of temporal sampling on evaluation of left ventricular ejection fraction by means of thallium-201 gated SPET: Comparison of 16- and 8-interval gating, with reference to equilibrium radionuclide angiography. *Eur J Nucl Med.* 2000;27:694–699.
7. Kumita S, Cho K, Nakajo H, et al. Assessment of left ventricular diastolic function with electrocardiography-gated myocardial perfusion SPECT: Comparison with multigated equilibrium radionuclide angiography. *J Nucl Cardiol.* 2001;8:568–574.
8. Germano G, Kavanagh PB, Slomka PJ, et al. Quantitation in gated perfusion SPECT imaging: The Cedars-Sinai approach. *J Nucl Cardiol.* 2007;14:433–454.
9. Pfisterer ME, Battler A, Zaret BL. Range of normal values for left and right ventricular ejection fraction at rest and during exercise assessed by radionuclide angiocardiography. *Eur Heart J.* 1985;6:647–655.
10. Jones RH, Johnson SH, Bigelow C, et al. Exercise radionuclide angiography predicts cardiac death in patients with coronary artery disease. *Circulation.* 1991;84:I52–I58.
11. Rozanski A, Nichols K, Yao SS, et al. Development and application of normal limits for left ventricular ejection fraction and volume measurements from 99mTc-sestamibi myocardial perfusion gated SPECT. *J Nucl Med.* 2000;41:1445–1450.
12. Moss AJ, Zareba W, Hall WJ, et al. Prophylactic implantation of a defibrillator in patients with myocardial infarction and reduced ejection fraction. *N Engl J Med.* 2002;346:877–883.
13. Bellenger NG, Burgess MI, Ray SG, et al. Comparison of left ventricular ejection fraction and volumes in heart failure by echocardiography, radionuclide ventriculography and cardiovascular magnetic resonance. Are they interchangeable? *Eur Heart J.* 2000;21:1387–1396.
14. Kliner D, Wang L, Winger D, Follansbee WP, Soman P. A prospective evaluation of the repeatability of left ventricular ejection fraction measurement by gated SPECT. *J Nucl Cardiol.* 2015;22:1237–1243.
15. Ather S, Iqbal F, Gulotta J, et al. Comparison of three commercially available softwares for measuring left ventricular perfusion and function by gated SPECT myocardial perfusion imaging. *J Nucl Cardiol.* 2014;21:673–681.
16. Wackers FJ, Berger HJ, Johnstone DE, et al. Multiple gated cardiac blood pool imaging for left ventricular ejection fraction: Validation of the technique and assessment of variability. *Am J Cardiol.* 1979;43:1159–1166.
17. Vallejo E, Dione DP, Bruni WL, et al. Reproducibility and accuracy of gated SPECT for determination of left ventricular volumes and ejection fraction: Experimental validation using MRI. *J Nucl Med.* 2000;41:874–882; discussion 83–86.
18. Knollmann D, Winz OH, Meyer PT, et al. Gated myocardial perfusion SPECT: algorithm-specific influence of reorientation on calculation of left ventricular volumes and ejection fraction. *J Nucl Med.* 2008;49:1636–1642.
19. Xu Y, Hayes S, Ali I, et al. Automatic and visual reproducibility of perfusion and function measures for myocardial perfusion SPECT. *J Nucl Cardiol.* 2010;17:1050–1057.
20. Mahmarian JJ, Moye L, Verani MS, et al. Criteria for the accurate interpretation of changes in left ventricular ejection fraction and cardiac volumes as assessed by rest and exercise gated radionuclide angiography. *J Am Coll Cardiol.* 1991;18:112–119.
21. Wackers FT. Has LVEF changed beyond chance? Limits of agreement of radiotracer-derived LVEF. *J Nucl Cardiol.* 2015:1–3.
22. DePuey EG, Rozanski A. Using gated technetium-99m-sestamibi SPECT to characterize fixed myocardial defects as infarct or artifact. *J Nucl Med.* 1995;36:952–955.
23. Taillefer R, DePuey EG, Udelson JE, et al. Comparative diagnostic accuracy of Tl-201 and Tc-99m-sestamibi SPECT imaging (perfusion and ECG-gated SPECT) in detecting coronary artery disease in women. *J Am Coll Cardiol.* 1997;29:69–77.
24. Smanio PE, Watson DD, Segalla DL, et al. Value of gating of technetium-99m-sestamibi single-photon emission computed tomographic imaging. *J Am Coll Cardiol.* 1997;30:1687–1692.
25. Chae SC, Heo J, Iskandrian AS, et al. Identification of extensive coronary artery disease in women by exercise single-photon emission computed tomographic (SPECT) thallium imaging. *J Am Coll Cardiol.* 1993;21:1305–1311.
26. Rehn T, Griffith LS, Achuff SC, et al. Exercise thallium-201 myocardial imaging in left main coronary artery disease: Sensitive but not specific. *Am J Cardiol.* 1981;48:217–223.
27. Christian TF, Miller TD, Bailey KR, et al. Noninvasive identification of severe coronary artery disease using exercise tomographic thallium-201 imaging. *Am J Cardiol.* 1992;70:14–20.
28. Sharir T, Bacher-Stier C, Dhar S, et al. Identification of severe and extensive coronary artery disease by postexercise regional wall motion abnormalities in Tc-99m-sestamibi gated single-photon emission computed tomography. *Am J Cardiol.* 2000;86:1171–1175.
29. Yamagishi H, Shirai N, Yoshiyama M, et al. Incremental value of left ventricular ejection fraction for detection of multivessel coronary artery disease in exercise (201)Tl gated myocardial perfusion imaging. *J Nucl Med.* 2002;43:131–139.
30. Emmett L, Iwanochko RM, Freeman MR, et al. Reversible regional wall motion abnormalities on exercise technetium-99m-gated cardiac single photon emission computed tomography predict high-grade angiographic stenoses. *J Am Coll Cardiol.* 2002;39:991–998.
31. Sharir T, Germano G, Kavanagh PB, et al. Incremental prognostic value of post-stress left ventricular ejection fraction and volume by gated myocardial perfusion single photon emission computed tomography. *Circulation.* 1999;100:1035–1042.
32. Sharir T, Germano G, Kang X, et al. Prediction of myocardial infarction versus cardiac death by gated myocardial perfusion SPECT: Risk stratification by the amount of stress-induced ischemia and the poststress ejection fraction. *J Nucl Med.* 2001;42:831–837.
33. Kroll D, Farah W, McKendall GR, et al. Prognostic value of stress-gated Tc-99m-sestamibi SPECT after acute myocardial infarction. *Am J Cardiol.* 2001;87:381–386.

34. Danias PG, Ahlberg AW, Clark BA, 3rd, et al. Combined assessment of myocardial perfusion and left ventricular function with exercise technetium-99m-sestamibi gated single-photon emission computed tomography can differentiate between ischemic and nonischemic dilated cardiomyopathy. *Am J Cardiol.* 1998;82:1253–1258.
35. Nagueh SF. Mechanical dyssynchrony in congestive heart failure: diagnostic and therapeutic implications. *J Am Coll Cardiol.* 2008;51:18–22.
36. Poole JE, Singh JP, Birgersdotter-Green U. QRS Duration or QRS Morphology: What Really Matters in Cardiac Resynchronization Therapy? *J Am Coll Cardiol.* 2016;67:1104–1117.
37. Zareba W, Klein H, Cygankiewicz I, et al. Effectiveness of cardiac resynchronization therapy by QRS morphology in the multicenter automatic defibrillator implantation trial-cardiac resynchronization therapy (MADIT-CRT). *Circulation.* 2011; 123:1061–1072.
38. Fauchier L, Marie O, Casset-Senon D, et al. Interventricular and intraventricular dyssynchrony in idiopathic dilated cardiomyopathy: A prognostic study with fourier phase analysis of radionuclide angioscintigraphy. *J Am Coll Cardiol.* 2002; 40:2022–2030.
39. Malhotra S, Pasupula D, Sharma R, et al. Left ventricular dyssynchrony predicts ventricular tachyarrhythmias in patients with severely reduced left ventricular systolic function. *J Am Coll Cardiol.* 2013;61.
40. Hawkins NM, Petrie MC, MacDonald MR, et al. Selecting patients for cardiac resynchronization therapy: Electrical or mechanical dyssynchrony? *Eur Heart J.* 2006;27:1270–1281.
41. Chung ES, Leon AR, Tavazzi L, et al. Results of the Predictors of Response to CRT (PROSPECT) trial. *Circulation.* 2008;117:2608–2616.
42. Ruschitzka F, Abraham WT, Singh JP, et al. Cardiac-resynchronization therapy in heart failure with a narrow QRS complex. *N Engl J Med.* 2013;369:1395–1405.
43. Galt JR, Garcia EV, Robbins WL. Effects of myocardial wall thickness on SPECT quantification. *IEEE Trans Med Imaging.* 1990;9:144–150.
44. Soman P, Chen J. Left Ventricular Dyssynchrony Assessment Using Myocardial Single-Photon Emission CT. *Semin Nucl Med.* 2014;44:314–319.
45. Chen J, Boogers MJ, Bax JJ, et al. The use of nuclear imaging for cardiac resynchronization therapy. *Curr Cardiol Rep.* 2010;12:185–191.
46. Chen J, Garcia EV, Folks RD, et al. Onset of left ventricular mechanical contraction as determined by phase analysis of ECG-gated myocardial perfusion SPECT imaging: Development of a diagnostic tool for assessment of cardiac mechanical dyssynchrony. *J Nucl Cardiol.* 2005;12:687–695.
47. Trimble MA, Velazquez EJ, Adams GL, et al. Repeatability and reproducibility of phase analysis of gated single-photon emission computed tomography myocardial perfusion imaging used to quantify cardiac dyssynchrony. *Nucl Med Commun.* 2008;29:374–381.
48. Lin X, Xu H, Zhao X, Chen J. Sites of latest mechanical activation as assessed by SPECT myocardial perfusion imaging in ischemic and dilated cardiomyopathy patients with LBBB. *Eur J Nucl Med Mol Imaging.* 2014;41:1232–1239.
49. Nakajima K, Okuda K, Matsuo S, et al. Comparison of phase dyssynchrony analysis using gated myocardial perfusion imaging with four software programs: Based on the Japanese Society of Nuclear Medicine working group normal database. *J Nucl Cardiol.* 2016.
50. Van Kriekinge SD, Nishina H, Ohba M, et al. Automatic global and regional phase analysis from gated myocardial perfusion SPECT imaging: Application to the characterization of ventricular contraction in patients with left bundle branch block. *J Nucl Med.* 2008;49:1790–1797.
51. Henneman MM, Chen J, Dibbets-Schneider P, et al. Can LV dyssynchrony as assessed with phase analysis on gated myocardial perfusion SPECT predict response to CRT? *J Nucl Med.* 2007;48:1104–1111.
52. Kiso K, Imoto A, Nishimura Y, et al. Novel algorithm for quantitative assessment of left ventricular dyssynchrony with ECG-gated myocardial perfusion SPECT: Useful technique for management of cardiac resynchronization therapy. *Ann Nucl Med.* 2011;25:768–776.
53. Mukherjee A, Patel CD, Naik N, et al. Quantitative assessment of cardiac mechanical dyssynchrony and prediction of response to cardiac resynchronization therapy in patients with nonischaemic dilated cardiomyopathy using gated myocardial perfusion SPECT. *Nucl Med Commun.* 2015;36:494–501.
54. Toussaint JF, Lavergne T, Kerrou K, et al. Basal asynchrony and resynchronization with biventricular pacing predict long-term improvement of LV function in heart failure patients. *Pacing Clin Electrophysiol.* 2003;26:1815–1823.
55. Lishmanov Y, Minin S, Efimova I, et al. The possible role of nuclear imaging in assessment of the cardiac resynchronization therapy effectiveness in patients with moderate heart failure. *Ann Nucl Med.* 2013;27:378–385.
56. Adelstein EC, Saba S. Scar burden by myocardial perfusion imaging predicts echocardiographic response to cardiac resynchronization therapy in ischemic cardiomyopathy. *Am Heart J.* 2007;153:105–112.
57. Ypenburg C, Schalij MJ, Bleeker GB, et al. Impact of viability and scar tissue on response to cardiac resynchronization therapy in ischaemic heart failure patients. *Eur Heart J.* 2007;28:33–41.
58. Xu YZ, Cha YM, Feng D, et al. Impact of myocardial scarring on outcomes of cardiac resynchronization therapy: extent or location? *J Nucl Med.* 2012;53:47–54.
59. Abu Daya H, Alam MB, Adelstein E, et al. Echocardiography-guided left ventricular lead placement for cardiac resynchronization therapy in ischemic vs nonischemic cardiomyopathy patients. *Heart Rhythm.* 2014;11:614–619.
60. Saba S, Marek J, Schwartzman D, et al. Echocardiography-guided left ventricular lead placement for cardiac resynchronization therapy: Results of the Speckle Tracking Assisted Resynchronization Therapy for Electrode Region trial. *Circ Heart Fail.* 2013;6:427–434.
61. Boogers MJ, Chen J, van Bommel RJ, et al. Optimal left ventricular lead position assessed with phase analysis on gated myocardial perfusion SPECT. *Eur J Nucl Med Mol Imaging.* 2011;38:230–238.
62. Zhou W, Hou X, Piccinelli M, et al. 3D fusion of LV venous anatomy on fluoroscopy venograms with epicardial surface on

SPECT myocardial perfusion images for guiding CRT LV lead placement. *JACC Cardiovasc Imaging.* 2014;7:1239–1248.
63. Malhotra S, Pasupula D, Khanna M, et al. Is left bundle branch block related to the mechanism of left ventricular dyssynchrony? *J Am Coll Cardiol.* 2014;63:A1121.
64. Friehling M, Chen J, Saba S, et al. A prospective pilot study to evaluate the relationship between acute change in left ventricular synchrony after cardiac resynchronization therapy and patient outcome using a single-injection gated SPECT protocol. *Circ Cardiovasc Imaging.* 2011;4:532–539.
65. Saba S, Marek J, Schwartzman D, et al. Echocardiography-guided left ventricular lead placement for cardiac resynchronization therapy: Results of the speckle tracking assisted resynchronization therapy for electrode region (STARTER) trial. *Circ Heart Fail.* 2013;6:427–434.
66. Khan FZ, Virdee MS, Palmer CR, et al. Targeted left ventricular lead placement to guide cardiac resynchronization therapy: The TARGET study: A randomized, controlled trial. *J Am Coll Cardiol.* 2012;59:1509–1518.

Interpretation and Reporting of SPECT Myocardial Perfusion Imaging

CHAPTER 12

Eve Vasutakarn Chongthammakun and Robert C. Hendel

INTERPRETATION

The review and interpretation of myocardial perfusion images are perhaps the key duty of a nuclear cardiologist. It is critical that image interpretation be performed in a systematic fashion so as to maximize the clinical value of the study and to ensure the highest-quality result of the entire procedure, providing optimal clinical information and assisting in clinical decision making. As discussed extensively in Chapter 5, the quality of the study must be reviewed and technical abnormalities be recognized. A comprehensive evaluation of all available imaging data must then be performed so as not to exclude potentially vital information.

A number of guidelines and tools have been recommended for the interpretation of myocardial perfusion studies.[1-5] These policies and guidelines have been developed by experts in the field and should be used as a guide to the successful interpretation of myocardial perfusion imaging (MPI). This chapter will provide suggestions for approaches for interpretation based upon these recommendations. Of note, as single-photon emission computed tomography (SPECT) imaging is performed in the vast majority of patients undergoing radionuclide imaging, this chapter focuses on the tomographic evaluation of perfusion and function with SPECT MPI, although the methods recommended in this chapter are largely applicable to PET imaging.

The sequence of imaging should include (1) review of the raw planar images, (2) analysis of the tomographic slices, (3) interpretation of gated SPECT data, and (4) incorporation of clinical data (Table 12-1).

Image Display

It is highly recommended that myocardial perfusion images be reviewed on a computer monitor as opposed to x-ray film or paper. While other media may provide useful information, the resolution of a computer monitor screen and the flexibility in adjusting a variety of parameters, including contrast, thresholds, and colors, makes this the medium that is greatly preferred. The practice of interpreting only "hard copy" images is discouraged, especially in view of the dynamic data, which is available by use of a workstation.

The patient's body habitus should be considered when interpreting images, as this information may support the artifactual nature of apparent perfusion defects. Therefore, data regarding height, weight, and gender should be provided to the interpreting

Table 12-1
Sequence of SPECT Myocardial Image Interpretation
Review raw planar images
Evaluate tomographic slices
Analyze gated SPECT data
Incorporate clinical data

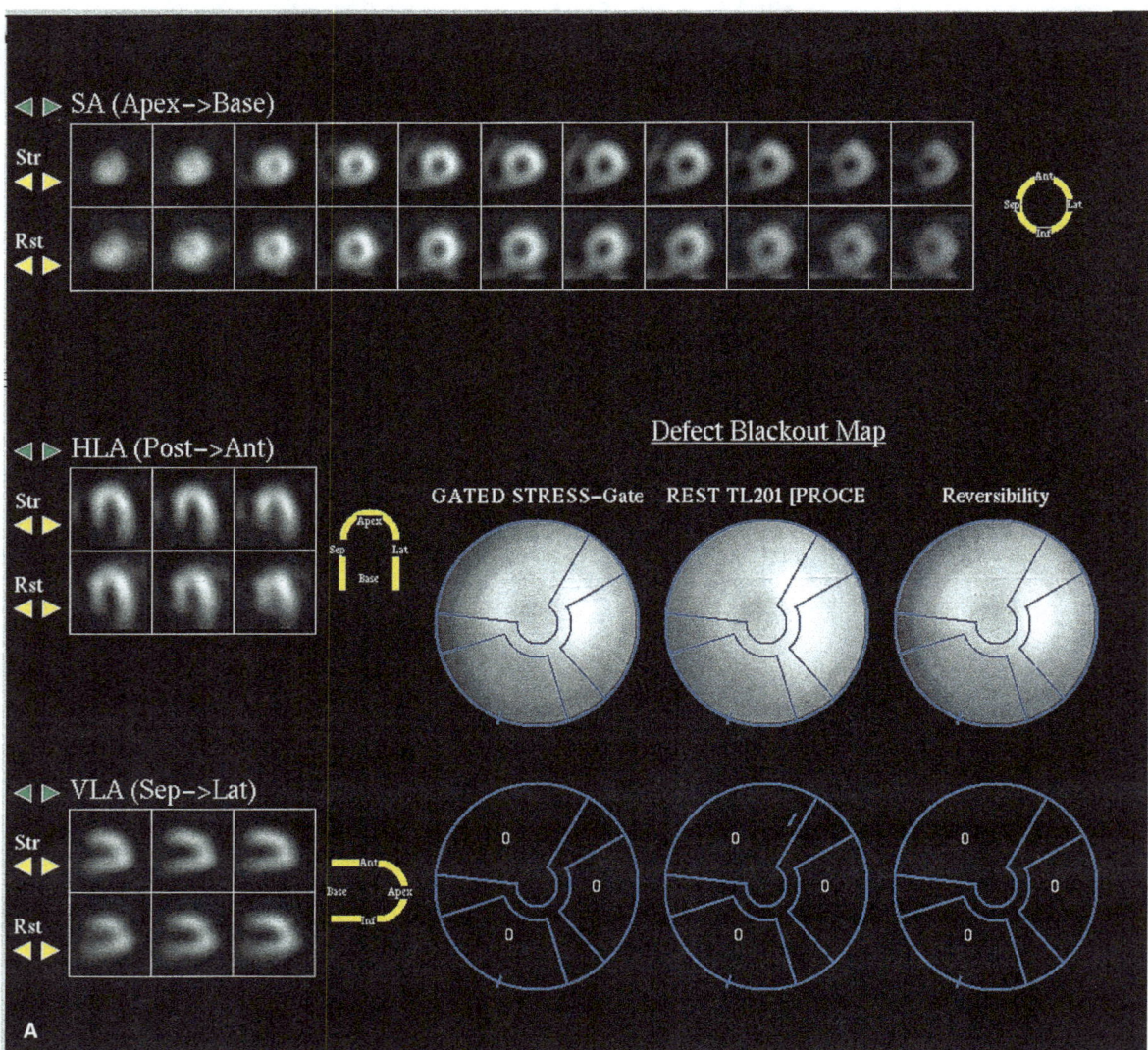

FIGURE 12-1 Exercise/rest dual-isotope myocardial perfusion images (thallium-201 for rest and technetium-99m-sestamibi for stress) in a 69-year-old man who presented with atypical chest pain. The myocardial perfusion images were felt to be normal except for the presence of soft tissue attenuation in the inferior and infraseptal regions. These images demonstrate the impact of varying tables. **(A)** Gray scale (exponential).

physician. Additional details, such as chest and bra size and the presence of a mastectomy or breast prostheses, may also be useful.

A linear color table is recommended for the interpretation of perfusion images. While linear gray scale is preferred and is recommended by many imaging guidelines, other continuous, linear color tables such as hot body/hot iron revised may also be used effectively (Fig. 12-1). A great variety of other color tables are available. It is critical that the interpreter understands the workings of these various color tables. It is usually recommended to avoid color tables with an abrupt transition between each color, for <10% change in tracer activity. Furthermore, it is critical that when a specific color table is used, the scaling should be linear, not exponential, as this will further enhance the appearance of artifacts potentially leading to false-positive results. Irrespective of the color table selected, the most important aspect of the use of these displays is that the operator

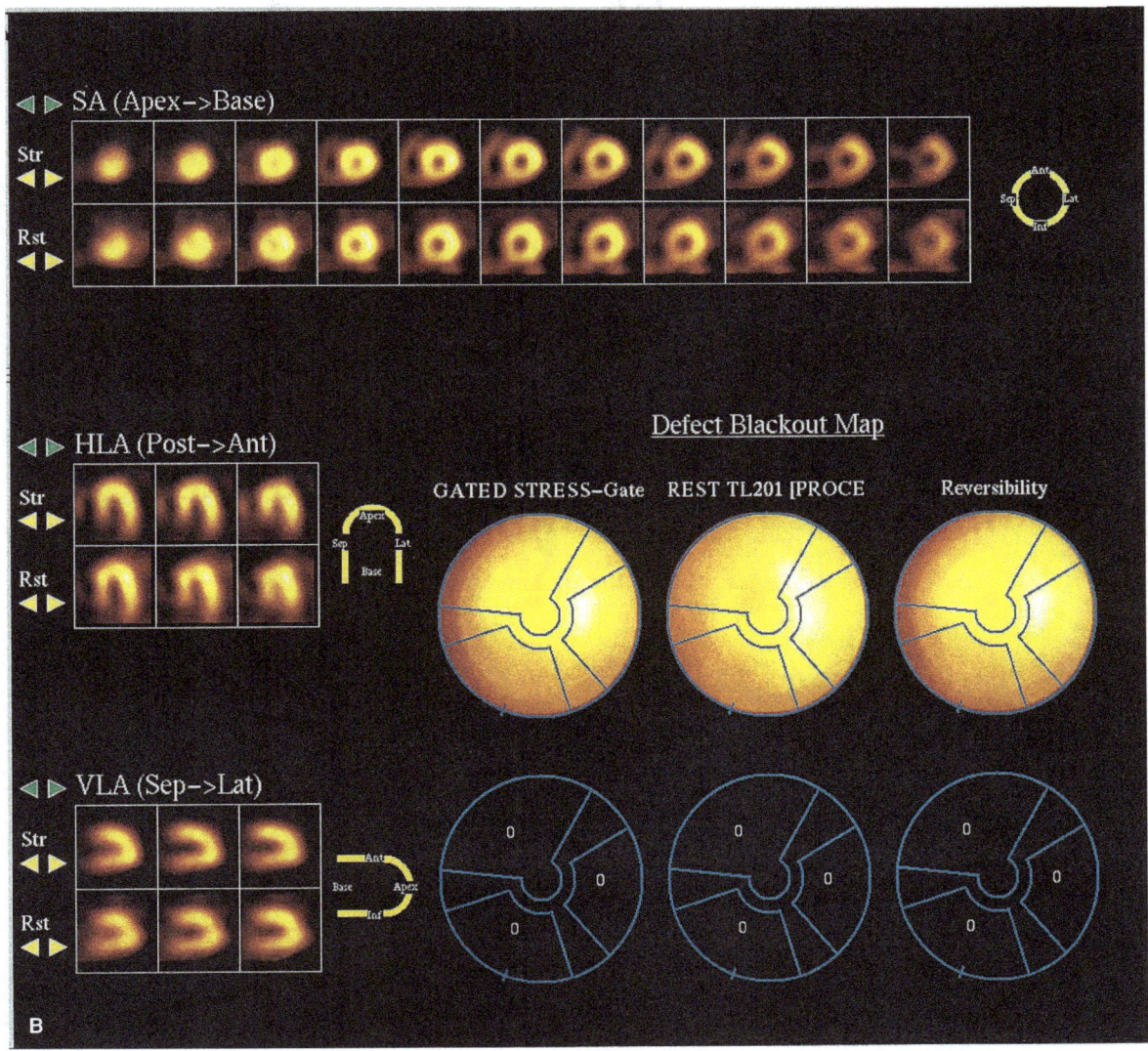

FIGURE 12-1 *(Continued)* **(B)** Hot body (or thermal) (exponential). *(continued)*

be very familiar with the one selected. A bar delineating the color table should also be displayed on screen.

Care should be taken in the review of images to ensure that the particular tomographic slices are aligned. By convention, the stress study is placed in the top row with the resting study below. It is now well accepted that the display of images should be in a specific format, as more than 10 years ago, the Joint Guidelines from the American Heart Association, the American College of Cardiology, and the Society of Nuclear Medicine stated the manner in which SPECT images should be displayed.[6]

The top row should present the short-axis views, which are obtained by slicing perpendicular to the long-axis of the lower left ventricle. By convention, the septum is on the left, with the lateral wall on the right. The slices should be displayed from apex to base (left to right). The long-axis should also be presented, demonstrating the data by slicing in a vertical plane (vertical long-axis) and a horizontal plane (horizontal long-axis). The vertical long-axis views should be displayed with the septal slices positioned on the left and progressing to the lateral wall on the right. The horizontal long-axis should be displayed with the

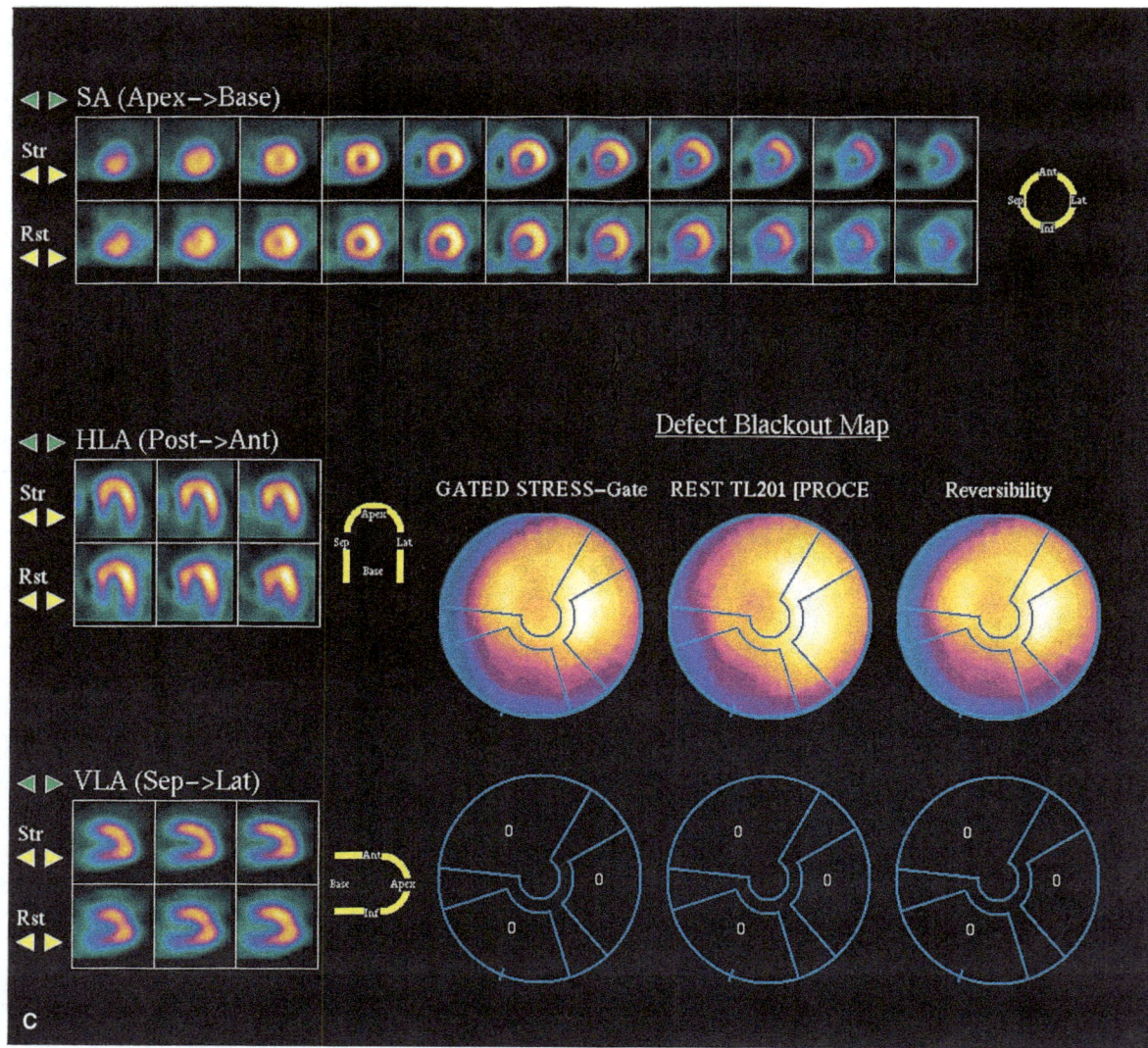

FIGURE 12-1 *(Continued)* **(C)** Warm metal (or CEqual) (linear).

inferior slices on the left and moving to the anterior location on the right. All images on the SPECT study should be normalized usually to the brightest pixel in the entire left ventricle within a series of slices (stress or rest). This is called series normalization.[4] Flexibility in display software should permit such scaling. Individual frame normalization may optimize image quality but lead to erroneous interpretation.

▶ Artifact Recognition

Although image artifacts may be recognized in several ways, the raw (unprocessed) projection images often provide the most useful information. Therefore, a critical aspect of the interpretation of tomographic data is the review of these rotating planar images.[3] All modern camera systems permit such a review often on the same screen as the SPECT slices.

Count Density

Adequate count data are essential to avoid "splotchy" data, which may easily be confused with perfusion defects. The reasons for low count density include: the dose and type of radiotracer, mode of stress, energy window, collimation, and attenuation. Beyond

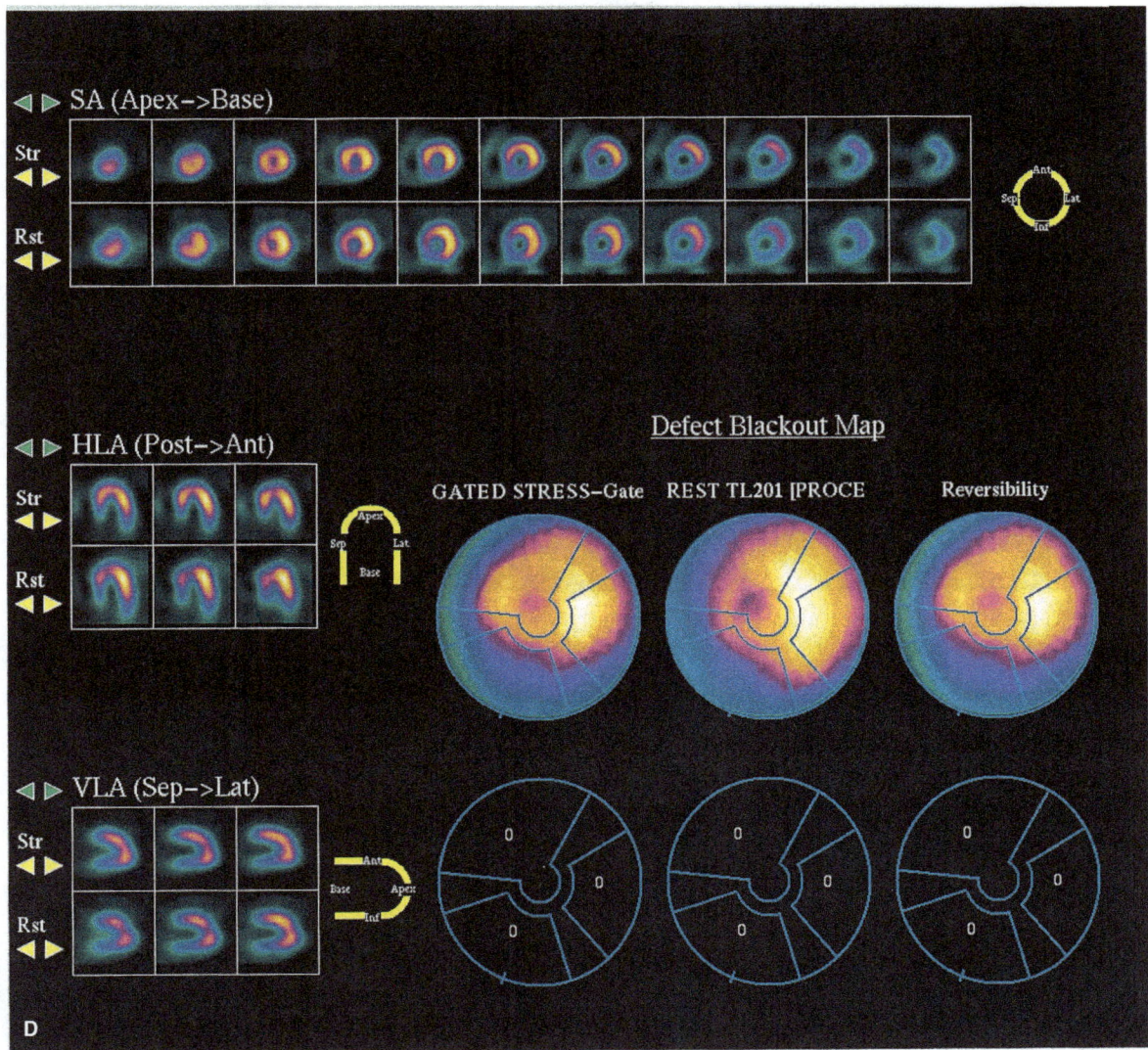

FIGURE 12-1 *(Continued)* **(D)** Warm metal (exponential). As can be noted, certain tables must be used with a linear scale, not an exponential relationship (**C** and **D**).

the visual assessment of rotating planar images or tomographic slices, quantitative assessment of the anterior planar project may be performed, with the requirement for peak pixel count of 100 and 200 for thallium-201 and Tc-99m, respectively.[4]

Patient Motion

While a sinogram (Fig. 12-2) or linogram has frequently been used to demonstrate motion and is composed of a sum of the planar data, this method for quality assessment is not ideal and is not recommended. The preferred approach is a review of a cine loop of both the stress and rest planar images usually simultaneously with the tomographic slices. It is often helpful to place a horizontal line beneath the inferior margin of the left ventricle for both rest and stress to better assess subtle but perhaps significant motion.

A patient motion-related artifact may be present in up to 15% of all SPECT studies.[7] A review of the rotating images provides clear evidence when there is patient motion, in either a superior–inferior manner or laterally. If substantial motion is present (≥2 pixels), repeating the image acquisition is recommended.

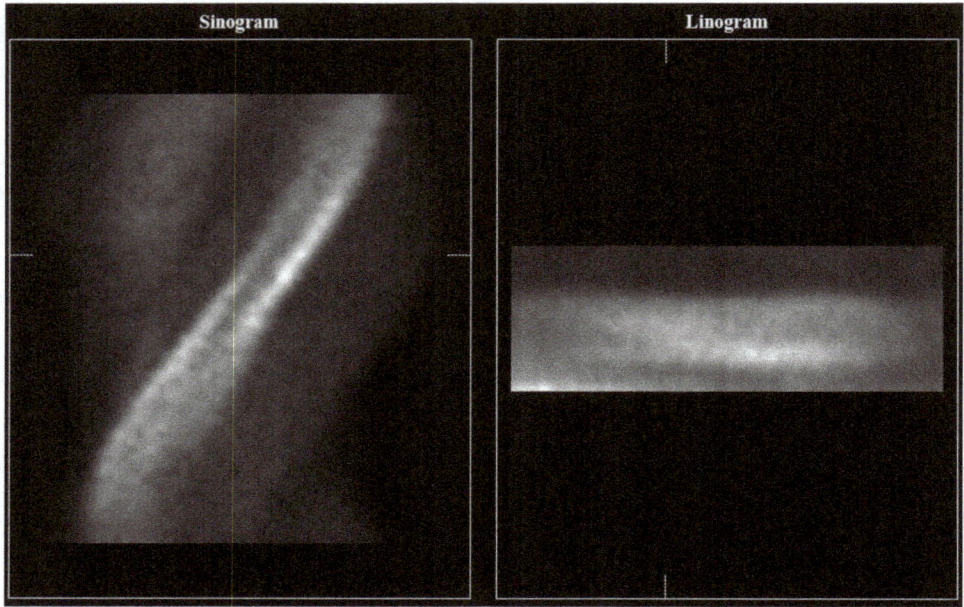

FIGURE 12-2 Example of a sonogram and a linogram. No patient motion is noted on this example as the borders of the lines are without displacement.

Motion correction algorithms may also be successfully applied,[8,9] but usually only when the patient motion is superior–inferior. Correction of lateral or rotational motion is challenging, but has been successfully incorporated into many software packages.

Multidetector systems may demonstrate abrupt motion on review of the rotating images. This is usually caused by temporal factors associated with a two-detector system and the fact that the last frame of acquisition for detector 1 is substantially later than the first frame obtained from detector 2. Thus, gradual motion throughout the acquisition is therefore accentuated when reviewing the rotating images.

The presence of patient motion may produce artifacts and therefore reduce diagnostic accuracy.[10] Not only do these artifacts resemble ischemic heart disease, but also patient motion may create the appearance of multivessel disease. "Upward creep" may also be detected by reviewing the rotating images. This phenomenon occurs when imaging is performed soon after strenuous exercise and results from the repositioning of the cardiac structures as the respiratory excursion decreases following exercise. The "upward creep" artifact may be avoided if imaging is delayed for about 15 minutes after exercise. Prominent patient motion may also be noted on the tomographic slices, producing a characteristic defect such as the "hurricane" sign and "flame" that occurs near the apex, as shown in Figure 12-3.[11]

Extracardiac Activity

The rotating planar images should be reviewed for the presence of abnormal activity beyond the boundaries of the myocardial structures. Skin or clothing

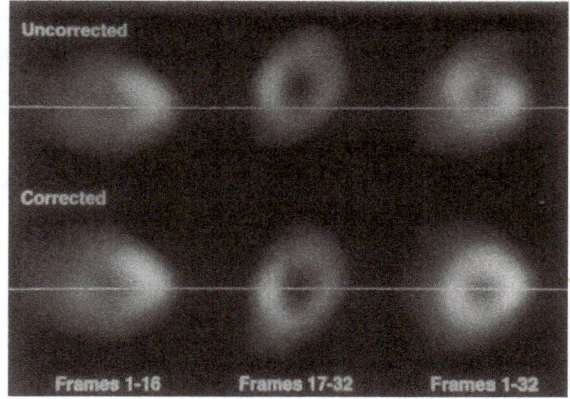

FIGURE 12-3 Hurricane sign, indicative of patient motion, as described in the original report. (Reproduced with permission from Sorrell V, Figueroa B, Hansen CL. The "hurricane sign": evidence of patient motion artifact on cardiac single-photon emission computed tomographic imaging. *J Nucl Cardiol.* 1996;3(1):86–88.)

contamination may mask or mimic a true perfusion abnormality but should be identifiable on the rotating images. The presence of intense subdiaphragmatic activity, emanating either from the liver or from the gastrointestinal (GI) tract, may confound image interpretation. Once such activity is present, it may cause a negative lobe artifact, also known as a ramp filter artifact. Intense adjacent activity may cause this reconstruction artifact, for which there is no reliable correction, although iterative reconstruction (as opposed to filtered backprojection) may help.[4] This type of abnormality may create an artifactual perfusion abnormality or may mask the presence of a true abnormality (Fig. 12-4). Ideally, when substantial activity is noted especially in the liver or adjacent bowel loop, image acquisition should be repeated to eliminate this type of artifact.

The interpretation of SPECT images should not be restricted only to the myocardium. A variety of neoplastic lesions may also be detected with commonly used radiopharmaceuticals.[3,12] These may reflect either primary or metastatic tumors and include the following types of neoplastic growths: lung, breast, sarcoma, lymphoma, thymoma, parathyroid tumor, thyroid abnormality, and kidney and hepatic tumors. Incidentally discovered clinical thyrotoxicosis can be detected by careful evaluation of the rotating planar images and may aid in the early detection of thyroid disease.[13]

Finally, the rotating images may reveal contamination by the radiopharmaceutical, occurring on either the skin or clothing, which once again may confound the SPECT image interpretation. In addition, it is usually possible to distinguish between a neoplastic growth and contamination by reviewing the rotating images.

Attenuation

Soft tissue, overlying cardiac structures, may confound image interpretation. Breasts/chest soft tissue, or that related to subdiaphragmatic structures, may reduce the specificity for coronary artery disease (CAD) detection and is present in up to 40% of all studies.

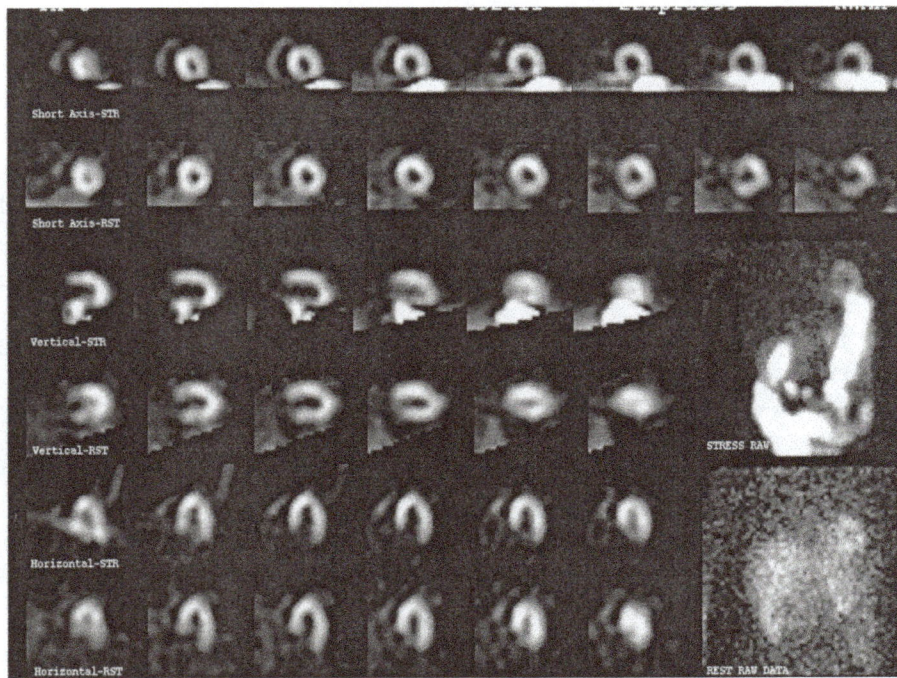

FIGURE 12-4 Dual-isotope myocardial perfusion images of a patient felt to be at low risk for coronary artery disease. **(A)** Prominent activity is noted in a bowel loop immediately adjacent to the infralateral wall on the resting images. This is clearly visible on the resting planar image. These images also demonstrate an apparent reversible inferior wall perfusion defect. (Used with permission from Thomas Holly, MD.) *(continued)*

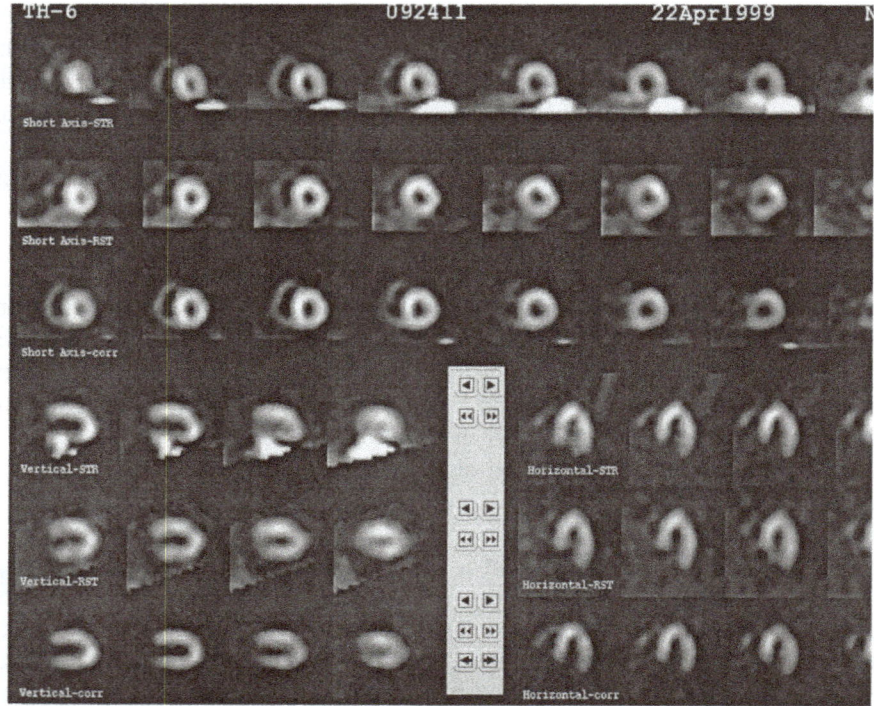

FIGURE 12-4 *(Continued)* **(B)** The stress and rest images are again shown on the first two rows in the short-axis, vertical long-axis, and horizontal long-axis images. The third row represents repeat image acquisition of the poststress images following food consumption, defecation, and waiting approximately 2 additional hours. With the subdiaphragmatic/bowel loop activity now removed, there is no perfusion abnormality noted in the inferior wall. (Used with permission from Thomas Holly, MD.)

Photopenic areas may be noted from overlapping breast tissue even when the size of the breast is relatively small. It is often possible to appreciate where the reduction of photons may occur on the SPECT slices by reviewing the cine images (Fig. 12-5).

In addition, soft tissue attenuation from the diaphragm may obscure the inferior wall, causing a false impression of an inferior wall abnormality. This occurs most commonly in men. Recognition of the superior-placed diaphragm is helpful in the interpretation of images and the enhanced recognition of a potential artifact. When such an abnormality is present, prone imaging may be helpful. In patients with large BMI, whose defect in the apical-inferior region may be diagnostically challenged, the addition of prone acquisition has been shown to improve diagnostic confidence, and when applied to stress-only MPI can reduce the need for unnecessary rest scans.[14,15]

Obviously, gated SPECT[16,17] and attenuation correction[18] methodologies may also be of substantial

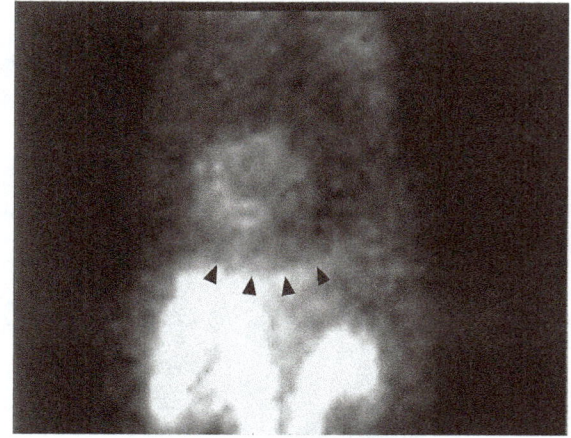

FIGURE 12-5 An individual frame of the rotating planar images demonstrating prominent soft tissue attenuation from the breast as depicted by the photopenic area (*arrowheads*). (Reproduced with permission from Hendel RC, Gibbons RJ, Bateman TM. Use of rotating (cine) planar projection images and the interpretation of a tomographic myocardial perfusion study. *J Nucl Cardiol.* 1999;6(2):234–240.)

use in the correct interpretation of soft tissue abnormalities. Differential soft tissue attenuation may occur when the overlying soft tissue is present in different positions on the rest and stress images, thereby leading to the appearance of an apparently reversible perfusion defect. This challenging scenario is not helped by gated SPECT, as true reversible defects (ischemia) may demonstrate normal left ventricular (LV) function.

▶ Analysis of Planar Images

Although tomographic MPI is considered the preferred modality for assessment of myocardial perfusion, planar imaging may be an alternative option in certain circumstances, such as in claustrophobic or critically ill patients where rapid acquisition is required, or in morbidly obese patients that do not qualify for the SPECT camera table. ECG-gated planar images can also be acquired. Regardless of whether the tomographic MPI is performed, planar images should always be inspected first preferably on a linear gray scale. Soft tissue attenuation by breast tissue, diaphragm, or other sources should be noted. Breast marker has been shown to be useful in identifying true perfusion defects from breast attenuation on planar images.

Similarly to the analysis of tomographic slices, segmental analysis of myocardial perfusion can be performed. The standard views for imaging positions and standardized nomenclature for myocardial segmental perfusion evaluation on planar images have been described in the ASNC myocardial perfusion planar imaging guideline.[19] For qualitative assessment, the severity of perfusion defect can be classified as mild, moderate, or severe and the extent of defect as small, medium, or large. A five-point segmental scoring system can be applied for semiquantitative evaluation, which is further described later in this chapter. If a quantitative analysis is to be performed on planar imaging, background subtraction must be applied to the images. Reversibility may also be reported from planar images.

▶ Analysis of Tomographic Slices

Image Quality

The first task is to determine whether or not adequate count statistics are present. A number of quality assurance tools are available from most manufacturers that assist in this process. The study should be graded based on overall image quality (uninterpretable, poor, fair, good, and excellent). Factors related to body habitus should be considered.

Cardiac and Lung Activity

The projection data also provide an assessment of cardiac size. Left ventricular hypertrophy (LVH) may be suspected when a reduced LV cavity:wall thickness ratio is noted. Prominent right ventricular uptake may be noted on the raw images or tomographic slices and may indicate right ventricular hypertrophy such as seen in pulmonary hypertension. However, no criterion other than subjective visual impression is available for this diagnosis.

Prominent lung activity may be present, which frequently is present in the setting of severe LV dysfunction or extensive ischemia. However, while abnormal lung activity is an important finding associated with thallium-201 scintigraphy, there is no consensus as to its meaning with technetium-99m imaging.[4]

LV cavity size may be assessed first by reviewing the rotating planar images. However, the overall cavity-to-wall-thickness ratio may be qualitatively determined by looking at the SPECT slices. In addition, it should be noted if the poststress images reveal a larger LV cavity than noted on the resting study (Fig. 12-6). This would be consistent with transient cavity dilation (TCD) also known as transient ischemic dilation (TID) of the LV cavity. The presence of TCD is a marker of proximal LAD and/or multivessel disease and a worsened prognosis.[20] The upper limits of normal TID values vary by protocols and types of isotopes used in the study (Table 12-2). Usually, about a 20% increase is required when using the dual-isotope protocol.[20] When using a single-isotope study, a lesser amount of cavity enlargement (approximately 5–10%) is felt to be abnormal.[21,22] Pharmacological MPI typically results in higher upper normal TID ratios when compared to exercise MPI as illustrated in Table 12-2. Gender difference for TID thresholds has also been noted, and should be taken into consideration when interpreting TID ratios.[23] In addition to the visual assessment, quantitative analysis of the TID ratio is available on most software packages.

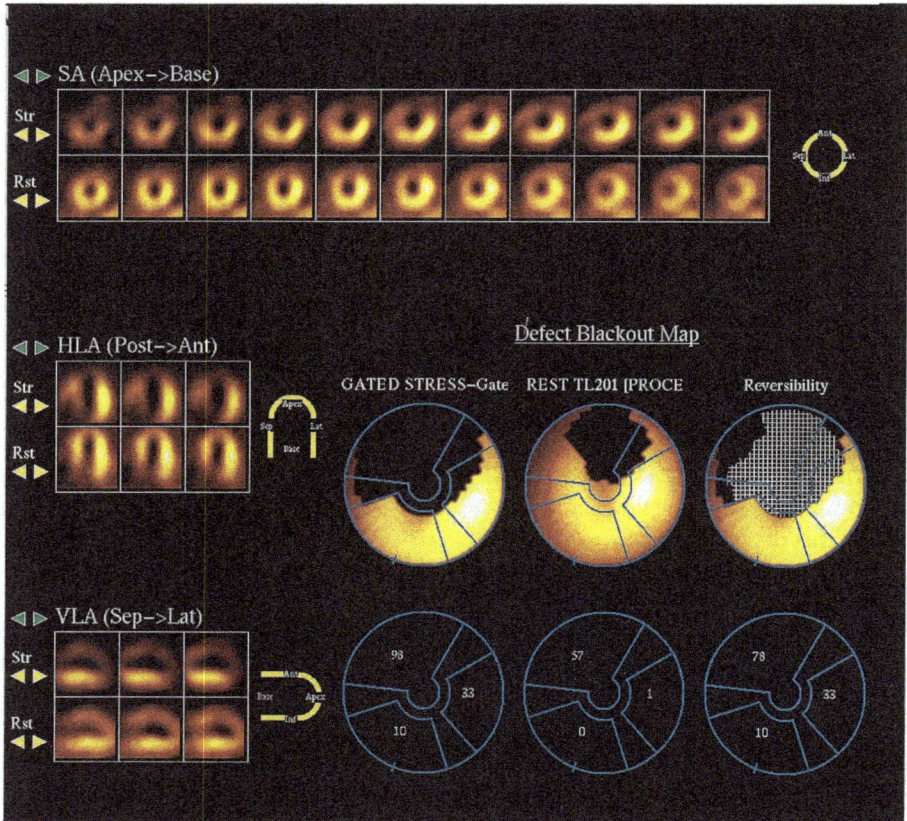

FIGURE 12-6 Perfusion images from a 31-year-old man with new onset of chest pain, who had limited exercise capacity and developed marked ST-segment changes during the stress test. The stress images reveal an extensive, severe defect in the anterior, septal, and apical regions, with substantial reversibility noted on the resting images. In addition, there is transient enlargement of the left ventricular cavity on the poststress images, relative to the resting study. The transient cavity dilation is most notable on the vertical and horizontal long-axis images; the TID ratio was 1.4.

Perfusion Defect

Defect severity is often described in a qualitative fashion (mild, moderate, and severe). A mild abnormality is one in which the clinical significance of the defect is unknown. Such an abnormality may reflect an equivocal finding. This often represents only a 10% reduction of peak tracer activity for a particular study. Moderate and severe defects carry more important diagnostic and prognostic value. In addition, the extent of the perfusion abnormality may also be qualitatively described as small, medium, or large (Figs. 12-7 and 12-8). Although these descriptions are relative, they may be based on objective information from quantitative programs.

In an attempt to describe the severity and extent as a combined value, a variety of scoring systems have been designed, the most popular being the summed stress and summed rest scores. These scores are derived by adding the point value using the range of "0" for normal perfusion to "4" for absent activity for each segment of the 17-segment model.[1] A mild, moderate, or severe reduction in count should be scored as 1, 2, or 3, respectively. The difference between the summed stress score and the summed rest score is called the summed difference score and is a measure of reversibility. Usually, individual segments with a ≥2-grade improvement on the resting study are felt to represent substantial ischemia. The size of the defect should be noted, as small, moderate, or large (Table 12-3).

Table 12-2

Abnormal TID Cutoffs for Different Protocols and Types of Isotope Used

Protocol	TID Threshold
Rest Tl-201/exercise stress Tc-99m sestamibi[20]	1.22
Rest Tl-201/exercise stress Tc-99m sestamibi[24]	1.23
Rest Tl-201/pharmacologic stress Tc-99m sestamibi	
Dipyridamole[25]	1.27
Adenodine[25]	1.35
Adenosine[26]	1.36
Regadenoson[27]	1.39
Dobutamine[25]	1.40
Exercise stress/rest Tc-99m sestamibi[24]	1.14
Rest/exercise stress Tc-99m sestamibi[21]	1.19
Gated rest/exercise stress Tc-99m sestamibi (end-diastolic volume)[21]	1.23
Regadenoson stress/rest Tc-99m sestamibi[28]	1.33
Rest/regadenoson stress Tc-99m tetrofosmin[22]	1.31
Dipyridamole stress/rest Tc-99m sestamibi (2-day)[29]	1.19
Gated stress/rest Tc-99m tetrofosmin (2-day; end-diastolic volume)[30]	1.25

The type of perfusion abnormality should also be described. A fixed perfusion defect (i.e., one that is the same on both the post stress and rest images) is often equated to a myocardial scar, especially when the abnormality is of severe intensity. However, a fixed perfusion abnormality may also reflect severe myocardial ischemia and the presence of myocardial viability. A reversible abnormality is a perfusion abnormality noted on the poststress images, but largely normalizes on the resting images. In many cases, some interpreters may use the term partially reversible. It is critical to determine whether it is a predominantly reversible defect or only a minimally reversible abnormality. Quantitatively, reversibility has a variety of definitions, but is often associated with a 20% to 30% improvement in regional activity.

"Reverse redistribution" describes a pattern where a defect noted on the rest images is either not present or less severe on the stress images. This finding may be noted in the setting of a subendocardial (nontransmural) scar and provides evidence of viability.[31] Although well described with thallium-201 scintigraphy, when this pattern is present with Tc-99m sestamibi or tetrofosmin, an artifact should be suspected. This finding likely relates to low count density of the resting study especially with a same day rest/stress protocol and does not correlate with significant coronary artery lesions.[32]

The perfusion abnormalities should also be identified by their location. Standard terminology has now been accepted.[1] The 17-segment model should be used for reference with regard to the nomenclature of such abnormalities (Fig. 12-9). However, in general terms, perfusion abnormalities should be described as being present in the apical, anterior, inferior, or lateral walls/regions. The term "posterior" should not be used. The perfusion abnormality may also be described as occurring within a specific vascular distribution. Obviously, the distribution of an individual coronary artery is highly variable. However, by convention, the 17 segments have been assigned specific vascular distributions so as to standardize interpretation and reporting. As a general rule, the lateral wall is assigned to the circumflex distribution, the anterior and anteroseptal regions to the left anterior descending coronary artery, the inferoseptal and inferior walls to the right coronary artery, and the apex is usually assigned to the left anterior descending distribution, although this is highly variable.

Table 12-3

Semiquantitative Defect Analysis

	Percent of Left Ventricle	Number of Segments[a]
Small	5–10	1–2
Moderate	15–20	3–4
Large	>20	≥5

[a]Data from Hendel RC, Budoff MJ, Cardella JF, et al. ACC/AHA/ACR/ASE/ASNC/HRS/ NASCI/RSNA/SAIP/SCAI/SCCT/SCMR/SIR. Key data elements and definitions for cardiac imaging. *J Am Coll Cardiol.* 2009;53:91–124.

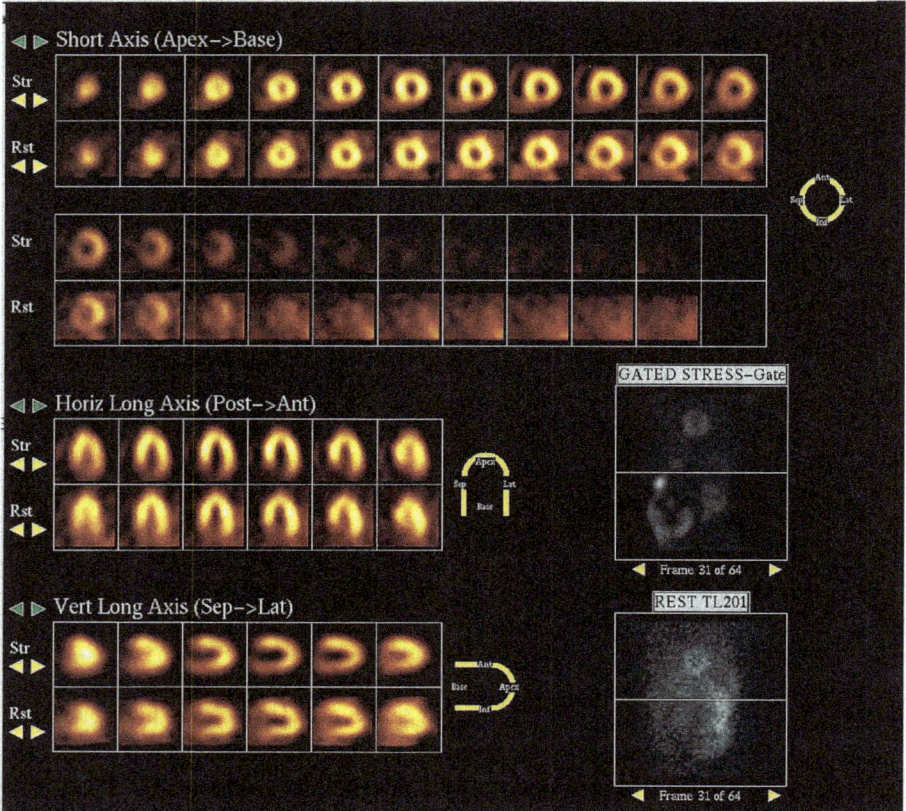

FIGURE 12-7 Exercise/rest dual-isotope myocardial perfusion images from a 69-year-old man with a history of hypertension, hyperlipidemia, and diabetes who presents with exertional chest pain. There is a small-sized defect of moderate severity involving the basal portion of the inferior wall. This perfusion abnormality appears completely reversible and is consistent with the significant stenosis in the right coronary artery. Subsequent coronary angiography confirms the presence of a 95% right coronary artery stenosis.

Quantitative Analysis

A variety of software tools are presently available, including the following products that are commercially available. These quantitative programs usually reference an individual patient's data to a normal reference profile. The comparison of individual studies to such a reference is often displayed as a polar map. The "blacked-out" segments usually reflect an area of activity that is below the threshold deemed as normal (Fig. 12-10). In many cases, it may represent a value such as 2.5 standard deviations below the mean value for a normal patient population; individual programs have specific thresholds. These thresholds and normal reference files are often different depending on the radiopharmaceutical. Furthermore, additional techniques, such as attenuation correction, may also alter the profiles. Most important, however, is that the normal reference files are gender specific unless attenuation correction methodology is employed. In addition to the polar map or bull's-eye projection, circumferential profiles may also be created again demonstrating where the count density falls below a specific threshold and is, therefore, deemed abnormal.

Quantitative analysis for most of the software programs has been validated in multiple studies and usually published in peer-reviewed journals,[33,34] which is further discussed in Chapter 9. However, it is advised that the quantitative analysis be used as a tool and guide, serving as a "second observer." These quantitative computer-assisted tools should not be used for primary analysis. Following the visual inspection of

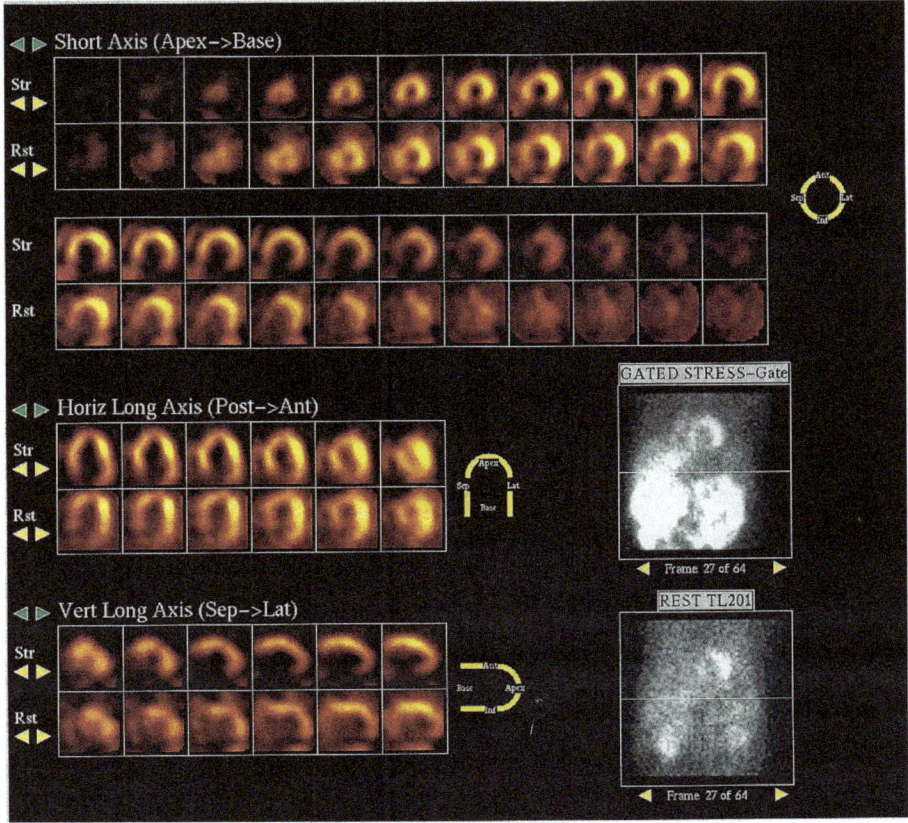

FIGURE 12-8 Adenosine/rest dual-isotope myocardial perfusion imaging in a 75-year-old man with a history of known coronary artery disease and status postmyocardial infarction. He is currently asymptomatic. The perfusion images demonstrate a large area of severely reduced activity in the inferior and inferoseptal walls, with a moderately severe abnormality noted in the septum and apical regions. No reversibility (ischemia) is noted.

the tomographic slices, quantitative interpretation may be examined. Any discrepancies or previously unrecognized abnormalities may then be reviewed. However, the individual interpreter must "overread" the computer-assisted interpretations, as many technical problems may develop and lead to false results. Therefore, quantitative analysis is not a substitute for an expert interpretation but should be used as an adjunct to assist the interpreter.

Gated SPECT

It is now recommended that gated SPECT be employed for essentially all myocardial perfusion SPECT imaging studies[35] with a standardized approach for the interpretation of gated SPECT data. This critical component of contemporary perfusion imaging is discussed in detail in Chapter 11. The gated SPECT data are often displayed in different fashions, depending on the software. Irrespective of the display, the most critical information is often demonstrated in the mid-ventricular slices from each of the orthogonal axes. Gated SPECT should be displayed as a cine loop, and the interpreter should observe the images for overall global function, examining the endocardial surfaces and their excursion. In addition to the motion of the endocardial walls, myocardial thickening may be determined by the increase in brightness noted on gated SPECT display resulting from the partial volume effect. It is possible that the thickening (brightening) may be normal, although the excursion is abnormal. This is

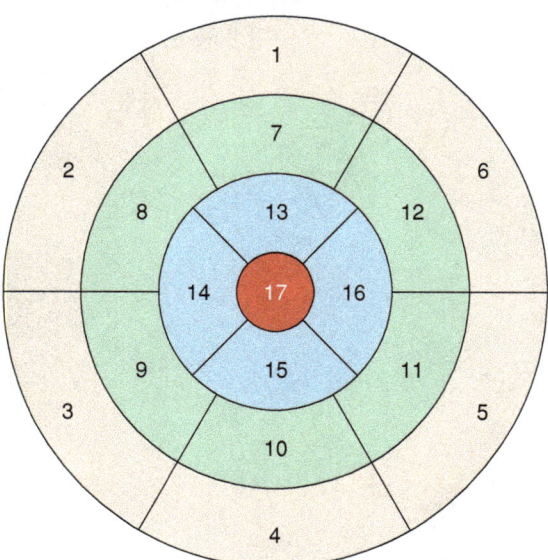

Left ventricular segmentation

1. Basal anterior
2. Basal anteroseptal
3. Basal inferoseptal
4. Basal inferior
5. Basal inferolateral
6. Basal anterolateral
7. Mid anterior
8. Mid anteroseptal
9. Mid inferoseptal
10. Mid inferior
11. Mid inferolateral
12. Mid anterolateral
13. Apical anterior
14. Apical septal
15. Apical inferior
16. Apical lateral
17. Apex

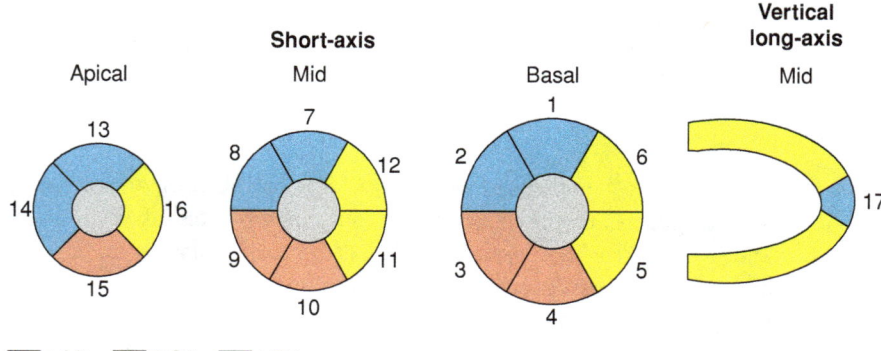

FIGURE 12-9 **(A)** A polar-plot depiction of left ventricular segmentation according to the 17-segment model. The recommended nomenclature is noted for each segment below. **(B)** The 17-segment model, obtained by three individual short-axis slices as well as one mid-cavity vertical long-axis slice. A depiction of the coronary artery distribution is also noted. (Reproduced with permission from Cerqueira MD, Weissman NJ, Dilsizian V, et al. Standardized myocardial segmentation and nomenclature for tomographic imaging of the heart: a statement for healthcare professionals from the Cardiac Imaging Committee of the Council on Clinical Cardiology of the American Heart Association. *Circulation.* 2002;105(4):539–542.)

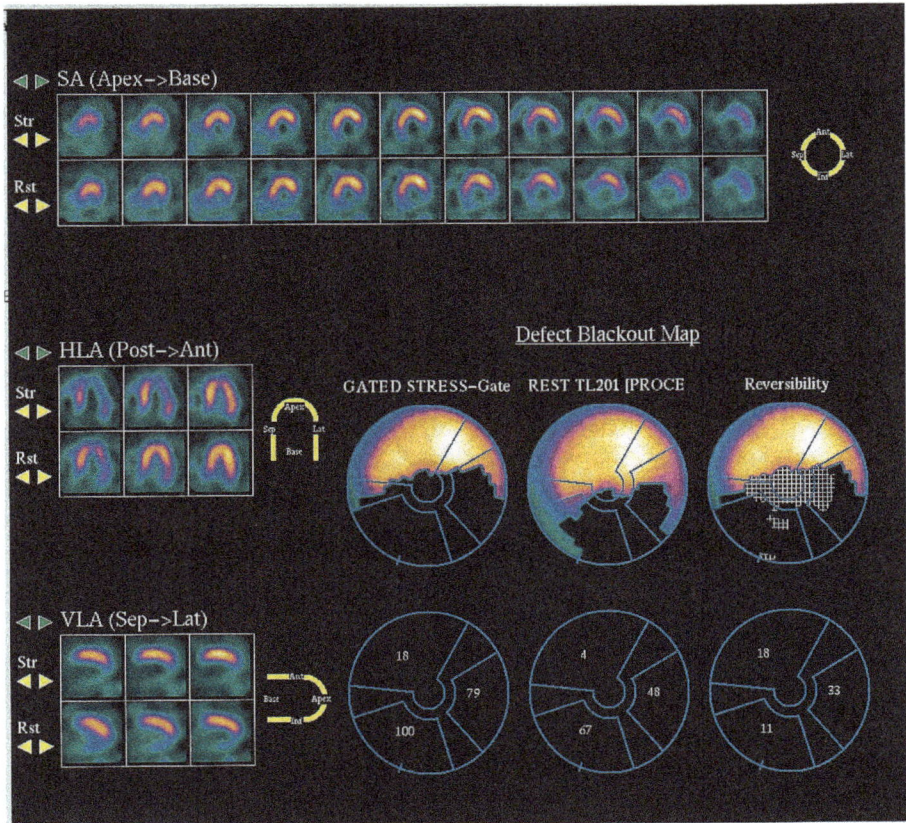

FIGURE 12-10 Stress/rest perfusion imaging demonstrates a large inferior, interoseptal, and interolateral defect, which has a small area of reversibility (ischemic) in the apex. The polar plots demonstrate the large extent of the defect, with the hatched region indicating reversibility.

often seen in settings such as following previous cardiac surgery, where the septum appears dyskinetic or akinetic, but thickens (brightens) normally. If there is difficulty localizing the endocardial surfaces, most software will provide "contours" where the computer will provide a line for what it believes to be the endocardial surface (Fig. 12-11). This may be used to assist the interpreter in evaluation of endocardial motion. Regional abnormalities may also be determined especially by examining multiple axes. Similar geographic schema to that noted for perfusion imaging should be employed when describing regional wall motion abnormalities.

A great variety exists with regard to the use of displays for gated SPECT information. While black and white or "hot body/thermal" may demonstrate brightening very effectively, a number of different color tables have also been used to assist in evaluating myocardial brightening or increases in count intensity. Overall, however, the monochromatic color tables are usually recommended.

Gated SPECT Quality

It is critical to have sufficient count density to examine for the accurate interpretation of gated SPECT data. A number of software programs analyze each of the frames to determine if the count density is adequate. The overall image quality should help the interpreter determine whether or not the study is interpretable. Another concern is that of poor gating, which is manifested as a flashing on the rotating planar images. This is due to variation in the beat–beat interval. For the most part, however, the overall global function data, including the ejection fraction, is still well preserved. If anything, cardiac arrhythmias more

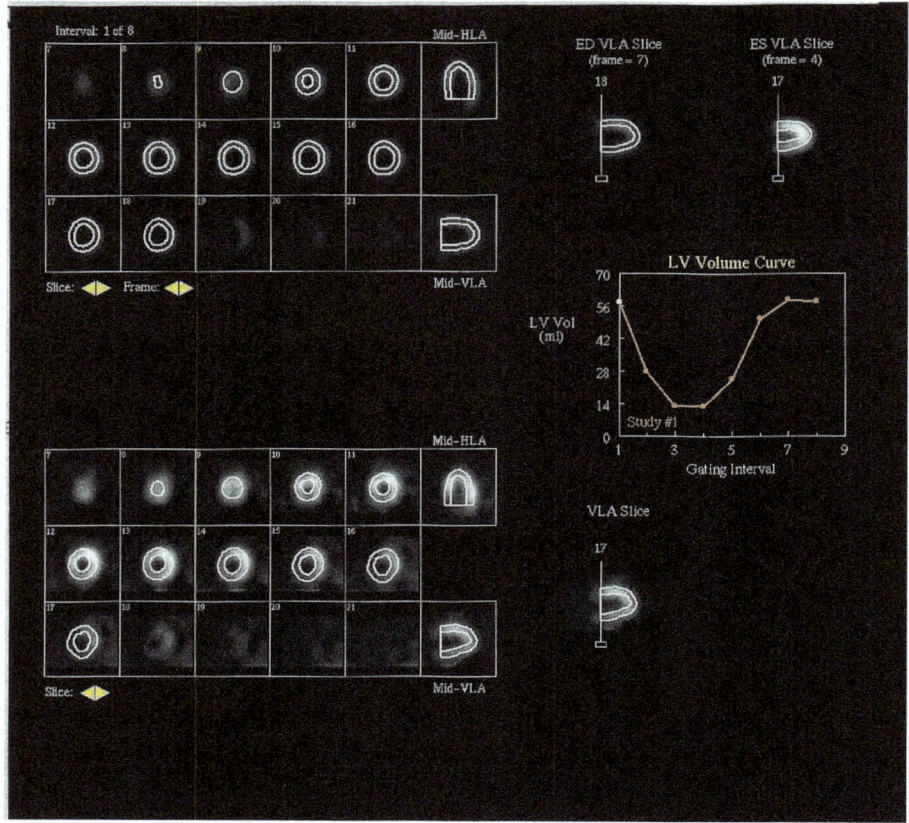

FIGURE 12-11 Computer-assisted detection of the endocardial surfaces on gated SPECT with the "contours" demonstrating the boundaries of the endocardial and epicardial surfaces (4 D-M SPECT™).

often affect the myocardial perfusion data than they do the gated SPECT information and its impact on functional information. The use of a heart rate histogram may be useful in this setting to explain apparent count "drop out" (Fig. 12-12).

Semiquantitative Description

Global and regional wall motion abnormalities should be defined as normal, hypokinetic, akinetic, or dyskinetic. It is possible to further subdivide the hypokinesis, although it may be difficult to differentiate between mild and moderate hypokinesis. A five-point scoring system for thickening and wall motion has been described ranging from normal function to mild or moderate hypokinesis, to akinesis and dyskinesis. Usually, wall thickening correlates well with wall motion. However, following cardiac surgery, there is usually reduced excursion of the septum, with normal thickening, a finding that is a normal variant.

Quantitative Analysis

Global LV function may be accurately quantified and described specifically using an ejection fraction determination. Each software program has been well validated and reveals good correlation with other methodologies. When the ejection fraction is >70%, such as occurring in patients with small LV cavities, it is suggested to describe this as either "normal" or "≥70%," as it is somewhat nonsensical to describe an ejection fraction of 92%. More qualitative descriptions may also be used such as "normal function" or those studies possessing mild, moderate, or severely reduced LV systolic function. However, given the overall validation of cardiac software packages, it is recommended to quantitatively describe the ejection

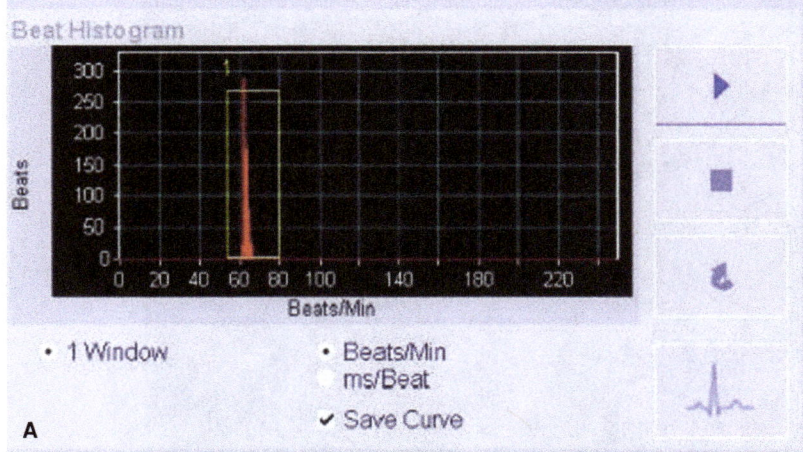

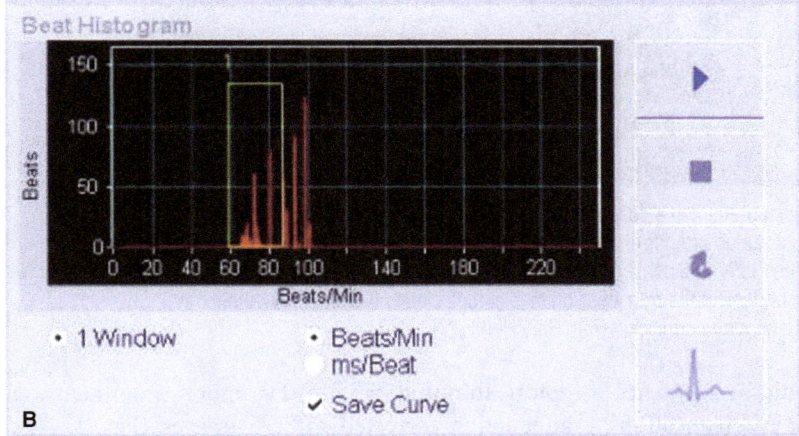

FIGURE 12-12 Histogram of patients with a regular rhythm and narrow range of beat rate (Panel **A**) and with an irregular rhythm with a substantial portion of beats lying outside of the R–R interval window (Panel **B**).

fraction. LV volumes, both end systolic and end diastolic, may also be noted.

Regional wall motion abnormalities and regional myocardial thickening have also been accurately determined using several cardiac software packages. This information is often graphically depicted as a three-dimensional plot. This may be used to assist the interpreter in determinations of abnormal function. However, most of these methods have been less well validated than the global ejection fraction determination. Therefore, the tools for regional determinations should be used as an adjunctive technique to assist the interpreter.

Attenuation Correction

A number of manufacturers possess well-validated methods for correcting soft tissue attenuation.[18] Although different techniques have been employed by most vendors, the literature now supports the conclusion that diagnostic specificity is improved. In addition, it appears that attenuation correction may assist in the improved detection of multivessel disease and left main stenosis. It is also likely that attenuation correction will assist in prognostic applications. It is, however, critical to understand the workings of each system, as they are widely different. The interpreter of myocardial perfusion SPECT imaging should note each system's benefits and potential limitations. All attenuation correction methods may cause artifacts, especially when used incorrectly. Therefore, the interpreter should know the specifics of such attenuation correction–derived artifacts as well as how effective it is in correcting soft tissue attenuation.

It is critical that the quality of the transmission map used for correcting the emission data be of high

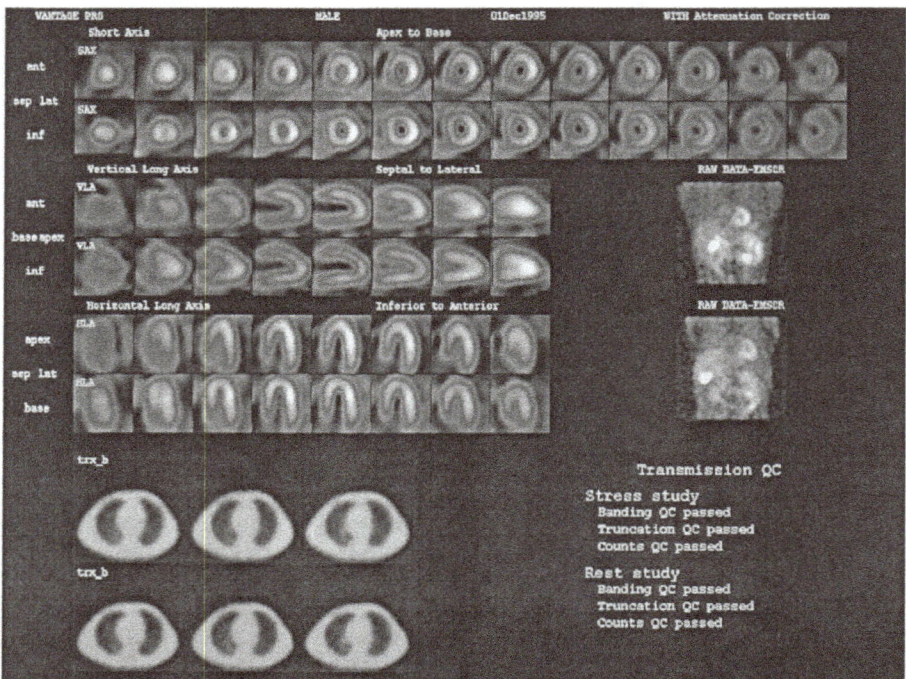

FIGURE 12-13 Stress images obtained in a 49-year-old man with a low likelihood for coronary artery disease. The top rows demonstrate an inferior and interoseptal wall perfusion abnormality. Following attenuation correction (Vantage Pro™, Philips), a more uniform appearance is present (bottom rows). The bottom portion of the figure depicts the transmission map, which clearly demonstrates the lungs and mediastinal structures. (Used with permission from Gary Heller, MD, PhD.)

quality (Fig. 12-13). The counts should be adequate, as determined by the manufacturer, and truncation should be absent or minimal. If the quality of the transmission scan is suboptimal, the attenuation-corrected images should not be used.

It is presently advised that the attenuation-corrected images be viewed in conjunction with the review of the uncorrected images. It is critical to understand how the correction occurred and its impact on the images. With the understandings of the benefits and limitations of each system, as well as comparing the uncorrected and corrected information, the interpreter can then gain the true value of attenuation-corrected perfusion imaging. Caution is often advised when there is prominent activity from overlying structures such as the bowel or liver. This can directly impact on the interpretation of an inferior wall abnormality. Specifically, if substantial hepatic or subdiaphragmatic activity is present, a true inferior wall perfusion abnormality may be masked by attenuation correction. Importantly,

apical thinning is also far more prominent on attenuation-corrected SPECT images (Fig. 12-14). It is, therefore, critical to understand the "normal" appearance of an attenuation-corrected image. Likewise, the right ventricle is far more prominent on attenuation-corrected SPECT imaging. This does not reflect right ventricular enlargement or hypertrophy, but instead improves visualization of the structure. Obviously, a "learning curve" is required to understand the impact of attenuation correction on the LV apex and right ventricle. It is recommended that the uncorrected SPECT images be examined in addition to the attenuation-corrected data.[4,5]

▶ Prone Imaging

In addition to the commercially available attenuation correction software, combined supine-prone myocardial perfusion SPECT without attenuation correction has been shown to minimize soft tissue attenuation and increase specificity and diagnostic

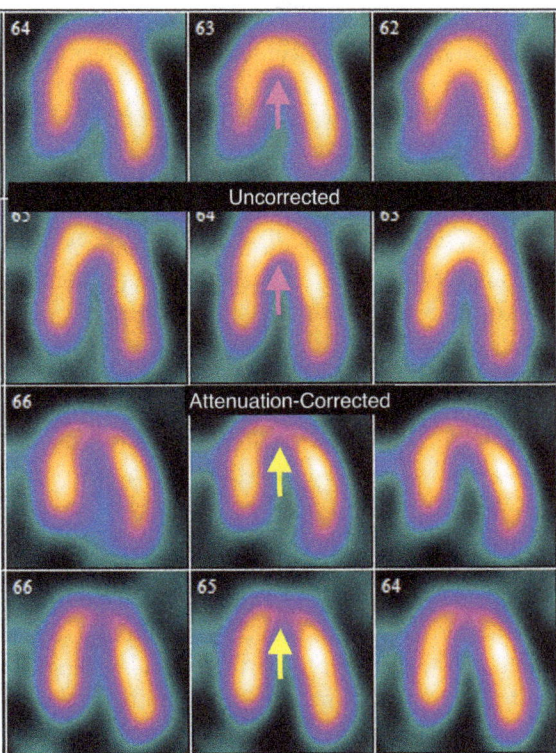

FIGURE 12-14 Horizontal long-axis images of a patient with normal myocardial perfusion. The top two rows depict standard, noncorrected stress and rest SPECT images, with the *pink arrow* pointed at the apex. The bottom two rows are following attenuation correction, demonstrating an apical defect (*yellow arrows*), which is due to apical thinning and commonly seen following attenuation correction.

accuracy in the detection of CAD, especially in women and obese patients.[14,15] By shifting the heart anteriorly and the diaphragm and subdiaphragmatic organs inferiorly, prone position improves inferior wall attenuation artifact. However, prone-only MPI is not recommended due to possible artifactual anterior and anteroseptal defects from the close proximity of the myocardium to anterior bony structures, for example, ribs and sternum, resulting in false-positive results.

The use of combined supine-prone MPI has similar prognostic values compared to attenuation-corrected MPI. The presence of perfusion defects on supine acquisitions but normal on prone images indicates a good prognosis and a low risk for subsequent cardiovascular events, similar to that of patients with normal supine-only studies.[14,15]

Incorporation of Clinical Data

Beyond information regarding the patient's body habitus, clinical data, including risk factors, may influence image interpretation. As such, these data should be considered only after careful image interpretation. How this information should be weighed with regard to final impression is controversial, although most experts recommend not including this in the final conclusion. However, data regarding prior cardiac events, including revascularization and myocardial infarction (MI), must be considered so as to add to the clinical relevance of the study.

Clinical Decision Support Systems

A clinical decision support systems (CDSS) is an interactive computer software developed to assist physicians and health care professionals with interpretation of imaging studies and to support clinical decision making in order to enable faster interpretation and more accurate diagnosis. With the aid of an artificial intelligence, subjectivity and intra- and interobserver variation in image interpretation are minimized, resulting in standardized high-level performance and more cost-effective care.

A CDSS has two basic components: (1) a dynamic knowledge base obtained from evidence-based medicine and expert opinions, and (2) an inferencing mechanism which is a navigational tool to reach a conclusion. Various methodologies and techniques used in MPI CDSS have been well described, such as bayesian networks, artificial neural networks, case-based reasoning, rule-based systems, data mining, and natural language processing.[36] After the images and clinical data are processed, a structured report is generated by the system, which allows the interpreter to edit or override the automated results from CDSS. The report generated by CDSS should meet the standardized reporting guidelines as further described in this chapter.

Despite the application of artificial intelligence to nuclear imaging, human interpreters will remain the role of primary diagnosticians, and results should be reviewed and confirmed by physicians. The development of integrated CDSS software will continue to ensure that nuclear cardiology remains the leader in the field of digital imaging.

▸ **Summary—Interpretation**

A systematic process of interpretation of myocardial perfusion SPECT images is critical for the highest level of accuracy and clinical utility. Attention must be paid to the quality of MPI data. In recent years, a variety of guidelines and position papers have focused on optimal techniques for image interpretation.[1–5,7,14,15,17–19] A complete listing of all items to be considered, including those that are standard, recommended, or optional, may be found in the most recent version of the ASNC guidelines for image interpretation.[4,5,19] A common vocabulary and format also ensures that high-quality interpretation and reporting is achieved. Advanced imaging technology, including quantitative analysis, gated SPECT, and attenuation correction, has improved the value of SPECT imaging, but the "reader" of such images must be cognizant of the advantages and pitfalls for these methods and understand the potential impact of these techniques on the final interpretation.

REPORTING

The final product of a nuclear cardiology procedure is the report. This directly reflects not only on the performance of the imaging study performed, but also on its interpretation. It is ultimately the critical piece of information that guides patient management. As such, it is essential that the report be inclusive yet clear in its meaning. The quality of the report reflects not only on the interpreting physician, but also on the nuclear cardiology laboratory and on the field of nuclear cardiology itself.

Many current nuclear cardiology reports fall far short of the mark of clarity. Words such as "suggestive of," "possible," and other qualifiers should be avoided. In addition, the unique descriptions of perfusion abnormalities such as describing the severity as ">2" or the use of words such as paradoxical should be removed. While the intent of the reader may be well known within one institution, significant problems may arise should the report migrate out of the individual laboratory's usual realm. In describing the location of various perfusion abnormalities, consistency must be present and words such as posterior are now not recommended. Finally, ubiquitous and somewhat insulting comments, such as "clinical correlation is suggested," should be avoided. The latter phrase need not be included, as the correlation of all imaging results should be performed with regard to the clinical history. Finally, descriptions such as "of unknown significance" or "equivocal" should be restricted to the most extreme of circumstances.

A number of publications have delineated the importance of a nuclear cardiology report[2,35,37] and guidelines have been proposed to define the components of the content of this report.[38,39] Obviously, individuality is critical, and reports will need to be adjusted to suit the laboratory as well as the individual nuclear cardiologist. However, some standardization is critical so as to optimize the information and to provide the most clinically relevant data to the referring physician.

Currently, reports are often variable in content and in form. While this is acceptable, ambiguity and a lack of an impression are not helpful to the patient, the referring physician, or nuclear cardiology. The most important goal of a nuclear cardiology report should be the communication of critical findings to the referring physician and their clinical implications. In addition, the report should serve to document information that is pertinent to reimbursement and accreditation licensure. The latter includes drug management and radiation safety.

Finally, certification and accreditation are based often on nuclear cardiology reports, and organizations such as IAC-Nuclear/PET (http://www.intersocietal.org/nuclear/) will review these reports to ensure that they are consistent with the standards of nuclear cardiology.[40] The key elements of the report, as mandated by IAC, are shown in Table 12-4. A majority of the nuclear laboratories across the nation were reported to be noncompliant, with the reporting standards in at least one element. However, compliance improved in laboratories that applied for accreditation in sequential cycles.[41] This topic is further discussed in Chapter 6.

▸ **Components of the Report**

Patient Data

Patient name and date of birth must be present, as well as name, contact information, and affiliation of the referring physician. Information that is important not only to the interpretation of the study, but also

Table 12-4
Reporting Standards-Mandatory Data Elements (Based on IAC Standards)[a]

1. Name, address, and phone number of imaging facility
2. Name of examination
3. Patient information including full name, gender, DOB, height/weight, or BMI
4. Requesting provider
5. Interpreting physician
6. Date of examination
7. Clinical indications and pertinent history
8. Procedural description, including radionuclide amount and route of administration, time from injection to imaging
9. Administered nonradioactive pharmaceuticals, include name, dose, and route, and timing
10. Anatomic area images
11. Views obtained, i.e., SPECT or SPECT CT
12. CT procedure, if applicable, including technique, dose, and contrast
13. Stress test results, if applicable, including protocol, duration, peak hemodynamic parameters, stress symptoms, ECG findings at rest and stress, and percent maximum predicted heart rate
14. Image quality and explanation of suboptimal studies
15. Image results including defect description as to size/extent, severity, location and type, as well as functional results including quantitative LVEF, global and regional wall motion.
16. Conclusion/Impression
17. Comparison to other imaging or nonimaging studies, or inclusion of statement that no prior studies were available.

[a]Intersocietal Accreditation Commission (IAC). The IAC standards and guidelines for nuclear/PET accreditation. http://www.intersocietal.org/nuclear/standards/IACNuclearPETStandards2016.pdf. Published September 9, 2016.

Table 12-5
Clinical Information

- Demographics (age, gender, race)
- Body habitus (height, weight)
- Symptoms
- Medications
- Cardiac risk factors
- Prior cardiac events
- Prior diagnostic tests
- Therapeutic cardiac procedures

Indications

The indication for the procedure should be fairly delineated to allow full understanding of why the study was performed, as well as to demonstrate the appropriateness of the study based on the previously described ACCF/ASNC appropriateness criteria for SPECT MPI and ACCF/AHA/ASE/ASNC/HFSA/HRS/SCAI/SCCT/SCMR/STS multimodality appropriate-use criteria for the detection and risk assessment of stable ischemic heart disease.[42–44] Ideally, this should be obtained from the report as well as from patient history. The key indications for the procedure include:

- diagnosis;
- assessment of the extent and severity of known CAD;
- risk assessment;
- determination of myocardial viability; and
- evaluation of acute chest pain syndrome.

The actual indication may also be referenced to a specific diagnostic code to assist in matters related to reimbursement. Many laboratories include the ICD10 codes directly in the report. If pharmacologic testing is performed, the reason why exercise testing was not performed should be included.

Procedures

Procedures should be well delineated in the report so as to provide a frame of reference for subsequent comparisons as well as to explain the testing results directly to the referring physician (Table 12-6). The mode of stress should be noted. If exercise, the specific protocol such as Naughton or Bruce should be

to provide clinical relevance must be included in the report (Table 12-5). This includes the age, gender, and body habitus of the patient. Height, weight, body surface area, and chest circumference are items that may be included. Relevant clinical information including past cardiac history such as MI or the performance of revascularization should be included. In addition, major cardiac risk factors should be noted. The patient's current medications should be included, as they may impact on the interpretation of the results. They also provide documentation of the current clinical status of the subject.

Table 12-6
Procedure
• Type and protocol of stress procedure
• Adequacy of results
• Symptoms during protocol
• Hemodynamic response (heart rate, blood pressure)
• ECG changes
• Reason for test termination
• Radiopharmaceuticals utilized (with dose)
• Imaging protocol
• Functional data
• Attenuation/scatter correction

noted. The duration of exercise should be stated as well as the protocol stage achieved. Finally, the number of metabolic equivalents (METS) should be specified. The adequacy of the test results should be stated, such as the target heart rate achieved in terms of the maximum predicted heart rate and the reasons for test termination, such as general fatigue or hypotension. If pharmacologic stress testing is performed, the agent and dose should be specified. In addition, whether adjunctive exercise was performed and its type should be mentioned.

The presence of symptoms, hemodynamic responses, as well as arrhythmias should be well delineated. The heart rate as well as blood pressure changes should be noted. Electrocardiographic changes, including those that deviate from the baseline electrocardiogram (ECG), should be mentioned. The resting ECG should be stated, especially if there are abnormalities noted such as left bundle branch block (LBBB), LVH, or nonspecific ST/T-wave abnormalities.

The content of the report may vary if separate reports are generated for the stress test and the perfusion imaging data. However, even when a separate stress test report is created, it is advised that the perfusion data be reported along with a minimum of stress data including: exercise duration, maximum heart rate and percent maximum predicted heart rate, blood pressure response, symptoms, and ECG findings.

The MPI agent and dose administered at peak stress and at rest should be noted. If the stress is continued after the radiopharmaceutical injection, the duration of the continuation of stress should be mentioned. The actual imaging protocol should also be stated. For example, planar or SPECT should be stated as well as whether the imaging was performed in a supine, prone, or upright position. The reason must be provided if the routine protocol was replaced with an alternative protocol (e.g., attenuation correction, patient motion, or body habitus). A 1- or 2-day protocol should be specified and single- or double-isotope studies should be noted. If gated SPECT or first-pass imaging was performed, again this should be well described and noted whether it was performed at stress or rest. If stress-only imaging was obtained, then it should be clearly stated. Finally, advanced imaging techniques such as attenuation correction should be noted.

Image Findings

The results or findings portion of the report should provide an in-depth discussion of all findings noted on review of the nuclear cardiology study. It should be comprehensive and attempt to describe all pertinent findings (Table 12-7).

The first portion of the results section should deal with image quality. This may be stated as excellent, good, fair, or poor quality, but at least inadequate quality should be noted. Extracardiac activity should also be described and correlated with any potential clinical information.

The perfusion defect characteristics should be carefully described. The well-defined 17-segment model should be used to describe the size and location of perfusion abnormalities (Fig. 12-9).[1] The location of the abnormality in terms of segmentation and vascular territory should also be described to the best of the interpreter's abilities and using standard nomenclature.[4,5] Clear delineation between single- and multivessel disease should be performed. Defect size should be noted as small (1–2 segments), moderate (3–4 segments), or large (≥5 segments).[45]

Table 12-7
Image Findings
• Study quality
• Defect description (size, reversibility, severity, location)
• Extensiveness (TID, lung activity, right ventricular activity)
• Left ventricular function (global, regional)
• Extracardiac activity

Further defect description should include the type (ischemic, reversible, persistent, and mixed) and severity (mild, moderate, and severe) of the finding. When compared with European guidelines, the European Association of Nuclear Medicine (EANM) and the European Association of Cardiovascular Imaging (EACVI) strongly recommended that reports should be written in simple language with limited use of technical terms and abbreviations, and qualitative descriptions (e.g., small, medium sized, large, or slightly, moderately, or severely reduced) should be replaced with quantitative assessment.[46]

Markers of extensive disease, such as multivessel distribution or the presence of abnormal tracer distribution in the lungs, should be carefully noted. In addition, the presence of cavity enlargement, either immediately following stress or on both stress and rest images, should be present. If TID is noted, the TID ratio should be described.

LV function assessment is a mainstay of MPI. Both global and regional function should be described qualitatively as well as quantitatively. The left ventricular ejection fraction (LVEF) should be stated if gated SPECT was performed. If the LVEF is between 50% and 70%, the interpreter may describe this as normal as well as report the quantitative value. Hyperdynamic function is defined as >70%, but it is well recognized that this finding is common with gated SPECT and is often related to small LV cavities. Defining function as "hyperdynamic" or >70% may be superior to nonsensical values, such as an LVEF of 91%. Mild, moderate, and severe LV dysfunctions are defined as 40% to 49%, 30% to 39%, and <30%, respectively. Both the rest and poststress functions should be noted, if available. Regional defects should be carefully described as hypokinetic, akinetic, or dyskinetic, and the location given. Optionally, images may be included in the final report if they clearly represent the finding and impression portions of the report without causing confusion to the clinician. A standardized scale should be used and only a limited number of images should be selected.[46]

Conclusion/Impression

The impression is frequently the only portion of the report read by the referring physician (Table 12-8).

Table 12-8

Impression

- Normal or abnormal (minimum use of "equivocal")
- Recognition of artifact, if relevant
- Global and regional LV function
- Summary and correlation of ECG findings
- Integration with clinical information
- Address the clinical indication for testing

It is critical that it be crisp in its meaning, and the final diagnosis must be clear. Most reports should begin the impression section with a statement that perfusion imaging is either normal or abnormal. The terms "equivocal," "possible," or "probable" should be used infrequently.[2,39] A study may still be interpreted as normal even if there are perfusion abnormalities noted in the results section (Tables 12-7 and 12-8). This discrepancy should be explained in the impression section briefly by commenting on whether or not this was believed to be due to an artifact, such as soft tissue, LBBB, or patient motion. The functional information should be incorporated in a brief manner describing whether LV function is reduced and whether regional wall motion abnormalities are present. The amount of LV dysfunction should be semiquantitated, such as stating that there is moderately reduced LV systolic function. Finally, the perfusion and function findings must be integrated in the final impression, as wall motion may help to distinguish between an attenuation artifact and a true fixed defect, consistent with scar.

In addition to conclusions about the perfusion ventricular function data, the "Impression" section must also summarize the results of stress testing, including the significance of electrocardiographic findings.

The "Conclusion" section is also the place for correlation of the perfusion imaging data with clinical information, data from the results of the stress test, and any correlation with angiographic data, as it is known. A comparison to prior studies should be undertaken, and a direct statement regarding any significant changes should be made. As the diagnostic accuracy of perfusion imaging is superior to that of ECG stress testing, an abnormal ECG response to exercise with normal perfusion images should be considered to be a false positive, especially in the setting of resting ST-segment abnormalities. Of note, however, is that ECG changes occurring during a vasodilator infusion may portend a worse prognosis, even in the setting of normal SPECT images.[47]

Finally, the impression must directly address the question that was asked. Therefore, specific comments should be made regarding the indications and reasons for performing the procedure. For example, many laboratories performing a diagnostic study will comment directly on the likelihood of CAD. Some practitioners, however, are concerned about the legal ramifications of such a statement and opt not to include this type of language. If the study is ordered for the delineation of risk, the prognostic value should be stipulated in the report. Following an MI, the findings of a second vascular distribution or peri-infarction ischemia should be noted and equated with an increased risk of subsequent cardiac events. Likewise, perioperative assessments should comment specifically in the report on whether an increased risk for perioperative cardiac complications is present based on the study. For acute imaging procedures, the interpreter should note whether there is any evidence of ongoing ischemia or MI.

Report Logistics

Once the report is prepared, it is critical that this information be disseminated to the referring physician as soon as possible. The reporting of preliminary results is discouraged, in deference to the viewpoint that the final results should be available within the same day of the study. A recent policy statement by ASNC recommends that all studies be interpreted within 1 business day of acquisition and that the final report should be disseminated within 2 business days.[48] These recommendations are in keeping with the standard of the IAC Nuclear/PET with the additional qualification that a final signed report is transmitted to the referring provider within 4 working days.[40]

The report may be transmitted to the referring physician by means of facsimile, e-mail, or intranet transfer. It may also be obtainable through hospital records. Telephone notification should occur, especially in the setting of high-risk findings. Many laboratories choose to notify the referring physician of all abnormal results. In fact, some laboratories contact all physicians with the results by telephone. High-risk findings should mandate the rapid communication of results to the referring physician.[39,48]

The final report may include copies of the images either embedded within the report or as an add-on. This provides for subsequent reference to future reports. Finally, the report should be data based and provided as an electronic record for rapid recall. Quality assurance information also may be obtained in this fashion.

Recently, great efforts have been made to attempt to standardize cardiac imaging language and report content. Furthermore, a recent multisociety health care policy statement encourages the development in implementation of structured reporting of cardiac imaging procedures, including SPECT MPI. The key aspects of such a structured reporting ensure portability standardization of content and output, compatibility, multimodality applications, and flexibility to be used in a variety of environments.[49]

Summary—Reporting

In conclusion, reporting should incorporate the "five C's":

- *Clarity*: Ambiguity must be minimized and the overall message of the report should come through loudly.
- *Completeness*: Symptoms, stress test results, perfusion data, and functional information should all be described within the report. In addition, it should be related to the clinical scenario as well as any additional cardiac testing data available.
- *Consistency*: The report should be consistent in terms of the individual reader's daily patterns as well as within a given laboratory. Group reading sessions should be undertaken so that all readers within a given laboratory adopt a similar manner of reading. This is critical, as a given reader is often not available to interpret a study on a subsequent visit.
- *Clinical relevancy*: The question that is asked should be directly answered.
- *Communication*: Rapid reporting of all results is critical to the performance of a successful laboratory. All physicians should be notified of critical values such as patients with multivessel disease or severe ischemia. Telephone contact or facsimile transmission of reports to physicians with patients who possess high-risk findings is highly encouraged.

SAMPLE TEMPLATE FOR EXERCISE MYOCARDIAL PERFUSION IMAGING
Stress/Rest (or Rest/Stress) Single-/Dual-Isotope SPECT Imaging with Exercise Stress and Gated SPECT Imaging

Indication
(select one)

- [ ] Diagnosis of coronary disease
- [ ] Evaluation of extent and severity of coronary artery disease
- [ ] Evaluation of myocardial viability
- [ ] Risk stratification—post-myocardial infarction MI/preoperative/general
- [ ] Assessment of acute chest pain

Clinical history

____ year old man/woman with (no) known coronary artery disease

Cardiac risk factors include: ____

Previous cardiac procedures include: ____

Current symptomatology includes: ____

Procedure

The patient performed treadmill exercise/bicycle exercise using a modified Bruce/Bruce/Naughton/ ____ protocol, completing ____ minutes and completing an estimated workload of ____ metabolic equivalents (METS). The test was terminated due to fatigue/shortness of breath/chest pain/___. The heart rate was ____ beats per minute at baseline and increased to ____ beats at peak exercise, which was ____% of the maximum predicted heart rate. The rest blood pressure was ___ mm/Hg and increased/ decreased to ___ mm/Hg, which is a normal/ hypotensive/hypertensive response. The patient did/ did not develop any symptoms other than fatigue during the procedure; specific symptoms include ____. The resting electrocardiogram demonstrated ____ and did/did not show ST-segment changes consistent with myocardial ischemia.

Myocardial perfusion imaging was performed at rest (____ minutes following the injection of ____ mCi of ____). At peak exercise, the patient was injected with ____ mCi of ____ and exercise was continued for ____ minute(s). Gating post-stress tomographic imaging was performed ____ minutes after stress (and rest).

Findings

The overall quality of the study is poor/fair/good/ excellent. Attenuation artifact was present/absent.

Left ventricular cavity is noted to be normal/enlarged on the rest(and/or stress) studies. There is evidence of abnormal lung activity. Additionally, the right ventricle is normal/abnormal (specify :____).

SPECT images demonstrate homogeneous tracer distribution through out the myocardium OR a small/moderate/large perfusion abnormality of mild/moderate/severe severity is present in the ____ (location) region on the stress images. The rest images reveal ____. Gated SPECT imaging reveals normal myocardial thickening and wall motion OR Gated SPECT imaging demonstrates hypokinesis/dyskinesis/akinesis of the ____ (location). The left ventricular ejection fraction was calculated to be ____% OR the left ventricular ejection fraction was normal (>60%).

Impression

Myocardial perfusion imaging is normal/abnormal. There is a small/moderate/large area of ischemia/infarction in the ____ location. Overall left ventricular systolic function was normal/abnormal with/without regional wall motion abnormalities (as noted above). Compared to the prior study from ____ (date), the current study reveals ____.

FIGURE 12-15 Sample template for reporting of exercise myocardial perfusion imaging. (Reproduced with permission from Tilkemeier PL, Cooke CD, Grossman GB, et al. ASNC imaging guidelines for nuclear cardiology procedures; standardized reporting of radionuclide myocardial perfusion and function. *J Nucl Cardiol* 2009;16(4):650.)

SAMPLE TEMPLATE FOR PHARMACOLOGIC MYOCARDIAL PERFUSION IMAGING
Stress/Rest (or Rest/Stress) Single-/Dual-Isotope SPECT Imaging with Pharmacologic Stress and Gated SPECT Imaging

Indication
(select one)

- [ ] Diagnosis of coronary disease
- [ ] Evaluation of extent and severity of coronary artery disease
- [ ] Evaluation of myocardial viability
- [ ] Risk stratification—post-MI/preoperative/general
- [ ] Assessment of acute chest pain

Clinical history

____ year old man/woman with (no)known coronary artery disease
Cardiac risk factors include :____
Previous cardiac procedures include :____
Current symptomatology includes :____

Procedure

Pharmacologic stress testing was performed with adenosine/dipyridamole/dobutamine/regadenoson at a rate of ____ for ____ minutes. Additionally, low-level exercise was performed along with the vasodilator infusion (specify :____). The heart rate was ____ at baseline and rose to ____ beats per minute during the adenosine/dipyridamole/dobutamine/regadenoson infusion. The rest blood pressure was ____ mm/Hg and increased/decreased to ____ mm/Hg, which is a normal/hypotensive/hypertensive response. The patient developed significant symptoms, which included____. The resting electrocardiogram demonstrated____ and did/did not show ST-segment changes consistent with myocardial ischemia.

Myocardial perfusion imaging was performed at rest (____ minutes following the injection of ____ mCi of ____). At peak pharmacologic effect, the patient was injected with ____ mCi of ____. Gating post-stress tomographic imaging was performed ____ minutes after stress (and rest).

Findings

The overall quality of the study is poor/fair/good/excellent. Attenuation artifact was present/absent.

Left ventricular cavity is noted to be normal/enlarged on the rest(and/or stress) studies. There is evidence of abnormal lung activity. Additionally, the right ventricle is normal/abnormal (specify :____).

SPECT images demonstrate homogeneous tracer distribution through out themyocardium OR a small/moderate/large perfusion abnormality of mild/moderate/severe severity is present in the ____ (location) region on the stress images. The rest images reveal ____. Gated SPECT imaging reveals normal myocardial thickening and wall motion OR Gated SPECT imaging demonstrates hypokinesis/dyskinesis/akinesis of the ____ (location). The left ventricular ejection fraction was calculated to be ____% OR the left ventricular ejection fraction was normal (>60%).

Impression

Myocardial perfusion imaging is normal/abnormal. There is a small/moderate/large area of ischemia/infarction in the ____ location. Overall left ventricular systolic function was normal/abnormal with/without regional wall motion abnormalities (as noted above). Compared to the prior study from ____ (date), the current study reveals ____.

FIGURE 12-16 Sample template for reporting of pharmacologic myocardial perfusion imaging. (Reproduced with permission from Tilkemeier PL, Cooke CD, Grossman GB, et al. ASNC imaging guidelines for nuclear cardiology procedures; standardized reporting of radionuclide myocardial perfusion and function. *J Nucl Cardiol* 2009;16(4):650.)

As described throughout this chapter, the report is probably the most critical aspect of the nuclear cardiology procedure. It provides a direct reflection of nuclear cardiology. Without a high-quality report, the value of the overall procedure may be negated. Therefore, all laboratories and individual readers should strive for the highest-quality report possible, conveying the maximum amount of clinical information. This will ensure continued referrals and the further development and growth of nuclear cardiology. Sample report templates, as previously approved by ASNC, are provided in Figures 12-15 and 12-16.[39]

REFERENCES

1. Cerqueira MD, Weissman NJ, Dilsizian V, et al. Standardized myocardial segmentation and nomenclature for tomographic imaging of the heart: a statement for healthcare professionals from the Cardiac Imaging Committee of the Council on Clinical Cardiology of the American Heart Association. *Circulation*. 2002;105:539–542.
2. Port SC, ed. Imaging guidelines for nuclear cardiology procedures, part II. American Society of Nuclear Cardiology. *J Nucl Cardiol*. 1999;6:G47–G84.
3. Hendel RC, Gibbons RJ, Bateman TM. Use of rotating (cine) planar projection images and the interpretation of a tomographic myocardial perfusion study. *J Nucl Cardiol*. 1999;6:234–240.
4. Hansen CL, Goldstein RA, Akinboboye AO, et al. ASNC imaging guidelines for nuclear cardiology procedures; myocardial perfusion and function: Single photon emission computed tomography. *J Nucl Cardiol*. 2007;14:e39–e60.
5. Holly TA, Abbott BG, Al-Mallah M, et al. ASNC imaging guidelines for nuclear cardiology procedures: Single photon-emission computed tomography. *J Nucl Cardiol*. 2010;17:941–973.
6. Standardization of cardiac tomographic imaging. The Cardiovascular Imaging Committee, American College of Cardiology; The Committee on Advanced Cardiac Imaging and Technology, Council on Clinical Cardiology, American Heart Association; and Board of Directors, Cardiovascular Council, Society of Nuclear Medicine. *J Am Coll Cardiol*. 1992;20:255–256.
7. Eisner RL. Sensitivity of thallium-201 SPECT to patient motion. *J Nucl Med*. 1992;33:1571.
8. Leslie WD, Dupont JO, McDonald D, et al. Comparison of motion correction algorithms for cardiac SPECT. *J Nucl Med*. 1997;38:785–790.
9. Matsumoto N, Berman DS, Kavanagh PB, et al. Quantitative assessment of motion artifacts and validation of a new motion-correction program for myocardial perfusion SPECT. *J Nucl Med*. 2001;42:687–694.
10. Fitzgerald J, Danias PG. Effect of motion on cardiac SPECT imaging: Recognition and motion correction. *J Nucl Cardiol*. 2001;8:701–706.
11. Sorrell V, Figueroa B, Hansen CL. The "hurricane sign": Evidence of patient motion artifact on cardiac single-photon emission computed tomographic imaging. *J Nucl Cardiol*. 1996;3:86–88.
12. Williams KA, Hill KA, Sheridan CM. Noncardiac findings on dual-isotope myocardial perfusion SPECT. *J Nucl Cardiol*. 2003;10:395–402.
13. Karacavus S, Ede H, Sarikaya S, et al. The importance of the incidental thyroid gland uptake during Tc-99m MIBI myocardial perfusion scintigraphy. *Eur Rev Med Pharmacol Sci*. 2015;19:2781–2785.
14. Berman DS, Kang Z, Nishina H, et al. Diagnostic accuracy of gated Tc-99m sestamibi stress myocardial perfusion SPECT with combined supine and prone imaging to detect coronary artery disease in obese and non-obese patients. *J Nucl Cardiol*. 2006;13:191–201.
15. Slomka PJ, Nishina H, Abidov A, et al. Combined quantitative supine-prone myocardial perfusion SPECT improves detection of coronary artery disease and normalcy rates in women. *J Nucl Cardiol*. 2007;14:44–52.
16. Taillefer R, DePuey EG, Udelson JE, et al. Comparative diagnostic accuracy of Tl-201 and Tc-99m sestamibi SPECT imaging (perfusion and ECG-gated SPECT) in detecting coronary artery disease in women. *J Am Coll Cardiol*. 1997;29:69–77.
17. Smanio PE, Watson DD, Segalla DL, et al. Value of gating of technetium-99m sestamibi single-photon emission computed tomographic imaging. *J Am Coll Cardiol*. 1997;30:1687–1692.
18. Hendel RC, Corbett JR, Cullom SJ, et al. The value and practice of attenuation correction for myocardial perfusion SPECT imaging: A joint position statement from the American Society of Nuclear Cardiology and the Society or Nuclear Medicine. *J Nucl Cardiol*. 2002;9:135–143.
19. Tilkemeier PL, Wackers FJ. ASNC imaging guideline: Myocardial perfusion planar imaging. *J Nucl Cardiol*. 2006;13:91–96.
20. Mazzanti M, Germano G, Kiat H, et al. Identification of severe and extensive coronary artery disease by automatic measurement of transient ischemic dilation of the left ventricular in dual-isotope myocardial perfusion SPECT. *J Am Coll Cardiol*. 1996;27:1612–1620.
21. Xu Y, Arsanjani R, Clond M, et al. Transient ischemic dilation for coronary artery disease in quantitative analysis of same-day sestamibi myocardial perfusion SPECT. *J Nucl Cardiol*. 2012;19:465–473.
22. Golzar Y, Olusanya A, Pe N, et al. The significance of automatically measured transient ischemic dilation in identifying severe and extensive coronary artery disease in regadenoson, single-isotope technetium-99m myocardial perfusion SPECT. *J Nucl Cardiol*. 2015;22:526–34.
23. Rivero A, Santana C, Folks RD, et al. Attenuation correction reveals gender-related differences in the normal values of transient ischemic dilation index in rest-exercise stress sestamibi myocardial perfusion imaging. *J Nucl Cardiol*. 2006;13:338–344.
24. Kritzman JN, Ficaro EP, Corbett JR. Post-stress LV dilation: The effect of imaging protocol, gender and attenuation correction [abstract]. *J Nucl Med*. 2001;42(supple):50P.
25. Williams K, Schnieder C. Transient ischemic dilation (TID) with pharmacological stress dual isotope SPECT [abstract]. *Circulation*. 2000;102:II–546.
26. Abidov A, Bax JJ, Hayes SW, et al. Integration of automatically measured transient ischemic dilation ratio into interpretation of adenosine stress myocardial perfusion SPECT for detection of severe and extensive CAD. *J Nucl Med*. 2004;45:1999–2007.

27. Katz JS, Ruisi M, Giedd KN, et al. Assessment of transient ischemic dilation (TID) ratio in gated SPECT myocardial perfusion imaging (MPI) using regadenoson, a new agent for pharmacologic stress testing. *J Nucl Cardiol.* 2012;19:727–734.
28. Lester D, El-Haji S, Farag AA, et al. Prognostic value of transient ischemic dilation with regadenoson myocardial perfusion imaging. *J Nucl Cardiol.* 2016;23:1147–1155.
29. Kakhki VR, Sadeghi R, Zakavi SR. Assessment of transient left ventricular dilation ratio via 2-day dipyridamole Tc-99m sestamibi nongated myocardial perfusion imaging. *J Nucl Cardiol.* 2007;14:529–536.
30. Bestetti A, Di Leo C, Alessi A, et al. Post-stress end-systolic left ventricular dilation. A marker of endocardial post-ischemic stunning. *Nucl Med Commun.* 2001;22:685–693.
31. Weiss AT, Maddahi J, Lew AS, et al. Reverse redistribution of thallium 201; a sign of nontransmural myocardial infarction with patency of the infarct-related coronary artery. *J Am Coll Cardiol.* 1986;7:61–67.
32. Smith EJ, Hussain A, Manoharan M, et al. A reverse perfusion pattern during Technetium-99m stress myocardial perfusion imaging does not predict flow limiting coronary artery disease. *Int J Cardiovasc Imaging.* 2004;20:321–326.
33. Slomka P, Xu Y, Berman D, Germano G. Quantitative analysis of perfusion studies: Strengths and pitfalls. *J Nucl Cardiol.* 2012;19:338–346.
34. Motwani M, Berman DS, Germano G, et al. Automated quantitative nuclear cardiology methods. *Cardiol Clin.* 2016;34:47–57.
35. Bateman TM, Berman DS, Heller GV, et al. American Society of Nuclear Cardiology position statement on electrocardiographic gating of myocardial perfusion SPECT scintigrams. *J Nucl Cardiol.* 1999;6:470–471.
36. Garcia EV, Klein JL, Taylor AT. Clinical decision support systems in myocardial perfusion imaging. *J Nucl Cardiol.* 2014;21:427–39
37. Cerqueira MD. The user-friendly nuclear cardiology report: What needs to be considered and what is included. *J Nucl Cardiol.* 1996;4:350–355.
38. Hendel RC, Wackers FJ, Berman DS, et al. American Society of Nuclear Cardiology consensus statement: Reporting of radionuclide myocardial perfusion imaging studies. *J Nucl Cardiol.* 2003;10:705–708.
39. Tilkemeier PL, Cooke CD, Grossman GB, et al. ASNC imaging guidelines for nuclear cardiology procedures; standardized reporting of radionuclide myocardial perfusion and function. *J Nucl Cardiol.* 2009;16:650.
40. Intersocietal Accreditation Commission (IAC). The IAC standards and guidelines for nuclear/PET accreditation. http://www.intersocietal.org/nuclear/standards/IACNuclearPET-Standards2016.pdf. Published September 9, 2016.
41. Tilkemeier PL, Serber ER, Farrell MB, et al. The nuclear cardiology report: problems, predictors, and improvement. A report from the ICANL database. *J Nucl Cardiol.* 2011;18:858–868.
42. Brindis RG, Douglas PS, Hendel RC, et al. ACCF/ASNC appropriateness criteria for single-photon emission computed tomography myocardial perfusion imaging (SPECT MPI): a report of the American College of Cardiology Foundation Quality Strategic Directions Committee Appropriateness Criteria Working Group and the American Society of Nuclear Cardiology endorsed by the American Heart Association. *J Am Coll Cardiol.* 2005;46:1587–1605.
43. Ward RP, Al-Mallah MH, Grossman GB, et al. American Society of Nuclear Cardiology review of the ACCF/ASNC appropriateness criteria for single-photon emission computed tomography myocardial perfusion imaging (SPECT MPI). *J Nucl Cardiol.* 2007;14:e26–e38.
44. Wolk MJ, Bailey SR, Doherty JU, et al. ACCF/AHA/ASE/ASNC/HFSA/HRS/SCAI/SCCT/SCMR/STS 2013 multimodality appropriate use criteria for the detection and risk assessment of stable ischemic heart disease: a report of the American College of Cardiology Foundation Appropriate Use Criteria Task Force, American Heart Association, American Society of Echocardiography, American Society of Nuclear Cardiology, Heart Failure Society of America, Heart Rhythm Society, Society for Cardiovascular Angiography and Interventions, Society of Cardiovascular Computed Tomography, Society for Cardiovascular Magnetic Resonance, and Society of Thoracic Surgeons. *J Am Coll Cardiol.* 2014;63:380–406.
45. Hendel RC, Budoff MJ, Cardella JF, et al. ACC/AHA/ACR/ASE/ASNC/HRS/NASCI/RSNA/SAIP/SCAI/SCCT/SCMR/SIR. Key data elements and definitions for cardiac imaging. *J Am Coll Cardiol.* 2009;53:91–124.
46. Trägårdh E, Hesse B, Knuuti J, et al. Reporting nuclear cardiology: a joint position paper by the European Association of Nuclear Medicine (EANM) and the European Association of Cardiovascular Imaging (EACVI). *Eur Heart J Cardiovasc Imaging.* 2015;16:272–279.
47. Abbott BG, Afshar M, Berger AK, et al. Prognostic significance of ischemic electrocardiographic changes during adenosine infusion in patients with normal perfusion imaging. *J Nucl Cardiol.* 2003;10:9–16.
48. Hendel RC, Ficaro EP, Williams KA. Timeliness of reporting results of nuclear cardiology procedures. *J Nucl Cardiol.* 2007;14:266.
49. Douglas PS, Hendel RC, Cummings JE, et al. ACC/ACR/AHA/ASE/ASNC/HRS/MITA/NASCI/RSNA/SAIP/SCCT/SCMR. Health policy statement on structured reporting in cardiovascular imaging. *J Am Coll Cardiol.* 2009;53:76–90.

SECTION 3

INDICATIONS AND APPLICATIONS OF MPI

CHAPTER 13

The Appropriate Use of Nuclear Cardiology Techniques

Camilo A. Gomez and Robert C. Hendel

INTRODUCTION

The past several decades have witnessed remarkable advances in medical care, including cardiac imaging. This rapid pace of technological development has provided a wealth of diagnostic and therapeutic tools that have impacted both quality and longevity of an individual's life.[1,2] Particularly notable are the advances in cardiac imaging, which have revolutionized how patients are diagnosed and treated, enhancing the sensitivity and specificity for the detection of ischemic heart disease and related these results to patient outcomes, thereby resulting in an impact on survival and quality of life.

However, the exuberance for nuclear cardiology, including single-photon emission tomography myocardial perfusion imaging (SPECT MPI) and positron emission tomography (PET), has resulted in a dramatic increase in its use and has contributed to the spiraling costs of health care cost.[3,4] Furthermore, unnecessary testing may result in additional diagnostic tests and potentially unjustified therapeutic intervention, further escalating costs but also potentially impacting on patient health. Furthermore, the use of nuclear cardiology procedures exposes patients who do not need the testing to avoidable risks, as related to ionizing radiation and stress testing.

The Medicare Payment Advisory Commission (Med-PAC) found that the rate of medical imaging between 1999 and 2002 far exceeded other medical services, with an annual increase by 10.1% during this time period (Fig. 13-1).[2,4] Although it was concluded that no determination of inappropriateness was possible to be made due to lack of credible data,[4] concern was raised as to the possible performance of unnecessary testing, which may have included financial motivation on the part of the providers. In addition to the excessive growth rate, SPECT/PET utilization demonstrated wide geographic variability across the United States, suggesting that differences in the volume of stress imaging procedures were unlikely a consequence of demographics or the prevalence of comorbid conditions alone,[2,7] as these data were corrected for disease severity. Possible contributing factors included the nonuniform distribution of specialized imaging centers, self-referral practice at specific centers, and variances in the understanding of the medical literature.[2]

Based on the concerns of overuse and misuse noted above, providers, regulators, and payers raised concern about overuse and misuse of radionuclide imaging, especially with regard to the negative economic consequences.[2,5] In response to this and in an effort to reduce spending, health plans began to use radiology benefits management (RBM) companies to act as procedural governors by developing mechanisms to constrain the exponential growth of imaging and limit associated costs.[2,3] The most common used programs included provider exclusion from imaging network and prior notification and precertification.[1,2] These RBM programs reflected a contract with payers and usually functioned with a model based on incentives to reduce volume and costs even though there was little

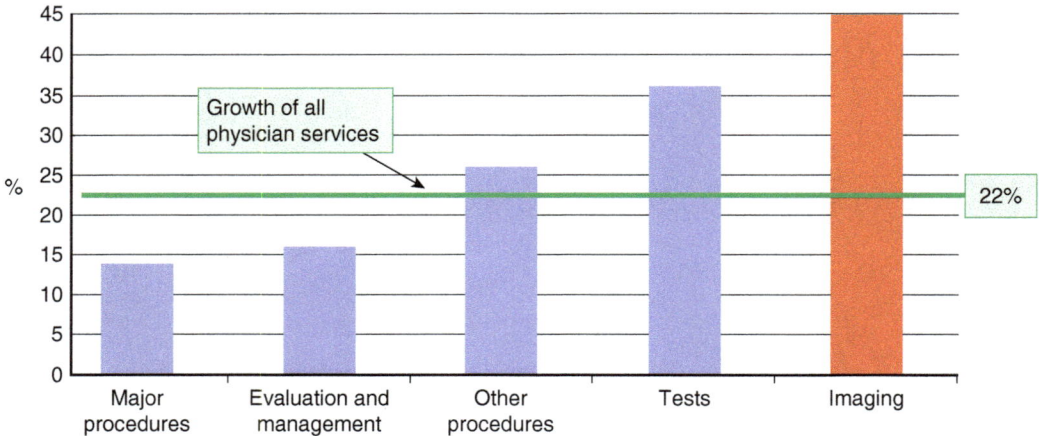

FIGURE 13-1 Comparison of the growth of medical imaging compared with other physician services between 1999 and 2002, demonstrating an approximate doubling of anticipated volume. (Data from MedPAC Analysis of Medicare Claims Data, March 17, 2005, Executive Director, Medicare Payment Advisory Commission, Mark Miller.)

evidence for the improvement of quality of care. The rules that governed the RBM were not necessarily literature based and often lacked transparency in informing providers of why a test was denied. This process varied from one RBM/health plan to another and caused delays in patient care, increased provider and staff work, and led to increased inefficiency. The mere presence of these onerous programs underscored the need for improved guidance regarding optimal patient selection for specific procedures.[6,7]

▶ Appropriate Use Criteria

In response to fiscal pressures and with the goal of optimizing test/patient selection to improve the utilization of cardiovascular procedures in an efficient and contemporary fashion,[1,3] appropriate use criteria (AUC) were developed by several organizations, including the American College of Cardiology Foundation (ACCF) and the American Society of Nuclear Cardiology (ASNC).[8-10] The first set of AUC was released in 2005, focused in the indications of cardiac radionuclide imaging[11] with an emphasis on the performance of the right test for the right patient at the right time. The appropriateness of a cardiovascular procedure or test is based on the definition showed in Table 13-1. A revised and expanded version of the AUC for radionuclide imaging was published in 2009.[12] However, the latest criteria were in the form of a multimodality testing document for use with stable ischemic heart disease published in 2013. The indications and ranking for SPECT and PET imaging were intended to replace the prior AUC documents for stable ischemic heart disease scenarios.[16] The goal of these 2013 multimodality AUC was to determine which testing modalities, if any, are reasonable for a specific indication. Importantly the new AUC introduced new definitions for categories of appropriate use, which include "may be appropriate" and "rarely appropriate" replacing

Table 13-1

Definition of Appropriate Use

An appropriate diagnostic or therapeutic procedure is one in which the expected clinical benefit exceeds the risks of the procedure by a sufficiently wide margin such that the procedure is generally considered acceptable or reasonable care.

Data from Hendel RC, Berman DS, Di Carli MF, et al. ACCF/ASNC/ACR/AHA/ASE/SCCT/SCMR/SNM 2009 Appropriate Use Criteria for Cardiac Radionuclide Imaging: A Report of the American College of Cardiology Foundation Appropriate Use Criteria Task Force, the American Society of Nuclear Cardiology, the American College of Radiology, the American Heart Association, the American Society of Echocardiography, the Society of Cardiovascular Computed Tomography, the Society for Cardiovascular Magnetic Resonance, and the Society of Nuclear Medicine. *J Am Coll Cardiol.* 2009;53(23):2201–2229.

Table 13-2

Categories of Appropriate Use

Appropriate Care

An appropriate option because the benefits generally outweigh the risks

May Be Appropriate Care

At times an appropriate option due to variable evidence or agreement regarding benefit/risk ration. May be reasonable for the indication.

Rarely Appropriate Care

Rarely an appropriate option due to lack of clear benefit/risk advantage. Not generally reasonable for the indication.

Data from Hendel RC, Patel MR, Allen JM, et al. Appropriate use of cardiovascular technology: 2013 ACCF appropriate use criteria methodology update: a report of the American College of Cardiology Foundation appropriate use criteria task force. *J Am Coll Cardiol.* 2013;61(12):1305–1317.

the prior terminology of "uncertain" and "inappropriate" (Table 13-2).[1] However, original and revised definitions of appropriate use should not be used interchangeably as each set of documents was created independently and the raters of the scenarios

Table 13-3

Differences between the Appropriateness Categorization Based on the 2009 Radionuclide Imaging AUC and the 2013 Multimodality AUC

Indication	2009 RNI[2]	2013 MM[3]
High CHD risk asymptomatic	A	M
Low CHD risk syncope	I	M
Worsening symptoms, normal prior study	U	A
High CHD risk, Agatston score 100–400	A	M
Agatston score >400	A	M
Preop assessment, intermediate-risk surgery, ≥1 risk factor with poor functional capacity	A	M
s/p CABG, asymptomatic, <5 years	U	R
s/p CABG, asymptomatic, ≥5 years	A	M

A, appropriate; M, may be appropriate; R, rarely appropriate; U, uncertain; I, inappropriate; Agaston score refers to CT-derived calcium scoring. Reproduced with permission from Hendel RC. The value and appropriateness of positron emission tomography: An evolving tale. *J Nucl Cardiol.* 2015;22(1):16–21.

were asked to utilize the specific definitions for these terms.

Although the 2009 and 2013 multimodality AUC ratings were similar for most indications, Table 13-3 shows the differences of appropriateness categorization between the 2009 radionuclide imaging AUC and the 2013 multimodality AUC.

▶ AUC Methodology

How the ratings for appropriate use were developed is important, in order to understand that there is a rigorous methodology behind these criteria. The methods for AUC have evolved since the first publication in 2005, but the process remains based in the application of the validated, prospectively based modified Delphi approach and previously published UCLA/RAND Appropriateness Method (Fig. 13-2).[13,14] Following the selection of a topic, and determination of definitions and assumptions, a writing group is created, clinical scenarios, definitions, and assumptions are created, which then undergo an external review. Subsequently, a literature review and guideline mapping is performed, a review panel of more than 30 members then provide feedback, and the writing group revises each of the indications and summary tables that are prepared for the indications raters. The rating panel composed of a variety of individuals with specific backgrounds rate each indication. A second rating is performed after the rating panel has a face-to-face meeting to scores the different scenarios. The final rating is then compiled with the appropriate use score of 7 to 9 as appropriate, 4 to 6 as may be appropriate, and 1 to 3 as rarely appropriate.[15] However, only the category of appropriate use is presented as the final rating, so as to avoid artificial comparisons among the testing modalities.

The indications are grouped under common headings in a structured approach, with the implementation of tables for diagnosis and risk assessment, symptomatology, prior testing, previous revascularization, evaluation for a change in clinical status, and consideration for special circumstances. A hierarchic approach of the indications is used to stratify a clinical situation to one of the indications.[3,16] This flowchart is designed to place clinical conditions into a hierarchy to help assess the appropriateness of a test

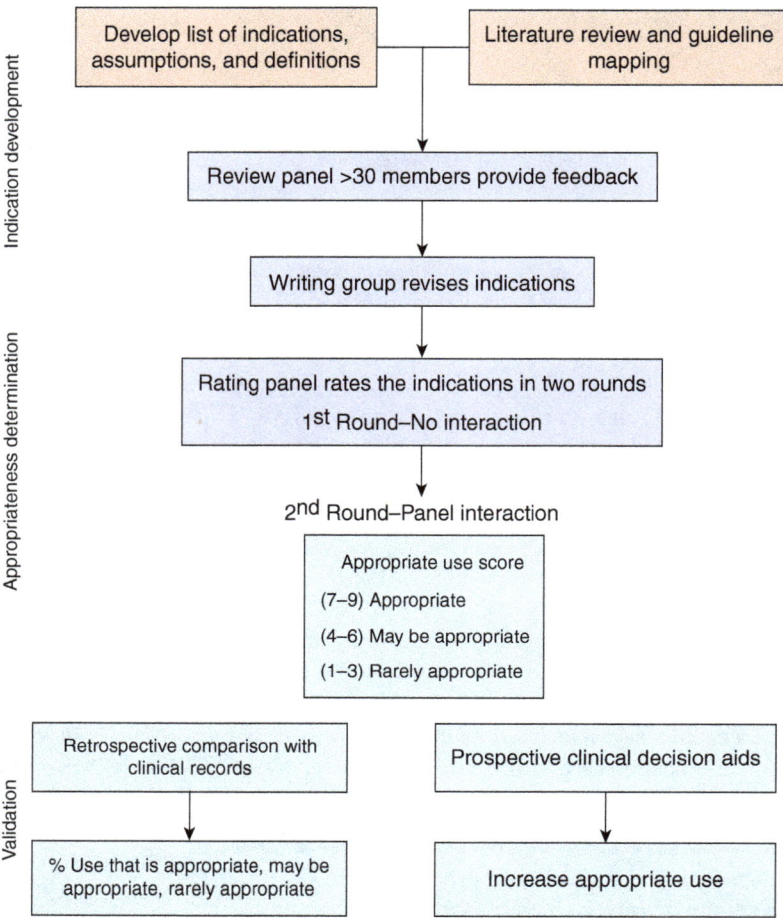

FIGURE 13-2 Methodology of ACCF appropriate use criteria construction, using the UCL/Rand method with a modified Delphi approach. (Reproduced with permission from Hendel RC, Patel MR, Allen JM, et al. Appropriate use of cardiovascular technology: 2013 ACCF appropriate use criteria methodology update: A report of the American College of Cardiology Foundation appropriate use criteria task force. *J Am Coll Cardiol*. 2013;61(12):1305–1317.)

(Fig. 13-3). The indications are not entirely comprehensive and are not intended to be, are meant to identify common clinical scenarios in the evaluation and follow-up of stable ischemic heart disease (SIHD) that could embrace the majority of contemporary practice, attempting to determine which testing modalities, may or may not be reasonable for a specific indication.[16]

The new multimodality AUC emphasizes not on which test is best for each indication but rather on whether a specific testing modality is reasonable for a specific indication. Seven different diagnostic procedures are presented including radionuclide imaging, in order to offer aid to clinical decision making for the detection and risk assessment of stable ischemic heart disease. Eighty indications were included in the most recent publication.[1]

▶ **AUC for Radionuclide Imaging**

Indications are often constructed based on pretest probability of CAD or global coronary heart disease (CHD) risk, exercise ability and electrocardiogram (ECG) interpretability (Appendix 13-1). The first subsection focuses on symptomatic patients where the clinicians should estimate the likelihood of coronary artery disease (CAD) before selecting testing based on age, sex and typical or atypical presentation based on the Diamond and Forrester pretest probability of CAD.[36] The next subsection is for asymptomatic patients and takes into account the global CHD risk estimating the probability of experience a cardiovascular event over a given period of time. The third subsection is related to newly diagnosed heart failure, evaluation of arrhythmias without ischemic

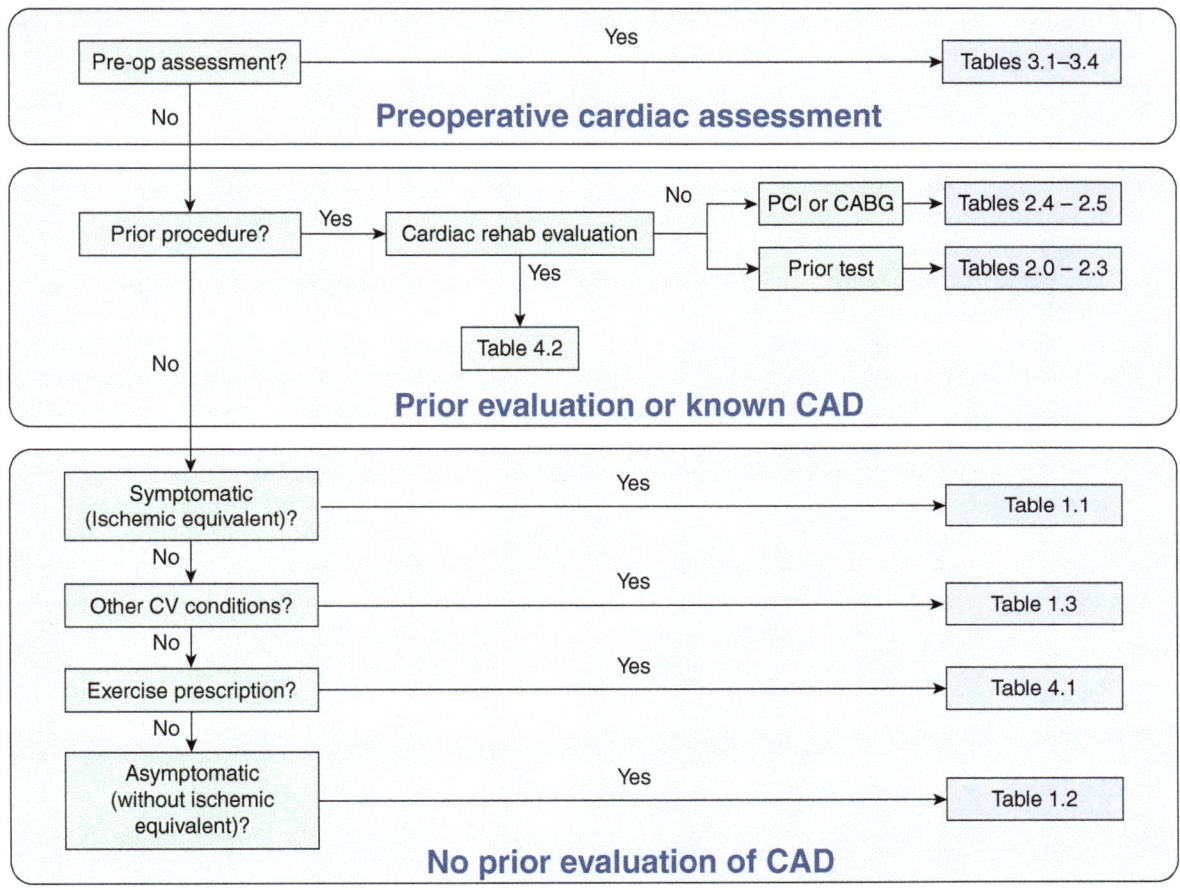

FIGURE 13-3 Suggested hierarchy for applying AUC when considering testing ordering. The tables cited within the figure are contained in the original publication; the figure is intended to show the hierarchical nature of the process. (Reproduced with permission from Wolk MJ, Bailey SR, Doherty JU, et al. ACCF/AHA/ASE/ASNC/HFSA/HRS/SCAI/SCCT/SCMR/STS 2013. Multimodality appropriate use criteria for the detection and risk assessment of stable ischemic heart disease. *J Am Coll Cardiol.* 2014;63(4):380–406.)

equivalent or prior cardiac evaluation, and syncope without ischemic equivalent.

The next part of the AUC is designed for patients with prior testing, with subsections for patients without previous intervening revascularization, as sequential testing, as follow-up testing in stable patients or with new or worsening symptoms, also includes another section for postrevascularized patients with percutaneous coronary intervention (PCI) or coronary artery bypass grafts (CABG), that are symptomatic or asymptomatic (Appendix 13-2). The third section is for preoperative evaluation of noncardiac surgery in view of the type of surgery, functional capacity, previous cardiac imaging, active cardiac conditions, and clinical risk factors.[16] This mimics the clinical practice guidelines and is discussed in detail in Chapter 16. The final section focuses on the value of testing to determine the exercise level prior to initiation of exercise prescription or cardiac rehabilitation in patients with and without revascularization, or heart failure.

The multimodality AUC provides several key conclusions:

- Guided by pretest probability, exercise ability and ECG interpretability stress radionuclide and echo imaging are appropriate for most categories.
- For asymptomatic patients, only exercise ECG is appropriate for high-risk patients who can exercise and had an interpretable ECG.
- Follow-up testing is largely inappropriate in asymptomatic patients or those with stable symptoms.

- Stress testing is appropriate for patients with syncope who have at least an intermediate likelihood of CAD.
- Among asymptomatic patients who have undergone revascularization, RNI is appropriate only for those with incomplete revascularization or when a substantial period of time has elapsed after coronary revascularization.
- For preoperative assessment, testing is indicated only for high-risk surgery in patients with poor or unknown functional capacity who also have ≥1 risk factor.
- In asymptomatic patients those with low and moderate global CHD risk but with an interpretable ECG and have ability to exercise testing is rarely appropriate.
- Those patients with prior testing less than 2 years ago and those with PCI or CABG less than 5 years ago, follow-up testing is rarely appropriate.
- As part of preoperatory evaluation before noncardiac surgery, testing is rarely appropriate prior to low-risk surgery, in asymptomatic patients with normal prior testing less than 1 year ago and in patients with moderate to good functional capacity or no clinical risk factors.
- Testing is rarely appropriate as part of evaluation prior to exercise prescription or cardiac rehabilitation, except in patients with heart failure.

AUC Implementation and Evaluation

The development of AUC is not likely sufficient alone to impact on changes in utilization. Appropriate utilization must be monitored, and this information used to impact on changes in practice. Numerous abstracts and papers focusing on the evaluation of appropriate use of radionuclide imaging have been published, clearly demonstrating that appropriateness is a metric that can be assessed. For radionuclide imaging, it appears that approximately 10% to 20% of the studies are performed for inappropriate indications (or rarely appropriate) (Table 13-4) and

Table 13-4
Classification of Appropriate Use for SPECT Myocardial Perfusion Imaging

Study	Year	n	Appropriate (%)	Uncertain (%)	Inappropriate (%)
Mehta et al.[18]	2008	1209	80	5	13
Gibbons et al.[19]	2008	284	64	11	14
Hendel et al.[20]	2010	6351	71	15	14
Carryer et al.[21]	2010	281	60	16	24
Gibbons et al.[22]	2010	284	66	15	7
Gholamrezanezhad et al.[23]	2011	291	75	5	14
Druz et al.[24]	2011	585	63	20	14
Koh et al.[25]	2011	1623	82	5	10
Gupta et al.[26]	2011	314	84	5	11
Aldweib et al.[27]	2013	1199	62	20	18
Doukky et al.[28]	2013	1511	52	3	46
Khawaja et al.[29]	2013	280	63	14	24
Moralidis et al.[30]	2013	3032	73	7	19
Medolago et al.[31]	2014	2134	84	9	7
Lalude et al.[32]	2014	420	77	10	13
Singh et al.[33]	2014	328	88	6	7

Percentage may not add to 100% due to unclassified studies or rounding errors.
Reproduced with permission from Hendel RC. The value and appropriateness of positron emission tomography: An evolving tale. *J Nucl Cardiol.* 2015;22(1):16–21.

Table 13-5

Most Common Inappropriate Indications

Indication	Inappropriate Studies (%)	Total Studies (%)
Detection of CAD Asymptomatic, low CHD risk[a]	44.5	6.4
Asymptomatic, postrevascularization <2 years after PCI, symptoms before PCI	23.8	3.4
Evaluation of chest pain, low probability Interpretable ECG and able to exercise	16.1	2.3
Asymptomatic/stable symptoms, known CAD <1 year after catheterization or abnormal prior SPECT	3.9	0.6
Preoperative assessment		
Low-risk surgery	3.7	0.5
Total[b]	92.0	13.2

[a]CHD risk was determined by the Framingham Risk score.
[b]The remaining 8% of inappropriate studies are contained among the remaining inappropriate indications.
Reproduced with permission from Hendel RC, Cerqueira M, Douglas PS, et al. A multicenter assessment of the use of single-photon emission computed tomography myocardial perfusion imaging with appropriateness criteria. *J Am Coll Cardiol.* 2010;55(2):156–162.

the most common reasons for inappropriate use of SPECT imaging are readily identifiable. In the largest multicenter study published with 6351 patients enrolled, the inappropriate use of MPI was noted in 14.4% of the patients, with a range of 4% to 22% at different sites. Importantly, this trial defined key categories of inappropriate SPECT use, as women and younger asymptomatic patients were more likely to undergo inappropriate testing. The most common indications of inappropriate SPECT use was in low-risk patients who had an interpretable ECG and were able to exercise, accounting for 44.5% of the inappropriate indications (Table 13-5).[20] In addition to the many studies examining the appropriateness of SPECT MPI, Winchester et al.[17] evaluated the appropriateness used criteria for MPI clinical utility use for PET and found that appropriate or uncertain indications for PET were present in 79.5% and 10.4%, respectively, with an inappropriate rate of 10.2%, demonstrating that the categorizations for PET appropriate use are similar to those for SPECT.[18–33]

A recent meta-analysis systematically review the literature on appropriate use criteria, with a total of 22,443 patients from 22 studies, showed that inappropriate studies are consistently less likely to be abnormal and lack ischemia than appropriate MPI, 15.6% versus 42%, respectively. However, multiple trials have described that even when SPECT MPI is performed for inappropriate or rarely appropriate indications, there remain a number of patients who have abnormal results (Table 13-6). These data raise the concern that the AUC may discourage performing a radionuclide examination and therefore miss important information. However, when the association of outcomes of patients with appropriateness categorization is compared, inappropriate studies carried far less associated risk even when abnormal.[41] In a large prospective study, Doukky et al.[28] evaluated the appropriateness of SPECT MPI related to its prognostic value and demonstrated that when SPECT MPI was performed for inappropriate indications, an abnormal perfusion imaging failed to predict major adverse cardiac events, in stark comparison to the excellent risk assessment provided by SPECT imaging when performed for appropriate indications. Inappropriate testing was associated with a higher revascularization rate but lacked effectiveness for risk stratification and had high societal costs and unnecessary radiation exposure. Conversely, when MPI was used for the appropriate indications, it demonstrated a high prognostic value with patients with higher rates of all-cause mortality and cardiac death. Another

Table 13-6

Abnormal SPECT Results and Event Rates Based on Appropriate Use Categories

	Year	n	A	U	I
Abnormal results					
Mehta et al.[18]	2008	1209	55%	47%	32%
Gholamrezanezhad et al.[23]	2011	291	33%	47%	11%
Koh et al.[25]	2011	1623	40%	21%	27%
Doukky et al.[28]	2013	1511	40%	21%	18%
Khawaja et al.[29]	2013	280	15%		7%
Medolago et al.[31]	2014	2134	58%	–	33%
Events					
Druz et al.[24]	2011	585	12%	7%	2%
Koh et al.[25]	2011	176	6%	–	1%
Aldweib et al.[27]	2013	1199	10%	4%	5%
Khawaja et al.[29]	2013	280	14%	0%	3%
Medolago et al.[31]	2014	2134	9%		3%

MI, death, revascularization, admission.
Perioperative 90-day major cardiac events.
Death.
Cardiac catheterization.
Reproduced with permission from Hendel RC. The value and appropriateness of positron emission tomography: An evolving tale. *J Nucl Cardiol.* 2015;22(1):16–21.

finding from the aforementioned meta-analysis is a trend from noncardiology physicians compared to cardiologist to order more inappropriate studies, consistent with similar findings in other studies.[30,49]

The development and publication of AUC is changing the practice patterns, supported by the development of tools for quality improvement. Many educational initiatives have been implemented. One of these strategies is the Choosing Wisely Campaign, a national program created with the goal to reduce waste in the health care system and avoid risks associated with unnecessary treatment, with a list of recommendations created by the ACC standing clinical councils, recommend procedures that should not be performed or rarely performed in specific circumstances. Four of the five items are based on AUC[37] and are shown in Table 13-7.

Also a variety of tools have been created that include web-based and portable device applications to foster the appropriate use of cardiovascular technology. There is an increasing trend of physicians that incorporate smartphones and tablets into their daily practice,[38] with the rate of smartphone usage among physicians has been reported as high as 75% and 81%.[39,40] An AUC smartphone app can be used

Table 13-7

Choosing Wisely

- Don't perform stress cardiac imaging or coronary angiography in patients without cardiac symptoms unless high-risk markers are present.
- Don't perform cardiac imaging for patients who are at low risk.
- Don't perform radionuclide imaging as part of routine follow-up in asymptomatic patients.
- Don't perform cardiac imaging as a preoperative assessment in patients scheduled to undergo low- or intermediate-risk noncardiac surgery.
- Use methods to reduce radiation exposure in cardiac imaging, whenever possible, including not performing such test when limited benefits are likely.

Data from Choosing Wisely. American College of Cardiology (ACC). http://www.choosingwisely.org/societies/american-college-of-cardiology/

to determine the level of appropriateness in less than a minute, demonstrating decision support in a time-effective manner, is free, convenient and easy to use, with the potential to promote the usage of AUC and possibly aid reduction of cost and radiation burden. (Fig. 13-4).[38] Internet-based instruments have also been created to reduce inappropriate imaging such as the FOCUS PMI (FOCUS: Formation of Optimal Cardiovascular Utilization Strategies, PMI: Imaging Performance Improvement Module), which is a national web-based community and quality improvement instrument created to increase use of the AUC and improve practice patterns. FOCUS has showed that the use of a self-directed quality improvement software and interactive community, makes possible for clinicians to decrease their proportion of test not meeting appropriateness of use.[34] Initial data from this program reveal that this tool resulted in a 50% reduction in the rate of inappropriate tests, from 10% to 5%, which was sustained during the follow-up period.[34]

Other interventions to reduce inappropriate testing include educational initiatives, peer review with feedback, and point-of-care decision support systems.[19,28,42,43] Overall, it appears that education alone seems insufficient to reduce inappropriate MPI, and that provider feedback and/or decision support systems are key in reducing unnecessary imaging.[44–46] A meta-analysis by Chaudhuri et al. designed to evaluate the quality improvement initiatives and its impact in appropriate testing showed that the presence of a physician audit and feedback mechanism is associated with lower odds of inappropriate testing (OR, 0.36 [95% CI, 0.31–0.41]; $p < 0.001$), while studies without this interventions had no significant

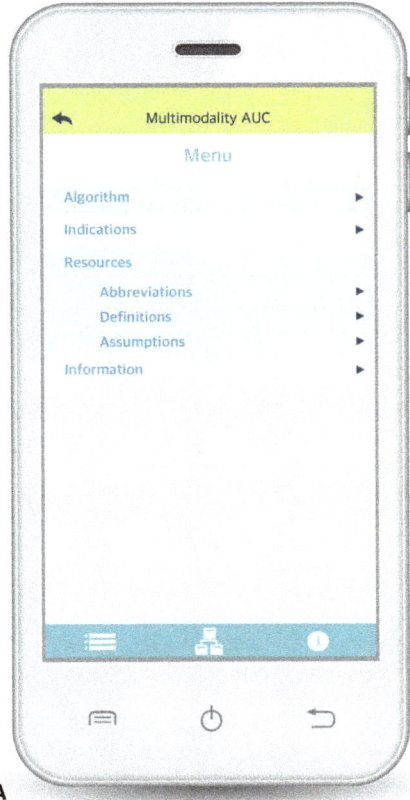
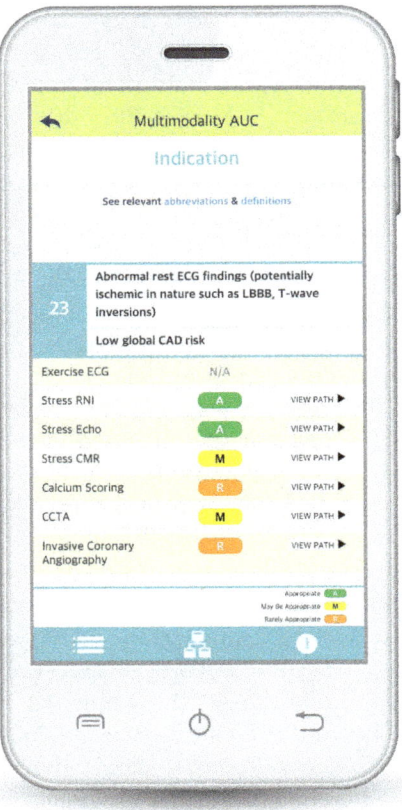

FIGURE 13-4 Smartphone app allowing for the rapid, point-of-care determination of appropriate use for a specific clinical indication. Panel **A** provides a means of search of the multimodality imaging appropriate use criteria via an algorithm or a specific indication. Panel **B** provides an example of appropriate use classification for multiple imaging modalities. (Reproduced with permission from Astellas Pharma US, Inc.)

impact on inappropriate testing (OR, 0.89 [95% CI, 0.61–1.29]; $p = 0.51$). This positions quality interventions with physician audit and feedback as an important process impacting the effectiveness of cardiovascular testing.[47] A prospective multicenter study by Lin et al. studied the use of a multimodality decision support tool and demonstrated that appropriate testing increased from 49% to 61%, and inappropriate testing was reduced from 22% to 6%, and required an average of 2 minutes to perform this consultation.[50] In contrast, a study which analyzed the alternative approach of prior authorization as frequently done by health insurance carriers, showed a lack of effect of this strategy on the rate of inappropriate MPI and physicians adherence to AUC.[48]

The AUC and various implementation strategies allow clinicians to optimize their use of cardiac imaging, by maximizing the clinical impact of cardiovascular technology and permitting cost reductions through the elimination of unnecessary tests and procedures.[1,3] Although adoption by private payers has been slow, the United States Congress passed legislation (Protecting Access to Medicare Act [PAMA]) in 2015 that mandates the use of the AUC for advance cardiac imaging, including nuclear cardiology, for all Medicare beneficiaries.[35] Following a 3-year period of data collection and self-evaluation of appropriateness patterns, physicians who demonstrate low adherence to the AUC may be required to obtain prior authorization before the performance of advanced cardiac imaging. The AUC developed by the American Colleague of Cardiology (ACC) will be included in this programs, as well several other provider lead entities, including the American College of Radiology (ACR).[52,53]

A recent study by Winchester et al.[53] examined differences between the ACC AUC and the ACR appropriateness criteria for radionuclide MPI. Notably, 52.2% of the indications of the ACC AUC could not be matched to an ACR rating, and 20.9% were in disagreement related to appropriateness. Further support for the use of the ACCF AUC is that the detection of myocardial ischemia was infrequent among patients rated as "inappropriate" by the ACC AUC (2.6%), whereas patients rated as "usually not appropriate" by the ACR AUC had ischemia noted in 17.5% of the patients. Thus, clear differences between criteria for appropriateness exist, which likely impact on the utility of these documents for clinical practice.

CONCLUSION

The appropriate use of radionuclide cardiac imaging, along with other applications of cardiovascular technologies, is of critical importance in the current era in order to maximize the value of such testing and to potentially reduce the costs and risks associated with unnecessary examinations. AUC were developed to promote change in utilization patterns and increase the value of cardiac imaging, including SPECT and PET. However, these documents must be incorporated into clinical practice in order to have an impact. The evaluation of clinician performance regarding technology utilization is paramount for the optimization of care and includes clinical decision support and audit/feedback mechanisms to allow for providers to continuously improve their practice.[51]

REFERENCES

1. Hendel RC. The value and appropriateness of positron emission tomography: An evolving tale. *J Nucl Cardiol*. 2015; 22:16–21.
2. Hendel RC. Utilization management of cardiovascular imaging pre-certification and appropriateness. *J Am Coll Cardiol*. 2008;1:241–248.
3. Hendel RC, Patel MR, Allen JM, et al. Appropriate use of cardiovascular technology: 2013 ACCF appropriate use criteria methodology update: A report of the American College of Cardiology Foundation appropriate use criteria task force. *J Am Coll Cardiol*. 2013;61(12):1305–1317.
4. Iglehart JK. The new era of medical imaging—Progress and pit-falls. *N Engl J Med*. 2009;360:1030–1037.
5. *Report to the Congress: Medicare Payment Policy*. Washington, DC: Medicare Payment Advisory Commission; 2009.
6. O'Connor GT, Quinton HB, Traven ND, et al. Geographic variation in the treatment of acute myocardial infarction: The Cooperative Cardiovascular Project. *JAMA*. 1999;627–633.
7. Wenberg JE. *The Darmouth Atlas of Cardiovascular Health Care. American Colleague of Cardiology, Society of Thoracic Surgeons*. Chicago, IL: AHA Press; 1999.
8. Mc Cardle BA, Dowsley TF, deKemp RA, et al. Does rubidium-82 PET have superior accuracy to SPECT perfusion imaging for the diagnosis of obstructive coronary disease: A systematic review and meta-analysis. *J Am Coll Cardiol*. 2012;60:1828–1837.
9. Parker MW, Iskandar A, Limone B, et al. Diagnostic accuracy of cardiac positron emission tomography versus single photon emission computed tomography for coronary artery disease: A bivariate meta-analysis. *Circ Cardiovasc Imaging*. 2012;5:700–707.
10. Bengel FM, Higuchi T, Javadi MS, et al. Cardiac positron emission tomography. *J Am Coll Cardiol*. 2009;54:1–15.
11. Brindis RG, Douglas PS, Hendel RC, et al. ACCF/ASNC appropriateness criteria for single-photon emission computed

tomography myocardial perfusion imaging (SPECT MPI): A report of the American College of Cardiology Foundation Quality Strategic Directions Committee Appropriateness Criteria Working Group and the American Society of Nuclear Cardiology. *J Am Coll Cardiol.* 2005;46:1587–1605.
12. Hendel RC, Berman DS, Di Carli MF, et al. ACCF/ASNC/ACR/AHA/ASE/SCCT/SCMR/SNM 2009 appropriate use criteria for cardiac radionuclide imaging: A report of the American College of Cardiology Foundation Appropriate Use Criteria Task Force, the American Society of Nuclear Cardiology, the American College of Radiology, the American Heart Association, the American Society of Echocardiography, the Society of Cardiovascular Computed Tomography, Journal of Nuclear Cardiology_ Hendel 19 Volume 22, Number 1;16–21 The value and appropriateness of positron emission tomography the Society for Cardiovascular Magnetic Resonance, and the Society of Nuclear Medicine. *J Am Coll Cardiol.* 2009;53:2201–2229.
13. Brook RH, Chassin MR, Fink A, et al. A method for the detailed assessment of the appropriateness of medical technologies. *Int J Technol Assess Health Care.* 1986;2:53–63.
14. Fitch K. *The RAND/UCLA Appropriateness Method User's Manual.* Santa Monica, CA: Rand; 2001.
15. Patel MR, Spertus JA, Brindis RG, et al. ACCF proposed method for evaluating the appropriateness of cardiovascular imaging. *J Am Coll Cardiol.* 2005;46:1606–1613.
16. Wolk MJ, Bailey SR, Doherty JU, et al. ACCF/AHA/ASE/ASNC/HFSA/HRS/SCAI/SCCT/SCMR/STS 2013. Multimodality appropriate use criteria for the detection and risk assessment of stable ischemic heart disease. *J Am Coll Cardiol.* 2014;63:380–406.
17. Winchester D, Randall M, Chauffe R, et al. Clinical utility of inappropriate positron emission tomography myocardial perfusion imaging: Test results and cardiovascular events. *J Nucl Cardiol.* 2014. doi: 10.1007/s12350- 014-9925-1.
18. Mehta R, Ward PR, Chandra S, et al. Evaluation of the American College of Cardiology Foundation/American Society of Nuclear Cardiology appropriateness criteria for SPECT myocardial perfusion imaging. *J Nucl Cardiol.* 2008;15:337–344.
19. Gibbons RJ, Miller TD, Hodges D, et al. Application of appropriateness criteria to stress single-photon emission computed tomography sestamibi studies and stress echocardiograms in an academic medical center. *J Am Coll Cardiol.* 2008;51:1283–1289.
20. Hendel RC, Cerqueira M, Douglas PS, et al. A multicenter assessment of the use of single-photon emission computed tomography myocardial perfusion imaging with appropriateness criteria. *J Am Coll Cardiol.* 2010;55:156–162.
21. Carryer DJ, Hodge DO, Miller TD, et al. Application of appropriateness criteria to stress single photon emission computed tomography sestamibi studies: A comparison of the 2009 revised appropriateness criteria to the 2005 original criteria. *Am Heart J.* 2010;160:244–249.
22. Gibbons RJ, Askew JW, Hodge D, et al. Temporal trends in compliance with appropriateness criteria for stress single-photon emission computed tomography sestamibi studies in an academic medical center. *Am Heart J.* 2010;159:484–489.
23. Gholamrezanezhad A, Shirafkan A, Mirpour S, et al. Appropriateness of referrals for single-photon emission computed tomography myocardial perfusion imaging (SPECT-MPI) in a developing community: A comparison between 2005 and 2009 versions of the ACCF/ASNC appropriateness criteria. *J Nucl Card.* 2011;18:1044.
24. Druz RS, Phillips LM, Sharifova G. Clinical evaluation of the appropriateness use criteria for single-photon emission computed tomography: Differences by patient population, physician specialty and patient outcomes. *ISRN Cardiol.* 2011;2011:798318.
25. Koh AS, Flores JL, Keng FY, et al. Evaluation of the American College of Cardiology Foundation/American Society of Nuclear Cardiology appropriateness criteria for SPECT myocardial perfusion imaging in an Asian tertiary cardiac center. *J Nucl Cardiol.* 2011;18:324–330.
26. Gupta A, Tsiara SV, Dunsiger SI, et al. Gender disparity and the appropriateness of myocardial perfusion imaging. *J Nucl Cardiol.* 2011;18:588–594.
27. Aldweib N, Negishi K, Seicean S, et al. Appropriate test selection for single-photon emission computed tomography imaging: Association with clinical risk, posttest management, and outcomes. *Am Heart J.* 2013;166:581–588.
28. Doukky R, Hayes K, Frogge N, et al. Impact of appropriate use on the prognostic value of single-photon emission computed tomography myocardial perfusion imaging. *Circulation.* 2013;128:1634–1643.
29. Khawaja FJ, Jouni H, Miller RD, et al. Downstream clinical implications of abnormal myocardial perfusion single-photon emission computed tomography based on appropriate use criteria. *J Nucl Cardiol.* 2013;20:1041–1048.
30. Moralidis E, Papadimitrious N, Stathaki M, et al. A multicenter evaluation of the appropriate use of single-photon emission tomography myocardial perfusion imaging in Greece. *J Nucl Cardiol.* 2013;20:275–283.
31. Medolago G, Marcassa C, Alkraisheh A, et al. Applicability of the appropriate use criteria for SPECT myocardial perfusion imaging in Italy: Preliminary results. *Eur J Nucl Med Mol Imaging.* 2014. doi: 10.1007/s00259-014- 2743-2745.
32. Lalude OO, Gutarra MF, Pollono EM, et al. Inappropriate utilization of SPECT myocardial perfusion imaging on the USA-Mexico border. *J Nucl Cardiol.* 2014;21:544–552.
33. Singh M, Babayan Z, Harjai KJ, et al. Utilization patterns of single-photon emission cardiac tomography myocardial perfusion imaging studies in a rural tertiary care setting. *Clin Cardiol.* 2014;37:67–72.
34. Saifi A, Taylor AJ, Allen J, et al. The use of the learning community and online evaluation of utilization for SPECT Myocardial Perfusion Imaging. *J Am Coll Cardiol.* 2013;6:823–829.
35. Text of the Protecting Access to Medicare Act of 2014. https://www.govtrack.us/congress/bills/113/hr4302/text. Accessed July 2, 2014.
36. Gibbons RJ, Balady GJ, Bricker JT, et al. ACC/AHA 2002 guideline update for exercise testing: summary article. A report of the American College of Cardiology/American Heart Association Task Force on Practice Guidelines (Committee to Update the 1997 Exercise Testing Guidelines). *J Am Coll Cardiol.* 2002;40:1531e40.
37. Choosing Wisely. ACC. http://www.cardiosource.org/news-media/media-center/news-releases/2014/09/choosing-wisely-statement.aspx. Accessed November 2016.
38. Mahajan A, Bal S, Hahn H. Myocardial perfusion imaging determination using an appropriate use smartphone application. *J Nucl Cardiol.* 2015;22:66–71.

39. http://industryreport.jacksoncoker.com/physician-career-resources/newsletters/monthlymain/des/apps.aspx. Accessed December 3, 2013.
40. Payne KB, Wharrad H, Watts K. Smartphone and medical related App use among medical students and junior doctors in the United Kingdom (UK): A regional survey. *BMC Med Inf Decis Mak*. 2012;12:121.
41. Elgendy IY, Mahmoud A, Shuster JJ, et al. Outcomes after inappropriate nuclear myocardial perfusion imaging: A meta-analysis. *J Nucl Cardiol*. 2016;23:680–689.
42. Johnson TV, Rose GA, Fenner DJ, et al. Improving appropriate use of echocardiography and single-photon emission computed tomographic myocardial perfusion imaging: A continuous quality improvement initiative. *J Am Soc Echocardiogr*. 2014;27:749–757.
43. Lin FY, Rosenbaum LR, Gebow D, et al. Cardiologist concordance with the American College of Cardiology appropriate use criteria for cardiac testing in patients with coronary artery disease. *Am J Cardiol*. 2012;110:337–44.
44. Dunne RM, Ip IK, Abbett S, et al. Effect of evidence-based clinical decision support on the use and yield of CT pulmonary angiographic imaging in hospitalized patients. *Radiology*. 2015;276:167–174.
45. Moriarity AK, Klochko C, O'Brien M, et al. The effect of clinical decision support for advanced inpatient imaging. *J Am Coll Radiol*. 2015;12:358–363.
46. Jenkins HJ, Hancock MJ, French SD, et al. Effectiveness of interventions designed to reduce the use of imaging for low-back pain: A systematic review. *CMAJ*. 2015;187:401–408.
47. Chaudhuri D, Montgomery A, Gulenchyn K, et al. Effectiveness of quality improvement interventions at reducing inappropriate cardiac imaging a systematic review and meta-analysis. *Circ Cardiovasc Qual Outcomes*. 2016;9:7–13.
48. Doukky R, Hayes K, Frogge N, et al. Impact of insurance carrier, prior authorization and socioeconomic status on appropriate use of SPECT myocardial perfusion imaging in private community-based office practice. *Clin Cardiol*. 2015;38:267–273.
49. Nelson KH, Willens HJ, Hendel RC. Utilization of radionuclide myocardial perfusion imaging in two health care systems: assessment with the 2009 ACCF/ASNC/AHA appropriateness use criteria. *J Nucl Cardiol*. 2012;19(1):37–42.
50. Lin FY. Dunning AM, Narula J, et al. Impact of an automated multimodality point-of-order decision support tool on rates of appropriate testing and clinical decision making for individuals with suspected coronary artery disease: A prospective multicenter study. *J Am Coll Cardiol*. 2013;62(4):308–316.
51. Hendel RC. Widespread Implementation of Appropriate Use Criteria for Cardiac Imaging—Which Are "Appropriate"? *JAMA Cardiol*. 2016;1(2):211–212.
52. Hoffmann U, Venkatesh V, White RD, et al. ACR Appropriateness Criteria acute nonspecific chest pain: Low probability of coronary artery disease. *J Am Coll Radiol*. 2012;9(10):745–750.
53. Winchester DE, Wolinsky D, Beyth RJ, et al. Discordance between appropriate use criteria for nuclear myocardial perfusion imaging from different specialty societies. *JAMA Cardiol*. 2016;1(2):207–210.

Appendix 13-1

Detection of CAD/Risk Assessment

Indication	Stress RNI
Symptomatic	
• Low pretest probability of CAD • ECG interpretable AND able to exercise	R
• Low pretest probability of CAD • ECG uninterpretable OR unable to exercise	A
• Intermediate pretest probability of CAD • ECG interpretable AND able to exercise	A
• Intermediate pretest probability of CAD • ECG uninterpretable OR unable to exercise	A
• High pretest probability of CAD • ECG interpretable AND able to exercise	A
• High pretest probability of CAD • ECG uninterpretable OR unable to exercise	A
Asymptomatic	
• Low global CHD risk • Regardless of ECG interpretability and ability to exercise	R
• Intermediate global CHD risk • ECG interpretable and able to exercise	R
• Intermediate global CHD risk • ECG uninterpretable OR unable to exercise	M
• High global CAD Risk • ECG interpretable and able to exercise	M
• High global CAD Risk • ECG uninterpretable OR unable to exercise	M
Other Cardiovascular Conditions	
Newly Diagnosed Heart Failure (Resting LV Function Previously Assessed but No Prior CAD Evaluation)	
• Newly diagnosed systolic heart failure	A
• Newly diagnosed diastolic heart failure	A
Evaluation of Arrhythmias	
Without Ischemic Equivalent (No Prior Cardiac Evaluation)	
• Sustained VT	A
• Ventricular Fibrillation	A
• Exercise induced VT or nonsustained VT	A
• Frequent PVCs	A
• Infrequent PVCs	M
• New-onset atrial fibrillation	M
• Prior to initiation of antiarrhythmia therapy in high global CAD risk patients	A
Syncope Without Ischemic Equivalent	
• Low global CAD Risk	M
• Intermediate or high global CAD risk	A

A, appropriate care; CHD, coronary heart disease; LV, left ventricular; M, may be appropriate care; PVC, premature ventricular complex; R, rarely appropriate care; VT, ventricular tachycardia.
Adapted from Wolk MJ, Bailey SR, Doherty JU, et al. ACCF/AHA/ASE/ASNC/HFSA/HRS/SCAI/SCCT/SCMR/STS 2013. Multimodality Appropriate Use Criteria for the Detection and Risk Assessment of Stable Ischemic Heart Disease. *J Am Coll Cardiol.* 2014;63:380–406.

Appendix 13-2

Prior Testing or Procedure

Indication	Stress RNI
Prior Testing Without Intervening Revascularization	
Sequential Testing (≤90 Days): Abnormal Prior Test/Study	
• Abnormal rest ECG findings (potentially ischemic in nature such as LBBB, T-wave inversions)	A
• Low global CAD risk	
• Abnormal rest ECG findings (potentially ischemic in nature such as LBBB, T-wave inversions)	A
• Intermediate to high global CAD risk	
• Abnormal prior exercise ECG test	A
• Abnormal prior stress imaging study (assumes not repeat of same type of stress imaging)	M
• Obstructive CAD on prior CCTA study	A
• Obstructive CAD on prior invasive coronary angiography	A
• Abnormal prior CCT calcium (Agatston score >100)	A
Sequential or Follow-Up Testing (≤90 Days): Uncertain Prior Results	
Equivocal, Borderline, or Discordant Prior Noninvasive Evaluation Where Obstructive CAD Remains a Concern	
• Prior exercise ECG test	A
• Prior stress imaging study (assumes not repeat of same type of stress imaging)	M
• Prior CCTA	A
Prior Coronary Angiography (Invasive or Noninvasive)	
• Coronary stenosis or anatomic abnormality of unclear significance found on cardiac CCTA	A
• Coronary stenosis or anatomic abnormality of unclear significance on previous coronary angiography	A
Follow-Up Testing (>90 Days): Asymptomatic or Stable Symptoms	
Abnormal Prior Exercise ECG Test	
Asymptomatic or Stable Symptoms	
• Last test <2 years ago	R
• Last test ≥2 years ago	M
Abnormal Prior Stress Imaging Study	
Asymptomatic or Stable Symptoms	
• Last test <2 years ago	R
• Last test ≥2 years ago	M
Obstructive CAD on Prior Coronary Angiography (Invasive or Noninvasive) Asymptomatic (Without Ischemic Equivalent) or Stable Symptoms	
• Last test <2 years ago	R
• Last test ≥2 years ago	M
Prior Coronary Calcium Agatston Score	
Asymptomatic (Without Ischemic Equivalent) or Stable Symptoms	
• Agatston score <100	R
• Low to intermediate global CAD risk Agatston score between 100 and 400	M
• High global CAD risk	M
• Agatston score between 100 and 400	
• Agatston score >400	M
Normal Prior Exercise ECG Test	
Asymptomatic (Without Ischemic Equivalent)	
• Low global CAD risk	R
• Intermediate to high global CAD risk	R
• Test <2 years ago	
• Intermediate to high global CAD risk	
• Test ≥2 years ago	M

Indication	Stress RNI
Prior Testing Without Intervening Revascularization	
Normal Prior Stress Imaging Study OR Nonobstructive CAD on Angiogram (Invasive or Noninvasive) Asymptomatic (Without Ischemic Equivalent)	
• Low global CAD risk	R
• Intermediate to high global CAD risk	R
• Test <2 years ago	
• Intermediate to high global CAD risk	M
• Test ≥2 years ago	
Normal Prior Exercise ECG Test Stable Symptoms	
• Low global CAD risk	R
• Intermediate to high global CAD risk	R
• Test <2 years ago	
• Intermediate to high global CAD risk	M
• Test ≥2 years ago	
Normal Prior Stress Imaging Study OR Nonobstructive CAD on Angiogram (Invasive or Noninvasive) Stable Symptoms	
• Low global CAD risk	R
• Intermediate to high global CAD risk	R
• Test <2 years ago	
• Intermediate to high global CAD risk	M
• Test ≥2 years ago	
Follow-Up Testing: New or Worsening Symptoms	
• Normal exercise ECG test	A
• Nonobstructive CAD on coronary angiography (invasive or noninvasive) OR normal prior stress imaging study	A
• Abnormal exercise ECG test	A
• Abnormal prior stress imaging study	M
• Obstructive CAD on CCTA study	A
• Obstructive CAD on invasive coronary angiography	A
• Abnormal CCTA calcium (Agatston score >100)	A
Postrevascularization (PCI or CABG)	
Symptomatic (Ischemic Equivalent)	
• Evaluation of ischemic equivalent	A
Asymptomatic (Without Ischemic Equivalent)	
• Incomplete revascularization	A
• Additional revascularization feasible	M
• Prior left main coronary stent	R
• <5 years after CABG	M
• ≥5 years after CABG	R
• <2 years after PCI	M
• ≥2 years after PCI	

A, appropriate care; CCTA, cardiac computed tomography angiography; CHD, coronary heart disease; LV, left ventricular; M, may be appropriate care; R, rarely appropriate care; VT, ventricular tachycardia.
Adapted from Wolk MJ, Bailey SR, Doherty JU, et al. ACCF/AHA/ASE/ASNC/HFSA/HRS/SCAI/SCCT/SCMR/STS 2013. Multimodality Appropriate Use Criteria for the Detection and Risk Assessment of Stable Ischemic Heart Disease. *J Am Coll Cardiol.* 2014;63:380–406.

Evaluation of Patients with Suspected Coronary Artery Disease Using Nuclear Myocardial Perfusion Imaging

CHAPTER 14

Sanjeev U. Nair and Gary V. Heller

BACKGROUND

The worldwide burden of coronary artery disease (CAD) remains substantial. Annually, an estimated 1.5% of the US population visits the primary care services with symptoms of chest pain.[1] Each year over 660,000 patients in the United States present to hospital with either a first myocardial infarction (MI) or sudden cardiac death (SCD) due to CAD.[2] Of these 305,000 will have had a recurrent MI. An estimated 160,000 will also suffer a silent first MI.[2] CAD is the leading cause of death across the world and is predicted to remain so for the next 20 years. Annually, approximately 3.8 million men and 3.4 million women die from CAD. The number is estimated to rise to 11.1 million deaths globally by 2020.[3] An estimated $108.9 billion is spent annually on treatment of CAD and is expected to exceed $320 billion by the year 2030.[2] Thus, means and methods to reduce the prevalence, morbidity, and mortality associated with CAD remain of great importance to health care providers.

For these reasons, a systematic approach for early diagnosis and risk stratification of CAD is important for patients to benefit from preventive and therapeutic strategies. Over the past two decades, radionuclide myocardial perfusion imaging (MPI) has become clinical mainstay for the noninvasive evaluation of CAD. In this chapter, the role of nuclear cardiac perfusion including both single-photon emission computed tomographic (SPECT) and positron emission tomography (PET) imaging will be discussed in relation to the diagnosis, risk stratification, and patient management decisions in patients with suspected CAD.

ASSESSMENT OF RISK FOR CAD

To optimize the use of testing for suspected CAD, the initial step involves stratifying the likelihood of such a patient to have underlying disease. Although a variety of tools are available for this purpose, the evaluation of risk factors and the nature of presenting chest pain and associated symptoms are often used to estimate the pretest likelihood of CAD in patients (Table 14-1).[4] Modifiable cardiac risk factors include hypercholesterolemia, tobacco smoking, hypertension, diabetes mellitus, physical inactivity, and obesity, while nonmodifiable risk factors are family history of CAD in first-degree relatives under the age of 60 years, advanced age, and male gender.[5,6] Multiple clinical prediction models have been developed to stratify asymptomatic patients into low, intermediate, and high risk for presence of CAD. The most commonly used risk score in the United States is the Framingham Risk Score (FRS) which predicts a 10-year risk for nonfatal MI and cardiac death based on the presence or absence of cardiac risk factors.[7] Using the FRS, patients can be categorized into low-risk (age-specific risk level below average; 10-year absolute risk of CAD <6%), intermediate-risk (age-specific risk level average or above average; 10-year absolute risk of CAD between 6% and 20%), or high-risk (patients with coronary risk equivalents; 10-year absolute risk >20%) groups. A modified

Table 14-1
Pretest Probability of Coronary Artery Disease by Age, Gender, and Symptoms

Age (Years)	Gender	Typical/Definite Angina Pectoris	Atypical/Probable Angina Pectoris	Nonanginal Chest Pain	Asymptomatic
30–39	Men	Intermediate	Intermediate	Low	Very low
	Women	Intermediate	Very low	Very low	Very low
40–49	Men	High	Intermediate	Intermediate	Low
	Women	Intermediate	Low	Very low	Very low
50–59	Men	High	Intermediate	Intermediate	Low
	Women	Intermediate	Intermediate	Low	Very low
60–69	Men	High	Intermediate	Intermediate	Low
	Women	High	Intermediate	Intermediate	Low

High: >90%; intermediate: 10–90%; low: <10%; very low: <5%.
Reproduced with permission from Gibbons RJ, Balady GJ, Beasley JW, et al. ACC/AHA Guidelines for Exercise Testing. A report of the American College of Cardiology/American Heart Association Task Force on Practice Guidelines (Committee on Exercise Testing). *J Am Coll Cardiol.* 1997;30(1):260–311.

---

version of the FRS has been incorporated into the Third Report of the National Cholesterol Education Program Expert Panel on Detection, Evaluation, and Treatment of High Blood Cholesterol in Adults (Adult Treatment Panel [ATP] III).[8] However, none of these models incorporated stroke, transient ischemic attack, claudication, and heart failure as outcomes, nor have the majority of models included family history of CAD. Additional models have also been developed including the following: (1) Framingham General CVD Score with a higher predictability for cardiovascular morbidity and mortality[9]; (2) Reynolds CVD Score which is gender specific and incorporates hemoglobin A1c, high-sensitivity CRP, and family history of MI[10]; (3) the ACC/AHA CVD risk calculator which is similar to the FRS[11]; and (4) the MESA risk calculator[12] which incorporates coronary calcium score.

SYMPTOM ASSESSMENT

Patients who present for evaluation of suspected CAD may have chest symptoms suggestive of angina or have no symptoms but have increased risk for CAD. Patients may also present for primary cardiac evaluation due to an upcoming surgical procedure. For symptomatic patients, the role of nuclear MPI is an important one. At the present time, MPI is considered appropriate care only in those asymptomatic patients who are at high cardiovascular disease risk based on standard ATP III criteria, or are at high cardiovascular disease risk with a moderately abnormal (100–400) or a severely abnormal (>400) coronary artery calcium score.[13,14] Stress testing may also be used in asymptomatic persons in high-risk jobs such as airline pilots or public transportation workers. This chapter will primarily focus on evaluation of symptomatic subjects.

Patients with classic angina have retrosternal chest pain, pressure, or discomfort which comes on with emotional or physical stress, may radiate to the shoulders, arms or jaw, and rarely below the epigastrium or above the mandible. The discomfort usually lasts for minutes, is relieved by cessation of activity or with sublingual nitroglycerin. When all three characteristics of angina are present (chest pain, exertion related, relieved with cessation or nitroglycerin), it is denoted as "typical." When only two out of the three characteristics are present, chest pain is considered "atypical" and when only one of the three characteristics is present the chest pain is likely "noncardiac." Using the characteristic of the presenting chest discomfort and the patient's age and gender, patients can thus be placed into low-, intermediate-, or high-risk categories for having significant CAD (Table 14-1).[15] It should be noted that many elderly and female patients who are eventually diagnosed with significant CAD present with atypical symptoms.

CHOOSING THE BEST DIAGNOSTIC TEST FOR THE PATIENT

The choice of diagnostic testing of patients with suspected CAD is based on a multitude of factors. The objective is to determine whether the patient has CAD as accurately as possible with the least harm, least discomfort, and cost involving the tests and procedures needed to do so. Other factors which are equally important in deciding the type of stress test include the patient's ability to perform adequate exercise, the presence of disqualifying abnormalities on the resting ECG and the patient's body habitus. In general, symptomatic patients who are in the category of lower pretest likelihood of CAD are referred for exercise tolerance testing (ETT) alone, while those in higher-risk categories are candidates for imaging procedures.

▶ Exercise Tolerance Testing

The simplest form of noninvasive stress testing is the ETT. While this chapter primarily focuses on nuclear imaging, it can be said that ETT should be a consideration in many patients who meet the criteria. This form of testing involves the patient exercising on a treadmill or stationary bicycle and can be an adequate test alone for certain patients without ancillary imaging. This procedure is discussed in detail in Chapter 8. For ETT, the patients should be able to achieve an adequate workload defined by peak heart rate and exercise duration to derive meaningful diagnostic and prognostic value from the test. In addition to the inability to exercise, the presence of left bundle branch block (LBBB), a paced rhythm, ST-T changes on ECG due to LVH or digoxin use, ventricular pre-excitation and ST depression of ≥1 mm on the resting ECG in such patients can render the testing ECGs nondiagnostic, and therefore not useful in such a patient.

Currently, exercise is the preferred stress modality with or without perfusion imaging since it provides prognostic information in the form of hemodynamic data, functional capacity, and evaluation of symptoms. The use of the Duke Treadmill Score which incorporates exercise duration, exercise-induced ST-segment changes, and stress-induced angina can risk stratify patients into low, intermediate, and high risk for likelihood of coronary artery stenosis of ≥75%, multivessel disease, and 1-year all-cause mortality.[16]

Various studies have shown the sensitivity and specificity of ETT is approximately 68% and 77%, respectively.[17] Thus, the diagnostic accuracy of ETT alone is moderate, indicating that the health care provider ordering the test needs to assume a modicum of inaccuracy. While a false-positive study can be resolved, a false-negative result is more difficult, since it is a normal result and dependent upon the clinical situation for further testing. Moreover, in women who tend to present with atypical symptoms, ETT has a lower accuracy to diagnose CAD as compared to men due to a lower prevalence of epicardial CAD in women, an increased likelihood of inadequate exercise especially in the elderly, and an increased incidence of false-positive ST depression on ECG during exercise in women.[17,18] The value of ETT in the elderly has been questioned. In a meta-analysis by Rai et al.[18] in patients ≥65 years of age, patients with abnormal and normal ETT results had similar cardiac event rates (OR 3.1, 95% confidence interval [CI] 0.8–11.5) following the procedure. In contrast, an abnormal stress MPI compared to normal stress MPI accurately stratified risk in these patients (OR 11.8, 95% CI 7.5–18.7). Thus in elderly patients, ETT may not be beneficial. A diagnostic study by Froelicher et al.[19] minimized referral bias by performing ETT and coronary angiography on all patients, irrespective of indication. In this predominantly male population, the ETT sensitivity was 45% and the specificity was 85%. Thus, ETT is primarily useful for patients at a lower risk of CAD in whom a true-negative test is much more likely than a false-negative test, and will be a reassuring finding.

Of note, despite data suggesting less accurate results in women, the most recent ACC/AHA guidelines recommend having a similar approach to the utilization of ETT for diagnosis of CAD regardless of gender.[20]

▶ Exercise Stress Testing with SPECT Myocardial Perfusion Imaging

A major limitation of ETT is its less than optimal diagnostic accuracy for detection of significant CAD. Studies have shown that the diagnostic accuracy of stress MPI is significantly higher than that of ETT alone and provides greater risk stratification for predicting future cardiac events. Thus, in a population of patients in which CAD is prevalent, stress MPI is a better choice than ETT alone. In an aging population, it is important to note that the accuracy of the ETT depends on a patient's ability to reach a predicted maximum heart rate. Patients with medical illness, debilitation, deconditioning, or musculoskeletal problems may be unable to perform an adequate ETT. MPI with pharmacologic stress using vasodilators (dipyridamole and adenosine) or dobutamine can be implemented in such patients. Pharmacologic stress with MPI is most advantageous in older patients who are at the highest risk of CAD, yet are likely to be the population least able to exercise adequately.

The addition of SPECT imaging to exercise stress testing is used to improve diagnostic accuracy and to provide valuable risk stratification. SPECT MPI is based on the principle of visualizing the effects of relative blood flow between the resting and stressed myocardium. If the perfusion abnormalities occur only on stress as compared to rest, it indicates ischemia in that territory whereas the presence of matched perfusion abnormalities in stress and rest images suggests areas of scar or prior infarction. Moreover, by incorporating ECG gating into the test, additional diagnostic and prognostic data in the form of left ventricular function and volume as well as wall thickening and motion can be obtained. The procedural aspects of SPECT imaging are described in Chapter 9.

The sensitivity of stress testing with SPECT imaging (87%) is substantially higher than that of exercise ECG testing without imaging (68%), as is specificity. A meta-analysis of SPECT accuracy reported a sensitivity of 88.3% and a specificity of 75% in analysis of 108 published studies.[21] A recent meta-analysis by Iskandar et al.[22] evaluating the effect of gender on the diagnostic accuracy of SPECT MPI yielded a mean sensitivity and specificity of 84.2% (95% CI 78.7–88.6%) and 78.7% (CI 70.0–85.3%) for SPECT MPI in women; and 89.1% (CI 84.0–92.7%) and 71.2% (CI 60.8–79.8%) for SPECT MPI in men. There was no significant difference in the sensitivity ($p = 0.15$) or specificity ($p = 0.23$) between male and female subjects, thus this test is equally effective in both genders (Fig. 14-1). The prognostic implications of stress

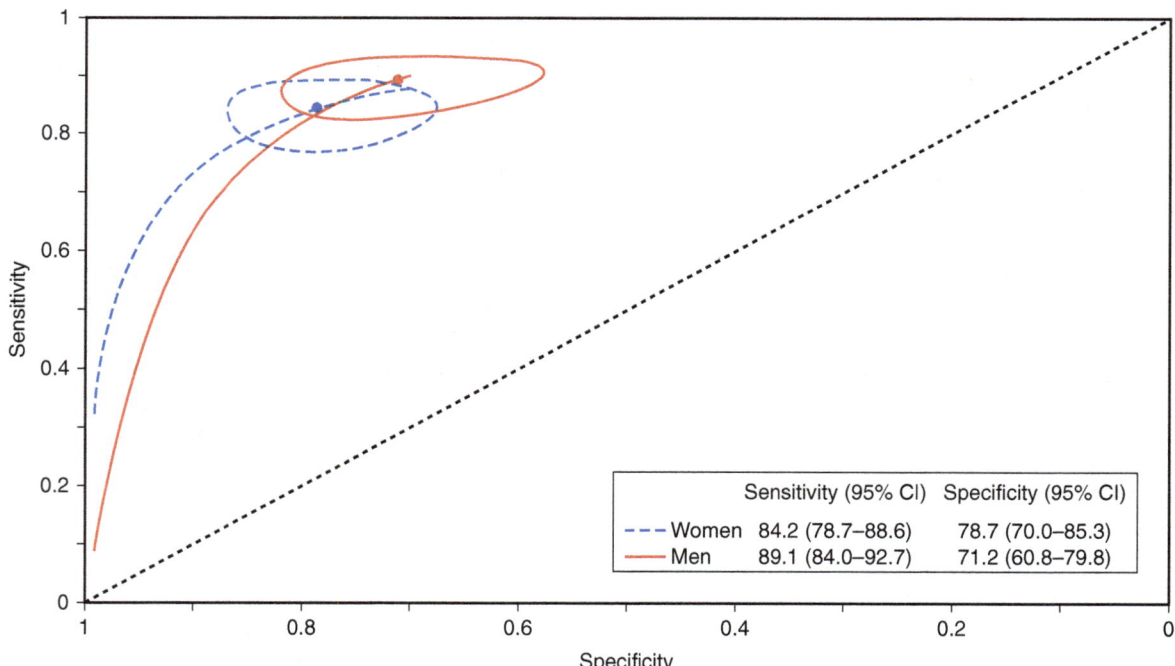

FIGURE 14-1 Receiver operating characteristic (ROC) curve from meta-analysis of diagnostic accuracy of SPECT, demonstrating high sensitivity and slightly lower specificity. There was no significant difference between genders. (Reproduced with permission from Iskandar A, Limone B, Parker MW, et al. Gender differences in the diagnostic accuracy of SPECT myocardial perfusion imaging: a bivariate meta-analysis. *J Nucl Cardiol*. 2013;20(1):53–63.)

MPI are discussed in Chapter 15. In summary, current literature demonstrates that diagnostic accuracy with SPECT is much higher than with ETT alone, and particularly useful in intermediate- to high-risk patients. In elderly patients, SPECT is particularly important in comparison to ETT.

▶ Pharmacologic Stress Testing with SPECT Myocardial Perfusion Imaging

One of the important advantages of MPI in assessing patients with suspected CAD is that patients who are unable to achieve adequate exercise for a diagnostic result can be studied using pharmacologic stress. It has been estimated that 40% to 50% of all stress MPI in the US is performed with pharmacologic agents, and the percentage increases annually. A detailed discussion regarding the use of pharmacologic stress testing may be found in Chapter 8. The two classes of pharmacologic agents are vasodilator (adenosine, dipyridamole, and more recently, a selective A2a agent, regadenoson) or inotropic stress (dobutamine). In brief, vasodilators, given intravenously, markedly increase coronary blood flow. This increased flow is less pronounced in arteries that are stenotic (flow restricted) due to atherosclerosis, as they are already maximally vasodilated. This causes heterogeneous myocardial perfusion, which can be identified using a radionuclide tracer that follows coronary blood flow. As an alternative to vasodilator stress in patients with contraindications to vasodilators, dobutamine works by increasing myocardial oxygen demand (through increased heart rate, systolic blood pressure, and myocardial contractility). This creates increased coronary blood flow, which results in heterogeneous blood flow due to stenotic arteries. An important marker of inotropic stress success is reaching at least 85% maximally predicted heart rate, similar to exercise stress. As in exercise MPI, scintigraphy images obtained at rest are compared to those obtained during peak pharmacologic stress to distinguish myocardial ischemia from infarction and normal.

The diagnostic accuracy of pharmacologic stress MPI has been examined, and results are similar to exercise stress MPI and do not differ substantially between pharmacologic agents. For example, dipyridamole planar scintigraphy has a reported sensitivity of 90% and a specificity of 70% for the detection of significant CAD, similar to exercise MPI.[23] The diagnostic accuracy of quantitative dipyridamole Tl-201 SPECT imaging was also comparable to exercise.[24] Similar results have been reported using adenosine stress SPECT (Fig. 14-2).[25]

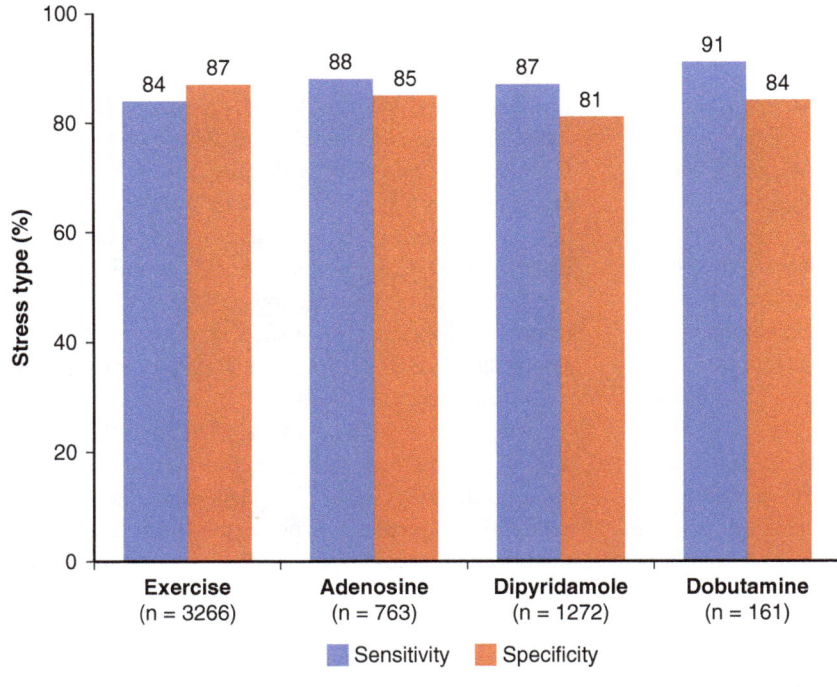

FIGURE 14-2 Comparison of diagnostic accuracy between exercise SPECT and various pharmacologic SPECT agents. (Adapted with permission from Leppo JA. Comparison of pharmacologic stress agents. J Nucl Cardiol. 1996;3(6 Pt 2):S22–6.)

Regadenoson is a newer selective A2A receptor agonist.[26] Multiple studies have shown that regadenoson is as efficacious in detecting perfusion abnormalities and has comparable diagnostic and prognostic value as adenosine in pharmacologic stress testing.[27-30] As mentioned above, dobutamine with imaging is used for patients who cannot exercise or have contraindications to vasodilator stress (primarily, reversible airway disease). Dobutamine stress using both planar and SPECT imaging has sensitivity and specificity comparable to vasodilators, even though the increase in coronary blood flow is less pronounced with dobutamine than with the vasodilators.[31,32] Moreover, as with exercise, the accuracy of dobutamine stress is heart-rate dependent.[33]

Comparative studies of diagnostic accuracy of Tc-99m imaging for angiographically significant CAD between exercise and pharmacologic stress are limited, but data that are available have not shown differences. Similarly, only small studies are available comparing vasodilator to inotropic stress. Marwick et al.[34] reported on 97 such patients without evidence of previous MI who were referred to coronary angiography for clinical reasons. This study demonstrated similar sensitivity and specificity of vasodilator and dobutamine Tc-99m-sestamibi MPI.

In conclusion, patients who are unable to exercise adequately and undergo pharmacologic stress have a similar diagnostic accuracy in comparison to exercise SPECT MPI, and this form of stress testing presents an important alternative.

▶ Factors Affecting Diagnostic Accuracy with SPECT MPI: Attenuation Artifact

Soft tissue attenuation of photons during the performance of SPECT MPI image acquisition has been a challenge for interpretation and achieving the best diagnostic accuracy. Attenuation artifacts are affected by body size and habitus, position of the heart in the body, gender of the patient, and the radionuclide tracer type and dose. Since these artifacts are potentially present in both rest and stress images, they potentially cause a fixed or reversible perfusion defect leading to false diagnosis of myocardial scar or, less commonly, ischemia.

Differentiation of a perfusion abnormality as consistent with artifact or true CAD is sometimes difficult, and without some method of adjudication, often leaves the interpreting physician with no choice to call the study abnormal, often leading to unnecessary catheterizations. Several methods to assist differentiation have been shown to be effective. First, and most commonly, assessing myocardial function in the area of a fixed defect using ECG-gated imaging, especially in the anterior or inferior regions is effective.[35-37] The assumption is that with a fixed defect in which wall motion is normal by ECG gating, the abnormality can be attributed to attenuation artifact. In contrast, if the wall motion is abnormal, the defect is consistent with CAD and scar. This assumption is negated if the abnormality is reversible or partially reversible, as an ischemic wall motion abnormality may have resolved by the time imaging is obtained (45–60 minutes later).

Gated SPECT MPI plays an important role in improving the diagnostic accuracy of MPI. Choi et al.[35] studied the impact of gated SPECT MPI on 109 patients who had equivocal fixed defects with perfusion imaging alone. The addition of gated data increased the diagnostic performance, with 66 patients determined disease negative and 25 patients as disease positive. Smanio et al.[36] studied 285 patients and found that the addition of gated data to Tc-99m-sestamibi imaging reduced the number of "borderline" interpretations from 89 to 29. More importantly, in the 137 patients with a <10% pretest likelihood of CAD, the percentage of images designated "normal" increased from 74% to 93%. Similarly, in the 49 patients with previous MI or known coronary artery stenosis of at least 70%, the percentage of "abnormal" image interpretations increased from 78% to 92%. Taillefer et al.[37] found that the addition of gated information to myocardial SPECT improved diagnostic accuracy in 85 patients with suspected CAD and 30 normal controls, particularly with specificity (Fig. 14-3).

Attenuation artifacts can also be identified with attenuation correction (AC) techniques. Using either computed tomography (CT) or an independent radionuclide line source, AC is performed with specialized software to process stress MPI images to reduce or remove attenuation artifacts from the final images. This form of processing is an effective means of distinguishing attenuation artifacts. Multiple studies

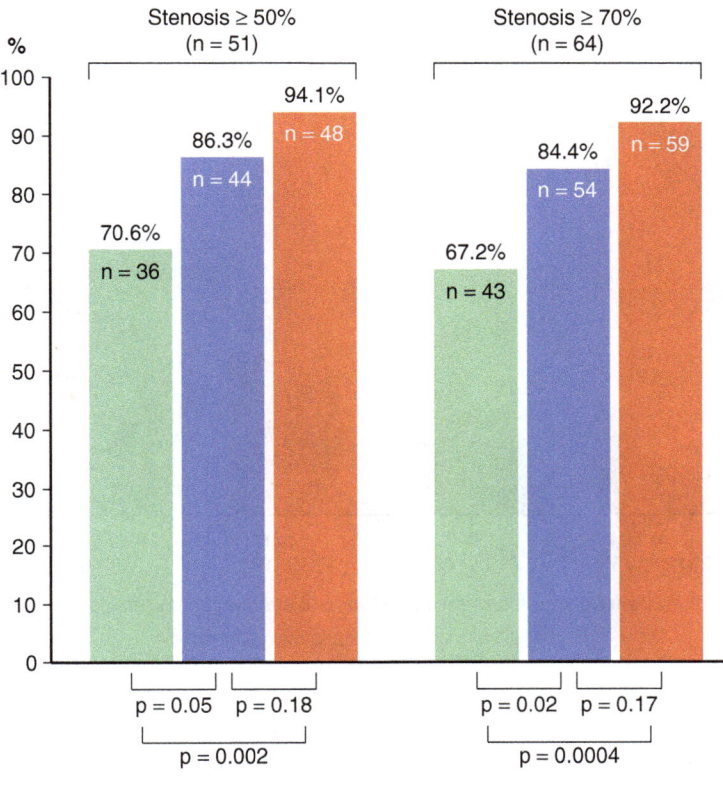

FIGURE 14-3 Impact of ECG gating on specificity for 50% and 70% stenosis. In both cases, specificity is improved with ECG gating. Green = Thallium-201; Blue = Technitium-99m sestamibi; Red = Technitium-99m sestamibi with gated SPECT. (Reproduced with permission from Taillefer R, Depuey EG, Udelson JE, et al. Comparative diagnostic accuracy of Tl-201 and Tc-99m sestamibi SPECT imaging (perfusion and ECG-gated SPECT) in detecting coronary artery disease in women. *J Am Coll Cardiol.* 1997;29(1):69–77.)

have shown AC to improve the study reader's confidence and diagnostic specificity. In an early study by Heller et al.[38] performed on 90 patients who underwent ECG-gated SPECT MPI stress imaging, the authors showed that the use of AC lead to improved diagnostic accuracy and reduced the need for rest imaging as compared to ECG-gated imaging alone and suggested that this may also lead to improved laboratory throughput. In a recent pooled analysis by Huang et al.[39] evaluating the diagnostic performance of AC in SPECT MPI using coronary angiography as a reference standard, the authors found that using AC as compared to non-AC lead to improved sensitivity (84% vs. 80%, respectively) and specificity (80% vs. 68%, respectively) of stress MPI studies. Several studies have also demonstrated value in risk stratification using line-source AC. Baghdasarian et al.[40] presented the concept that if the nuclear study was in the SSS 1 to 3 range, generally considered normal by SPECT, patients (495) were at an elevated risk compared to completely normal (SSS 0). In a much larger study, Ardestani et al.[41] confirmed accurate identification of low-, intermediate-, and high-risk patients with attenuation-corrected studies (Fig. 14-4).

Another means of reducing or eliminating soft tissue attenuation artifacts in SPECT MPI is prone imaging. The rationale for this type of imaging is that the heart (moves superior) and diaphragm (moves inferior) separate in prone position as compared to supine position leading to elimination of diaphragmatic inferior wall attenuation artifacts. Prone imaging can be performed either selectively only in those patients who have inferior wall fixed defects or in all patients undergoing SPECT MPI. In general, the stress part of the test undergoes the prone study. Various studies have shown the usefulness of prone imaging in improving specificity and thus diagnostic accuracy of SPECT MPI studies. Most recently, Taasan et al.[42] reported that the use of supine and prone imaging as compared to supine imaging alone leads to reduction of equivocal studies from 13% to 4% ($p < 0.001$). Moreover, the diagnostic accuracy was increased with the addition of prone imaging (the area under receiver operating curve being 0.8 with combined imaging as

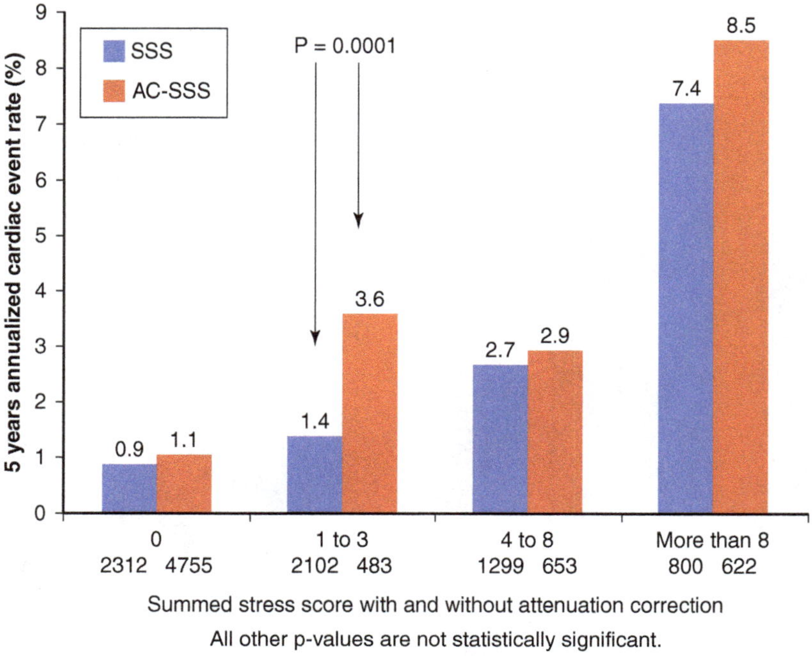

FIGURE 14-4 Annualized rate of cardiac death and nonfatal MI in relation to the Summed Stress Score with and without attenuation correction using the proposed cutoff with attenuation-corrected data. (Reproduced with permission from Ardestani A, Ahlberg AW, Katten DM, et al. Risk stratification using line source attenuation correction with rest/stress Tc-99m sestamibi SPECT myocardial perfusion imaging. *J Nucl Cardiol.* 2014;21(1):118–126.)

compared to 0.5 with supine imaging alone).[42] Prone imaging has been shown to have prognostic value as patients with no inferior wall attenuation artifacts on prone imaging have a low cardiac event rate similar to supine-only normal studies.[43]

While prone imaging has supportive data, there are also concerns. For example, in a recent report on stress-only imaging and prone acquisition to decide on further rest necessity, the percentage of patients requiring a rest study with prone imaging (39.1%) was substantially higher than similar studies with AC (8–10%).[44] Although prone imaging is not associated with additional cost, the additional imaging time for the prone acquisition requires an extra 10 to 15 minutes per patient, thus affecting laboratory throughput. It has also been found that some patients are not able to undergo prone due to body habitus and other issues. It has also been reported that patients experience more discomfort during prone positioning. Finally, there are instances when prone imaging leads to anterior wall defects and leads to false-positive interpretations. While these are cautionary thoughts, in the aggregate, if other forms of addressing attenuation artifact are not available, prone imaging should be a consideration.

Pharmacologic Stress Testing with PET Myocardial Perfusion Imaging

MPI using cardiac PET has been increasing in use as an alternative to SPECT imaging in many laboratories across the country. Recent estimates are that PET MPI is being performed in over 250 sites. The interest of this modality is based on several advantages such as high diagnostic accuracy, excellent image quality, rapid protocols, and low radiation exposure as well as added information such as regional and global myocardial blood flow. For a complete discussion of this modality, see Chapter 10. Pharmacologic stress is the primary form of stress for cardiac PET. The current tracers in use are rubidium-82 (Rb-82) and ^{13}N-ammonia. The half-life of Rb-82 is 75 seconds and therefore patients recommended for this procedure should only undergo pharmacologic stress. The half-life for ^{13}N-ammonia is 9.8 minutes and therefore exercise is possible, but difficult. Ammonia is cyclotron produced, and because of the short half-life it must be onsite or within close proximity, thus limiting its use to few centers.

The diagnostic accuracy of PET, particularly with pharmacologic stress has been extensively examined, and covered in detail in Chapter 10. Bateman et al.[45]

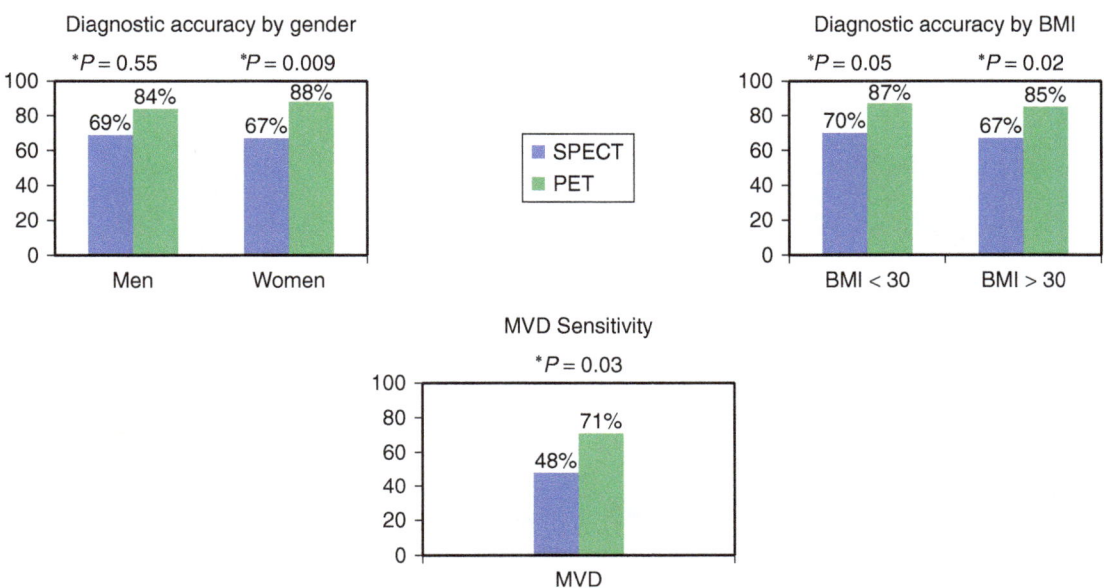

FIGURE 14-5 Comparison of diagnostic accuracy in similar patients between SPECT and cardiac PET in men and women as well as body mass index as well as identification of multivessel disease. In all three situations, PET was superior to SPECT. (Data from Bateman TM, Heller GV, McGhie AI, et al. Diagnostic accuracy of rest/stress ECG-gated Rb-82 myocardial perfusion PET: comparison with ECG-gated Tc-99m sestamibi SPECT. *J Nucl Cardiol.* 2006;13(1):24–33.)

compared Rb-82 PET and Tc-99m-sestamibi SPECT in two matched patient cohorts undergoing clinically indicated pharmacologic stress perfusion imaging using SPECT and PET.[47] Overall diagnostic accuracy using 70% angiographic threshold was higher for PET than for SPECT (89% vs. 79%, respectively). The diagnostic accuracy was maintained in nonobese patients and both genders (Fig. 14-5). In a meta-analysis evaluating the current literature, accuracy of Rb-82 PET for the diagnosis of obstructive CAD in comparison to SPECT, Mc Ardle et al.[46] reported that Rb-82 PET demonstrated sensitivity and specificity of 90% and 88%, respectively. In this study Rb-82 PET was demonstrated to have superior accuracy in comparison with Tc-99m SPECT with both ECG-gating and AC SPECT studies (Fig. 14-6). Similarly in a meta-analysis of 11,862 patients by Parker et al.,[21] MPI using PET demonstrated a higher sensitivity for CAD than SPECT although there was no difference in specificity (Fig. 14-7).

The inherent value of cardiac PET has recently been recognized by the American Society of Nuclear Cardiology and the Society of Nuclear Medicine

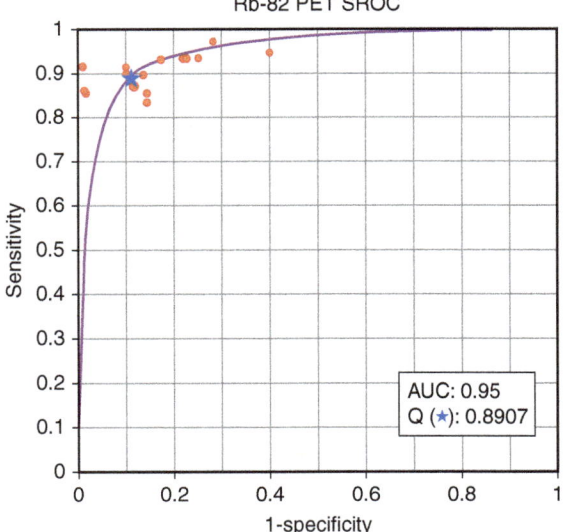

FIGURE 14-6 Diagnostic accuracy of cardiac PET: a recent meta-analysis demonstrates high sensitivity and specificity. (Reproduced with permission from Mc Ardle BA, Dowsley TF, deKemp RA, et al. Does rubidium-82 PET have superior accuracy to SPECT perfusion imaging for the diagnosis of obstructive coronary disease?: A systematic review and meta-analysis. *J Am Coll Cardiol.* 2012;60(18):1828–1837.)

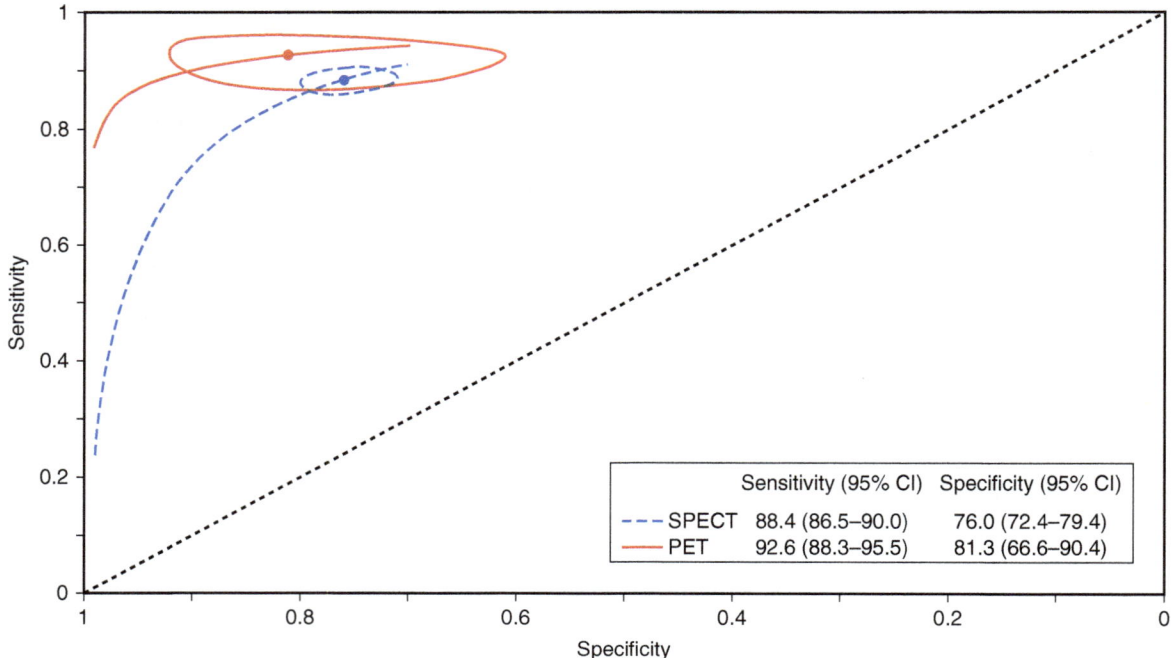

FIGURE 14-7 Summary ROC curves for SPECT and PET MPI. ROC, receiver-operating characteristic; SPECT, single-photon emission computed tomography; PET, positron emission tomography; MPI, myocardial perfusion imaging; CI, confidence interval. (Reproduced with permission from Parker MW, Iskandar A, Limone B, et al. Diagnostic accuracy of cardiac positron emission tomography versus single photon emission computed tomography for coronary artery disease: a bivariate meta-analysis. *Circ Cardiovasc Imaging*. 2012;5(6):700–707.)

and Molecular Imaging resulting in a Position Statement which opined that this was the "preferred" test for patients undergoing pharmacologic stress, and "recommended" for patients in whom body habitus might be a challenge, younger patients in which lowered radiation exposure is a high priority.[47] Thus, in laboratories in which cardiac PET is available, assessing patients with suspected CAD using this technique is a reasonable strategy with a high diagnostic accuracy and low radiation exposure.

IMPACT OF NEW TECHNOLOGIES FOR RADIONUCLIDE IMAGING

The development of semiconductor cadmium-zinc-telluride (CZT) cameras has raised the hopes of improving energy resolution and image quality as compared to conventional NaI SPECT Anger cameras. CZT cameras have been designed to work with the traditional software and collimation systems and improve count sensitivity and spatial resolution. These cameras lead to faster acquisition times and lower radiation to patients (and staff). However, solid-state CZT SPECT cameras are expensive, do not have AC, cannot be used to motion correct and can accentuate diaphragmatic attenuation artifacts. Moreover, their advantage over the traditional NaI SPECT cameras has been challenged with newer collimation techniques and recovery software using the traditional NaI SPECT cameras. There is however a growing body of literature supporting the value of CZT cameras as compared to the traditional NaI SPECT cameras.[48–51]

APPROACH TO THE USE OF STRESS MYOCARDIAL PERFUSION IMAGING FOR SUSPECTED CAD

The preceding sections presented data which aids in selection of testing procedures. What follows is a simplified stepwise approach to the patient suspected of having CAD. Several questions are important.

Question 1: Should My Patient Have a Radionuclide Test or Is ETT Sufficient?

The decision to order a stress MPI study should be based on the need for diagnosis and/or risk stratification. The decision to order a diagnostic study should be done only if the procedure significantly alters the pretest probability of disease or provides useful prognostic information. In general, patients with a low pretest risk for CAD will benefit from ETT alone as a first test. However, radionuclide testing would be appropriate in this category if a patient were unable to exercise, has an uninterpretable ECG, or has an abnormal ETT response.

Patients with a pretest intermediate or high risk of CAD benefit most from stress MPI. For patients with high pretest risk, nuclear imaging may be more useful in risk stratification rather than diagnosis, but may be helpful to guide therapies at catheterization. Although the probability of angiographically significant CAD is not altered dramatically by MPI in these patients, a negative or minimally abnormal MPI test portends an excellent prognosis in such patients.

Question 2: Which Type of Stress Should Be Used?

Exercise stress testing provides important diagnostic and prognostic information for patients being assessed for CAD, especially using the Duke Treadmill Score.[16] Furthermore, MPI provides additive information to the treadmill data.[52] Thus, any patient who can perform exercise should do so. If a patient is not capable of performing adequate stress, then vasodilator stress should be performed if there are no contraindications. In those unable to exercise and with contraindications to vasodilators, dobutamine stress should be considered.

Question 3: Which Type of Nuclear Study Should Be Used?

Growing evidence suggests that cardiac PET has a higher diagnostic accuracy than routine SPECT with better image quality, lower radiation exposure, and a faster protocol. The limitation to PET is the tracers which are best suited for pharmacologic stress. Current recommendations from the ASNC/SNMMI Position Statement recommends PET is preferred over SPECT in patients unable to exercise and recommended for patients with body habitus concerns that might interfere with diagnostic accuracy as well as patients with high risk for CAD in which a normal SPECT would not be helpful.[47]

CONCLUSIONS

In patients suspected of having CAD, a systematic approach to early diagnosis and accurate risk stratification is paramount to improve outcomes. While choosing the appropriate test for this purpose, one must take into account various factors such as age, gender, body mass index, the likelihood of having CAD, baseline ECG abnormalities, and the ability to exercise. Although newer modalities of imaging and stress testing are becoming more widely available, traditional forms of stress testing including MPI with nuclear tracers remain a mainstay for the diagnosis and risk stratification in patients with suspected CAD. The growing use of cardiac PET as the first choice has become an important aspect to evaluating patients with suspected CAD.

REFERENCES

1. Ruigómez A, Rodríguez LA, Wallander MA, Johansson S, Jones R. Chest pain in general practice: Incidence, comorbidity and mortality. *Fam Pract*. 2006;23(2):167–174.
2. Mozaffarian D, Benjamin EJ, Go AS, et al.; Writing Group Members; American Heart Association Statistics Committee; Stroke Statistics Subcommittee. Executive Summary: Heart Disease and Stroke Statistics—2016 Update: A Report From the American Heart Association. *Circulation*. 2016;133(4):447–454.
3. Mathers CD, Loncar D. Projections of global mortality and burden of disease from 2002 to 2030. *PLoS Med*. 2006;3(11):e442.
4. Diamond GA, Forrester JS. Analysis of probability as an aid in the clinical diagnosis of coronary-artery disease. *N Engl J Med*. 1979;300(24):1350–1358.
5. Kannel WB, McGee D, Gordon T. A general cardiovascular risk profile: the Framingham Study. *Am J Cardiol*. 1976;38(1):46–51.
6. Pryor DB, Shaw L, McCants CB, et al. Value of the history and physical in identifying patients at increased risk for coronary artery disease. *Ann Intern Med*. 1993;118(2):81–90.
7. D'Agostino RB Sr, Grundy S, Sullivan LM, Wilson P; CHD Risk Prediction Group. Validation of the Framingham coronary heart disease prediction scores: results of a multiple ethnic groups investigation. *JAMA*. 2001;286(2):180–187.

8. Third Report of the National Cholesterol Education Program (NCEP). Expert Panel on Detection, Evaluation, and Treatment of High Blood Cholesterol in Adults (Adult Treatment Panel III) final report. *Circulation.* 2002;106(25):3143–3421.
9. D'Agostino RB Sr, Vasan RS, Pencina MJ, et al. General cardiovascular risk profile for use in primary care: the Framingham Heart Study. *Circulation.* 2008;117(6):743–753.
10. Ridker PM, Paynter NP, Rifai N, Gaziano JM, Cook NR. C-reactive protein and parental history improve global cardiovascular risk prediction: the Reynolds Risk Score for men. *Circulation.* 2008;118(22):2243–2251.
11. Goff DC Jr, Lloyd-Jones DM, Bennett G, et al.; American College of Cardiology/American Heart Association Task Force on Practice Guidelines. 2013 ACC/AHA guideline on the assessment of cardiovascular risk: a report of the American College of Cardiology/American Heart Association Task Force on Practice Guidelines. *Circulation.* 2014;129(25 Suppl 2):S49–S73.
12. McClelland RL, Jorgensen NW, Budoff M, et al. 10-Year Coronary Heart Disease Risk Prediction Using Coronary Artery Calcium and Traditional Risk Factors: Derivation in the MESA (Multi-Ethnic Study of Atherosclerosis) With Validation in the HNR (Heinz Nixdorf Recall) Study and the DHS (Dallas Heart Study). *J Am Coll Cardiol.* 2015;66(15):1643–1653.
13. Hendel RC, Berman DS, Di Carli MF, et al.; ACCF/ASNC/ACR/AHA/ASE/SCCT/SCMR/SNM 2009 appropriate use criteria for cardiac radionuclide imaging: a report of the American College of Cardiology Foundation Appropriate Use Criteria Task Force, the American Society of Nuclear Cardiology, the American College of Radiology, the American Heart Association, the American Society of Echocardiography, the Society of Cardiovascular Computed Tomography, the Society for Cardiovascular Magnetic Resonance, and the Society of Nuclear Medicine. *Circulation.* 2009;119(22):e561–e587.
14. Wolk MJ, Bailey SR, Doherty JU, et al. ACCF/AHA/ASE/ASNC/HFSA/HRS/SCAI/SCCT/SCMR/STS 2013 multimodality appropriate use criteria for the detection and risk assessment of stable ischemic heart disease: a report of the American College of Cardiology Foundation Appropriate Use Criteria Task Force, American Heart Association, American Society of Echocardiography, American Society of Nuclear Cardiology, Heart Failure Society of America, Heart Rhythm Society, Society for Cardiovascular Angiography and Interventions, Society of Cardiovascular Computed Tomography, Society for Cardiovascular Magnetic Resonance, and Society of Thoracic Surgeons. *J Am Coll Cardiol.* 2014;63(4):380–406.
15. Gibbons RJ, Balady GJ, Bricker JT, et al. ACC/AHA 2002 guideline update for exercise testing: summary article: a report of the American College of Cardiology/American Heart Association Task Force on Practice Guidelines (Committee to Update the 1997 Exercise Testing Guidelines). *Circulation.* 2002;106(14):1883–1892.
16. Mark DB, Hlatky MA, Harrell FE Jr, Lee KL, Califf RM, Pryor DB. Exercise treadmill score for predicting prognosis in coronary artery disease. *Ann Intern Med.* 1987;106(6):793–800.
17. Gianrossi R, Detrano R, Mulvihill D, et al. Exercise-induced ST depression in the diagnosis of coronary artery disease. A meta-analysis. *Circulation.* 1989;80(1):87–98.
18. Rai M, Baker WL, Parker MW, Heller GV. Meta-analysis of optimal risk stratification in patients >65 years of age. *Am J Cardiol.* 2012;110(8):1092–1099.
19. Froelicher VF, Lehmann KG, Thomas R, et al. The electrocardiographic exercise test in a population with reduced workup bias: diagnostic performance, computerized interpretation, and multivariable prediction. Veterans Affairs Cooperative Study in Health Services #016 (QUEXTA) Study Group. Quantitative Exercise Testing and Angiography. *Ann Intern Med.* 1998;128(12 Pt 1):965–974.
20. Gibbons RJ, Balady GJ, Bricker JT, et al. ACC/AHA 2002 guideline update for exercise testing: summary article. A report of the American College of Cardiology/American Heart Association Task Force on Practice Guidelines (Committee to Update the 1997 Exercise Testing Guidelines). *J Am Coll Cardiol.* 2002;40(8):1531–1540.
21. Parker MW, Iskandar A, Limone B, et al. Diagnostic accuracy of cardiac positron emission tomography versus single photon emission computed tomography for coronary artery disease: a bivariate meta-analysis. *Circ Cardiovasc Imaging.* 2012;5(6):700–707.
22. Iskandar A, Limone B, Parker MW, et al. Gender differences in the diagnostic accuracy of SPECT myocardial perfusion imaging: a bivariate meta-analysis. *J Nucl Cardiol.* 2013;20(1):53–63.
23. Leppo JA. Dipyridamole-thallium imaging: the lazy man's stress test. *J Nucl Med.* 1989;30(3):281–287.
24. Borges-Neto S, Mahmarian JJ, Jain A, Roberts R, Verani MS. Quantitative thallium-201 single photon emission computed tomography after oral dipyridamole for assessing the presence, anatomic location and severity of coronary artery disease. *J Am Coll Cardiol.* 1988;11(5):962–969.
25. Leppo JA. Comparison of pharmacologic stress agents. *J Nucl Cardiol.* 1996;3(6 Pt 2):S22–S26.
26. Thomas GS, Tammelin BR, Schiffman GL, et al. Safety of regadenoson, a selective adenosine A2A agonist, in patients with chronic obstructive pulmonary disease: A randomized, double-blind, placebo-controlled trial (RegCOPD trial). *J Nucl Cardiol.* 2008;15(3):319–328.
27. Cerqueira MD, Nguyen P, Staehr P, Underwood SR, Iskandrian AE; ADVANCE-MPI Trial Investigators. Effects of age, gender, obesity, and diabetes on the efficacy and safety of the selective A2A agonist regadenoson versus adenosine in myocardial perfusion imaging integrated ADVANCE-MPI trial results. *JACC Cardiovasc Imaging.* 2008;1(3):307–316.
28. Iskandrian AE, Bateman TM, Belardinelli L, et al.; ADVANCE MPI Investigators. Adenosine versus regadenoson comparative evaluation in myocardial perfusion imaging: results of the ADVANCE phase 3 multicenter international trial. *J Nucl Cardiol.* 2007;14(5):645–658.
29. Mahmarian JJ, Peterson LE, Xu J, et al. Regadenoson provides perfusion results comparable to adenosine in heterogeneous patient populations: a quantitative analysis from the ADVANCE MPI trials. *J Nucl Cardiol.* 2015;22(2):248–261.
30. Hage FG, Ghimire G, Lester D, et al. The prognostic value of regadenoson myocardial perfusion imaging. *J Nucl Cardiol.* 2015;22(6):1214–1221.
31. Hays JT, Mahmarian JJ, Cochran AJ, Verani MS. Dobutamine thallium-201 tomography for evaluating patients with suspected coronary artery disease unable to undergo exercise or vasodilator pharmacologic stress testing. *J Am Coll Cardiol.* 1993;21(7):1583–1590.
32. Mason JR, Palac RT, Freeman ML, et al. Thallium scintigraphy during dobutamine infusion: nonexercise-dependent screening test for coronary disease. *Am Heart J.* 1984;107(3):481–485.

33. Shehata AR, Gillam LD, Mascitelli VA, et al. Impact of acute propranolol administration on dobutamine-induced myocardial ischemia as evaluated by myocardial perfusion imaging and echocardiography. *Am J Cardiol.* 1997;80(3):268–272.
34. Marwick T, Willemart B, D'Hondt AM, et al. Selection of the optimal nonexercise stress for the evaluation of ischemic regional myocardial dysfunction and malperfusion. Comparison of dobutamine and adenosine using echocardiography and 99mTc-MIBI single photon emission computed tomography. *Circulation.* 1993;87(2):345–354.
35. Choi JY, Lee KH, Kim SJ, et al. Gating provides improved accuracy for differentiating artifacts from true lesions in equivocal fixed defects on technetium 99m tetrofosmin perfusion SPECT. *J Nucl Cardiol.* 1998;5(4):395–401.
36. Smanio PE, Watson DD, Segalla DL, Vinson EL, Smith WH, Beller GA. Value of gating of technetium-99m sestamibi single-photon emission computed tomographic imaging. *J Am Coll Cardiol.* 1997;30(7):1687–1692.
37. Taillefer R, Depuey EG, Udelson JE, Beller GA, Latour Y, Reeves F. Comparative diagnostic accuracy of Tl-201 and Tc-99m sestamibi SPECT imaging (perfusion and ECG-gated SPECT) in detecting coronary artery disease in women. *J Am Coll Cardiol.* 1997;29(1):69–77.
38. Heller GV, Bateman TM, Johnson LL, et al. Clinical value of attenuation correction in stress-only Tc-99m sestamibi SPECT imaging. *J Nucl Cardiol.* 2004;11(3):273–281.
39. Huang JY, Huang CK, Yen RF, et al. Diagnostic performance of attenuation-corrected myocardial perfusion imaging for coronary artery disease: a systematic review and meta-analysis. *J Nucl Med.* 2016;57(12):1893–1898.
40. Baghdasarian SB, Noble GL, Ahlberg AW, Katten D, Heller GV. Risk stratification with attenuation-corrected stress Tc-99m sestamibi SPECT myocardial perfusion imaging in the absence of ECG-gating due to arrhythmias. *J Nucl Cardiol.* 2009;16(4):533–539.
41. Ardestani A, Ahlberg AW, Katten DM, et al. Risk stratification using line source attenuation correction with rest/stress Tc-99m sestamibi SPECT myocardial perfusion imaging. *J Nucl Cardiol.* 2014;21(1):118–126.
42. Taasan V, Wokhlu A, Taasan MV, et al. Comparative accuracy of supine-only and combined supine-prone myocardial perfusion imaging in men. *J Nucl Cardiol.* 2016;23(6):1470–1476.
43. Hayes SW, De LA, Hachamovitch R, et al. Prognostic implications of combined prone and supine acquisitions in patients with equivocal or abnormal supine myocardial perfusion SPECT. *J Nucl Med.* 2003;44(10):1633–1640.
44. Gutstein A, Bental T, Solodky A, Mats I, Zafrir N. Prognosis of stress-only SPECT myocardial perfusion imaging with prone imaging. *J Nucl Cardiol.* 2016.
45. Bateman TM, Heller GV, McGhie AI, et al. Diagnostic accuracy of rest/stress ECG-gated Rb-82 myocardial perfusion PET: comparison with ECG-gated Tc-99m sestamibi SPECT. *J Nucl Cardiol.* 2006;13(1):24–33.
46. Mc Ardle BA, Dowsley TF, deKemp RA, Wells GA, Beanlands RS. Does rubidium-82 PET have superior accuracy to SPECT perfusion imaging for the diagnosis of obstructive coronary disease?: A systematic review and meta-analysis. *J Am Coll Cardiol.* 2012;60(18):1828–1837.
47. Bateman TM, Dilsizian V, Beanlands RS, Depuey EG, Heller GV, Wolinsky DA. American Society of Nuclear Cardiology and Society of Nuclear Medicine and Molecular Imaging Joint Position Statement on the Clinical Indications for Myocardial Perfusion PET. *J Nucl Med.* 2016;57(10):1654–1656.
48. Gimelli A, Bottai M, Genovesi D, Giorgetti A, Di MF, Marzullo P. High diagnostic accuracy of low-dose gated-SPECT with solid-state ultrafast detectors: preliminary clinical results. *Eur J Nucl Med Mol Imaging.* 2012;39(1):83–90.
49. Lima R, Peclat T, Soares T, Ferreira C, Souza AC, Camargo G. Comparison of the prognostic value of myocardial perfusion imaging using a CZT-SPECT camera with a conventional anger camera. *J Nucl Cardiol.* 2017;24(1):245–251.
50. Oldan JD, Shaw LK, Hofmann P, et al. Prognostic value of the cadmium-zinc-telluride camera: A comparison with a conventional (Anger) camera. *J Nucl Cardiol.* 2016;23(6):1280–1287.
51. Sharir T, Slomka PJ, Hayes SW, et al. Multicenter trial of high-speed versus conventional single-photon emission computed tomography imaging: quantitative results of myocardial perfusion and left ventricular function. *J Am Coll Cardiol.* 2010;55(18):1965–1974.
52. Vanzetto G, Ormezzano O, Fagret D, Comet M, Denis B, Machecourt J. Long-term additive prognostic value of thallium-201 myocardial perfusion imaging over clinical and exercise stress test in low to intermediate risk patients: study in 1137 patients with 6-year follow-up. *Circulation.* 1999;100(14):1521–1527.

Risk Stratification with Myocardial Perfusion Imaging

CHAPTER 15

Javier Gomez and Rami Doukky

INTRODUCTION

In the past three decades, a great body of literature has established the use of radionuclide myocardial perfusion imaging (MPI), for risk stratification in patients with known or suspected coronary artery disease (CAD). The early studies have been reinforced and enhanced with the use of novel stress agents, modern single-photon emission tomography (SPECT) technologies, and the evolution of the appropriate use criteria (AUC). This chapter will review the use of stress radionuclide SPECT MPI for risk stratification in a general population and among patients with chronic CAD. Risk stratification for specific applications is discussed elsewhere in this book, including prior to major noncardiac surgery (Chapter 16), after therapeutic intervention (Chapter 17), in heart failure patients (Chapter 18), and for a variety of unique populations (Chapter 19).

▶ Risk Assessment

Risk stratification is of crucial importance for the practice of contemporary medicine. Appropriate management of CAD should include the assessment of the individual risk of future cardiac events, particularly cardiac death and myocardial infarction (MI).[1] Extending the paradigm of noninvasive cardiac testing beyond the detection of disease is especially important, as risk assessment permits patient management decisions to be formulated on an evidence-based approach. Patients who are identified as being at high risk for subsequent cardiac events should be considered for aggressive management, including cardiac catheterization and revascularization procedures that may improve their outcome. Conversely, the management of low-risk patients should be focused toward aggressive medical therapy and risk factor modification,[2,3] thus reserving invasive procedures for patients who fail medical management. Additional testing in this low-risk group should generally be avoided, thereby minimizing cost. An outcome-based risk assessment model strives for improved patient outcome and avoidance of complications from unnecessary procedures, and is cost-effective.

Risk strata are often defined in many ways; but when related to CAD events, specifically nonfatal MI and cardiac death, an annual event rate of <1% is accepted as a low risk, while an annual event rate of >3% is considered high risk and an annual event rate between 1% and 3% is an intermediate risk.[4]

Risk can be defined using clinical parameters, namely cardiac risk factors[5] and symptoms characterization, such as chest pain[4] or dyspnea.[6] However, risk assessment based only on clinical findings and resting ECG is often limited. Exercise tolerance test (ETT) without imaging and related risk indices, such as the Duke Treadmill Score, provide substantial prognostic value.[7] Unfortunately, in contemporary practice, many patients cannot undergo ETT due to aging, obesity, and other limiting comorbidities. Moreover, using clinical data and the Duke Treadmill Score, most patients with suspected CAD would fall in an intermediate-risk group which may necessitate additional risk stratification.[8]

While coronary angiography is considered the "gold standard" for the diagnosis of CAD, it does not provide information about the physiologic significance of atherosclerotic disease, especially in borderline lesions (50–70% stenosis) or when the culprit lesion cannot be determined by angiography data alone.[9] In fact, disparity often exists when comparing anatomic findings with physiologic data obtained with SPECT or fractional flow reserve (FFR).[9–15] Importantly, angiographic data do often not provide a clear marker of risk of adverse events, especially in patients with moderate disease severity.[11] However, functional information related to a coronary stenosis, including both noninvasive physiologic testing as well as invasive determinants of hemodynamic significance, is highly predictive of outcomes in patients with ischemic heart disease.[11–15]

RISK STRATIFICATION WITH SPECT MYOCARDIAL PERFUSION IMAGING

SPECT MPI is ideally suited for risk stratification among patients with known or suspected CAD (Table 15-1). This method detects ischemia and the presence of a scar, but importantly provides the physiologic significance of a known stenosis. In addition, it permits the determination of the location, extent, and severity of perfusion defects, which has important implications in clinical decision making. There is a clear association between the type of perfusion abnormalities and cardiac events, with reversible defects being associated with acute coronary syndromes and fixed abnormalities being predictive of death and heart failure.[16] SPECT MPI may also predict functional recovery of myocardial contractility as discussed in Chapter 21.

▶ Normal SPECT Imaging Study

The presence of a normal SPECT MPI study at a high level of stress (≥85% of maximum predicted heart rate) or adequate pharmacologic stress carries a benign prognosis, with mortality rate usually <1% per year. On the other hand, an abnormal perfusion study is associated with a multifold increase in the risk of nonfatal MI and/or cardiac death.[17,18] This finding has been reproduced in a multitude of studies in various clinical settings.[19–24] Pooling the results of SPECT imaging in >100,000 patients, Shaw and Iskandrian[24] demonstrated that the event rate (death or MI) for patients with normal MPI is 0.6% per year, whereas a moderate–severely abnormal study carries 5.9% per year event rate, an almost 10-fold increase in risk (Fig. 15-1). A meta-analysis of over 8000 patients demonstrated that a normal exercise SPECT MPI study had a negative predictive value of 98.8% and was associated with an annual event rate of 0.45%.[25] Moreover, a normal scan was associated with low rates of unstable angina and coronary revascularization.[25] Thus, a normal exercise stress SPECT MPI carries an excellent negative predictive value for adverse events.

The predictive value of SPECT MPI is independent of the radiopharmaceutical being used.[20,25] In a

Table 15-1

Rationale for the Use of SPECT MPI for Risk Assessment

- Widely available technology
- Identifies ischemia
- Quantitatively determines extent, severity, and location of altered coronary perfusion
- Associated with cardiac events
- Predicts functional recovery
- Impacts on medical decision making

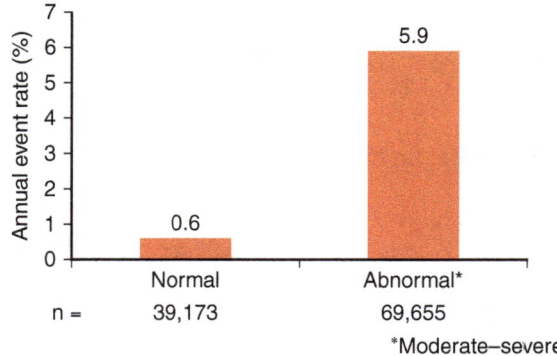

FIGURE 15-1 Differential risk of event rate in normal and abnormal myocardial perfusion imaging study. An abnormal SPECT study is associated with an almost 10-fold increase in event rate compared to a normal study. (Data from Shaw LJ, Iskandrian AE. Prognostic value of gated myocardial perfusion SPECT. *J Nucl Cardiol.* 2004;11(2):171–185.)

meta-analysis of published literature on prognostic value of normal SPECT MPI using various tracers (thallium-201 [Tl-201] and Tc-99m-sestamibi), Shaw et al.[20] confirmed similar excellent survival rates (99.3–99.7%) regardless of the radiopharmaceutical agent used. Similarly, the prognostic value of SPECT imaging is not dependent on the mode of stress. As with exercise SPECT, abnormal pharmacologic stress MPI is associated with several fold increase in risk compared to a normal scan. However, the risk of a cardiac event following a normal pharmacologic stress SPECT MPI is greater than the risk associated with normal exercise SPECT MPI[20,23,26]; that is likely due to selection of patients with greater comorbidities and higher pretest likelihood of disease for pharmacologic stress.[27,28] In other high-risk groups, such as the elderly and patients with diabetes, established CAD, or end-stage renal disease, a normal MPI still predicts lower risk than abnormal MPI. However, a normal scan in these patient populations carries greater risk than a normal scan in patients without these comorbidities.[28–32]

The favorable outcome associated with normal SPECT MPI has not only been demonstrated with exercise stress, but also with dipyridamole,[16,33,34] adenosine,[20,35,36] and dobutamine[26,37,38] stress modalities. Recent data with regadenoson (a selective A2A-adenosine receptor agonist), indicated that normal regadenoson SPECT MPI portrays low risk of adverse cardiac events, similar to normal adenosine MPI.[35] More recently, perfusion abnormalities produced by regadenoson has been shown to carry similar prognostic information to adenosine stress.[35,39] Furthermore, the excellent prognostic value of normal SPECT MPI has been demonstrated not only in tertiary care centers, but also in community-based cardiology and primary care office settings.[22,36]

When stress methods are combined, such as vasodilator stress with symptom-limited exercise, SPECT imaging permitted stratification of >2000 patients into low-, intermediate-, and high-risk groups on the basis of their functional capacity, perfusion defects, left ventricular ejection fraction (LVEF), and the presence or absence of transient ischemic dilation (TID).[40] The benign prognosis associated with a normal SPECT study appears to persist even in patients with positive ETT or angiographically significant coronary disease.[41,42] However, if an abnormal ECG response is noted with the infusion of dobutamine, adenosine, or regadenoson; the risk associated with a normal study increases significantly, suggesting that such patients should not be considered low risk.[26,43–45] Despite this increase in risk, patients with abnormal ECG response to pharmacologic stress and normal MPI are generally at lower risk than those with abnormal MPI.[45]

Most of the prognostic data for SPECT MPI were derived from conventional scintillation Anger cameras. However, the robust risk stratification value for SPECT MPI has been reproduced using modern SPECT cameras. A major recent advancement in SPECT technology has been the advent of cadmium-zinc-telluride (CZT) cameras, which implement semiconductors in photon detection. This and other recent advances in SPECT technology, such as modern attenuation correction methods (CT or fluorescence x-ray), cardiocentric collimation, and resolution recovery software, allow for marked improvement in count statistics, and special resolution. In a recent study in over 2000 patients, Oldan et al.[46] demonstrated that, compared to conventional Anger camera, images produced by modern CZT camera have a similar prognostic value in predicting events of death and MI. Therefore, the vast accumulated wealth of prognostic SPECT MPI data are applicable to CZT SPECT technology.[46,47]

Although the excellent prognostic value of SPECT MPI has been established based on conventional rest–stress protocols, data published in the past decade clearly demonstrated that normal stress-only SPECT scan carries similar excellent prognostic value. Chang et al.[48] analyzed data from over 16,000 patients and found that the mortality rates for patients with normal stress-only versus rest–stress protocols are similar, but patients who underwent stress-only imaging had a 61% reduction in radiation dose. Similarly in a cohort of over 10,000 patients, Duvall et al.[49] demonstrated that in patients with low pretest probability for CAD, the prognostic value of a negative stress-only MPI was similar to that of a rest–stress MPI protocol. Based on these findings, a stress-only protocol for appropriate patients is an option to consider in an effort to reduce radiation exposure and improve patient experience with the test.

In summary, the excellent prognostic value of a normal or near-normal stress myocardial perfusion study has been confirmed in numerous investigations

Table 15-2

Prognostic Indicators

- Perfusion defect
- Extensive and/or severe defect
- Multivessel distribution
- Reversibility
- Postinfarct ischemia
- Transient ischemic dilation (TID)
- Left ventricular dilation
- Left ventricular dysfunction
- Abnormal lung activity

using various radiopharmaceuticals and differing stress modalities.[10,16,17,19,20,26,36,38,50–56] These findings have been noted in different subsets of patients regardless of race,[57] clinical setting,[22,36] or CAD status,[58] and in important patient subgroups, including diabetics and women; these unique cohorts will be discussed in Chapter 19.

Abnormal SPECT Scan

An abnormal SPECT MPI study conveys a multifold increase in the risk of subsequent cardiac events compared to a normal scan. However, the presence of a perfusion defect is but one of the many variables that may provide important prognostic information (Table 15-2). The increased risk associated with abnormal MPI, compared to a normal scan, has been shown to be sustained for more than a decade after testing.[31,32,37,59]

The value of radionuclide MPI comes from its ability to identify and quantify the size and severity of scintigraphic abnormalities during stress, and thus place patients in more defined risk categories. The size of the perfusion abnormality provides powerful prognostic information and has been shown to directly relate to outcome,[21,50,60–63] as the larger the perfusion abnormality, the higher the mortality rate.[61–71] Ladenheim et al.[61] have demonstrated that the magnitude of ischemia (severity and extent) correlates well with cardiac events, and this relationship is not linear, but exponential (Fig. 15-2). Vanzetto et al.[50] have also shown a correlation between event rate (death, nonfatal MI, and revascularization) and the extent of ischemia, quantified by the number of ischemic segments on SPECT scan. Hage et al.[39] replicated these findings with regadenoson, demonstrating a stepwise increase in cardiac event rates with increasing

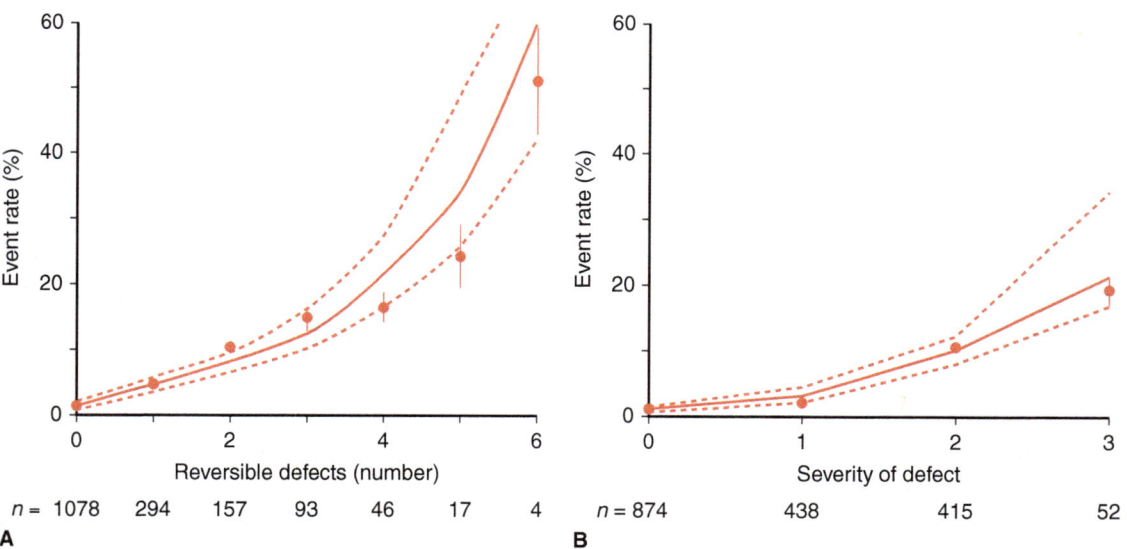

FIGURE 15-2 **(A)** Correlation between cardiac event rate on the vertical axis and number of reversible segmental defects on the horizontal axis (six-segment model using planar imaging employing thallium-201). **(B)** Correlation between event rate (vertical axis) and ischemic severity on the horizontal axis (four-point scale: 0, no defect; 1, mild defect; 2, moderate defect; and 3, severe defect). As ischemic extent or severity increases to moderate level, the event rate increases exponentially. (Reproduced with permission from Ladenheim ML, Pollock BH, Rozanski A, et al. Extent and severity of myocardial hypoperfusion as predictors of prognosis in patients with suspected coronary artery disease. *J Am Coll Cardiol.* 1986;7(3):464–471.)

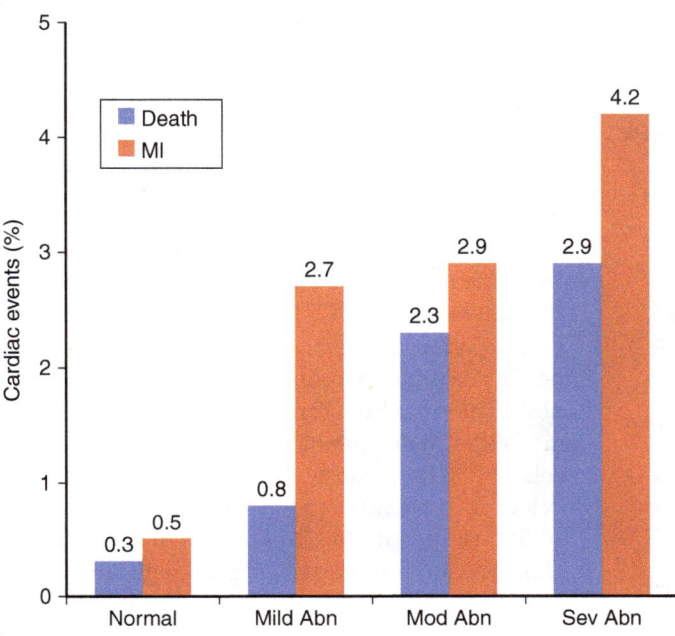

FIGURE 15-3 Cardiac events based on SPECT imaging results, differential stratification for risk of cardiac death, and myocardial infarction. Patients with mildly abnormal SPECT scan have an increased rate of nonfatal MI but maintain very low risk of cardiac death. (Reproduced with permission from Hachamovitch R, Berman DS, Shaw LJ, et al. Incremental prognostic value of myocardial perfusion single photon emission computed tomography for the prediction of cardiac death: differential stratification for risk of cardiac death and myocardial infarction. *Circulation*. 1998;97(6):535–543.)

percent myocardium affected by perfusion abnormalities. Moreover, among patients with dyspnea, the defect size correlates with mortality, as patients with a normal MPI study had 80% fewer events of death than those with severe perfusion defect.[64]

Even among asymptomatic patients without a prior diagnosis of ischemic heart disease, the presence of an ischemic defect of at least 7.5% of the myocardium identified a high-risk marker for cardiac death or MI.[65] This was confirmed in a second study of moderate-risk asymptomatic patients, which demonstrated a relationship between survival and the burden of perfusion abnormality by SPECT.[66]

Several studies have demonstrated that defect reversibility is an important predictor of type of cardiac events, as fixed perfusion defects are associated with cardiac death, whereas reversible perfusion defects are associated with nonfatal MI.[16,18,62,67] An examination of 7849 patients confirmed that the extent of ischemia correlated with event rates.[67] Moreover, Shaw et al.[67] demonstrated that resting perfusion defects also convey important prognostic information, as for each 1% defect on a rest study, there was a corresponding 3% increase in cardiac events. Rest defects also inversely correlated with LVEF. Overall, there is a synergy between rest and reversible defects, with both contributing to risk for subsequent cardiac events. Therefore, stress perfusion studies should be reported documenting defect severity (mild, moderate, and severe), size (small, moderate, and large), and reversibility in order to provide essential risk stratification information.[72] Moreover, Hachamovitch et al.[62] demonstrated a difference in the type of events predicted based on varying severity/extent of perfusion defects. As shown in Figure 15-3, a mildly abnormal study was associated with a very low mortality rate (0.8%) but a slightly higher risk of nonfatal MI (2.7%) than a normal scan (0.5%). In contrast, the most common event in patients with severe perfusion abnormalities was found to be cardiac death, not MI. These findings have important management implications, as coronary artery bypass grafting and percutaneous coronary intervention have not been shown to reduce the rates of nonfatal MI, whereas statins effectively reduce event rate of death and MI. Thus, medical therapy such as statins and angiotensin-converting enzyme inhibitors, rather than revascularization procedures, should be the mainstay in the management of patients with mildly abnormal MPI.[68,73,74]

Hachamovitch et al.[69] further extended the predictive value of SPECT MPI by demonstrating that the burden of inducible ischemia is not only predictive of event-free survival, but may also indicate whether medical therapy or coronary revascularization should

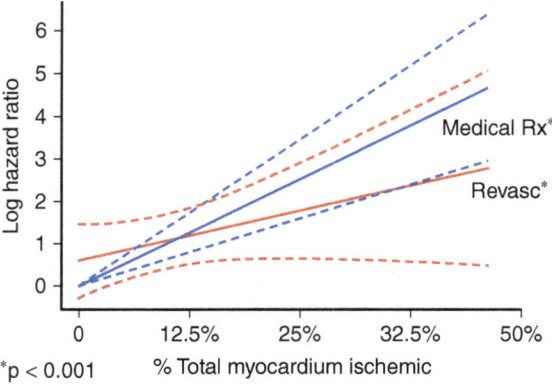

FIGURE 15-4 The relationship between ischemic myocardium and the log of the hazard ratio for revascularization versus medical therapy. The intersection of these lines (around 12% ischemic myocardium) defines the ischemic burden above which a survival benefit is achieved with revascularization. (Reproduced with permission from Hachamovitch R, Hayes SW, Friedman JD, et al. Comparison of the short-term survival benefit associated with revascularization compared with medical therapy in patients with no prior coronary artery disease undergoing stress myocardial perfusion single photon emission computed tomography. *Circulation*. 2003;107(23):2900–2907.)

be undertaken. A survival advantage was shown in patients with no or mild ischemia (<10% ischemic myocardium) undergoing medical therapy while those with moderate or severe ischemia (>12.5% ischemic myocardium) had a survival benefit with coronary revascularization, as compared with medical therapy alone (Fig. 15-4).

The use of optimal medical therapy as the mainstay of management in patients with mild perfusion abnormality is supported by the COURAGE trial which did not demonstrate an overall benefit from PCI beyond optimal medical therapy.[68] However, the nuclear substudy of the COURAGE trial suggests that among patients with moderate–severe ischemia on SPECT MPI, those treated with PCI in addition to optimal medical therapy had a greater reduction of ischemic events (33%) than medical therapy alone (19%).[75] The ISCHEMIA trial, which is an ongoing multicenter, randomized controlled trial planning to enroll 8000 patients with at least moderate ischemia on stress imaging, will compare a routine invasive strategy with complete revascularization when feasible versus optimal medical therapy only; it is the hope that this trial will provide evidence to help guide management in patients with stable ischemic heart disease.

Incremental Prognostic Value

The prognostic value of the SPECT scan is not simply a substitute but a valuable addition to prognostic data derived from clinical findings or stress testing. Iskandrian et al.[70] and others[50,71,76–78] have shown the additive value of SPECT MPI to clinical data and ETT, especially if the burden of perfusion abnormalities is taken into account.[50] The incremental prognostic value has been confirmed using various stress modalities, radiopharmaceutical agents, and protocols.[8,58,79–84] In a cohort of 2200 patients, Hachamovitch et al.[8] demonstrated that gated SPECT provided additional prognostic information irrespective of Duke Treadmill Score risk category (high, intermediate, and low). The added prognostic value of SPECT was most notable in the intermediate Duke Treadmill Score (55% of the cohort), in whom MPI effectively separated between low-risk patients with normal perfusion and high-risk patients with abnormal perfusion.[8] However, the added prognostic value of MPI in patients with low-risk Duke Treadmill Score was modest, as most of these patients had normal- or low-risk scan with low event rates. On the other hand, the added prognostic value of MPI in patients with high-risk Duke Treadmill Score was also limited, as these patients had increased event rates, irrespective of MPI.[8] Thus, MPI provides the highest incremental prognostic value in patients who are not fully risk stratified by ETT. Based on these observations, Bourque et al.[85] prospectively examined the incremental diagnostic yield of MPI in a cohort of 1056 patients on the basis of workload achieved during ETT. Among 430 patients who reached a workload of ≥10 METs without exercise-induced ST-segment depression, none had ≥10% left ventricular (LV) ischemia. In contrast, the prevalence of ≥10% LV ischemia was highest in the patients achieving <10 METs with ST-segment depression (19.4%).[85] In a separate investigation, the same group demonstrated that in patients at intermediate risk for CAD or with known CAD, achieving ≥10 METs is associated with very low rates of cardiac mortality (0.1% per year) and nonfatal MI (0.3% per year), irrespective of heart rate achieved. These results suggest that patients who attain ≥10 METs during ETT have an excellent intermediate-term prognosis, regardless of peak exercise heart rate achieved. Thus, the added value of MPI to standard exercise ECG testing in this population is limited.[86] Based on the aforementioned findings, these investigators proposed a provisional SPECT MPI imaging protocol, in which patients undergoing exercise stress MPI would receive the stress radiotracer injection only if they fail to achieve ≥10 METs or if they develop ischemic ST-segment changes.[87] However, deploying such protocol in the clinical setting possesses some logistic and financial challenges.

Moreover, SPECT perfusion imaging is a better predictor of cardiac events than cardiac catheterization.[60,70] SPECT MPI, when added to stress and clinical data, has shown a greater incremental prognostic value than cardiac catheterization, which in fact failed to produce incremental information beyond MPI.[70] In fact, multiple studies have demonstrated excellent correlation between MPI and invasive assessment of coronary physiology, such as coronary flow reserve, relative coronary flow velocity reserve, and FFR.[88–93] Even when angiographically insignificant disease is noted, the presence of an abnormal perfusion study is associated with a worse outcome, suggesting that these findings do not necessarily indicate a "false-positive" result, but rather a dissociation between anatomy and physiology.[12,94] On the other hand, Yokota et al.[95] investigated "false-negative" SPECT MPI in selected patients who underwent coronary angiography after normal MPI; of those, 36% had significant CAD (≥70% or ≥50% left main stenosis). The majority of patients with significant CAD had single vessel disease. Left main or three vessel disease, causing "balanced ischemia," is a less common cause of false-negative MPI. Irrespective of the underlying coronary anatomy, the prognostic value of normal SPECT MPI remains excellent. The patients analyzed in the report by Yokota et al. were selected to undergo coronary angiography despite normal MPI, likely due to ominous clinical presentation.

The incremental value of physiologic assessment in predicting outcome and guiding revascularization decisions has been confirmed in the FAME trials.[9,11,14] In these trials, the physiologic significance of coronary lesions was assessed using FFR, which is a calculated ratio of the measured pressure distal to a coronary lesion to the pressure proximal to the lesion during vasodilator-induced hyperemia (typically with adenosine). An FFR ≤0.8 is considered to represent significant ischemia. In the FAME trial, patients who were randomized to undergo an FFR-guided PCI had a significant reduction in the composite end point of death, nonfatal MI, and repeat revascularization compared to patients randomized to PCI guided by angiography alone.[9,14] In the FAME II trial, patients with CAD and significant coronary stenosis (FFR ≤0.80), FFR-guided PCI plus best medical therapy decreased the composite end point of death, nonfatal MI, or urgent revascularization, as compared with the best medical therapy alone. In patients without significantly reduced FFR (>0.80), the outcome appeared to be favorable with the best medical therapy alone.[11] These trials confirmed the incremental prognostic and decision-making value of physiologic data derived from MPI which were established nearly two decades earlier. These studies and others indicate that, in patients with stable CAD, physiologic information, such as MPI, remains the main gatekeeper to coronary revascularization rather than purely anatomic data derived from invasive and noninvasive coronary angiography.[12,69,96–98]

SPECT MPI delivers incremental prognostic value even when used in conjunction with vasodilator stress testing.[94,99] The prognostic value of vasodilator MPI can be further enhanced by incorporating MPI data into a risk score that encompasses patient's age, heart rate, ECG findings, the presence of dyspnea, and the percentage of ischemic and scarred myocardium.[99] In a study of 5873 subjects undergoing adenosine stress SPECT MPI, this prognostic score successfully placed patients into low-, intermediate-, and high-risk categories, with observed cardiac death rates of 0.9%, 3.3%, and 9.5%, respectively. This score was superior to SPECT data alone and is likely useful in subsequent decision making.[99] The aforementioned score has not been validated for other vasodilator stress agents.

ANCILLARY DATA ASSOCIATED WITH SPECT MYOCARDIAL PERFUSION IMAGING

Left Ventricular Dysfunction

The availability of Tc-99m–based agents (i.e., Tc-99m sestamibi and Tc-99m tetrofosmin) has facilitated the widespread use of ECG-gated acquisition of myocardial perfusion studies. Gated SPECT allows the evaluation of global and regional wall motion and an accurate computation of LVEF.[78,100] The assessment of global and regional myocardial contractility not only increases the specificity of SPECT MPI,[101–103] but also provides incremental prognostic value.[71,104] Sharir et al.[71] demonstrated an incremental prognostic value of LVEF when added to SPECT perfusion imaging data. In this study, LVEF <45% or an end-systolic volume of >70 mL was independently predictive of adverse outcome irrespective of the severity of perfusion abnormalities (Fig. 15-5). Similarly, in an evaluation of gated SPECT imaging in a community setting, for every 1% decrease in LVEF, there was an increase in the cardiac event rate.[22] Furthermore, Emmett et al.[56] demonstrated that reversible regional wall motion abnormalities in patients undergoing exercise stress Tc-99m–gated SPECT MPI were highly specific for severe coronary stenosis and correlated well with CAD anatomy. Even when the LVEF is preserved, poststress regional wall motion abnormalities are incrementally predictive of cardiac death and MI to reversible perfusion defects alone.[105] The drop in poststress LVEF is considered to represent myocardial stunning or severe and extensive subendocardial ischemia.[106,107] This phenomenon has been observed not only with exercise but also with vasodilator stress.[56,108–112] The mechanism of myocardial stunning with vasodilator stress is not entirely understood, as these agents do not increase myocardial oxygen demand.[107,113,114] It is likely that ischemia with vasodilator stress is mediated by coronary steal phenomenon, since it is often associated with ST-segment shifts.[45] Irrespective of the mechanism, a drop in LVEF or stress-induced regional wall motion abnormalities has been generally correlated with extensive CAD and poor outcome.

A recent software innovation in gated SPECT applications has been the advent of phase analysis for the assessment of LV mechanical dyssynchrony. The degree of heterogeneity in the distribution of these time intervals (phase standard deviation) and the time during which 95% of the LV pixels initiate contraction (phase bandwidth) serve as measures of LV dyssynchrony.[115] Measures of LV mechanical dyssynchrony have been shown to provide additional prognostic value in patients with heart failure as well as asymptomatic patients with end-stage renal disease under evaluation for renal transplant.[116,117]

▶ Transient Ischemic Dilation (also known as Transient Cavity Dilation)

TID is the appearance of a larger LV cavity volume on the poststress perfusion images when compared

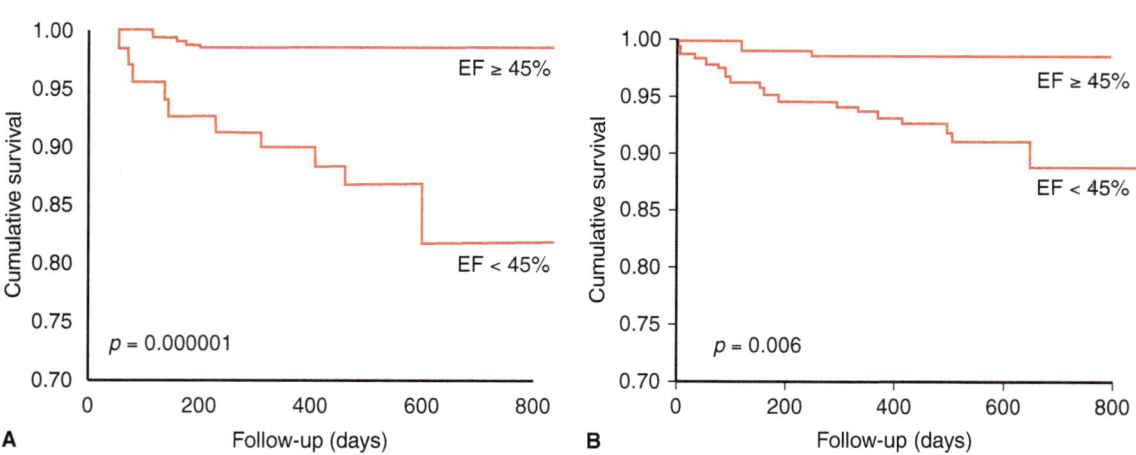

FIGURE 15-5 Incremental prognostic value for LVEF evaluation by gated SPECT. Cumulative survival in: **(A)** patients with mild/moderate perfusion abnormalities and **(B)** patients with severe perfusion abnormalities, stratified into ejection fraction ≥45% and <45%. (Reproduced with permission from Sharir T, Germano G, Kavanagh PB, et al. Incremental prognostic value of post-stress left ventricular ejection fraction and volume by gated myocardial perfusion single photon emission computed tomography. *Circulation.* 1999;100(10):1035–1042.)

with the resting study. TID is expressed as a ratio of the stress-to-rest LV volumes. It is thought to be predominantly due to stress-induced subendocardial myocardial hypoperfusion leading to the appearance of cavity dilation (Fig. 15-6).[118] Other proposed mechanisms include poststress myocardial stunning and actual LV dilation.[118] However, a true stress-induced cavity dilation is rare, as the stress scan is acquired 20 to 60 minutes poststress (with Tc-99m radiotracers), by which time true ischemic dilation typically resolves.[118,119] Notably, TID can be produced by several disease processes other than CAD, as it has been reported with conditions associated with elevated end-diastolic pressure such as hypertensive heart disease, aortic stenosis, and hypertrophic cardiomyopathy. It is hypothesized that elevated LV end-diastolic pressure is a culprit for subendocardial ischemia (without CAD) leading to the appearance of TID.[112,118,120] Thus, some experts prefer using the term "transient cavity dilation," as not all cases of "TID" are due to ischemia or CAD.

A TID threshold of 1.19 or more was reported to be abnormal for 1-day rest/exercise stress Tc-99m protocol and a cutoff of 1.31 was reported for 1-day

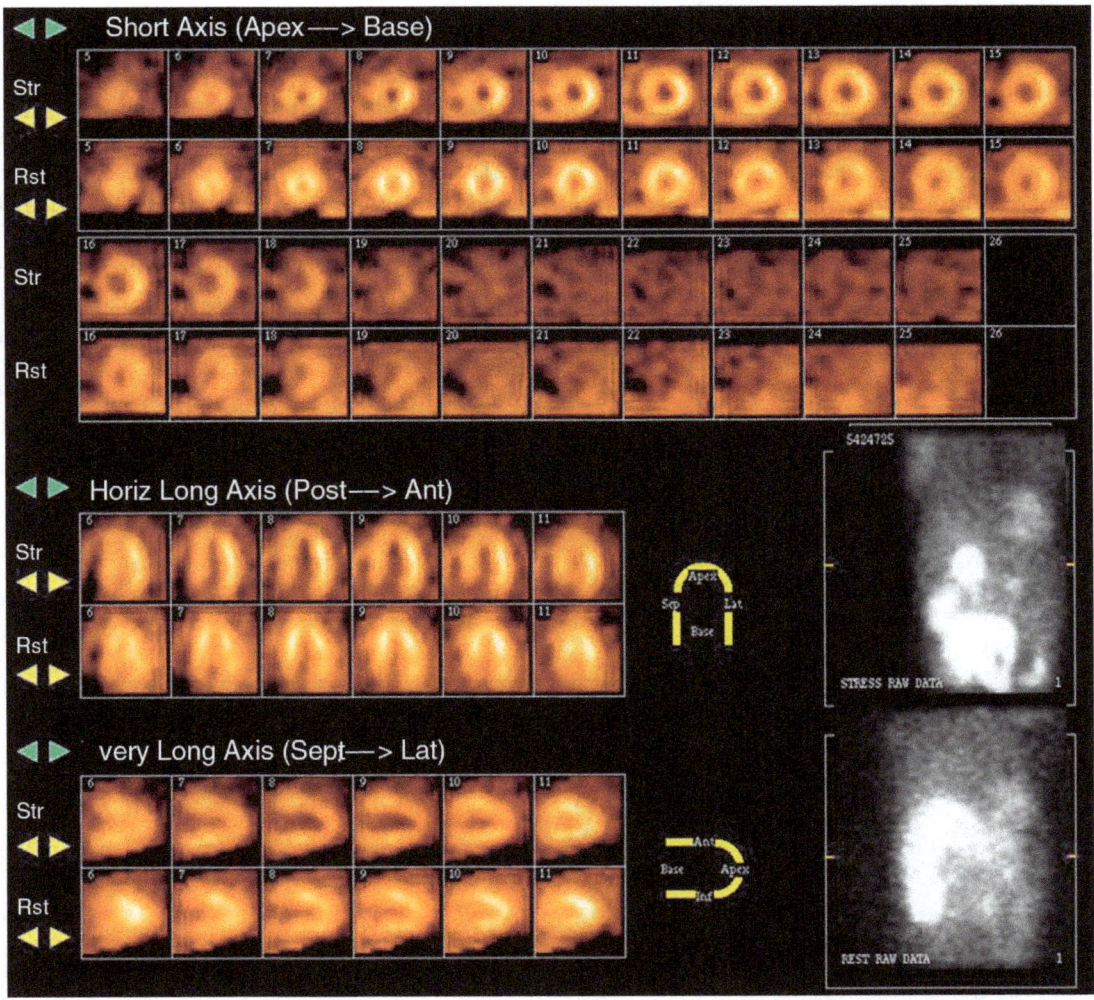

FIGURE 15-6 Exercise (top rows) SPECT myocardial perfusion imaging demonstrating a large perfusion defect in the septal, anterior, and apical walls, which appears to be completely reversible on the rest images (bottom rows). Prominent transient cavity enlargement is present, with a TID ratio of 1.45.

Table 15-3
Abnormal TID Cutoffs for Different Protocols and Types of Isotope Used

Protocol	TID Threshold
Rest Tl-201/exercise stress Tc-99m sestamibi[125]	1.22
Rest Tl-201/exercise stress Tc-99m sestamibi[127]	1.23
Rest Tl-201/pharmacologic stress Tc-99m sestamibi	
Dipyridamole[128]	1.27
Adenodine[128]	1.35
Adenosine[129]	1.36
Regadenoson[130]	1.39
Dobutamine[128]	1.40
Exercise stress/rest Tc-99m sestamibi[127]	1.14
Rest/exercise stress Tc-99m sestamibi[121]	1.19
Gated rest/exercise stress Tc-99m sestamibi (end-diastolic volume)[121]	1.23
Regadenoson stress/rest Tc-99m sestamibi[131]	1.33
Rest/regadenoson stress Tc-99m tetrofosmin[112]	1.31
Dipyridamole stress/rest Tc-99m sestamibi (2-day)[132]	1.19
Gated stress/rest Tc-99m tetrofosmin (2-day; end-diastolic volume)[133]	1.25

rest/regadenoson stress Tc-99m protocol.[112,121,122] As a general principle, dual-isotope protocol generally produces higher abnormal TID threshold than a single-isotope protocol, and vasodilator stress modality produces higher abnormal TID threshold than exercise stress.[111,112,121–126] Table 15-3, which is also included in Chapter 12 on reporting, outlines specific abnormal TID cutoffs for different stress modalities and imaging protocols.

In the presence of abnormal myocardial perfusion, this finding is predictive of severe and extensive CAD, such as left main, proximal left anterior descending coronary artery stenosis or three-vessel disease. In addition, TID is associated with a significantly increased incidence of cardiac events,[123–126] irrespective of the radiotracer or stress modality used.[122] There is an agreement in the literature that in patients with perfusion abnormalities, TID represents a high-risk feature for severe and extensive CAD and adverse outcome. Therefore, these patients should undergo coronary angiography in consideration for coronary revascularization (Fig. 15-7).

The value of TID in patients without perfusion defects is controversial. A study by Valdiviezo et al.[135] showed that the presence of TID without any other perfusion abnormalities was not associated with an increase in CAD severity or adverse outcomes.[134,135] However, other investigations by Abidov et al.[136]

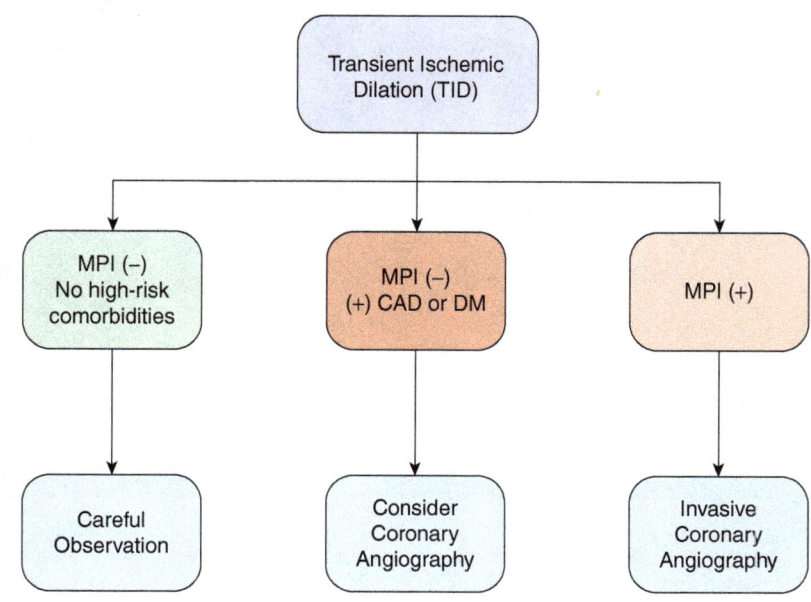

FIGURE 15-7 Suggested algorithm to approaching patients with transient ischemic dilation. TID, transient ischemic dilation; MPI, myocardial perfusion imaging; CAD, coronary artery disease; DM, diabetes mellitus.

and Doukky et al.[111] demonstrated that TID with an otherwise normal myocardial perfusion is associated with increased risk of adverse cardiac events, particularly among high-risk patients, such as those with known CAD or diabetes. Figure 15-7 illustrates a proposed approach to patients with TID. There is a general agreement in the literature that patients with TID, normal MPI, and no high-risk comorbidities, such as CAD and diabetes can be carefully observed. On the other hand, patients with TID and normal MPI but who have high-risk comorbidities, such as CAD and diabetes, should be considered for coronary angiography. The same consideration should be given to patients with typical ischemic symptoms. It has been suggested that coronary calcium score may help identify high-risk patients with TID and normal MPI.[137]

Increased Lung Uptake

An increase in the lung activity of Tl-201 identified on planar imaging is a surrogate of stress-induced LV dysfunction, as it represents an increase in the pulmonary capillary wedge pressure and pulmonary congestion. Increased lung uptake (lung–heart ratio [LHR]) has also been shown to predict severe disease and subsequent adverse events.[138-140] A quantitative and/or automated approach improves the discriminatory value of this marker.[141,142] This finding appears to be more reliable in the setting of exercise testing than vasodilatory stress[141] and with Tl-201. Although the lung activity of Tc-99m sestamibi has been shown some correlation with extensive disease,[143] there has been limited support for this as a prognostic marker as it is highly dependent on the timing of imaging.

SERIAL IMAGING

An advantage for SPECT MPI is the availability of quantitative software capable of fully automated assessment of myocardial perfusion, function, and other variables, which allows for highly reproducible perfusion images, eliminating the subjectivity of visual analysis.[144-146] Using quantitative analysis in the ADVANCE-MPI trials, Mahmarian et al.[144] demonstrated the reproducibility of SPECT MPI not only with the same vasodilator stress agent (adenosine), but also when different vasodilator stress agents are used (adenosine and regadenoson).[144,147]

Certain high-risk populations, particularly those with established CAD, diabetics, and the elderly are at increased risk for adverse cardiac events.[29,148] Hachamovitch et al.[29] demonstrated that the "warranty" period of a normal MPI is shorter in these high-risk populations. Thus, a case could be made for serial MPI testing in high-risk patients in order to detect disease progression, anticipate cardiac events, and perhaps intervene to modify risk. Indeed, serial MPI testing has been widely used to monitor response to medical and revascularization therapies as well as novel interventions such as gene and stem cell therapy.[149,150] Despite the large body of clinical evidence supporting the use of MPI for risk assessment, there is a paucity of information related to follow-up testing, such as how often to retest patients with known CAD or at risk for the disease, especially when asymptomatic. It is agreed that routine testing of asymptomatic patients or those with stable symptoms is generally not justified.[1] However, serial testing may be useful in reclassifying patients' risk for subsequent cardiovascular events.[149] Farzaneh-Far et al.[151] followed 1425 patients with angiographically documented CAD who underwent at least 2 SPECT MPI scans; patients were divided into 3 groups based on intervention received, medical therapy, and revascularization therapy. After a mean follow-up of 5.8 years, ischemic worsening by ≥5% was a significant and independent predictor of death or MI and resulted in a significant improvement in risk reclassification. Moreover, although the COURAGE trial failed to demonstrate a benefit of PCI beyond that obtained with optimal medical therapy, it was suspected that subpopulations might benefit from revascularization.[68] The nuclear sub-study of the COURAGE trial[75] suggests that serial SPECT MPI after the institution of medical therapy may identify such a high-risk subset, which should be considered for coronary revascularization. Among patients with moderate–severe ischemia on SPECT MPI, those treated with PCI in addition to optimal medical therapy had a greater reduction of ischemic events (33%) than those treated with medical therapy alone (19%). More importantly, the reduction in ischemia was associated with a lower risk of death and MI, as none of the patients without residual ischemia had any events, but 39.3% of patients with ≥10% ischemic myocardium had a cardiac event.[75]

APPROPRIATE USE CRITERIA FOR RISK ASSESSMENT WITH SPECT MYOCARDIAL PERFUSION IMAGING

The AUC were developed for SPECT MPI[152,153] by the American College of Cardiology and other professional societies as the first in a series of documents aimed at guiding clinicians, patients, and payers on the effective use of cardiac imaging and other cardiac procedures. The latest iteration of AUC addressed all cardiac imaging modalities used in the assessment of patients with known or suspected stable CAD.[154] With regard to risk assessment in asymptomatic patients, SPECT MPI is "rarely appropriate" in those who are at low global CHD risk or those at intermediate risk with an interpretable ECG and able to exercise (Table 15-4), whereas patients with intermediate global CHD risk, patients with uninterpretable ECG, and those with high global CHD risk were considered "may be appropriate" for SPECT MPI. When equivocal or discordant findings are noted in other studies, SPECT imaging is generally appropriate. Repeat SPECT imaging is rarely appropriate within 2 years of prior testing if symptoms are stable. However, if new ischemic equivalent symptoms develop, then SPECT would be appropriate if the prior study was normal.[154]

Recently, the appropriate use of SPECT MPI has been shown to improve the acumen of SPECT MPI in risk assessment. In a prospective, community-based cohort of 1511 patients followed for >2 years, Doukky et al.[155] assessed the impact of appropriate use on the prognostic value of SPECT MPI. As illustrated in Figure 15-8, among patients referred for appropriate MPI, abnormal scans predicted a multifold increase in the rates of adverse cardiac events. However, among subjects who underwent inappropriate (rarely appropriate) testing, abnormal MPI failed to effectively predict risk,[156] though it was associated with a high revascularization rate. Moreover, appropriate MPI use provided an incremental prognostic value beyond myocardial perfusion and ejection fraction data. Thus, rarely appropriate use seems to impair the value of SPECT MPI in risk

Table 15-4
Appropriate Use Criteria for Radionuclide Imaging: Risk Assessment

Clinical Indication	Appropriateness
Symptomatic, low CHD risk, interpretable ECG	R
Symptomatic, intermediate, or high CHD risk	A
Asymptomatic, low CHD risk	R
Asymptomatic, intermediate CHD risk, interpretable ECG	R
Asymptomatic, intermediate CHD risk, uninterpretable ECG	M
Asymptomatic, high CHD risk	M
Newly diagnosed heart failure	A
New-onset atrial fibrillation	M
Ventricular fibrillation	A
Sustained ventricular tachycardia	A
Syncope, low CHD risk	M
Syncope, intermediate, or high CHD risk	A
Equivocal or discordant prior testing if CAD still a concern • Prior stress imaging study • Prior exercise ECG or CCTA	 M A
Coronary stenosis of uncertain significance	A
Stable symptoms, normal stress ECG or imaging <2 years ago	R
Stable symptoms, normal stress ECG or imaging ≥2 years ago • Low CHD risk • High CHD risk	 R M
Stable symptoms, abnormal stress ECG or imaging <2 years ago	R
Stable symptoms, abnormal stress ECG or imaging ≥2 years ago	M
New/worsening symptoms with abnormal prior study	A
New/worsening symptoms with normal prior study	M

A, appropriate; M, may be appropriate; R, rarely appropriate.
Data from Kapetanopoulos A, Ahlberg AW, Taub CC, et al. Regional wall-motion abnormalities on post-stress electrocardiographic-gated technetium-99m sestamibi single-photon emission computed tomography imaging predict cardiac events. *J Nucl Cardiol.* 2007;14(6):810–817

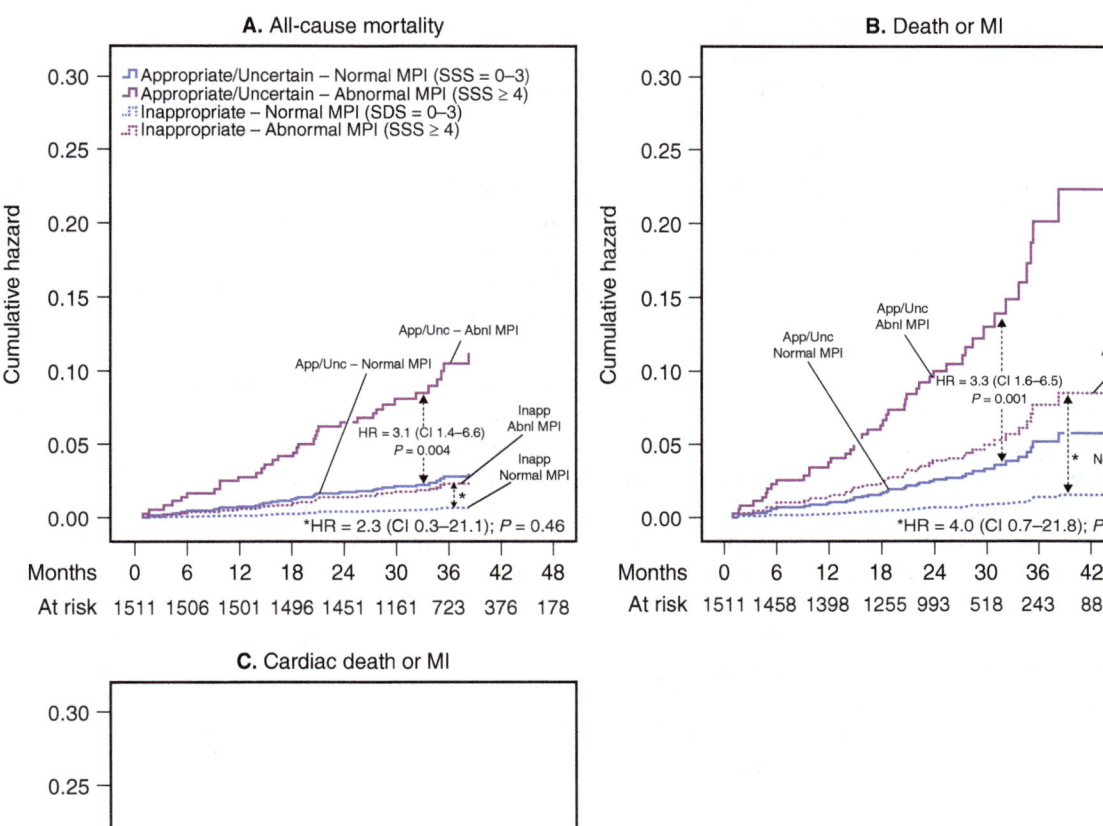

FIGURE 15-8 Impact of appropriate use on the prognostic value of MPI. In patients who underwent appropriate/uncertain (may be appropriate) use testing, MPI provided significant prognostic value. However, in patients who underwent inappropriate (rarely appropriate) testing, MPI failed to predict risk. (Reproduced with permission from Doukky R, Hayes K, Frogge N, et al. Impact of appropriate use on the prognostic value of single-photon emission computed tomography myocardial perfusion imaging. *Circulation*. 2013;128(15):1634–1643.)

assessment.[155,156] Data from the same cohort demonstrated that appropriate use has a similar impact on the diagnostic and prognostic utility of MPI in men and women.[157] A meta-analysis by Elgendy et al.[158] demonstrates that inappropriate (rarely appropriate) MPI studies are less likely to yield abnormal results or demonstrate myocardial ischemia. Moreover, recent data has shown that appropriate use is associated with significant direct cost savings[159] and a significant reduction in the estimated radiation risk, particularly among women.[160] The volume of SPECT MPI performed in the United States has significantly declined since it peaked in 2006.[161] Most of the decline occurred in patients undergoing exercise stress MPI,[161] suggesting a reduction in unnecessary MPI studies in which patients may be candidates for ECG-only stress testing. Notably, the reported adherence to AUC in the published literature has not substantially changed since their inception in 2005.[158,162] However, AUC reports in the literature only represent practices from which they originated (often academic centers) and may be subject to publication bias.

SPECT MPI is highly correlated with clinical outcomes and test results may be used in decision making regarding coronary revascularization. However, in a study examining predictors of elective percutaneous coronary intervention in Medicare recipients, only 44.5% of patients underwent stress testing prior to PCI; thus, the majority of patients underwent revascularization without objective evidence of myocardial ischemia.[163] This is in contradiction with AUC for percutaneous and surgical coronary revascularization which consider documented myocardial ischemia an integral component of decision making for revascularization.[164,165] Thus, SPECT MPI should be strongly considered for demonstrating ischemia prior to revascularization. Moreover, observational data suggest that inappropriate (rarely appropriate) MPI use has low yield for lesions that require revascularization procedure.[166]

COST-EFFICIENCY OF RADIONUCLIDE IMAGING FOR RISK ASSESSMENT

Increased scrutiny of costs related to medical imaging has led, in recent years, to heightened interest in examining the comparative cost-effectiveness of various strategies for CAD evaluation. As SPECT imaging can identify patients at risk for subsequent cardiac events, perfusion imaging may be used to guide further testing and revascularization therapies, thus functioning as a gatekeeper for more resource-intense procedures.[167] Nallamothu et al.[76] demonstrated that SPECT imaging may help guide which patients should undergo coronary angiography and thereby reduce "unnecessary" cardiac catheterizations. The European EMPIRE study compared four different strategies for detection of CAD.[168] When stress MPI was utilized, an overall saving of 23% to 34% was observed compared to angiography-based approach, while clinical outcomes were similar.

In perhaps the most detailed analysis of the financial implications of perfusion imaging versus angiography, the Economics of Noninvasive Diagnosis (END) study by Shaw et al.[98] evaluated 11,372 consecutive patients with stable angina gathered from several sites. In this cohort-matched study, the investigators compared direct catheterization ("cath-all") with selective catheterization based on the results of SPECT MPI. Event rates of death and nonfatal MI were similar in both cohorts. The only significant difference was in the rate of revascularization procedures, which was reduced by nearly 50% in the MPI cohort, as shown in Figure 15-9. Most notably, there was a substantial (31–50%) reduction in costs using MPI with selective catheterization strategy.

ETT (without imaging) has also been compared with exercise SPECT MPI as an initial strategy.[169] For low-likelihood patients, ETT alone was less costly than SPECT MPI. However, for intermediate or high-likelihood patients there was no difference between the two approaches. In the randomized WOMEN trial of 824 low-risk exercising women, Shaw et al.[170] demonstrated that an approach that uses ETT versus exercise MPI yields similar 2-year posttest outcomes while providing significant diagnostic cost savings. The authors concluded that ETT with selective follow-up testing should be considered as the initial strategy in symptomatic women at low risk for CAD. In addition, Bourque et al.[85,86] demonstrated that the incremental diagnostic and prognostic value of MPI is limited in patients who achieve a workload of ≥10 METs during ETT. Thus, MPI may not be cost-effective in patients who can undergo high level of exercise. Moreover, Shaw et al.[171] examined the prognostic value and cost-effectiveness of exercise echocardiography versus exercise SPECT MPI in over 9000 stable patients with chest pain. These investigators demonstrated that stress echocardiography was more cost-effective in low-risk patients, whereas higher-risk patients benefited from referral to SPECT MPI.

In the SPARC study, Hlatky et al.[172] demonstrated in propensity-matched cohorts that 2-year

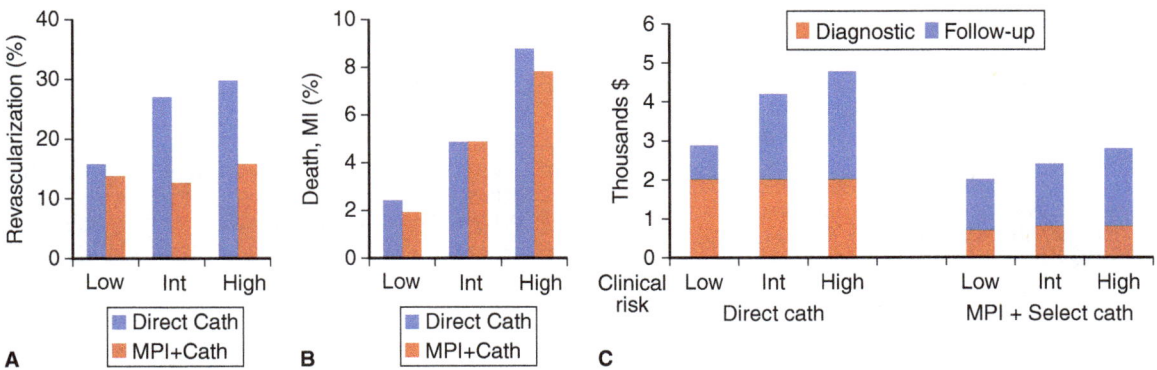

FIGURE 15-9 Direct catheterization approach versus selective catheterization based on the result of MPI study, as noted in the END study. Selective catheterization approach resulted in 50% reduction in revascularization procedures (PTCA and CABG), **(A)** but no significant difference in cardiac events of death or MI between the two groups. **(B)** Selective catheterization approach was associated with 30% to 40% cost reduction compared to direct catheterization approach. **(C)** These findings were demonstrated in patients with all levels of pretest clinical risk (low, intermediate, or high). (Reproduced with permission from Shaw LJ, Hachamovitch R, Berman DS, et al. The economic consequences of available diagnostic and prognostic strategies for the evaluation of stable angina patients: an observational assessment of the value of precatheterization ischemia. Economics of Noninvasive Diagnosis (END) Multicenter Study Group. *J Am Coll Cardiol.* 1999;33(3):661–669.)

costs of care were highest after positron emission tomography (PET) MPI, intermediate after coronary CT angiography, and lowest after SPECT MPI. After multivariable adjustment, CTA costs were 15% higher than SPECT ($p < 0.01$), and PET costs were 22% higher than SPECT ($p < 0.0001$). Two-year mortality was 0.7% after CTA, 1.6% after SPECT, and 5.5% after PET. Given the observational design, and despite propensity-matching and multivariable adjustments, some of the observed differences in costs and outcomes may be related to selection biases, such that lowest-risk patients may have been selected for coronary CT angiography, while PET was reserved for highest-risk patients.

More recently, the PROMISE trial demonstrated that there was no significant difference in outcomes for symptomatic patients with suspected CAD, who were evaluated with a strategy of anatomical testing with coronary CT angiography, compared to a functional testing strategy of stress MPI, stress echocardiography, or ETT.[173] In patients who underwent subsequent cardiac catheterization, there was a higher rate of nonobstructive CAD in the functional testing group. However, in the anatomic testing group, there was an increased rate of coronary revascularization with a slight, but statistically insignificant, increase in overall cost.[174]

In summary, available evidence supports the use of radionuclide MPI for cost-effective risk stratification of patients with known or suspected CAD. For low-risk patients, no testing or the use of ETT or exercise echocardiography is likely the most cost-effective strategy, while for intermediate- and high-risk patients with stable or suspected CAD, the use of SPECT imaging as an initial strategy of evaluation is not only clinically valuable but also a cost-effective approach.

CONCLUSION

A wealth of literature supports the use of radionuclide MPI for risk stratification in patients with known or suspected CAD. A normal perfusion study portends an excellent prognosis, even in the setting of known ischemic heart disease. Furthermore, an abnormal perfusion study predicts subsequent cardiac events such as cardiac death or MI. The ability of SPECT imaging to localize and define the extent and severity of disease adds incremental prognostic value. The prognostic applications of perfusion imaging are germane to managing physicians, as these methods may be used to guide subsequent tests and treatments. Thus, MPI significantly impacts management decisions and the cost-effective utilization of health care dollars.

REFERENCES

1. Fihn SD, Gardin JM, Abrams J, et al. 2012 ACCF/AHA/ACP/AATS/PCNA/SCAI/STS Guideline for the Diagnosis and Management of Patients With Stable Ischemic Heart Disease: Executive Summary: A Report of the American College of Cardiology Foundation/American Heart Association Task Force on Practice Guidelines, and the American College of Physicians, American Association for Thoracic Surgery, Preventive Cardiovascular Nurses Association, Society for Cardiovascular Angiography and Interventions, and Society of Thoracic Surgeons. *J Am Coll Cardiol.* 2012;60(24):2564–2603.
2. Gibbons RJ, Abrams J, Chatterjee K, et al. ACC/AHA 2002 guideline update for the management of patients with chronic stable angina—summary article: a report of the American College of Cardiology/American Heart Association Task Force on practice guidelines (Committee on the Management of Patients With Chronic Stable Angina). *J Am Coll Cardiol.* 2003;41(1):159–168.
3. Solomon AJ, Gersh BJ. Management of chronic stable angina: medical therapy, percutaneous transluminal coronary angioplasty, and coronary artery bypass graft surgery. Lessons from the randomized trials. *Ann Intern Med.* 1998;128(3):216–223.
4. Gibbons RJ, Balady GJ, Bricker JT, et al. ACC/AHA 2002 guideline update for exercise testing: summary article. A report of the American College of Cardiology/American Heart Association Task Force on Practice Guidelines (Committee to Update the 1997 Exercise Testing Guidelines). *J Am Coll Cardiol.* 2002;40(8):1531–1540.
5. Grundy SM, Pasternak R, Greenland P, Smith S Jr, Fuster V. Assessment of cardiovascular risk by use of multiple-risk-factor assessment equations: a statement for healthcare professionals from the American Heart Association and the American College of Cardiology. *Circulation.* 1999;100(13):1481–1492.
6. Abidov A, Rozanski A, Hachamovitch R, et al. Prognostic significance of dyspnea in patients referred for cardiac stress testing. *N Engl J Med.* 2005;353(18):1889–1898.
7. Mark DB, Hlatky MA, Harrell FE Jr, Lee KL, Califf RM, Pryor DB. Exercise treadmill score for predicting prognosis in coronary artery disease. *Ann Intern Med.* 1987;106(6):793–800.
8. Hachamovitch R, Berman DS, Kiat H, et al. Exercise myocardial perfusion SPECT in patients without known coronary artery disease: incremental prognostic value and use in risk stratification. *Circulation.* 1996;93(5):905–914.
9. Tonino PA, De Bruyne B, Pijls NH, et al.; FAME Study Investigators. Fractional flow reserve versus angiography for guiding percutaneous coronary intervention. *N Engl J Med.* 2009;360(3):213–224.
10. Schuijf JD, Wijns W, Jukema JW, et al. Relationship between noninvasive coronary angiography with multi-slice computed tomography and myocardial perfusion imaging. *J Am Coll Cardiol.* 2006;48(12):2508–2514.
11. De Bruyne B, Pijls NH, Kalesan B, et al.; FAME 2 Trial Investigators Fractional flow reserve-guided PCI versus medical therapy in stable coronary disease. *N Engl J Med.* 2012;367(11):991–1001.
12. Gould KL, Johnson NP, Bateman TM, et al. Anatomic versus physiologic assessment of coronary artery disease. Role of coronary flow reserve, fractional flow reserve, and positron emission tomography imaging in revascularization decision-making. *J Am Coll Cardiol.* 2013;62(18):1639–1653.
13. Meijboom WB, Van Mieghem CA, van Pelt N, et al. Comprehensive assessment of coronary artery stenoses: computed tomography coronary angiography versus conventional coronary angiography and correlation with fractional flow reserve in patients with stable angina. *J Am Coll Cardiol.* 2008;52(8):636–643.
14. Pijls NH, Fearon WF, Tonino PA, et al.; FAME Study Investigators. Fractional flow reserve versus angiography for guiding percutaneous coronary intervention in patients with multivessel coronary artery disease: 2-year follow-up of the FAME (Fractional Flow Reserve Versus Angiography for Multivessel Evaluation) study. *J Am Coll Cardiol.* 2010;56(3):177–184.
15. Gimelli A, Marzullo P, Rovai D. Physiologic risk assessment in stable ischemic heart disease: still superior to the anatomic angiographic approach. *J Nucl Cardiol.* 2009;16(5):697–700.
16. Hendel RC, Whitfield SS, Villegas BJ, Cutler BS, Leppo JA. Prediction of late cardiac events by dipyridamole thallium imaging in patients undergoing elective vascular surgery. *Am J Cardiol.* 1992;70(15):1243–1249.
17. Berman DS, Hachamovitch R, Kiat H, et al. Incremental value of prognostic testing in patients with known or suspected ischemic heart disease: a basis for optimal utilization of exercise technetium-99m sestamibi myocardial perfusion single-photon emission computed tomography. *J Am Coll Cardiol.* 1995;26(3):639–647.
18. Iskander S, Iskandrian AE. Risk assessment using single-photon emission computed tomographic technetium-99m sestamibi imaging. *J Am Coll Cardiol.* 1998;32(1):57–62.
19. Brown KA, Altland E, Rowen M. Prognostic value of normal technetium-99m-sestamibi cardiac imaging. *J Nucl Med.* 1994;35(4):554–557.
20. Shaw LJ, Hendel R, Borges-Neto S, et al.; Myoview Multicenter Registry. Prognostic value of normal exercise and adenosine (99m)Tc-tetrofosmin SPECT imaging: results from the multicenter registry of 4,728 patients. *J Nucl Med.* 2003;44(2):134–139.
21. Heller GV, Brown KA. Prognosis of acute and chronic coronary artery disease by myocardial perfusion imaging. *Cardiol Clin.* 1994;12(2):271–287.
22. Thomas GS, Miyamoto MI, Morello AP, 3rd, et al. Technetium 99m sestamibi myocardial perfusion imaging predicts clinical outcome in the community outpatient setting. The Nuclear Utility in the Community (NUC) Study. *J Am Coll Cardiol.* 2004;43(2):213–223.
23. Navare SM, Mather JF, Shaw LJ, Fowler MS, Heller GV. Comparison of risk stratification with pharmacologic and exercise stress myocardial perfusion imaging: A meta-analysis. *J Nucl Cardiol.* 2004;11(5):551–561.
24. Shaw LJ, Iskandrian AE. Prognostic value of gated myocardial perfusion SPECT. *J Nucl Cardiol.* 2004;11(2):171–185.
25. Metz LD, Beattie M, Hom R, Redberg RF, Grady D, Fleischmann KE. The prognostic value of normal exercise myocardial perfusion imaging and exercise echocardiography: a meta-analysis. *J Am Coll Cardiol.* 2007;49(2):227–237.
26. Calnon DA, McGrath PD, Doss AL, Harrell FE Jr, Watson DD, Beller GA. Prognostic value of dobutamine stress technetium-99m-sestamibi single-photon emission computed tomography myocardial perfusion imaging: stratification

27. Poulin MF, Alexander S, Doukky R. Prognostic implications of stress modality on mortality risk and cause of death in patients undergoing office-based SPECT myocardial perfusion imaging. *J Nucl Cardiol.* 2016;23(2):202–211.
28. Rozanski A, Gransar H, Hayes SW, Friedman JD, Hachamovitch R, Berman DS. Comparison of long-term mortality risk following normal exercise vs. adenosine myocardial perfusion SPECT. *J Nucl Cardiol.* 2010;17(6):999–1008.
29. Hachamovitch R, Hayes S, Friedman JD, et al. Determinants of risk and its temporal variation in patients with normal stress myocardial perfusion scans: what is the warranty period of a normal scan? *J Am Coll Cardiol.* 2003;41(8):1329–1340.
30. Doukky R, Fughhi I, Campagnoli T, Wassouf M, Ali A. The prognostic value of regadenoson SPECT myocardial perfusion imaging in patients with end-stage renal disease. *J Nucl Cardiol.* 2017;24(1):112–118..
31. Ottenhof MJ, Wai MC, Boiten HJ, et al. 12-year outcome after normal myocardial perfusion SPECT in patients with known coronary artery disease. *J Nucl Cardiol.* 2013;20(5):748–754.
32. Rozanski A, Gransar H, Min JK, et al. Long-term mortality following normal exercise myocardial perfusion SPECT according to coronary disease risk factors. *J Nucl Cardiol.* 2014;21(2):341–350.
33. Hendel RC, Layden JJ, Leppo JA. Prognostic value of dipyridamole thallium scintigraphy for evaluation of ischemic heart disease. *J Am Coll Cardiol.* 1990;15(1):109–116.
34. Lette J, Bertrand C, Gossard D, et al. Long-term risk stratification with dipyridamole imaging. *Am Heart J.* 1995;129(5):880–886.
35. Iqbal FM, Hage FG, Ahmed A, et al. Comparison of the prognostic value of normal regadenoson with normal adenosine myocardial perfusion imaging with propensity score matching. *JACC Cardiovasc Imaging.* 2012;5(10):1014–1021.
36. Doukky R, Frogge N, Balakrishnan G, et al. The prognostic value of cardiac SPECT performed at the primary care physician's office. *J Nucl Cardiol.* 2013;20(4):519–528.
37. Boiten HJ, van Domburg RT, Valkema R, Schinkel AF. Eleven-year prognostic value of dobutamine stress (99m)Tc-sestamibi myocardial perfusion imaging in patients with limited exercise capacity. *Am J Cardiol.* 2015;115(7):884–889.
38. Schinkel AF, Elhendy A, van Domburg RT, Bax JJ, Roelandt JR, Poldermans D. Prognostic value of dobutamine-atropine stress (99m)Tc-tetrofosmin myocardial perfusion SPECT in patients with known or suspected coronary artery disease. *J Nucl Med.* 2002;43(6):767–772.
39. Hage FG, Ghimire G, Lester D, et al. The prognostic value of regadenoson myocardial perfusion imaging. *J Nucl Cardiol.* 2015;22(6):1214–1221.
40. Ahlberg AW, Baghdasarian SB, Athar H, et al. Symptom-limited exercise combined with dipyridamole stress: prognostic value in assessment of known or suspected coronary artery disease by use of gated SPECT imaging. *J Nucl Cardiol.* 2008;15(1):42–56.
41. Brown KA, Rowen M. Prognostic value of a normal exercise myocardial perfusion imaging study in patients with angiographically significant coronary artery disease. *Am J Cardiol.* 1993;71(10):865–867.
42. Schalet BD, Kegel JG, Heo J, Segal BL, Iskandrian AS. Prognostic implications of normal exercise SPECT thallium images in patients with strongly positive exercise electrocardiograms. *Am J Cardiol.* 1993;72(15):1201–1203.
43. Abbott BG, Afshar M, Berger AK, Wackers FJ. Prognostic significance of ischemic electrocardiographic changes during adenosine infusion in patients with normal myocardial perfusion imaging. *J Nucl Cardiol.* 2003;10(1):9–16.
44. Klodas E, Miller TD, Christian TF, Hodge DO, Gibbons RJ. Prognostic significance of ischemic electrocardiographic changes during vasodilator stress testing in patients with normal SPECT images. *J Nucl Cardiol.* 2003;10(1):4–8.
45. Doukky R, Olusanya A, Vashistha R, et al. Diagnostic and prognostic significance of ischemic electrocardiographic changes with regadenoson-stress myocardial perfusion imaging. *J Nucl Cardiol.* 2015;22(4):700–713.
46. Oldan JD, Shaw LK, Hofmann P, et al. Prognostic value of the cadmium-zinc-telluride camera: A comparison with a conventional (Anger) camera. *J Nucl Cardiol.* 2016;23(6);1280–1287.
47. Lima R, Peclat T, Soares T, Ferreira C, Souza AC, Camargo G. Comparison of the prognostic value of myocardial perfusion imaging using a CZT-SPECT camera with a conventional anger camera. *J Nucl Cardiol.* 2017;24(1):245–251.
48. Chang SM, Nabi F, Xu J, Raza U, Mahmarian JJ. Normal stress-only versus standard stress/rest myocardial perfusion imaging: similar patient mortality with reduced radiation exposure. *J Am Coll Cardiol.* 2010;55(3):221–230.
49. Duvall WL, Wijetunga MN, Klein TM, et al. The prognosis of a normal stress-only Tc-99m myocardial perfusion imaging study. *J Nucl Cardiol.* 2010;17(3):370–377.
50. Vanzetto G, Ormezzano O, Fagret D, Comet M, Denis B, Machecourt J. Long-term additive prognostic value of thallium-201 myocardial perfusion imaging over clinical and exercise stress test in low to intermediate risk patients: study in 1137 patients with 6-year follow-up. *Circulation.* 1999;100(14):1521–1527.
51. Soman P, Parsons A, Lahiri N, Lahiri A. The prognostic value of a normal Tc-99m sestamibi SPECT study in suspected coronary artery disease. *J Nucl Cardiol.* 1999;6(3):252–256.
52. Groutars RG, Verzijlbergen JF, Muller AJ, et al. Prognostic value and quality of life in patients with normal rest thallium-201/stress technetium 99m-tetrofosmin dual-isotope myocardial SPECT. *J Nucl Cardiol.* 2000;7(4):333–341.
53. Levine MG, Ahlberg AW, Mann A, et al. Comparison of exercise, dipyridamole, adenosine, and dobutamine stress with the use of Tc-99m tetrofosmin tomographic imaging. *J Nucl Cardiol.* 1999;6(4):389–396.
54. Heller GV, Herman SD, Travin MI, Baron JI, Santos-Ocampo C, McClellan JR. Independent prognostic value of intravenous dipyridamole with technetium-99m sestamibi tomographic imaging in predicting cardiac events and cardiac-related hospital admissions. *J Am Coll Cardiol.* 1995;26(5):1202–1208.
55. Farzaneh-Far A, Shaw LK, Dunning A, Oldan JD, O'Connor CM, Borges-Neto S. Comparison of the prognostic value of regadenoson and adenosine myocardial perfusion imaging. *J Nucl Cardiol.* 2015;22(4):600–607.
56. Emmett L, Iwanochko RM, Freeman MR, Barolet A, Lee DS, Husain M. Reversible regional wall motion abnormalities on exercise technetium-99m-gated cardiac single photon emission computed tomography predict high-grade angiographic stenoses. *J Am Coll Cardiol.* 2002;39(6):991–998.

57. Akinboboye OO, Idris O, Onwuanyi A, Berekashvili K, Bergmann SR. Incidence of major cardiovascular events in black patients with normal myocardial stress perfusion study results. *J Nucl Cardiol*. 2001;8(5):541–547.
58. Galassi AR, Azzarelli S, Tomaselli A, et al. Incremental prognostic value of technetium-99m-tetrofosmin exercise myocardial perfusion imaging for predicting outcomes in patients with suspected or known coronary artery disease. *Am J Cardiol*. 2001;88(2):101–106.
59. Boiten HJ, van der Sijde JN, Ruitinga PR, et al. Long-term prognostic value of exercise technetium-99m tetrofosmin myocardial perfusion single-photon emission computed tomography. *J Nucl Cardiol*. 2012;19(5):907–913.
60. Marie PY, Danchin N, Durand JF, et al. Long-term prediction of major ischemic events by exercise thallium-201 single-photon emission computed tomography. Incremental prognostic value compared with clinical, exercise testing, catheterization and radionuclide angiographic data. *J Am Coll Cardiol*. 1995;26(4):879–886.
61. Ladenheim ML, Pollock BH, Rozanski A, et al. Extent and severity of myocardial hypoperfusion as predictors of prognosis in patients with suspected coronary artery disease. *J Am Coll Cardiol*. 1986;7(3):464–471.
62. Hachamovitch R, Berman DS, Shaw LJ, et al. Incremental prognostic value of myocardial perfusion single photon emission computed tomography for the prediction of cardiac death: differential stratification for risk of cardiac death and myocardial infarction. *Circulation*. 1998;97(6):535–543.
63. Machecourt J, Longère P, Fagret D, et al. Prognostic value of thallium-201 single-photon emission computed tomographic myocardial perfusion imaging according to extent of myocardial defect. Study in 1,926 patients with follow-up at 33 months. *J Am Coll Cardiol*. 1994;23(5):1096–1106.
64. Marwick TH. Dyspnea and risk in suspected coronary disease. *N Engl J Med*. 2005;353(18):1963–1965.
65. Zellweger MJ, Hachamovitch R, Kang X, et al. Threshold, incidence, and predictors of prognostically high-risk silent ischemia in asymptomatic patients without prior diagnosis of coronary artery disease. *J Nucl Cardiol*. 2009;16(2):193–200.
66. Khandaker MH, Miller TD, Chareonthaitawee P, Askew JW, Hodge DO, Gibbons RJ. Stress single photon emission computed tomography for detection of coronary artery disease and risk stratification of asymptomatic patients at moderate risk. *J Nucl Cardiol*. 2009;16(4):516–523.
67. Shaw LJ, Hendel RC, Heller GV, Borges-Neto S, Cerqueira M, Berman DS. Prognostic estimation of coronary artery disease risk with resting perfusion abnormalities and stress ischemia on myocardial perfusion SPECT. *J Nucl Cardiol*. 2008;15(6):762–773.
68. Boden WE, O'Rourke RA, Teo KK, et al.; COURAGE Trial Research Group. Optimal medical therapy with or without PCI for stable coronary disease. *N Engl J Med*. 2007;356(15):1503–1516.
69. Hachamovitch R, Hayes SW, Friedman JD, Cohen I, Berman DS. Comparison of the short-term survival benefit associated with revascularization compared with medical therapy in patients with no prior coronary artery disease undergoing stress myocardial perfusion single photon emission computed tomography. *Circulation*. 2003;107(23):2900–2907.
70. Iskandrian AS, Chae SC, Heo J, Stanberry CD, Wasserleben V, Cave V. Independent and incremental prognostic value of exercise single-photon emission computed tomographic (SPECT) thallium imaging in coronary artery disease. *J Am Coll Cardiol*. 1993;22(3):665–670.
71. Sharir T, Germano G, Kavanagh PB, et al. Incremental prognostic value of post-stress left ventricular ejection fraction and volume by gated myocardial perfusion single photon emission computed tomography. *Circulation*. 1999;100(10):1035–1042.
72. Tilkemeier PL, Cooke CD, Ficaro EP, et al. American Society of Nuclear Cardiology information statement: Standardized reporting matrix for radionuclide myocardial perfusion imaging. *J Nucl Cardiol*. 2006;13(6):e157–e171.
73. Yusuf S, Sleight P, Pogue J, Bosch J, Davies R, Dagenais G. Effects of an angiotensin-converting-enzyme inhibitor, ramipril, on cardiovascular events in high-risk patients. Heart Outcomes Prevention Evaluation Study Investigators. *N Engl J Med*. 2000;342(3):145–153.
74. Pitt B, Waters D, Brown WV, et al. Aggressive lipid-lowering therapy compared with angioplasty in stable coronary artery disease. Atorvastatin versus Revascularization Treatment Investigators. *N Engl J Med*. 1999;341(2):70–76.
75. Shaw LJ, Berman DS, Maron DJ, et al.; COURAGE Investigators. Optimal medical therapy with or without percutaneous coronary intervention to reduce ischemic burden: results from the Clinical Outcomes Utilizing Revascularization and Aggressive Drug Evaluation (COURAGE) trial nuclear substudy. *Circulation*. 2008;117(10):1283–1291.
76. Nallamothu N, Ghods M, Heo J, Iskandrian AS. Comparison of thallium-201 single-photon emission computed tomography and electrocardiographic response during exercise in patients with normal rest electrocardiographic results. *J Am Coll Cardiol*. 1995;25(4):830–836.
77. Pollock SG, Abbott RD, Boucher CA, Beller GA, Kaul S. Independent and incremental prognostic value of tests performed in hierarchical order to evaluate patients with suspected coronary artery disease. Validation of models based on these tests. *Circulation*. 1992;85(1):237–248.
78. Germano G, Berman DS. On the accuracy and reproducibility of quantitative gated myocardial perfusion SPECT. *J Nucl Med*. 1999;40(5):810–813.
79. Amanullah AM, Berman DS, Erel J, et al. Incremental prognostic value of adenosine myocardial perfusion single-photon emission computed tomography in women with suspected coronary artery disease. *Am J Cardiol*. 1998;82(6):725–730.
80. Kang X, Berman DS, Lewin HC, et al. Incremental prognostic value of myocardial perfusion single photon emission computed tomography in patients with diabetes mellitus. *Am Heart J*. 1999;138(6 Pt 1):1025–1032.
81. Schinkel AF, Elhendy A, van Domburg RT, et al. Incremental value of exercise technetium-99m tetrofosmin myocardial perfusion single-photon emission computed tomography for the prediction of cardiac events. *Am J Cardiol*. 2003;91(4):408–411.
82. Hachamovitch R, Berman DS, Kiat H, Cohen I, Friedman JD, Shaw LJ. Value of stress myocardial perfusion single photon emission computed tomography in patients with normal resting electrocardiograms: an evaluation of incremental prognostic value and cost-effectiveness. *Circulation*. 2002;105(7):823–829.

83. Zerahn B, Jensen BV, Nielsen KD, Møller S. Increased prognostic value of combined myocardial perfusion imaging and exercise electrocardiography in patients with coronary artery disease. *J Nucl Cardiol.* 2000;7(6):616–622.
84. Hachamovitch R, Berman DS, Kiat H, et al. Incremental prognostic value of adenosine stress myocardial perfusion single-photon emission computed tomography and impact on subsequent management in patients with or suspected of having myocardial ischemia. *Am J Cardiol.* 1997;80(4):426–433.
85. Bourque JM, Holland BH, Watson DD, Beller GA. Achieving an exercise workload of > or = 10 metabolic equivalents predicts a very low risk of inducible ischemia: does myocardial perfusion imaging have a role? *J Am Coll Cardiol.* 2009;54(6):538–545.
86. Bourque JM, Charlton GT, Holland BH, Belyea CM, Watson DD, Beller GA. Prognosis in patients achieving ≥10 METS on exercise stress testing: was SPECT imaging useful? *J Nucl Cardiol.* 2011;18(2):230–237.
87. Smith L, Myc L, Beller GA, Bourque JM. A high exercise workload of ≥10 METs predicts a very low risk of significant ischemia in patients of advanced age. *J Nucl Cardiol.* 2015;22(4):776 [Abstract].
88. Joye JD, Schulman DS, Lasorda D, Farah T, Donohue BC, Reichek N. Intracoronary Doppler guide wire versus stress single-photon emission computed tomographic thallium-201 imaging in assessment of intermediate coronary stenoses. *J Am Coll Cardiol.* 1994;24(4):940–947.
89. Miller DD, Donohue TJ, Younis LT, et al. Correlation of pharmacological 99mTc-sestamibi myocardial perfusion imaging with poststenotic coronary flow reserve in patients with angiographically intermediate coronary artery stenoses. *Circulation.* 1994;89(5):2150–2160.
90. Deychak YA, Segal J, Reiner JS, et al. Doppler guide wire flow-velocity indexes measured distal to coronary stenoses associated with reversible thallium perfusion defects. *Am Heart J.* 1995;129(2):219–227.
91. Voudris V, Avramides D, Koutelou M, et al. Relative coronary flow velocity reserve improves correlation with stress myocardial perfusion imaging in assessment of coronary artery stenoses. *Chest.* 2003;124(4):1266–1274.
92. Pijls NH, De Bruyne B, Peels K, et al. Measurement of fractional flow reserve to assess the functional severity of coronary-artery stenoses. *N Engl J Med.* 1996;334(26):1703–1708.
93. De Bruyne B, Bartunek J, Sys SU, Heyndrickx GR. Relation between myocardial fractional flow reserve calculated from coronary pressure measurements and exercise-induced myocardial ischemia. *Circulation.* 1995;92(1):39–46.
94. Alqaisi F, Albadarin F, Jaffery Z, et al. Prognostic predictors and outcomes in patients with abnormal myocardial perfusion imaging and angiographically insignificant coronary artery disease. *J Nucl Cardiol.* 2008;15(6):754–761.
95. Yokota S, Ottervanger JP, Mouden M, Timmer JR, Knollema S, Jager PL. Prevalence, location, and extent of significant coronary artery disease in patients with normal myocardial perfusion imaging. *J Nucl Cardiol.* 2014;21(2):284–290.
96. Hachamovitch R, Di Carli MF. Nuclear cardiology will remain the "gatekeeper" over CT angiography. *J Nucl Cardiol.* 2007;14(5):634–644.
97. Min JK, Shaw LJ, Berman DS. The present state of coronary computed tomography angiography a process in evolution. *J Am Coll Cardiol.* 2010;55(10):957–965.
98. Shaw LJ, Hachamovitch R, Berman DS, et al. The economic consequences of available diagnostic and prognostic strategies for the evaluation of stable angina patients: an observational assessment of the value of precatheterization ischemia. Economics of Noninvasive Diagnosis (END) Multicenter Study Group. *J Am Coll Cardiol.* 1999;33(3):661–669.
99. Hachamovitch R, Hayes SW, Friedman JD, Cohen I, Berman DS. A prognostic score for prediction of cardiac mortality risk after adenosine stress myocardial perfusion scintigraphy. *J Am Coll Cardiol.* 2005;45(5):722–729.
100. Germano G, Kavanagh PB, Kavanagh JT, Wishner SH, Berman DS, Kavanagh GJ. Repeatability of automatic left ventricular cavity volume measurements from myocardial perfusion SPECT. *J Nucl Cardiol.* 1998;5(5):477–483.
101. DePuey EG, Rozanski A. Using gated technetium-99m-sestamibi SPECT to characterize fixed myocardial defects as infarct or artifact. *J Nucl Med.* 1995;36(6):952–955.
102. Taillefer R, DePuey EG, Udelson JE, Beller GA, Latour Y, Reeves F. Comparative diagnostic accuracy of Tl-201 and Tc-99m sestamibi SPECT imaging (perfusion and ECG-gated SPECT) in detecting coronary artery disease in women. *J Am Coll Cardiol.* 1997;29(1):69–77.
103. Smanio PE, Watson DD, Segalla DL, Vinson EL, Smith WH, Beller GA. Value of gating of technetium-99m sestamibi single-photon emission computed tomographic imaging. *J Am Coll Cardiol.* 1997;30(7):1687–1692.
104. Sharir T, Germano G, Kang X, et al. Prediction of myocardial infarction versus cardiac death by gated myocardial perfusion SPECT: risk stratification by the amount of stress-induced ischemia and the poststress ejection fraction. *J Nucl Med.* 2001;42(6):831–837.
105. Kapetanopoulos A, Ahlberg AW, Taub CC, Katten DM, Heller GV. Regional wall-motion abnormalities on post-stress electrocardiographic-gated technetium-99m sestamibi single-photon emission computed tomography imaging predict cardiac events. *J Nucl Cardiol.* 2007;14(6):810–817.
106. Hida S, Chikamori T, Tanaka H, et al. Diagnostic value of left ventricular function after stress and at rest in the detection of multivessel coronary artery disease as assessed by electrocardiogram-gated SPECT. *J Nucl Cardiol.* 2007;14(1):68–74.
107. Druz RS, Akinboboye OA, Grimson R, Nichols KJ, Reichek N. Postischemic stunning after adenosine vasodilator stress. *J Nucl Cardiol.* 2004;11(5):534–541.
108. Johnson LL, Verdesca SA, Aude WY, et al. Postischemic stunning can affect left ventricular ejection fraction and regional wall motion on post-stress gated sestamibi tomograms. *J Am Coll Cardiol.* 1997;30(7):1641–1648.
109. Paul AK, Hasegawa S, Yoshioka J, et al. Characteristics of regional myocardial stunning after exercise in gated myocardial SPECT. *J Nucl Cardiol.* 2002;9(4):388–394.
110. Toba M, Kumita S, Cho K, Ibuki C, Kumazaki T, Takano T. Usefulness of gated myocardial perfusion SPECT imaging soon after exercise to identify postexercise stunning in patients with single-vessel coronary artery disease. *J Nucl Cardiol.* 2004;11(6):697–703.
111. Doukky R, Frogge N, Bayissa YA, et al. The prognostic value of transient ischemic dilatation with otherwise normal SPECT myocardial perfusion imaging: a cautionary note in patients with diabetes and coronary artery disease. *J Nucl Cardiol.* 2013;20(5):774–784.

112. Golzar Y, Olusanya A, Pe N, et al. The significance of automatically measured transient ischemic dilation in identifying severe and extensive coronary artery disease in regadenoson, single-isotope technetium-99m myocardial perfusion SPECT. *J Nucl Cardiol.* 2015;22(3):526–534.
113. Hashimoto J, Kubo A, Iwasaki R, et al. Gated single-photon emission tomography imaging protocol to evaluate myocardial stunning after exercise. *Eur J Nucl Med.* 1999;26(12):1541–1546.
114. del Val Gómez M, Gallardo FG, San Martín MA, Garcia A, Terol I. Ischaemic related transitory left ventricular dysfunction in 201Tl gated SPECT. *Nucl Med Commun.* 2005;26(7):601–605.
115. Chen J, Garcia EV, Folks RD, et al. Onset of left ventricular mechanical contraction as determined by phase analysis of ECG-gated myocardial perfusion SPECT imaging: development of a diagnostic tool for assessment of cardiac mechanical dyssynchrony. *J Nucl Cardiol.* 2005;12(6):687–695.
116. Aggarwal H, AlJaroudi WA, Mehta S, et al. The prognostic value of left ventricular mechanical dyssynchrony using gated myocardial perfusion imaging in patients with end-stage renal disease. *J Nucl Cardiol.* 2014;21(4):739–746.
117. Pazhenkottil AP, Buechel RR, Husmann L, et al. Long-term prognostic value of left ventricular dyssynchrony assessment by phase analysis from myocardial perfusion imaging. *Heart.* 2011;97(1):33–37.
118. McLaughlin MG, Danias PG. Transient ischemic dilation: a powerful diagnostic and prognostic finding of stress myocardial perfusion imaging. *J Nucl Cardiol.* 2002;9(6):663–667.
119. Henzlova MJ, Duvall WL, Einstein AJ, Travin MI, Verberne HJ. ASNC imaging guidelines for SPECT nuclear cardiology procedures: Stress, protocols, and tracers. *J Nucl Cardiol.* 2016;23(3):606–639.
120. Elhabyan AK, Reyes BJ, Hallak O, et al. Subendocardial ischemia without coronary artery disease: is elevated left ventricular end diastolic pressure the culprit? *Current Med Res Opin.* 2004;20(5):773–777.
121. Xu Y, Arsanjani R, Clond M, et al. Transient ischemic dilation for coronary artery disease in quantitative analysis of same-day sestamibi myocardial perfusion SPECT. *J Nucl Cardiol.* 2012;19(3):465–473.
122. Slomka PJ, Berman DS, Germano G. Normal limits for transient ischemic dilation with 99mTc myocardial perfusion SPECT protocols. *J Nucl Cardiol.* 2016.
123. Weiss AT, Berman DS, Lew AS, et al. Transient ischemic dilation of the left ventricle on stress thallium-201 scintigraphy: a marker of severe and extensive coronary artery disease. *J Am Coll Cardiol.* 1987;9(4):752–759.
124. McClellan JR, Travin MI, Herman SD, et al. Prognostic importance of scintigraphic left ventricular cavity dilation during intravenous dipyridamole technetium-99m sestamibi myocardial tomographic imaging in predicting coronary events. *Am J Cardiol.* 1997;79(5):600–605.
125. Mazzanti M, Germano G, Kiat H, et al. Identification of severe and extensive coronary artery disease by automatic measurement of transient ischemic dilation of the left ventricle in dual-isotope myocardial perfusion SPECT. *J Am Coll Cardiol.* 1996;27(7):1612–1620.
126. Kinoshita N, Sugihara H, Adachi Y, et al. Assessment of transient left ventricular dilatation on rest and exercise on Tc-99m tetrofosmin myocardial SPECT. *Clin Nucl Med.* 2002;27(1):34–39.
127. Kritzman JN, Ficaro EP, Corbett JR. Post-stress LV dilation: The effect of imaging protocol, gender and attenuation correction. *J Nucl Med.* 2001;42(5):50P.
128. Williams KA, Schnieder CM, Jain A. Transient ischemic dilation (TID) with pharmacological stress dual isotope SPECT [Abstract]. *Circulation.* 2000;102(suppl 2):546.
129. Abidov A, Bax JJ, Hayes SW, et al. Integration of automatically measured transient ischemic dilation ratio into interpretation of adenosine stress myocardial perfusion SPECT for detection of severe and extensive CAD. *J Nucl Med.* 2004;45(12):1999–2007.
130. Katz JS, Ruisi M, Giedd KN, Rachko M. Assessment of transient ischemic dilation (TID) ratio in gated SPECT myocardial perfusion imaging (MPI) using regadenoson, a new agent for pharmacologic stress testing. *J Nucl Cardiol.* 2012;19(4):727–734.
131. Lester D, El-Hajj S, Farag AA, et al. Prognostic value of transient ischemic dilation with regadenoson myocardial perfusion imaging. *J Nucl Cardiol.* 2016;23(5):1147–1155.
132. Kakhki VR, Sadeghi R, Zakavi SR. Assessment of transient left ventricular dilation ratio via 2-day dipyridamole Tc-99m sestamibi nongated myocardial perfusion imaging. *J Nucl Cardiol.* 2007;14(4):529–536.
133. Bestetti A, Di Leo C, Alessi A, Triulzi A, Tagliabue L, Tarolo GL. Post-stress end-systolic left ventricular dilation: a marker of endocardial post-ischemic stunning. *Nucl Med Commun.* 2001;22(6):685–693.
134. Abidov A, Germano G, Berman DS. Transient ischemic dilation ratio: a universal high-risk diagnostic marker in myocardial perfusion imaging. *J Nucl Cardiol.* 2007;14(4):497–500.
135. Valdiviezo C, Motivala AA, Hachamovitch R, et al. The significance of transient ischemic dilation in the setting of otherwise normal SPECT radionuclide myocardial perfusion images. *J Nucl Cardiol.* 2011;18(2):220–229.
136. Abidov A, Bax JJ, Hayes SW, et al. Transient ischemic dilation ratio of the left ventricle is a significant predictor of future cardiac events in patients with otherwise normal myocardial perfusion SPECT. *J Am Coll Cardiol.* 2003;42(10):1818–1825.
137. Bourque JM. Contemporary relevance of TID: Based on the company it keeps. *J Nucl Cardiol.* 2015;22(3):535–538.
138. Gibson RS, Watson DD, Carabello BA, Holt ND, Beller GA. Clinical implications of increased lung uptake of thallium-201 during exercise scintigraphy 2 weeks after myocardial infarction. *Am J Cardiol.* 1982;49(7):1586–1593.
139. Boucher CA, Zir LM, Beller GA, et al. Increased lung uptake of thallium-201 during exercise myocardial imaging: clinical, hemodynamic and angiographic implications in patients with coronary artery disease. *Am J Cardiol.* 1980;46(2):189–196.
140. Kamínek M, Myslivecek M, Skvarilová M, et al. Increased prognostic value of combined myocardial perfusion SPECT imaging and the quantification of lung Tl-201 uptake. *Clinical Nucl Med.* 2002;27(4):255–260.
141. Cox JL, Wright LM, Burns RJ. Prognostic significance of increased thallium-201 lung uptake during dipyridamole myocardial scintigraphy: comparison with exercise scintigraphy. *Can J Cardiol.* 1995;11(8):689–694.
142. Daou D, Delahaye N, Lebtahi R, et al. Diagnosis of extensive coronary artery disease: intrinisic value of increased lung 201 Tl uptake with exercise SPECT. *J Nucl Med.* 2000;41(4):567–574.

143. Bacher-Stier C, Sharir T, Kavanagh PB, et al. Postexercise lung uptake of 99mTc-sestamibi determined by a new automatic technique: validation and application in detection of severe and extensive coronary artery disease and reduced left ventricular function. *J Nucl Med.* 2000;41(7):1190–1197.
144. Mahmarian JJ, Cerqueira MD, Iskandrian AE, et al. Regadenoson induces comparable left ventricular perfusion defects as adenosine: a quantitative analysis from the ADVANCE MPI 2 trial. *JACC Cardiovasc Imaging.* 2009;2(8):959–968.
145. Berman DS, Kang X, Gransar H, et al. Quantitative assessment of myocardial perfusion abnormality on SPECT myocardial perfusion imaging is more reproducible than expert visual analysis. *J Nucl Cardiol.* 2009;16(1):45–53.
146. Iskandrian AE, Garcia EV, Faber T, Mahmarian JJ. Automated assessment of serial SPECT myocardial perfusion images. *J Nucl Cardiol.* 2009;16(1):6–9.
147. Mahmarian JJ, Peterson LE, Xu J, et al. Regadenoson provides perfusion results comparable to adenosine in heterogeneous patient populations: A quantitative analysis from the ADVANCE MPI trials. *J Nucl Cardiol.* 2015;22(2):248–261.
148. Giri S, Shaw LJ, Murthy DR, et al. Impact of diabetes on the risk stratification using stress single-photon emission computed tomography myocardial perfusion imaging in patients with symptoms suggestive of coronary artery disease. *Circulation.* 2002;105(1):32–40.
149. Iskandrian AE, Hage FG, Shaw LJ, Mahmarian JJ, Berman DS. Serial myocardial perfusion imaging: defining a significant change and targeting management decisions. *JACC Cardiovasc Imaging.* 2014;7(1):79–96.
150. Losordo DW, Vale PR, Hendel RC, et al. Phase 1/2 placebo-controlled, double-blind, dose-escalating trial of myocardial vascular endothelial growth factor 2 gene transfer by catheter delivery in patients with chronic myocardial ischemia. *Circulation.* 2002;105(17):2012–2018.
151. Farzaneh-Far A, Phillips HR, Shaw LK, et al. Ischemia change in stable coronary artery disease is an independent predictor of death and myocardial infarction. *JACC Cardiovasc Imaging.* 2012;5(7):715–724.
152. Brindis RG, Douglas PS, Hendel RC, et al. ACCF/ASNC appropriateness criteria for single-photon emission computed tomography myocardial perfusion imaging (SPECT MPI): a report of the American College of Cardiology Foundation Quality Strategic Directions Committee Appropriateness Criteria Working Group and the American Society of Nuclear Cardiology endorsed by the American Heart Association. *J Am Coll Cardiol.* 2005;46(8):1587–1605.
153. Hendel RC, Berman DS, Di Carli MF, et al. ACCF/ASNC/ACR/AHA/ASE/SCCT/SCMR/SNM 2009 Appropriate Use Criteria for Cardiac Radionuclide Imaging: A Report of the American College of Cardiology Foundation Appropriate Use Criteria Task Force, the American Society of Nuclear Cardiology, the American College of Radiology, the American Heart Association, the American Society of Echocardiography, the Society of Cardiovascular Computed Tomography, the Society for Cardiovascular Magnetic Resonance, and the Society of Nuclear Medicine. Endorsed by the American College of Emergency Physicians. *J Am Coll Cardiol.* 2009;53(23):2201–2229.
154. Wolk MJ, Bailey SR, Doherty JU, et al. ACCF/AHA/ASE/ASNC/HFSA/HRS/SCAI/SCCT/SCMR/STS 2013 multimodality appropriate use criteria for the detection and risk assessment of stable ischemic heart disease: a report of the American College of Cardiology Foundation Appropriate Use Criteria Task Force, American Heart Association, American Society of Echocardiography, American Society of Nuclear Cardiology, Heart Failure Society of America, Heart Rhythm Society, Society for Cardiovascular Angiography and Interventions, Society of Cardiovascular Computed Tomography, Society for Cardiovascular Magnetic Resonance, and Society of Thoracic Surgeons. *J Am Coll Cardiol.* 2014;63(4):380–406.
155. Doukky R, Hayes K, Frogge N, et al. Impact of appropriate use on the prognostic value of single-photon emission computed tomography myocardial perfusion imaging. *Circulation.* 2013;128:1634–1643.
156. Alexander S, Doukky R. Effective risk stratification of patients on the basis of myocardial perfusion SPECT is dependent on appropriate patient selection. *Curr Cardiol Rep.* 2015;17(1):549.
157. Doukky R, Hayes K, Frogge N. Appropriate use criteria for SPECT myocardial perfusion imaging: Are they appropriate for women? *J Nucl Cardiol.* 2016;23(4):695–705.
158. Elgendy IY, Mahmoud A, Shuster JJ, Doukky R, Winchester DE. Outcomes after inappropriate nuclear myocardial perfusion imaging: A meta-analysis. *J Nucl Cardiol.* 2016;23(4):680–689.
159. Dos Santos MA, Santos MS, Tura BR, Félix R, Brito AS, De Lorenzo A. Budget impact of applying appropriateness criteria for myocardial perfusion scintigraphy: The perspective of a developing country. *J Nucl Cardiol.* 2016;23(5):1160–1165.
160. Doukky R, Frogge N, Appis A, et al. Impact of appropriate use on the estimated radiation risk to men and women undergoing radionuclide myocardial perfusion imaging. *J Nucl Med.* 2016;57(8):1251–1257.
161. AMR/Arlington Medical Resources Inc. Myocardial Study Market Guide, 2012.
162. Fonseca R, Negishi K, Otahal P, Marwick TH. Temporal changes in appropriateness of cardiac imaging. *J Am Coll Cardiol.* 2015;65(8):763–773.
163. Lin GA, Dudley RA, Lucas FL, Malenka DJ, Vittinghoff E, Redberg RF. Frequency of stress testing to document ischemia prior to elective percutaneous coronary intervention. *JAMA.* 2008;300(15):1765–1773.
164. Levine GN, Bates ER, Blankenship JC, et al. 2011 ACCF/AHA/SCAI Guideline for Percutaneous Coronary Intervention. A report of the American College of Cardiology Foundation/American Heart Association Task Force on Practice Guidelines and the Society for Cardiovascular Angiography and Interventions. *J Am Coll Cardiol.* 2011;58(24):e44–e122.
165. Hillis LD, Smith PK, Anderson JL, et al. 2011 ACCF/AHA Guideline for Coronary Artery Bypass Graft Surgery. A report of the American College of Cardiology Foundation/American Heart Association Task Force on Practice Guidelines. Developed in collaboration with the American Association for Thoracic Surgery, Society of Cardiovascular Anesthesiologists, and Society of Thoracic Surgeons. *J Am Coll Cardiol.* 2011;58(24):e123–e210.
166. Khawaja FJ, Jouni H, Miller TD, Hodge DO, Gibbons RJ. Downstream clinical implications of abnormal myocardial perfusion single-photon emission computed tomography based on appropriate use criteria. *J Nucl Cardiol.* 2013;20(6):1041–1048.

167. Brown KA. Cardiac risk defined by stress myocardial perfusion imaging: Impact on physician decision making and cost savings. *J Nucl Cardiol.* 2002;9(1):124–126.
168. Underwood SR, Godman B, Salyani S, Ogle JR, Ell PJ. Economics of myocardial perfusion imaging in Europe–the EMPIRE Study. *Eur Heart J.* 1999;20(2):157–166.
169. Sabharwal NK, Stoykova B, Taneja AK, Lahiri A. A randomized trial of exercise treadmill ECG versus stress SPECT myocardial perfusion imaging as an initial diagnostic strategy in stable patients with chest pain and suspected CAD: cost analysis. *J Nucl Cardiol.* 2007;14(2):174.
170. Shaw LJ, Mieres JH, Hendel RH, et al.; WOMEN Trial Investigators. Comparative effectiveness of exercise electrocardiography with or without myocardial perfusion single photon emission computed tomography in women with suspected coronary artery disease: results from the What Is the Optimal Method for Ischemia Evaluation in Women (WOMEN) trial. *Circulation.* 2011;124(11):1239–1249.
171. Shaw LJ, Marwick TH, Berman DS, et al. Incremental cost-effectiveness of exercise echocardiography vs. SPECT imaging for the evaluation of stable chest pain. *Eur Heart J.* 2006;27(20):2448–2458.
172. Hlatky MA, Shilane D, Hachamovitch R, Dicarli MF. Economic outcomes in the study of myocardial perfusion and coronary anatomy imaging roles in coronary artery disease registry: the SPARC Study. *J Am Coll Cardiol.* 2014;63(10):1002–1008.
173. Douglas PS, Hoffmann U, Patel MR, et al. Outcomes of anatomical versus functional testing for coronary artery disease. *N Engl J Med.* 2015;372(14):1291–1300.
174. Mark DB, Federspiel JJ, Cowper PA, et al. Economic outcomes with anatomical versus functional diagnostic testing for coronary artery disease. *Ann Intern Med.* 2016;165(2):94–102.

Preoperative Risk Assessment for Noncardiac Surgery

CHAPTER 16

Sumeet S. Mitter and Thomas A. Holly

INTRODUCTION

Cardiovascular disease is the leading cause of death worldwide. Of the 200 million patients who undergo noncardiac surgery each year the world over, approximately 10 million have a major perioperative cardiac complication within 30 days.[1] Taken by itself, perioperative death constitutes the third leading cause of death in the United States and myocardial injury after noncardiac surgery is associated with a population attributable risk of 34% for death at 30 days in a recent international cohort analysis.[2,3] With an aging and increasingly comorbid population, these numbers are expected to grow.

Cardiovascular perioperative risk assessment has become a vital tool for evaluating patients prior to surgery to optimize their cardiovascular safety and initiate lifestyle modifications that coupled together provide short- and long-term benefits. Myocardial perfusion imaging (MPI) can play an important role in this process. The American College of Cardiology/American Heart Association (ACC/AHA) task force committee created guidelines for the perioperative risk assessment of cardiovascular disease for noncardiac surgery. Since the last iteration of the guidelines in 2007, data on perioperative cardiac risk factor modification and management have significantly changed, and the guidelines were subsequently updated in 2014.[4]

▶ Goals of Preoperative Evaluation

As a physician evaluates a patient prior to noncardiac surgery, several goals should be kept in mind:

1. Identify unstable patients who are at high risk for perioperative cardiac events.
2. Identify the risk of the proposed surgery (Table 16-1).

Table 16-1
Surgery-Specific Cardiac Risk

High-risk surgery (reported cardiac risk >5%)
Emergent major operation (particularly in the elderly)
Aortic and other major vascular
Peripheral vascular
Anticipated prolonged surgical procedures associated with large fluid shifts and/or blood loss

Intermediate-risk surgery (reported risk <5%)
Carotid endarterectomy
Head and neck
Intraperitoneal and intrathoracic
Orthopedic
Prostate

Low-risk surgery (reported risk <1%)
Endoscopic procedures
Superficial procedures
Cataract
Breast

3. Assess risk for major adverse perioperative cardiovascular events using a validated risk prediction tool.
4. Determine the patient's functional capacity.
5. Perform diagnostic testing and interventions to reduce perioperative morbidity and mortality or cancel the planned procedure.
6. Intervene to reduce long-term cardiovascular morbidity and mortality.
7. Follow-up with the patient postoperatively, when most perioperative cardiac events occur.

CLINICAL EVALUATION

The preoperative evaluation begins with a thorough history with special emphasis on the need to identify clinical markers of perioperative risk as well as to assess functional capacity.

In 2002, the ACC/AHA guidelines delineated major, intermediate, and minor risk factors for perioperative cardiac events. In 2007, the guidelines sought to identify patients at high risk for complications with surgery due to serious cardiac conditions such as unstable coronary syndromes, severe angina, recent myocardial infarction (MI), decompensated heart failure (HF), significant arrhythmias, and severe valvular disease that require urgent evaluation regardless of impending surgery. The most recent update in 2014 reflects a paradigm shift in the methodology of guidelines preparation that continues to evolve.[4,5] In estimating risk, they dichotomize combined clinical and surgical risk into low (major adverse cardiac event [MACE] probability <1%) and elevated (MACE probability ≥1%).

The revised cardiac risk index (RCRI), devised and validated by Lee et al., remains the predominantly used and recommended tool for the estimation of MACE risk in the updated guidelines.[6] The RCRI defined six independent risk correlates of cardiac risk for stable patients undergoing nonurgent major noncardiac surgery: high-risk surgery, history of ischemic heart disease, history of congestive HF, history of cerebrovascular disease, preoperative treatment with insulin, and preoperative serum creatinine >2.0 mg/dL. The rates of major cardiac complications with 0, 1, 2, or >3 in the validation cohort of 1422 patients were 0.4%, 0.9%, 7%, and 11%, respectively.[6] The updated guidelines also highlight two newer tools developed by the American College of Surgeons National Surgical Quality and Improvement Program (NSQIP)—the MI and cardiac arrest risk prediction tool and the surgical risk calculator—but note that they have not been externally validated and use definitions of MI and assessments of physical status that are not standardized. Furthermore, the updated guidelines highlight a growing interest in the use of clinical biomarkers for multivariate risk prediction, but also note that information on how to treat based on such serologic tests still requires further investigation.[4,7,8]

The assessment of functional capacity is critical for preoperative evaluation (Table 16-2). Poor functional capacity in patients with known CAD or prior MI is associated with an increased risk of subsequent cardiac events.[9] Multiple investigators have studied the importance of functional capacity assessment for preoperative risk stratification.[10–12] These and other studies suggest that poor functional status identifies patients at high risk for perioperative complications. Therefore, it is extremely important to determine the patient's maximal activity during daily activities and assess his or her functional capacity. This also could be assessed by treadmill exercise stress testing. Patients with poor functional capacity may require further evaluation, including MPI in multiple clinical situations as detailed later in this chapter.

Based on the above information a stepwise approach in the updated ACC/AHA guidelines can be used to determine if a patient needs perioperative cardiac assessment for coronary artery disease (Fig. 16-1).[4]

Table 16-2

Functional Capacity and Estimated Energy Requirements for Various Activities

1 MET
Eat, dress, or use the toilet
Walk indoors around the house
Walk on level ground at 2 mph (3.2 km/h)
Do light housework such as washing dishes
4 METs
Climb a flight of stairs
Walk on level ground at 4 mph (6.4 km/h)
Run a short distance
Heavy work such as vacuuming or lifting heavy furniture
Play sports such as golf or doubles tennis
>10 METs
Participate in strenuous activities such as swimming, singles tennis, basketball, or skiing

MET, metabolic equivalent.

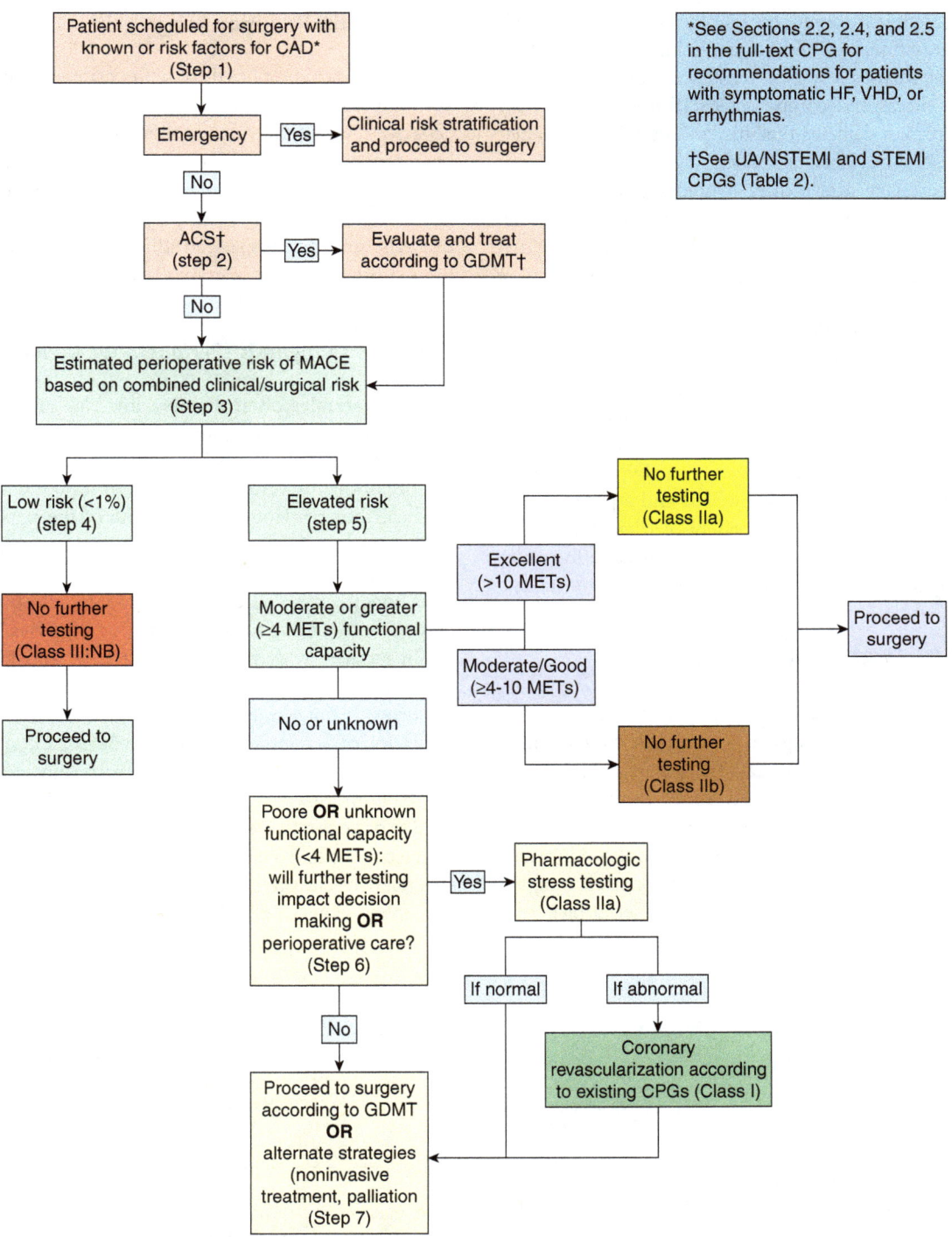

FIGURE 16-1 ACC/AHA task force guidelines for cardiac evaluation before noncardiac surgery. The sections of text and Table 16-2 cited in the figure are contained in the published guidelines. (Reproduced with permission from Fleisher LA, Fleischmann KE, Auerbach AD, et al. 2014 ACC/AHA guideline on perioperative cardiovascular evaluation and management of patients undergoing noncardiac surgery: A report of the American College of Cardiology/American Heart Association Task Force on practice guidelines. *J Am Coll Cardiol*. 2014;64(22):e77–e137.)

Emphasis should be placed on identifying evidence of disease states that might impact perioperative events, such as severe aortic stenosis, other severe valvular diseases, decompensated HF, unstable coronary syndromes, diabetes mellitus, and peripheral vascular disease. The aforementioned algorithm for assessing coronary artery disease preoperatively does not account for nonischemic cardiovascular events such as HF, valvular heart disease, pulmonary vascular disease and arrhythmias, which are beyond the scope of this chapter, but are otherwise addressed separately in the updated guidelines.[13,14] Briefly, nonetheless, the updated perioperative guidelines recommend addressing clinically significant moderate or severe valvular heart disease prior to elective noncardiac surgery, a continuation of targeted therapy for chronic pulmonary vascular disease and/or assessment by a pulmonary hypertension specialist as needed and a perioperative plan for management of a patient's cardiac implantable electronic device should he or she have one to reduce perioperative cardiovascular morbidity and mortality.[4]

PREOPERATIVE TESTING

Although indicated less often in current practice, noninvasive cardiac testing can be a valuable component of the preoperative evaluation. The expertise of the local laboratory in identifying advanced coronary disease is probably more important than the particular type of test. However, there are certain contraindications to exercise, dobutamine, or vasodilator stress imaging tests that should be considered before selecting a test.

▶ Myocardial Perfusion Imaging

Thus far, this chapter has dealt with perioperative risk assessment using primarily clinical data and exercise capacity. Despite the value of this information, it has been recognized that further data may be beneficial in selected patients. Landmark studies demonstrated that stress MPI could stratify patients into low- or high-risk groups. This risk stratification is helpful for both short-term (perioperative) and long-term prediction of cardiac events.

Short-Term Prognosis (Perioperative Period)

Clinical variables often define a low-risk group for whom no further testing may be needed and a high-risk group that may need further assessment with the intention for revascularization and/or intensive medical therapy. However, for some of the patients in the intermediate-risk group, further assessment with noninvasive testing would be needed. Radionuclide imaging is a well-established tool to risk stratify patients undergoing major noncardiac surgeries.

In studies by Eagle et al. both low- and high-risk patients were identified by clinical variables.[11,12] However, the intermediate-risk group had a 15.5% likelihood of developing perioperative cardiac complication. This group was further classified by dipyridamole thallium into patients with no ischemia who had a 3.2% perioperative event rate. In contrast, patients with ischemia had a 29.6% event rate (Fig. 16-2). This effectively reclassified the intermediate-risk group into either a low- or a high-risk group.

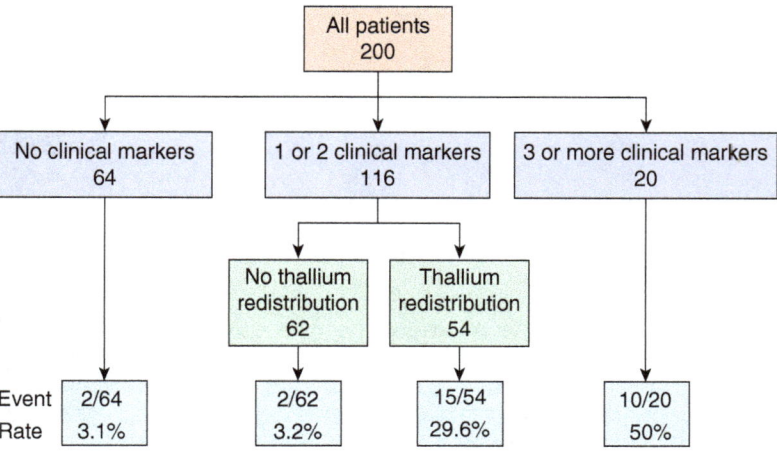

FIGURE 16-2 Clinical markers of risk and thallium redistribution. (Reproduced with permission from Eagle KA, Coley CM, Newell JB, et al. Combining clinical and thallium data optimizes preoperative assessment of cardiac risk before major vascular surgery. *Ann Intern Med.* 1989;110(11):859–866.)

Further evidence to support selective use of preoperative dipyridamole thallium comes from L'Italien et al.[15] In a multicenter study, they developed a prediction model in 567 patients on the basis of clinical variables (age >70 years, angina, history of MI, diabetes mellitus, history of congestive HF, and prior revascularization). A second model was developed from dipyridamole-thallium imaging. The models were then validated in a separate cohort of 514 patients. The observed and predicted cardiac event rates were similar for both patient sets. The addition of dipyridamole-thallium data reclassified more than 80% of the intermediate-risk patients into low-risk (3% event rate) and high-risk (19% event rate) categories. However, it provided no further stratification for patients previously classified as low- or high-risk by the clinical model. Thus, clinical markers reliably stratify risk in patients undergoing vascular surgery, and the selective use of myocardial imaging provides additional risk stratification in patients classified as intermediate risk.

The presence of ischemia on MPI identifies patients at higher risk, as noted earlier. The extent of ischemia can further classify this group of patients. Shaw et al. performed a meta-analysis of 15 studies that have available cardiac event rates after vascular surgery.[16] Ten studies using dipyridamole thallium were identified (1994 patients). The perioperative event rates (death or MI) were 3% for patients with normal results, 7% for patients with fixed defects, and 9% for patients with reversible defects. Dipyridamole-induced ECG ST-segment depression occurred in 7% of patients and was associated with a cardiac event (death or MI) in 14% of patients. Furthermore, higher event rates were associated with larger perfusion defects. The event rate was 14% in patients with one or more reversible defects versus 30% in patients with two or more reversible defects. Therefore, patients with larger perfusion defects or evidence of multivessel ischemia have a worse prognosis.

The predictive value of thallium redistribution (ischemia) for death or MI ranged from 4% to 20% in reports that were selected in the ACC/AHA task force report on preoperative testing.[17] The positive predictive value has decreased over time for MPI as this information is used to guide therapeutic interventions, such as intensive medical therapy or coronary revascularization. Moreover, the results of radionuclide imaging may lead to the performance of less extensive procedures or even cancellation of surgery. Nonetheless, the negative predictive value is very high (approximately 99%), and the prognosis associated with a normal scan is excellent.[17]

Fewer studies are available with technetium-99m agents, which are the contemporary standard. Stratmann et al. reported on the value of dipyridamole Tc-99m-sestamibi scintigraphy in 285 consecutive patients being considered for major and minor nonvascular surgery and in 229 consecutive patients being considered for vascular surgery.[18,19] Perioperative cardiac events included unstable angina, ischemic pulmonary edema, nonfatal MI, or cardiac death. Twelve events (4%) occurred in the whole cohort with 1 occurring in the 89 patients undergoing minor procedures and 11 occurring in the 140 patients undergoing major procedures.[18] Perioperative cardiac events occurred in 4% of patients with a normal study, 24% with evidence of ischemia, and 37% with a fixed defect. In the second study by the same authors, the event rate was 3% in patients with a normal scan, 5% with an abnormal scan, and 6% with evidence of ischemia.[19] Similar perioperative risk was reported in the group of patients who were identified to have ischemia and had intensive medical therapy or revascularization in comparison to those who had no ischemia. Thus, preoperative evaluation appears equally effective using Tc-99m sestamibi or thallium-201. In addition, although many of the studies utilized planar imaging, SPECT imaging has been documented to be effective in this role as well.[20]

Long-Term Prognosis

It is well recognized that stress testing has considerable value in predicting cardiac events over a 2- to 3-year period in patients assessed for known or suspected CAD.[21] This is further extended to patients undergoing surgical procedures. Hendel et al. evaluated 360 patients, of whom 327 underwent vascular surgery, wherein a cardiac event (cardiac death or MI) occurred in 14.4% of patients who had transient thallium defects and only in 1% of patients with a normal result.[22] The late cardiac event rate was 4.9% in those with a normal dipyridamole-thallium scan compared with 24% in patients with a fixed perfusion defect, with this abnormality being the most powerful predictor of late events, increasing the relative risk fivefold.

Shaw et al. in a meta-analysis showed that late cardiac event rates were largely comparable in patients with fixed or reversible defects, with approximately one-third of patients with either defect pattern experiencing a cardiac event 2 to 3 years after vascular surgery.[16] Therefore, intensive medical therapy, risk modification, and close follow-up of patients with evidence of CAD is likely the optimal approach.

Summary of Preoperative MPI

MPI can provide valuable information regarding perioperative risk, short-term risk prognosis, and long-term prognosis. These data contribute to decision making regarding choice of operation and perioperative management. Patients with normal- or low-risk test results can usually proceed with the planned procedure. Those with high-risk findings (such as large perfusion defects, transient cavity dilatation, or decreased left ventricular ejection fraction) should be considered for further evaluation and treatment as in the nonpreoperative setting.

Dobutamine Echocardiography

Dobutamine echocardiography is also a useful tool for preoperative risk assessment, although fewer data are available in comparison with MPI. In the meta-analysis by Shaw et al., of the 173 patients with a dobutamine-induced new or worsening wall motion response, 40 (23%) had a perioperative ischemic event compared with 1 (0.37%) of 270 patients with a normal stress echocardiographic response. The positive predictive value of testing was 13% for cardiac death or MI and 26% for any cardiac event. The negative predictive value of a normal dobutamine echocardiographic response was 99%. The long-term (1-year) cardiac event rate was 2.9% for 69 patients with normal and 15% for 20 patients with abnormal stress echocardiographic result. Summary odds ratios were greater for dobutamine echocardiography (14.0–27.0) than for dipyridamole thallium (3.7–4.0). These data suggest that preoperative evaluation with dobutamine echocardiography is useful when performed by experienced individuals.

Coronary Computed Tomography Angiography

The latest perioperative guidelines and multimodality imaging appropriate use criteria (AUC) offer no clear indication for the use of coronary computed tomography angiography (CCTA) for preoperative cardiovascular risk stratification due to a paucity of data.[4,23] In a single-center study, Hwang et al. were able to show that in 844 patients undergoing elective surgery with at least one clinical risk factor for ischemic heart disease, CCTA revealed incremental 4- to 17-fold higher risk for major adverse cardiovascular events in individuals with ≥50% stenosis in one, two, and three vessels compared to individuals with <50% stenosis in all coronary beds. Furthermore, CCTA improved risk prediction for major adverse cardiovascular events in individuals with an RCRI score of 2 to 3 when comparing those with significant to those without significant computed tomography findings.[24] However, although the large, multicenter CTA VISION study showed that increasing severity of coronary disease seen on CCTA was associated with higher hazard ratios for the primary outcome of cardiac death or nonfatal MI within 30 days after surgery, the findings on CCTA were more than five times as likely to lead to an inappropriate overestimation of risk among patients who will not experience such a cardiac event.[25] Further research is needed before CCTA becomes a more routinely accepted technique for preoperative evaluation.

Invasive Coronary Angiography

Routine preoperative coronary angiography is not recommended in the updated ACC/AHA perioperative guidelines.[4] The indications for coronary angiography are similar to those identified for the nonoperative setting and include:

1. High risk of adverse outcome based on noninvasive test results.
2. Angina unresponsive to medical therapy.
3. Unstable angina.
4. Equivocal noninvasive test results in patients at high clinical risk undergoing high-risk surgery.

It is important to emphasize that coronary angiography should be performed in the appropriate clinical context on the basis of unstable angina or noninvasive test results that indicate large zones of ischemia and should not be performed for limited ischemia without other significant clinical findings.

ACC/AHA GUIDELINES—STEPWISE APPROACH

On the basis of current knowledge, the ACC/AHA task force developed guidelines for cardiac evaluation before noncardiac surgery.[4] A general strategy for preoperative cardiac risk assessment is summarized in Figure 16-1.

Step 1. Determine the urgency of noncardiac surgery. Preoperative risk assessment may be inappropriate for patients who must undergo emergency surgery.

Step 2. Determine if the patient has an acute coronary syndrome. In patients being considered for elective noncardiac surgery, the presence of an acute coronary syndrome should lead to evaluation prior to surgery and usually leads to cancellation or delay of surgery until the cardiac problem has been clarified and treated appropriately.

Step 3. Estimate the combined clinical/surgical risk of a perioperative major adverse cardiovascular event using a validated risk prediction tool.

Step 4. If the patient is at a low combined clinical/surgical risk (<1%) no further preoperative testing is needed and the patient may proceed to surgery.

Step 5. If there is an elevated combined clinical/surgical risk (≥1%), determine the functional capacity (Table 16-2). In excellent or moderately functional asymptomatic patients, management will rarely be changed on the basis of results of any further cardiovascular testing. It is therefore appropriate to proceed with the planned surgery.

Step 6. If the patient has poor or unknown functional capacity and if it is thought that further testing will impact decision making or perioperative care, then noninvasive pharmacologic stress testing can be performed for further risk stratification for ischemic heart disease.

Step 7. If further testing will not affect decision making or perioperative care, then the patient may proceed to surgery according to guideline-directed medical therapy or pursue alternative management strategies (including noninvasive treatment and/or palliation).

▶ Multimodality Appropriate Use Criteria and Special Scenarios

The American College of Cardiology Foundation, along with several subspecialty societies updated AUC for the use of cardiac stress testing and anatomical imaging for stable ischemic heart disease patients in 2013.[23] The AUC reinforce that stress testing and imaging are rarely appropriate in those with a good functional capacity, prior normal testing within 1 year or those undergoing low-risk surgeries. Stress MPI or echocardiography is only appropriate in individuals with unknown or low functional capacity undergoing vascular surgery with ≥1 clinical risk factor or undergoing kidney or liver transplantation (Table 16-3). This latter group of patients, however, deserves special attention as preoperative ischemic evaluations are not only part of a patient's surgical workup for kidney or liver transplantation, but also help in assessing the long-term outcomes in these special patient populations.

The ACCF and the American Heart Association Guidelines provide a Class IIB recommendation (level of evidence C) for noninvasive testing in end-stage renal disease (ESRD) and end-stage liver disease (ESLD) patients without active cardiac issues if there are cardiovascular risk factors.[26] There is, however, no validated number of clinical risk factors needed to elicit such testing in ESRD or ESLD patients. Presently, the AUC consider radionuclide imaging appropriate in the setting of ESRD and ESLD prior to transplantation. Wide variability in sensitivity (0.29–0.92) and specificity (0.67–0.89) regarding the detection of significant coronary artery disease for MPI is present in ESRD patients. Similar variability is notable for dobutamine stress echocardiography. Nonetheless, a meta-analysis assessing the use of MPI or dobutamine stress echocardiography in ESRD patients were notable for almost six times the risk of myocardial ischemia and four times the risk of cardiac death among those with inducible ischemia. Fixed defects were associated with five times the risk for cardiac death.[27] In comparing the modalities,

Table 16-3
Preoperative Multimodality Imaging for Noncardiac Surgery Appropriate Use Criteria

Indication Text	Exercise ECG	Stress MPI	Stress Echo	Stress CMR	Calcium Scoring	CCTA	Invasive Coronary Angiography
Moderate-to-Good Functional Capacity (≥4 METs) OR No Clinical Risk Factors							
Any surgery	R	R	R	R	R	R	R
Asymptomatic AND < 1 Year Post Any of the Following: Normal CCTA or Invasive Angiogram, Normal Stress Test for CAD, or Revascularization							
Any surgery	R	R	R	R	R	R	R
Poor or Unknown Functional Capacity (<4 METs)							
Low-risk surgery and ≥1 clinical risk factor	R	R	R	R	R	R	R
Intermediate-risk surgery and ≥1 clinical risk factor	M	M	M	M	R	R	R
Vascular surgery and ≥1 clinical risk factor	M	A	A	M	R	R	R
Kidney transplant	M	A	A	M	R	R	M
Liver transplant	M	A	A	M	R	R	M

Appropriate use key: A, appropriate; M, may be appropriate; R, rarely appropriate.
General Key: CAD, coronary artery disease; CCTA, coronary computed tomography angiography; CMR, cardiac magnetic resonance; ECG, electrocardiogram; Echo, echocardiography; METs, metabolic equivalents; MPI, myocardial perfusion imaging.
Adapted with permission from Wolk MJ, Bailey SR, Doherty JU, et al. ACCF/AHA/ASE/ASNC/HFSA/HRS/SCAI/SCCT/SCMR/STS 2013 multimodality appropriate use criteria for the detection and risk assessment of stable ischemic heart disease: A report of the American College of Cardiology Foundation Appropriate Use Criteria Task Force, American Heart Association, American Society of Echocardiography, American Society of Nuclear Cardiology, Heart Failure Society of America, Heart Rhythm Society, Society for Cardiovascular Angiography and Interventions, Society of Cardiovascular Computed Tomography, Society for Cardiovascular Magnetic Resonance, and Society of Thoracic Surgeons. *J Am Coll Cardiol.* 2014;63(4):380–406.

there is recent evidence that MPI may have higher diagnostic accuracy versus dobutamine echocardiography and also lead to a cost savings as well; however the data is limited to a single center.[28] In ESLD patient, MPI has limited correlation with findings on cardiac catheterization and cardiac events after liver transplantation due to poor specificity. The presence of baseline coronary vasodilation in this population may also be a factor with regard to diagnostic sensitivity.[26,29,30]

Preoperative cardiac evaluation in patients undergoing bariatric surgery provides certain challenges as these patients can be difficult to evaluate noninvasively due to their body habitus. Although perioperative mortality and cardiac event rates with these procedures are low,[31] there are times when preoperative cardiac evaluation is indicated. The data on such evaluations are sparse. Gemignani et al. examined 383 stress MPI studies performed on patients who planned to undergo bariatric surgery at their institution.[32] MPI failed to predict 1-year survival, and postoperative cardiac event rates were low.

Cardiac PET stress testing is an option for these patients given its greater accuracy in obese patients,[33] but there are no systematic studies published in the area of evaluation prior to bariatric surgery. Issues with PET imaging in this setting include some patients exceeding the weight limit of the scanner and some being unable to physically fit in the scanner.

PERIOPERATIVE RISK REDUCTION

▶ Use of Beta-Blockers

The latest perioperative guidelines for noncardiac surgery reflect a re-examination of the data on the use of beta-blockers around the time of noncardiac surgery. Owing to debate regarding the legitimacy of prior evidence favoring the initiation of beta-blockers prior to cardiac surgery to reduce perioperative major adverse cardiovascular events, the current guidelines have increased the recommended threshold for starting beta-blockers to those patients who exhibit ischemia during preoperative risk stratification and to those individuals with at least three or more clinical risk factors.[4] Notably, beta-blockers should be initiated long enough in advance to assess safety and tolerability, at least 1 day prior to surgery and patients who were previously on beta-blockers should continue them around the time of surgery.[4]

The new recommendations draw largely from a systematic review that examined the evidence for use when initiating beta blockade within 45 days prior to noncardiac surgery, and cautioned against beta-blocker use at the time of surgery.[34,35] This recent systematic review noted a net 28% reduction in the hazard for nonfatal MI but a 79% and 30% increase in the hazards for stroke and all-cause mortality, respectively.[34]

▶ Use of Statins

Increasing evidence shows that statin therapy can reduce the risk of perioperative major adverse cardiovascular events for noncardiac nonvascular and vascular surgeries.[36–40] In the case of nonvascular surgery, a 49% reduction in a combined 30-day endpoint of all-cause mortality, atrial fibrillation, and nonfatal MI among statin users was noted.[37] Multiple additional studies have found statins to be beneficial in this population,[38] including a study by Desai et al. showing that statins conferred a greater benefit compared to beta-blockers in reducing perioperative MI and all-cause mortality in patients undergoing noncardiac vascular surgery.[39]

▶ Use of Coronary Revascularization

Percutaneous Coronary Intervention (PCI) and Stent Implantation

Coronary angiography should be performed prior to noncardiac surgery only if the initial evaluation raises concern for perioperative cardiac complications, as there are limited data supporting this approach in order to reduce major adverse cardiovascular events.

Early evidence from Kałuza et al. found a high rate of stent thrombosis and bleeding events in patients receiving coronary artery stenting less than 2 to 4 weeks ahead of noncardiac surgery also leading to high rate of death.[41] In the light of these details, the current guidelines recommend that percutaneous coronary intervention (PCI) should only be performed ahead of noncardiac surgery in patients with acute coronary syndromes who would benefit from an early invasive strategy and those with left main coronary artery disease in whom comorbidities would preclude coronary artery bypass grafting.[4] Furthermore, based on the time frame of a nonurgent noncardiac surgery, the guidelines recommend consideration of a bare-metal stent during PCI to reduce bleeding complications during future surgery by decreasing the recommended duration of dual antiplatelet therapy and reducing the risk for late stent thrombosis, compared to a drug-eluting stent, in the event surgery needs to be performed sooner. This recommendation may change with newer generation, zotarolimus-eluting stents.[42,43] A recent focused update on the duration of dual antiplatelet therapy recommends optimally delaying noncardiac surgery 6 months after drug-eluting stent implantation, and consideration of only a 3-month delay if the risk of delaying surgery is considered greater than the expected risks of stent thrombosis.[44]

Coronary Artery Bypass Grafting

There are limited data to support coronary artery bypass grafting ahead of noncardiac surgery to reduce intra- and postoperative cardiac events. Manske et al. reported the results of a randomized trial in which patients with CAD who were scheduled to undergo renal transplantation were assigned to receive CABG surgery or medical therapy.[45] Revascularized patients had a 57% reduction in cardiac events but value of this study was limited due to small sample size and loss to follow-up. Eagle at al. evaluated 24,959 participants in the Coronary Artery Surgery Study (CASS) database including 1961 patients undergoing higher-risk surgery.[46] Prior CABG was associated with fewer postoperative deaths and MIs compared with medically managed coronary disease.

However, those undergoing intermediate- and low-risk surgery had mortality of <1% regardless of prior coronary treatment.

As a result of these limited data, current recommendations for preoperative CABG are only for instances already supported by existing clinical practice guidelines.[47] Examples include patients with the following conditions: acceptable coronary revascularization risk and suitable viable myocardium with left main stenosis, severe three-vessel disease, two-vessel disease involving severe left anterior descending artery obstruction, and intractable coronary ischemia despite maximal medical therapy.

CONCLUSION

Clinical markers, physical examination, and functional capacity are the most important elements of estimating perioperative risk. Noninvasive testing is helpful in the group of patients estimated to be at intermediate risk, who have limited functional capacity and are being evaluated for high-risk surgery. MPI has a long history of clinical utility for such patients. Coronary angiography should be limited to patients with evidence of unstable coronary disease or evidence of extensive ischemia on noninvasive testing. Perioperative beta-blockers should be initiated in high-risk patients with stress-induced ischemia undergoing high-risk surgery. The perioperative evaluation also represents an opportunity to initiate or modify cardiac care, including primary and secondary preventative measures, which will be beneficial long after the surgical procedure (Table 16-4).

Table 16-4

Shortcut to Consider Noninvasive Testing in Preoperative Patients if All Three Present[a]

1. Poor functional capacity (<4 METs)
2. One or more clinical risk factors[b]
3. Intermediate- or high-risk surgery

[a]Emergency major operations may require immediately proceeding to surgery without sufficient time for noninvasive testing or preoperative interventions.
[b]Clinical risk factors include ischemic heart disease, compensated or prior heart failure, diabetes mellitus, renal insufficiency, and cerebrovascular disease.

REFERENCES

1. Devereaux PJ, Sessler DI. Cardiac complications in patients undergoing major noncardiac surgery. *NEJM*. 2015;373:2258–2269.
2. Bartels K, Karhausen J, Clambey ET, et al. Perioperative organ injury. *Anesthesiology*. 2013;119:1474–1489.
3. Botto F, Alonso-Coello P, Chan MT, et al. Myocardial injury after noncardiac surgery: A large, international, prospective cohort study establishing diagnostic criteria, characteristics, predictors, and 30-day outcomes. *Anesthesiology*. 2014;120:564–578.
4. Fleisher LA, Fleischmann KE, Auerbach AD, et al. 2014 ACC/AHA guideline on perioperative cardiovascular evaluation and management of patients undergoing noncardiac surgery: A report of the American College of Cardiology/American Heart Association Task Force on practice guidelines. *J Am Coll Cardiol*. 2014;64:e77–137.
5. Jacobs AK, Anderson JL, Halperin JL. The evolution and future of ACC/AHA clinical practice guidelines: A 30-year journey: A report of the American College of Cardiology/American Heart Association Task Force on Practice Guidelines. *J Am Coll Cardiol*. 2014;64:1373–1384.
6. Lee TH, Marcantonio ER, Mangione CM, et al. Derivation and prospective validation of a simple index for prediction of cardiac risk of major noncardiac surgery. *Circulation*. 1999;100:1043–1049.
7. Gupta PK, Gupta H, Sundaram A, et al. Development and validation of a risk calculator for prediction of cardiac risk after surgery. *Circulation*. 2011;124:381–387.
8. Cohen ME, Ko CY, Bilimoria KY, et al. Optimizing ACS NSQIP modeling for evaluation of surgical quality and risk: Patient risk adjustment, procedure mix adjustment, shrinkage adjustment, and surgical focus. *J Am Coll Surg*. 2013;217:336–346.e1.
9. Morris CK, Ueshima K, Kawaguchi T, et al. The prognostic value of exercise capacity: A review of the literature. *Am Heart J*. 1991;122:1423–1431.
10. Cutler BS, Wheeler HB, Paraskos JA, et al. Applicability and interpretation of electrocardiographic stress testing in patients with peripheral vascular disease. *Am J Surg*. 1981;141:501–506.
11. Eagle KA, Coley CM, Newell JB, et al. Combining clinical and thallium data optimizes preoperative assessment of cardiac risk before major vascular surgery. *Ann Intern Med*. 1989;110:859–866.
12. Eagle KA, Singer DE, Brewster DC, et al. Dipyridamole-thallium scanning in patients undergoing vascular surgery. Optimizing preoperative evaluation of cardiac risk. *JAMA*. 1987;257:2185–2189.
13. van Diepen S, Bakal JA, McAlister FA, et al. Mortality and readmission of patients with heart failure, atrial fibrillation, or coronary artery disease undergoing noncardiac surgery: An analysis of 38047 patients. *Circulation*. 2011;124:289–296.
14. Healy KO, Waksmonski CA, Altman RK, et al. Perioperative outcome and long-term mortality for heart failure patients undergoing intermediate- and high-risk noncardiac surgery: Impact of left ventricular ejection fraction. *Congest Heart Fail*. 2010;16:45–49.
15. L'Italien GJ, Paul SD, Hendel RC, et al. Development and validation of a Bayesian model for perioperative cardiac risk assessment in a cohort of 1,081 vascular surgical candidates. *J Am Coll Cardiol*. 1996;27:779–786.

16. Shaw LJ, Eagle KA, Gersh BJ, et al. Meta-analysis of intravenous dipyridamole-thallium-201 imaging (1985 to 1994) and dobutamine echocardiography (1991 to 1994) for risk stratification before vascular surgery. *J Am Coll Cardiol.* 1996;27:787–798.
17. Eagle KA, Berger PB, Calkins H, et al. ACC/AHA guideline update for perioperative cardiovascular evaluation for noncardiac surgery—executive summary: A report of the American College of Cardiology/American Heart Association Task Force on Practice Guidelines (Committee to Update the 1996 Guidelines on Perioperative Cardiovascular Evaluation for Noncardiac Surgery). *J Am Coll Cardiol.* 2002;39:542–553.
18. Stratmann HG, Younis LT, Wittry MD, et al. Dipyridamole technetium 99m sestamibi myocardial tomography for preoperative cardiac risk stratification before major or minor nonvascular surgery. *Am Heart J.* 1996;132:536–541.
19. Stratmann HG, Younis LT, Wittry MD, et al. Dipyridamole technetium-99m sestamibi myocardial tomography in patients evaluated for elective vascular surgery: Prognostic value for perioperative and late cardiac events. *Am Heart J.* 1996;131:923–929.
20. Koutelou MG, Asimacopoulos PJ, Mahmarian JJ, et al. Preoperative risk stratification by adenosine thallium 201 single-photon emission computed tomography in patients undergoing vascular surgery. *J Nucl Cardiol.* 1995;2:389–394.
21. Beller GA, Zaret BL. Contributions of nuclear cardiology to diagnosis and prognosis of patients with coronary artery disease. *Circulation.* 2000;101:1465–1478.
22. Hendel RC, Whitfield SS, Villegas BJ, et al. Prediction of late cardiac events by dipyridamole thallium imaging in patients undergoing elective vascular surgery. *Am J Cardiol.* 1992;70:1243–1249.
23. Wolk MJ, Bailey SR, Doherty JU, et al. ACCF/AHA/ASE/ASNC/HFSA/HRS/SCAI/SCCT/SCMR/STS 2013 multimodality appropriate use criteria for the detection and risk assessment of stable ischemic heart disease: A report of the American College of Cardiology Foundation Appropriate Use Criteria Task Force, American Heart Association, American Society of Echocardiography, American Society of Nuclear Cardiology, Heart Failure Society of America, Heart Rhythm Society, Society for Cardiovascular Angiography and Interventions, Society of Cardiovascular Computed Tomography, Society for Cardiovascular Magnetic Resonance, and Society of Thoracic Surgeons. *J Am Coll Cardiol.* 2014;63:380–406.
24. Sheth T, Butler C, Chow B, et al. The coronary CT angiography vision protocol: A prospective observational imaging cohort study in patients undergoing non-cardiac surgery. *BMJ Open.* 2012;2:e001474.
25. Hwang JW, Kim EK, Yang JH, et al. Assessment of perioperative cardiac risk of patients undergoing noncardiac surgery using coronary computed tomographic angiography. *Circ Cardiovasc Imaging.* 2015;8:e002582–e002582.
26. Lentine KL, Costa SP, Weir MR. Cardiac disease evaluation and management among kidney and liver transplantation candidates: A scientific statement from the American Heart Association and the American College of Cardiology Foundation. *J Am Coll Cardiol.* 2012;60:434–480.
27. Rabbat CG, Treleaven DJ, Russell JD, et al. Prognostic value of myocardial perfusion studies in patients with end-stage renal disease assessed for kidney or kidney-pancreas transplantation: A meta-analysis. *JASN.* 2003;14:431–439.
28. Thai JN, Abidov A, Jie T, et al. Nuclear myocardial perfusion imaging versus stress echocardiography in the preoperative evaluation of patients for kidney transplantation. *J Nucl Med Technol.* 2015;43:201–205.
29. Baker S, Chambers C, McQuillan P, et al. Myocardial perfusion imaging is an effective screening test for coronary artery disease in liver transplant candidates. *Clin Transplant.* 2015;29:319–326.
30. Aydinalp A, Bal U, Atar I, et al. Value of stress myocardial perfusion scanning in diagnosis of severe coronary artery disease in liver transplantation candidates. *Transplantation Proceedings.* 2009;41:3757–3760.
31. Santry HP, Gillen DL, Lauderdale DS. Trends in bariatric surgical procedures. *JAMA.* 2005;294(15):1909–1917.
32. Gemignani AS, Muhlebach SG, Abbott BG, et al. Stress-only or stress/rest myocardial perfusion imaging in patients undergoing evaluation for bariatric surgery. *J Nucl Cardiol.* 2011;18(5):886–892.
33. Bateman TM, Heller GV, McGhie AI, et al. Diagnostic accuracy of rest/stress ECG-gated Rb-82 myocardial perfusion PET: Comparison with ECG-gated Tc-99m sestamibi SPECT. *J Nucl Cardiol.* 2006;13(1):24–33.
34. Wijeysundera DN, Duncan D, Nkonde-Price C, et al. Perioperative beta blockade in noncardiac surgery: A systematic review for the 2014 ACC/AHA guideline on perioperative cardiovascular evaluation and management of patients undergoing noncardiac surgery: A report of the American College of Cardiology/American Heart Association Task Force on practice guidelines. *J Am Coll Cardiol.* 2014;64:2406–2425.
35. POISE Study Group, Devereaux PJ, Yang H, et al. Effects of extended-release metoprolol succinate in patients undergoing non-cardiac surgery (POISE trial): A randomised controlled trial. *Lancet.* 2008;371:1839–1847.
36. Lindenauer PK, Pekow P, Wang K, et al. Lipid-lowering therapy and in-hospital mortality following major noncardiac surgery. *JAMA.* 2004;291:2092–2099.
37. Raju MG, Pachika A, Punnam SR, et al. Statin therapy in the reduction of cardiovascular events in patients undergoing intermediate-risk noncardiac, nonvascular surgery. *Clin Cardiol.* 2013;36:456–461.
38. Durazzo AE, Machado FS, Ikeoka DT, et al. Reduction in cardiovascular events after vascular surgery with atorvastatin: A randomized trial. *J Vasc Surg.* 2004;39:967–975, discussion 975-6.
39. Desai H, Aronow WS, Ahn C, et al. Incidence of perioperative myocardial infarction and of 2-year mortality in 577 elderly patients undergoing noncardiac vascular surgery treated with and without statins. *Arch Gerontol Geriatr.* 2010;51:149–151.
40. Sanders RD, Nicholson A, Lewis SR, et al. Perioperative statin therapy for improving outcomes during and after noncardiac vascular surgery. Lewis SR, editor. *Cochrane Database Syst Rev.* 2013:CD009971.
41. Kałuza GL, Joseph J, Lee JR, et al. Catastrophic outcomes of noncardiac surgery soon after coronary stenting. *J Am Coll Cardiol* 2000;35:1288–1294.
42. Valgimigli M, Patialiakas A, Thury A, et al. Zotarolimus-eluting versus bare-metal stents in uncertain drug-eluting stent candidates. *J Am Coll Cardiol.* 2015;65:805–815.
43. Ariotti S, Adamo M, Costa F, et al. Is bare-metal stent implantation still justifiable in high bleeding risk patients

undergoing percutaneous coronary intervention?: A Pre-Specified Analysis From the ZEUS Trial. *JACC Cardiovasc Interv.* 2016;9:426–436.

44. Levine GN, Bates ER, Bittl JA, et al. 2016 ACC/AHA Guideline Focused Update on Duration of Dual Antiplatelet Therapy in Patients With Coronary Artery Disease: A Report of the American College of Cardiology/American Heart Association Task Force on Clinical Practice Guidelines: An Update of the 2011 ACCF/AHA/SCAI Guideline for Percutaneous Coronary Intervention, 2011 ACCF/AHA Guideline for Coronary Artery Bypass Graft Surgery, 2012 ACC/AHA/ACP/AATS/PCNA/SCAI/STS Guideline for the Diagnosis and Management of Patients With Stable Ischemic Heart Disease, 2013 ACCF/AHA Guideline for the Management of ST-Elevation Myocardial Infarction, 2014 AHA/ACC Guideline for the Management of Patients With Non-ST-Elevation Acute Coronary Syndromes, and 2014 ACC/AHA Guideline on Perioperative Cardiovascular Evaluation and Management of Patients Undergoing Noncardiac Surgery. *Circulation.* 2016;134(10):e123–55

45. Manske CL, Wang Y, Rector T, et al. Coronary revascularisation in insulin-dependent diabetic patients with chronic renal failure. *The Lancet.* 1992;340:998–1002.

46. Eagle KA, Rihal CS, Mickel MC, et al. Cardiac risk of noncardiac surgery: Influence of coronary disease and type of surgery in 3368 operations. CASS Investigators and University of Michigan Heart Care Program. Coronary Artery Surgery Study. *Circulation.* 1997;96:1882–1887.

47. Hillis LD, Smith PK, Anderson JL, et al. 2011 ACCF/AHA Guideline for Coronary Artery Bypass Graft Surgery. A report of the American College of Cardiology Foundation/American Heart Association Task Force on Practice Guidelines. Developed in collaboration with the American Association for Thoracic Surgery, Society of Cardiovascular Anesthesiologists, and Society of Thoracic Surgeons. *J Am Coll Cardiol.* 2011;58:e123–210.

Evaluation of Patients with Known Coronary Artery Disease

CHAPTER 17

Javier Gomez and Rami Doukky

INTRODUCTION

In the last 40 years, there has been a dramatic decline in cardiovascular mortality. Over the past decade alone, the rate of death attributable to cardiovascular disease has decreased by 30%.[1] This trend is credited primarily to the development and implementation of effective treatment strategies including medical therapy, interventions such as coronary artery bypass graft surgery (CABG) and percutaneous coronary interventions (PCIs), and successful treatment for acute myocardial infarction (MI). The decision to undergo myocardial perfusion imaging (MPI) evaluation following the diagnosis of ischemic heart disease is an important one, particularly in asymptomatic patients. This chapter will evaluate the role of stress MPI in patients with known CAD in a variety of settings, including medical therapy, postinterventions, and following MI.

MYOCARDIAL PERFUSION IMAGING AND CHRONIC ISCHEMIC HEART DISEASE

▶ Indications for Stress Myocardial Perfusion Imaging

Stress testing is an important tool in the longitudinal assessment of patients with known coronary disease, especially when there is a change in the frequency or pattern of symptoms. However, several factors may preclude the use of exercise tolerance testing (ETT) without imaging to make management decisions, as discussed in Chapters 8 and 26. The American College of Cardiology/American Heart Association (ACC/AHA) guidelines for ETT strongly recommend an imaging study as part of the evaluation in patients unable to exercise and in those with baseline EGG abnormalities (pre-excitation, paced ventricular rhythm, ≥1 mm resting ST-segment depression, and complete left bundle branch block [LBBB]).[2] The use of digoxin, presence of left ventricular hypertrophy (LVH), or any resting ST-segment depression decreases the specificity of exercise testing while sensitivity may remain unaffected.[2] Importantly, several other subsets of patients benefit incrementally with the use of radionuclide imaging, including patients with previous MI and/or coronary revascularization procedures (CABG or PCI), patients with prior angiography demonstrating significant disease (where identification of the lesion causing myocardial ischemia is important), individuals with high risk for future events (e.g., diabetics), and patients with a previous positive MPI.[2-6]

▶ Timing of Imaging of Follow-Up in Patients with Stable Coronary Artery Disease

Many patients with CAD undergo stress MPI for postinterventional assessment. Stress MPI is indicated as part of initial risk assessment and/or prior to planning PCI or CABG. It is also performed during follow-up after revascularization (PCI or CABG) or modification of medical therapy.

The role of stress MPI in stable CAD is linked to an effort to identify individuals at higher or lower risk for future cardiac events. Unless cardiac catheterization is indicated, patients with known CAD who present with changing symptoms suggestive of ischemia should likely first undergo stress imaging, to assess the risk of future events.[2] Furthermore, localization of ischemia, identification of extent and severity of ischemic burden, and assessment of left ventricular performance are desirable for most patients who are being evaluated for intervention or titration of medical therapy.[7] Despite some limitations in the setting of multivessel disease,[8] MPI remains the test of choice for identifying the culprit lesion causing ischemic symptoms. Routine testing in patients with stable symptoms and in patients with severe comorbidities that limit life expectancy or preclude revascularization is not supported by the literature.[2]

Although studies in nuclear cardiology have provided substantial data regarding prognosis and risk stratification, there is limited evidence regarding the widespread practice of follow-up or serial MPI testing. Clinicians must use their best judgment to answer important questions: What constitutes a "definite" change that is outside the limit of reproducibility of the test? What constitutes a "clinically significant" improvement or worsening? What degree of improvement should be expected after medical management or intervention? If the patient does improve symptomatically on medical therapy, does this portray a favorable prognosis? Nonetheless, a worsening in myocardial ischemic burden by ≥5% seems to correlate with adverse outcome. Farzaneh-Far et al. followed 1425 patients with angiographically documented CAD who underwent at least two SPECT MPI scans; patients were divided into three groups based on intervention received, medical therapy, and revascularization therapy. After a mean follow-up of 5.8 years, ischemic worsening by ≥5% was a significant and independent predictor of death or MI. Importantly, worsening ischemia of ≥5% provided improvement in risk classification compared to known risk predictors.[9]

To address some of the issues related to management strategy in patients with stable ischemic heart disease, the COURAGE trial compared outcomes of patients treated with PCI plus optimal medical therapy (OMT) versus OMT alone.[10] The trial confirmed that, in low-risk patients, the hard endpoints of death and MI were relatively infrequent and were not reduced by PCI when compared with OMT alone.[11] The nuclear substudy of the COURAGE trial compared outcomes of patients with baseline stress MPI and a repeat stress MPI after 6 to 18 months of treatment.[12] These analyses demonstrated that PCI added to OMT was more effective in reducing ischemia and improving angina than OMT alone, particularly in patients with moderate-to-severe pretreatment ischemia. Improvement in the ischemic burden on stress MPI occurred in 33% of patients in the PCI plus OMT arm, compared with 19% of patients in the OMT-alone group. Patients with moderate-to-severe pretreatment ischemia had a 78% improvement in ischemia, compared with 52% in those who had mild pretreatment ischemia ($p = 0.007$). Furthermore, ischemia reduction was associated with a lower risk of death/MI, whereas residual ischemia was associated with a higher risk of death/MI regardless of the treatment strategy (Fig. 17-1). There was a graded relationship between event risk and residual ischemic burden: none (0%) of the patients with no ischemia had death or MI events, while 39.3% of the patients with ≥10% ischemic myocardium had events during follow-up. These data suggest that patients with known CAD and moderate-to-severe perfusion abnormalities would benefit from both OMT and, when appropriate, coronary revascularization. Thus, MPI may be useful in determining the need for coronary revascularization so as to hopefully improve outcomes.

MYOCARDIAL PERFUSION IMAGING AFTER REVASCULARIZATION PROCEDURES

The timing of MPI after revascularization has traditionally been dependent on the presence or absence of symptoms suggestive of myocardial ischemia. The role of MPI for risk stratification in patients who have stable symptoms or those who are asymptomatic is controversial. Shah et al.[13] evaluated the patterns of stress MPI utilization after revascularization in community practices, and determined that out of 28,177 patients who underwent revascularization (21,046 PCI and 7131 CABG); 59% had at least 1 cardiac stress

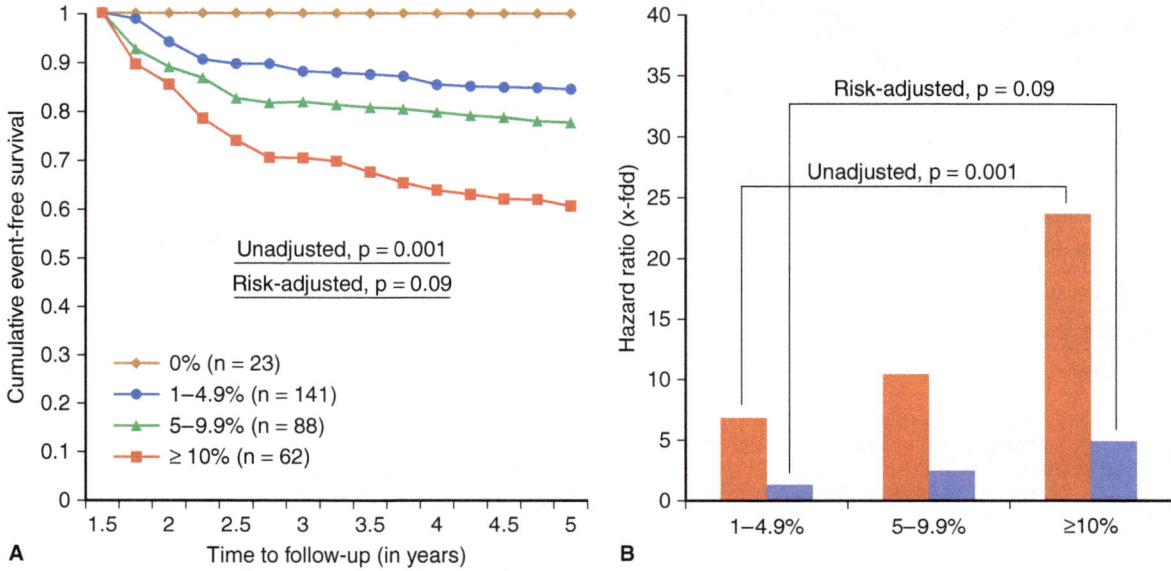

FIGURE 17-1 (**A**) Kaplan–Meier survival for patients by residual ischemia including 0%, 1% to 4.9%, 5% to 9.9%, and ≥10% ischemic myocardium, respectively, after 6 to 18 months of PCI + OMT or OMT. Overall event-free survival was 100%, 84.4%, 77.7%, and 60.7%, respectively, for 0%, 1% to 4.9%, 5% to 9.9%, and ≥10% ischemic myocardium ($p = 0.001$). In a risk-adjusted Cox model (controlling for randomized treatment), this difference was not significant ($p = 0.09$). (**B**) Unadjusted (*red bars*) and risk-adjusted (*blue bars*) hazard ratios for the extent and severity of residual ischemia at 6 to 18 months of follow-up. (Reproduced with permission from Shaw LJ, Berman DS, Maron DJ, et al. Optimal medical therapy with or without percutaneous coronary intervention to reduce ischemic burden: Results from the Clinical Outcomes Utilizing Revascularization and Aggressive Drug Evaluation (COURAGE) trial nuclear substud. *Circulation*. 2008;117(10):1283–1291.)

test within 24 months. As shown in Figure 17-2, the incidence of testing spiked at 6 and 12 months after revascularization, suggesting an association with elective follow-up visits or revascularization anniversary; 11% of those tested underwent subsequent cardiac catheterization and only 5% had repeat revascularization. These findings highlight the low yield of routine testing after revascularization and are aligned

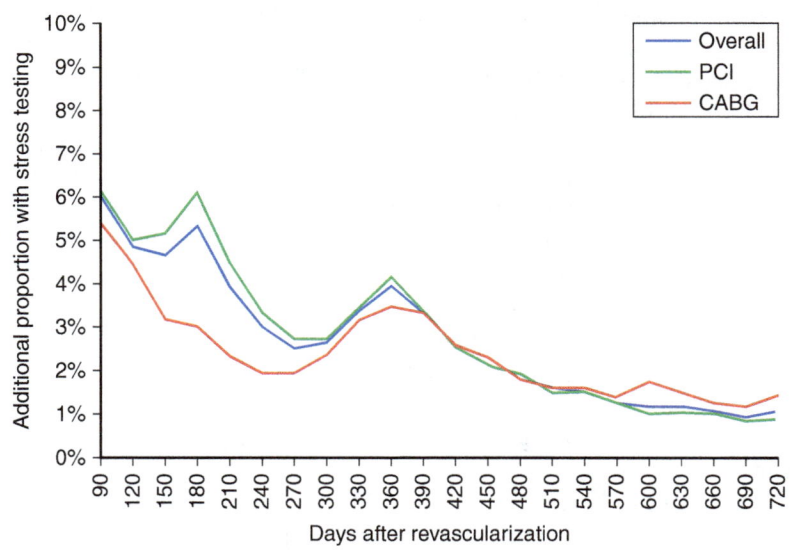

FIGURE 17-2 Graph showing proportion of patients undergoing stress testing after coronary revascularization. Note spikes in testing at 6 and 12 months after revascularization. CABG, coronary artery bypass grafting; PCI, percutaneous coronary intervention. (Reproduced with permission from Shah BR, Cowper PA, O'Brien SM, et al. Patterns of cardiac stress testing after revascularization in community practice. *J Am Coll Cardiol*. 2010;56(16):1328–1334.)

Table 17-1

ACCF/AHA/ASNC Appropriateness Criteria for SPECT MPI Postrevascularization

Evaluation of ischemic equivalent	A
Asymptomatic with incomplete revascularization	A
Prior left main coronary stent	M
Asymptomatic, <5 years, s/p CABG	R
Asymptomatic, ≥5 years, s/p CABG	M
Asymptomatic, <2 years s/p PCI	R
Asymptomatic, ≥2 years s/p PCI	M

A, appropriate; M, may be appropriate; R, rarely appropriate; CABG, coronary artery bypass graft; PCI, percutaneous coronary intervention. Data from Wolk MJ, Bailey SR, Doherty JU, et al. ACCF/AHA/ASE/ASNC/HFSA/HRS/SCAI/SCCT/SCMR/STS 2013 multimodality appropriate use criteria for the detection and risk assessment of stable ischemic heart disease: a report of the American College of Cardiology Foundation Appropriate Use Criteria Task Force, American Heart Association, American Society of Echocardiography, American Society of Nuclear Cardiology, Heart Failure Society of America, Heart Rhythm Society, Society for Cardiovascular Angiography and Interventions, Society of Cardiovascular Computed Tomography, Society for Cardiovascular Magnetic Resonance, and Society of Thoracic Surgeons. *J Am Coll Cardiol.* 2014;63(4):380–406.

with the latest iteration of the ACCF/AHA/American Society of Nuclear Cardiology (ASNC) multimodality AUC for risk assessment of stable ischemic heart disease in which repeat stress imaging studies were deemed "appropriate" for patients with new/worsening symptoms or incomplete revascularization but "rarely appropriate" in asymptomatic patients <2 years post-PCI and "may be appropriate" ≥2 years after PCI (Table 17-1).[14-17] These data suggest that too many stress MPI studies have been performed too soon following revascularization, thus highlighting the importance of adhering to evidence-based practice guidelines and AUC. The value of stress MPI in risk assessment is greatest in symptomatic patients to identify those who would benefit from coronary revascularization.[15]

Coronary Artery Bypass Graft Surgery

CABG is the most commonly performed cardiac surgery.[18,19] The long-term effectiveness of this procedure is limited by graft occlusion and progression of native disease. Evaluation of post-CABG patients with stress MPI depends on the presence or absence of symptoms as well as timing from the surgical procedure.[20]

In a study of 294 patients ≥5 years post-CABG, Palmas et al. demonstrated that Tl-201 reversibility score (a global measure of ischemic burden) and increased lung uptake added significant prognostic information to a clinical model.[6] Similarly, in a study of 1765 post-CABG patients (mean 7.1 ± 5.0 years) who underwent SPECT MPI, Zellweger et al. demonstrated that patients >5 years post-CABG, irrespective of symptoms, and symptomatic patients ≤5 years post-CABG, benefited from MPI testing, as the assessment of ischemia provided a guide to appropriate therapy.[21] However, asymptomatic patients ≤5 years post-CABG have a low cardiac death rate (1.3%) and did not benefit from MPI. Mortality rates were significantly higher in patients with moderate (2.1%) and severely (3.1%) abnormal summed stress score (Fig. 17-3). In addition, in a cohort of 362 patients who underwent SPECT MPI after CABG, Acampa et al. found that event-free survival was 96% in patients with normal SPECT MPI, 86% in those with abnormal MPI without ischemia, and 70% in those with myocardial ischemia ($p = 0.008$), suggesting that SPECT MPI may be a useful tool for risk stratification 5 years after CABG.[22] However, the question remains as to whether coronary revascularization in asymptomatic patients post-CABG can improve patients' outcomes.

Based on these data, the most recent 2013 multimodality AUC for stable ischemic heart disease considered MPI to be "appropriate" for the evaluation of symptomatic patients any time after revascularization as well as asymptomatic patients with incomplete revascularization (Table 17-1).[14] On the other hand, MPI use was considered "may be appropriate" for the evaluation of asymptomatic patients ≥5 years post-CABG, but "rarely appropriate" for asymptomatic patients <5 years post-CABG (Table 17-1). Current multimodality appropriate use criteria (AUC) for radionuclide imaging therefore argue against routine testing of asymptomatic patients, but in selected cases testing may be appropriate in asymptomatic patients >5 years post-CABG.[14,22,23]

Percutaneous Coronary Intervention

The explosion of PCI use in increasingly complex lesions and higher-risk patients with single- or

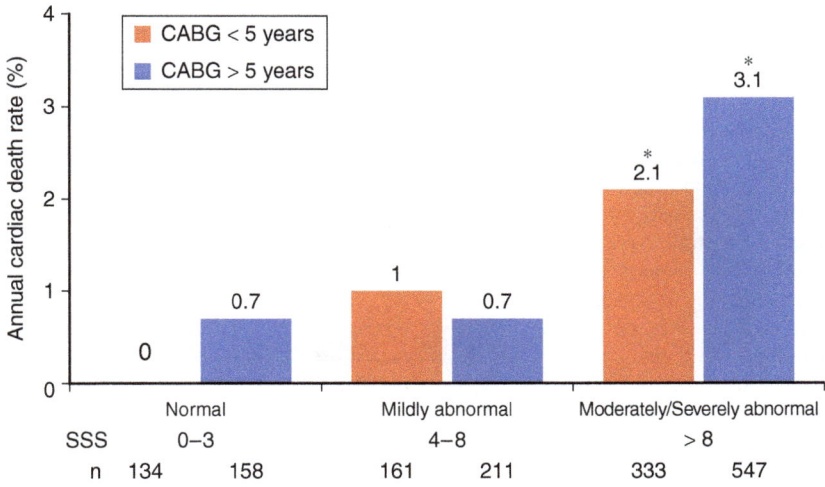

FIGURE 17-3 Annual cardiac death (CD) rates as a function of SSS in patients ≤5 and >5 years post-CABG (n = 1544). Statistically significant increase as a function of SSS ($p = 0.049$ and 0.005 for ≤5 and >5 years, respectively). CABG, coronary artery bypass graft surgery; SSS, summed stress score. (Reproduced with permission from Zellweger MJ, Lewin HC, Lai S, et al. When to stress patients after coronary artery bypass surgery? Risk stratification in patients early and late post-CABG using stress myocardial perfusion SPECT: implications of appropriate clinical strategies. *J Am Coll Cardiol.* 2001;37(1):144–152.)

multivessel disease has created a necessity for detection of restenosis and disease progression as well as risk assessment. A number of clinical studies have documented the usefulness of stress SPECT MPI for identifying restenosis in patients after PCI.[24,25] The optimal time of performing SPECT imaging after PCI is somewhat controversial.[14] Initial studies in the era of balloon angioplasty reported a high frequency of false-positive transient perfusion defects when SPECT imaging was performed in the first few weeks after angioplasty.[26,27] Currently, MPI is considered reasonable in patients with atypical symptoms within a few weeks post-PCI, or those in whom additional ischemia detection is warranted due to incomplete revascularization. Patients with typical symptoms following PCI are best evaluated in the catheterization laboratory. Studies by Giedd et al.[28] and Zellweger et al.[29] suggested that when performed ≥6 months following PCI, MPI can reliably identify patients most at risk for poor long-term outcome. However, there are no randomized clinical data to support this. Peterson et al. evaluated a cohort of 1848 patients who had PCI, of whom 241 were asymptomatic when they had follow-up SPECT MPI. Among those who had the study within the first 2 years (n = 138), no patient required revascularization, whereas in those who had the study after 2 years (n = 103), two patients underwent revascularization. These results suggest that routine stress testing after PCI in asymptomatic patients has low yield, especially within the first 2 years.[30]

When performed shortly after PCI, MPI can identify problems related to the target vessel. Zellweger et al. investigated a cohort of 476 patients who underwent SPECT MPI 6 months after PCI and followed for a mean of 1 year. As shown in Figure 17-4, those who had target vessel ischemia had significantly higher rate of major adverse cardiac events, mostly driven by an increase in target vessel revascularization.[17] In this cohort, ischemia was silent in 68% of patients. However, the impact of coronary revascularization on the outcomes of patients with silent target vessel ischemia is not established.

In contrast, when performed late after PCI, SPECT MPI often identifies CAD in remote arteries, rather than in the target vessel. In a cohort of patients who underwent routine SPECT MPI 5 years after PCI, Zellweger et al. demonstrated that abnormal

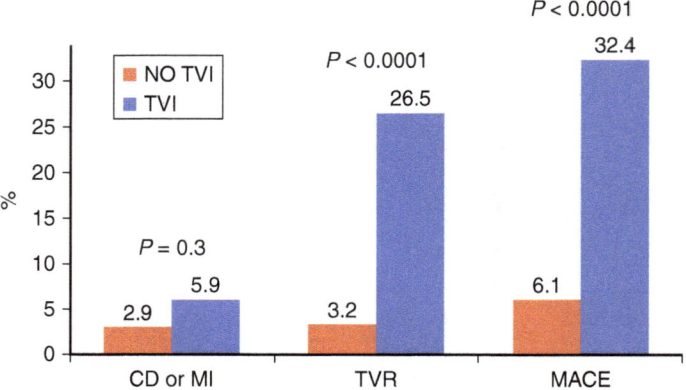

FIGURE 17-4 Event rates in patients with target-vessel ischemia versus patients without. TVI, target vessel ischemia; CD, cardiac death; MI, myocardial infarction; TVR, target revascularization; MACE, major adverse cardiac events (CD, MI, TVR). (Reproduced with permission from Zellweger MJ, Kaiser C, Brunner-La Rocca HP, et al. Value and limitations of targetvessel ischemia in predicting late clinical events after drug-eluting stent implantation, *J Nucl Med.* 2008;49(4):550–556.)

perfusion imaging was frequent irrespective of symptoms, and its utility lies in the detection of persistent or progressive CAD in remote vessel areas rather than in the diagnosis of late intervention-related problems in the treated vessels.[23] These findings are consistent with our understanding of the timeline of in-stent restenosis and PCI-related complications which tend to occur within the first year after intervention.

MYOCARDIAL PERFUSION IMAGING IN ACUTE CORONARY SYNDROME PATIENTS

Thrombolytic Therapy for Acute ST-Segment Elevation Myocardial Infarction (STEMI)

The most effective therapy for patients experiencing STEMI is timely reperfusion therapy with primary PCI. Unfortunately, this is not possible in every setting, and in these cases thrombolytic therapy has been shown to improve myocardial salvage and reduce mortality rate compared to patients not receiving reperfusion therapy. However, even after successful thrombolytic therapy, patients may remain at risk for future events. Post-thrombolysis MPI provides valuable prognostic information by quantifying the infarcted myocardium and the myocardium at risk. Basu et al. demonstrated that reversible perfusion abnormality (ischemia) post-lytic therapy predicts adverse events (death, reinfarction, CHF, and unstable angina) during follow-up (range, 8–32 months) with a hazard ratio of 8.1 (95% CI: 2.7–23.8, $p < 0.001$).[31] Similarly, Dakik et al. showed the esti-mated cardiac event rate after thrombolytic therapy doubled with every 10% decrease in LVEF and 10% increase in MPI defect size.[32] Based on these data, select uncomplicated STEMI patients who receive successful thrombolytic therapy are reasonable candidates for stress MPI.

ST-Elevation Myocardial Infarction without Reperfusion Therapy

Patients who survive STEMI without receiving any reperfusion therapy are also at risk for re-infarction, heart failure, and cardiac death. Thus, they are candidates for risk stratification. Clinically unstable post-STEMI patients (heart failure, arrhythmias, hemodynamic instability) and those with clinical or electrocardiographic evidence of recurrent ischemia need to undergo coronary angiography to determine further management. However, those with uncomplicated STEMI may be candidate for noninvasive risk assessment. Pharmacologic stress MPI has been shown to be superior to conventional submaximal ETT with modified Bruce protocol as a risk stratification tool in these patients.[33-37] Stress testing with dipyridamole, adenosine, or regadenoson may be performed safely as early as 2 to 4 days following an uncomplicated MI. This approach can shorten hospital stay, and more importantly, it has been shown to have an excellent prognostic value, as patients with low-risk myocardial perfusion scan (i.e., without evidence of reversible perfusion defect) have low risk for cardiac events.[33-35] Mahmarian et al. showed that a large area of myocardial ischemia (>10% of the left ventricle) on adenosine stress MPI following noncomplicated MI is superior to coronary angiography in separating patients at increased risk for cardiac events from those at low risk.[35] These data paved the way for the INSPIRE trial.[38] In this multicenter prospective study, Mahmarian et al. enrolled 728 clinically stable survivors of acute MI (ST-elevation and non–ST-elevation ACS) who did not receive coronary revascularization and underwent adenosine SPECT MPI within 10 days of admission. Three risk groups were prospectively defined based on perfusion defect size (PDS) and ischemia perfusion defect size (IPDS); low risk (PDS <20%), intermediate risk (PDS >20% and IPDS <10%), and high risk (PDS >20% and IPDS >10%). The study also prospectively defined discharge and treatment strategies on the basis of MPI risk group and ejection fraction. The cardiac events/death and reinfarction rates were 5.4%, 1.8% in the low-risk, 14%, 9.2% in the intermediate-risk, and 18.6%, 11.6% in the high-risk group ($p < 0.0001$), demonstrating a significant increase in event rates with increasing burden of perfusion abnormalities. Furthermore, the study established the value of commonly measured MPI variables to improve the precision for assessing risk beyond TIMI risk score and ejection fraction, as shown in Figure 17-5.[38] More importantly, the study prospectively demonstrated that low-risk patients are candidates for safe early discharge, whereas patients in the intermediate and high-risk groups should be considered for early invasive management. Moreover, in the high-risk group, coronary revascularization was associated with significant reduction in the cardiac event rate (10% vs. 32%, $p = 0.049$). Thus, the INSPIRE trial demonstrated that MPI not only defines risk, but can also guide patient management. These findings may also be relevant in patients who present late after an ST-elevation MI.[38]

▶ Non–ST-Elevation Acute Coronary Syndrome

It is generally accepted that intermediate- and high-risk patients with non–ST-elevation acute coronary syndrome (ACS) benefit from early invasive strategy aimed at early coronary revascularization.[39] However, low-risk non–ST-elevation ACS, such as those with low TIMI risk score and negative biomarkers, are candidates for a noninvasive risk assessment, especially if they respond well to initial medical management.[40–42] In addition, noninvasive risk stratification prior to invasive testing should be considered in ACS patients with a relative contraindication for coronary angiography, such as those with bleeding diatheses or chronic kidney disease.[43]

Exercise or pharmacologic stress MPI can be used safely to assess risk for cardiac events (death or MI) in patients with unstable angina following the initial response to medical management.[44–46] The safety of

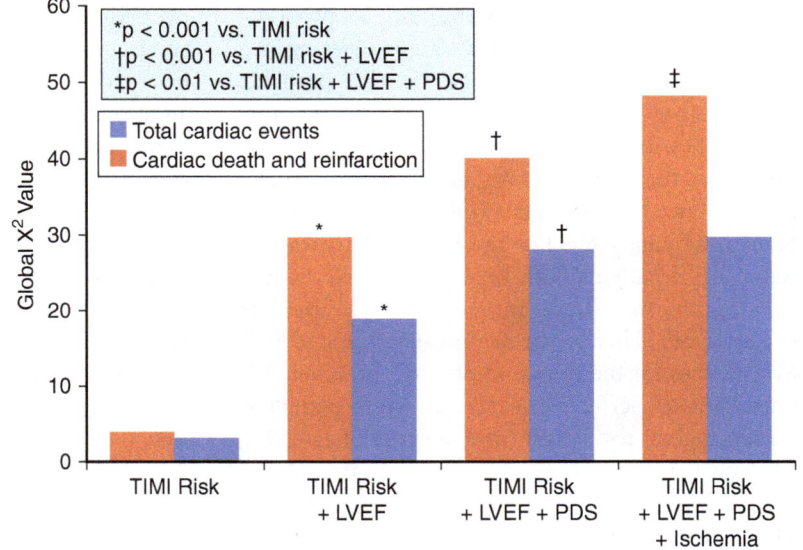

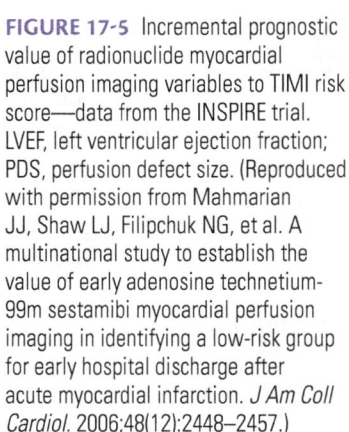

FIGURE 17-5 Incremental prognostic value of radionuclide myocardial perfusion imaging variables to TIMI risk score—data from the INSPIRE trial. LVEF, left ventricular ejection fraction; PDS, perfusion defect size. (Reproduced with permission from Mahmarian JJ, Shaw LJ, Filipchuk NG, et al. A multinational study to establish the value of early adenosine technetium-99m sestamibi myocardial perfusion imaging in identifying a low-risk group for early hospital discharge after acute myocardial infarction. *J Am Coll Cardiol.* 2006;48(12):2448–2457.)

adenosine and dipyridamole vasodilator stress performed 2 to 7 days after ACS is well established.[33–36] More recently, regadenoson vasodilator stress has been shown to be associated with similarly low adverse event rates among patients undergoing in-hospital MPI for the assessment of ACS or elevated cardiac biomarkers.[37]

SPECT MPI has been shown to be safe and effective for risk stratification in patients presenting with ACS. Brown et al. and Stratmann et al. demonstrated that stress MPI can effectively risk stratify patients with unstable angina for long-term adverse cardiac events, and thus identifying patients with inducible ischemia as candidates for coronary angiography and revascularization.[44,46] However, with demonstrated effectiveness of early invasive management of ACS, the role of stress MPI in the risk stratification of ACS patients in the modern era has significantly diminished. Nonetheless, there may be a role for MPI in the risk assessment of low-risk non–ST-elevation ACS and those with relative contraindication for coronary angiography.[39]

MYOCARDIAL PERFUSION IMAGING TO ASSESS EFFICACY OF MEDICAL THERAPY

Intensive medical therapy with risk factor modification is essential in the management of patients with coronary artery disease. While high-risk patients gain a survival benefit from CABG, low- and moderate-risk patients have equivalent outcomes with respect to mortality with either approach (medical management or revascularization). Appropriate medical therapy would include antiplatelet agents, beta-blockers, lipid-lowering agents, and probably angiotensin-converting enzyme (ACE) inhibitors in diabetics and patients with impaired LV function. Since the degree and extent of ischemia predict future events, MPI has been used to assess the impact of medical management on the burden of myocardial ischemia in patients with known coronary disease. Importantly, the use of antianginal medications is usually avoided before performing diagnostic SPECT MPI studies for the detection of CAD, however, it is important to perform the studies while patient is on antianginal regimen for the purpose of assessing prognosis and response to therapy. Data from Mahmarian et al. demonstrated that quantitative exercise Tl-201 MPI is highly reproducible and can be used to accurately interpret temporal changes in MPI in individual patients.[47] Moreover, in the ADVANCE MPI trials, Mahmarian et al. demonstrated, in same patient controls, that adenosine and regadenoson produce similar perfusion defects; thus temporal changes with repeat testing can be followed when either of these vasodilator stress agents is used.[48]

The beneficial impact of various pharmacologic interventions on the clinical outcomes of patients with CAD has been well established. Medical therapy has been associated with improvement in myocardial perfusion defects as a result of either decreased oxygen demand (beta blockers)[49–51] or improved coronary blood flow (nitrates, calcium channel blockers [CCBs], and statins).[52–54] In asymptomatic patients with CAD and known myocardial perfusion abnormalities, the 2013 ACCF/AHA/ASNC multimodality AUC for radionuclide MPI deem stress testing "rarely appropriate" when last stress imaging study was done <2 years prior, but "may be appropriate" if previous stress imaging was performed ≥2 years prior.[40]

▶ Beta Blockers

Among the antianginal medications, beta-blockers have been shown in multiple studies to markedly decrease the burden of exercise-induced ischemia or even normalize the test.[49,55] The anti-ischemic effect of beta-blockers is mediated primarily by decreasing the heart rate, prolonging diastole, increasing coronary perfusion time and myocardial oxygen extraction, and decreasing myocardial oxygen consumption in ischemic tissue.[50] At the cellular level, beta blockers alter myocyte metabolism providing additional myocardial protection against ischemia. One week of oral propranolol treatment has been shown to improve MPI abnormalities in men with established CAD.[49] Similarly, acute propranolol administration in patients with dobutamine-induced reversible perfusion abnormalities has been shown to dampen heart rate response (peak heart rate 83 ± 18 vs. 125 ± 17, $p < 0.001$), rate–pressure product (14,169 ± 4,248 vs. 19,894 ± 3,985; $p < 0.001$), and myocardial ischemia score (6.9 ± 5.8 vs. 10.1 ± 7.1, $p = 0.047$) despite a higher infusion dose.[50] The extent of perfusion abnormalities has been shown to be significantly reduced with beta blockers even with the use of vasodilator stress.[55]

Nitrates

The anti-ischemic effect of nitroglycerin has been attributed to the redistribution of blood flow from normal to ischemic myocardium through dilation of collateral vessels. In addition, nitroglycerine reduces myocardial oxygen consumption by producing a systemic venodilation leading to a reduction in systemic venous return, left ventricular dimensions, and myocardial wall stress.

Either in conjunction with beta blockers[51] or alone,[52,54] both of these agents decrease the size of reversible defects (particularly in patients with large ischemic perfusion defects). Mahmarian et al. prospectively evaluated whether short-term (6.1 ± 1.8 days) transdermal nitroglycerin patches could limit the extent of exercise-induced LV ischemia as assessed by quantitative Tl-201 tomography. Patients randomized to receive active patch therapy had a significant reduction in their total perfusion defect size (−8.9 ± 11.1%) compared with placebo-treated patients (−1.8 ± 6.1%, $p = 0.04$). The reduction in perfusion defect size was most apparent in those with the largest (≥20%) baseline perfusion defects (−11.4 ± 13.4% vs. 1.0 ± 3.6%, respectively, $p < 0.02$). Nitrate therapy did not significantly reduce heart rate, blood pressure, or double product, in consistence with its known mechanisms of action.[54]

Calcium Channel Blockers

The primary benefit of CCBs seems to be a reduction in myocardial oxygen demand, which is achieved by decreasing arterial tone, peripheral vascular resistance, intraventricular pressure, and wall stress. CCBs also enhance myocardial perfusion through their effects on myocardial microcirculation and metabolism. They improve coronary flow in CAD by selectively dilating larger arterioles and may prevent coronary spasm.[52]

Limited data suggest that acute administration of nifedipine before exercise planar MPI resulted in significant improvement in perfusion (defined as >20% increase) in approximately one-half of patients and in one-fourth of segments compared with no CCB administration. Chronic administration of nifedipine and nicorandil in two separate studies before exercise SPECT reduced the defect extent and severity.[52]

Lipid-lowering Agents

The impact of lipid-lowering agents in the secondary prevention of coronary disease has been demonstrated in multiple large studies, such as CARE,[53] CTT,[56] 4S,[57] TNT,[58] PROVE-IT,[59] and JUPITER.[60] Statins improve endothelial function and preserve coronary perfusion independent of their reduction in cholesterol. They increase smooth muscle relaxation, decrease oxidative stress, and prevent vascular inflammation. Although statins may halt the progression or cause a regression of atherosclerosis as assessed by coronary angiography and intravascular ultrasound, the degree of regression is slight compared with the substantial improvement in clinical outcomes which is likely related to plaque stabilization. Using rest-dipyridamole positron emission tomography (PET), Gould et al. demonstrated that there were statistically significant improvements in size and severity of perfusion abnormalities after intensive 90-day cholesterol lowering compared to baseline control.[61] Thus, short-term intensive cholesterol lowering improves myocardial perfusion before anatomic regression of stenosis occurs. Schwartz et al. used SPECT imaging in patients with CAD and hypercholesterolemia to assess serial changes in myocardial perfusion associated with cholesterol-lowering therapy.[62] Following improvement in total cholesterol (pretreatment: 223 ± 51, posttreatment: 147 ± 33, $p < 0.001$), the stress defect score (% ischemic myocardium) was significantly improved (pretreatment: 19 ± 16, posttreatment: 9 ± 13, $p = 0.022$). Furthermore, the same investigators studied the effect of short-term (6 weeks) or long-term (6 months) pravastatin in dyslipidemic patients with baseline MPI ischemic defects.[63,64] Despite a significant reduction of low-density lipoprotein (LDL) at 6 weeks (33%, $p < 0.001$), myocardial perfusion scores were reduced only at 6 months (12.6 ± 5.7 at baseline, 9.4 ± 6.2 at 6 months, $p < 0.01$). The time course of reduced perfusion abnormalities, rather than LDL reduction, paralleled documented clinical benefit.[53,57,61,65]

Angiotensin-Converting Enzyme Inhibitors

There is notable evidence that ACE inhibitors exert a beneficial effect in patients with known coronary disease. The mechanism for ACE inhibitors benefit is complex (improved endothelial function, vasodilation and reduced afterload, antiplatelet effect, and inhibition of neurohormonal activation). There is no large study to examine their direct anti-ischemic mechanism using MPI. In two studies, ACE inhibition was associated with improved epicardial[66] and microvascular blood flow[67]; the mechanism is predominantly endothelium mediated. After 12 weeks of treatment, enalapril delayed the onset of ischemic ST-segment depression during ETT (5.6 ± 1.9 minutes in the enalapril group vs. 4.4 ± 1.3 minutes in the placebo group, $p < 0.05$) without affecting the double product.[68] Further studies are needed to elucidate a direct anti-ischemic mechanism of ACE inhibitors and explore the role of MPI in monitoring such an effect.

▶ Lifestyle Modifications

The widespread interest in the noninvasive management of coronary atherosclerosis has brought new attention to the impact of various lifestyle changes on the prognosis of coronary disease. Diet, exercise, and behavioral interventions are generally advised for patients with documented coronary disease. The impact of these changes on the extent of atherosclerosis, as determined by angiography, is modest. However, after 5 years of intensive risk factor modification, the size and severity of perfusion abnormalities on rest-dipyridamole PET imaging improved in the intervention group compared to controls.[69]

CONCLUSIONS

The value of stress MPI is well established in patients with CAD for both risk stratification and clinical decision making. This has grown to include risk assessment after coronary revascularization procedures and medical therapies and in patients with ACS. The decision regarding when to repeat testing is difficult and somewhat controversial. Appropriate indications for imaging include any patients who develop new or worsening symptoms or in those with incomplete revascularization when additional revascularization is feasible. Repeat stress MPI "may be appropriate" in asymptomatic patients ≥5 years after CABG or ≥2 years after PCI; imaging before these periods in asymptomatic patients is considered "rarely appropriate."

REFERENCES

1. Writing Group Members, Mozaffarian D, Benjamin EJ, Go AS, et al. Heart Disease and Stroke Statistics-2016 Update: A Report From the American Heart Association. *Circulation*. 2016;133(4):e38–360.
2. Gibbons RJ, Balady GJ, Bricker JT, et al. ACC/AHA 2002 guideline update for exercise testing: summary article. A report of the American College of Cardiology/American Heart Association Task Force on Practice Guidelines (Committee to Update the 1997 Exercise Testing Guidelines). *J Am Coll Cardiol*. 2002;40(8):1531–1540.
3. Lee TH, Boucher CA. Clinical practice. Noninvasive tests in patients with stable coronary artery disease. *N Engl J Med*. 2001;344(24):1840–1845.
4. Vanzetto G, Halimi S, Hammoud T, et al. Prediction of cardiovascular events in clinically selected high-risk NIDDM patients. Prognostic value of exercise stress test and thallium-201 single-photon emission computed tomography. *Diabetes Care*. 1999;22(1):19–26.
5. Hecht HS, Shaw RE, Chin HL, Ryan C, Stertzer SH, Myler RK. Silent ischemia after coronary angioplasty: Evaluation of restenosis and extent of ischemia in asymptomatic patients by tomographic thallium-201 exercise imaging and comparison with symptomatic patients. *J Am Coll Cardiol*. 1991;17(3):670–677.
6. Palmas W, Bingham S, Diamond GA, et al. Incremental prognostic value of exercise thallium-201 myocardial single-photon emission computed tomography late after coronary artery bypass surgery. *J Am Coll Cardiol*. 1995;25(2):403–409.
7. Klocke FJ, Baird MG, Lorell BH, et al. ACC/AHA/ASNC guidelines for the clinical use of cardiac radionuclide imaging–executive summary: a report of the American College of Cardiology/American Heart Association Task Force on Practice Guidelines (ACC/AHA/ASNC Committee to Revise the 1995 Guidelines for the Clinical Use of Cardiac Radionuclide Imaging). *J Am Coll Cardiol*. 2003;42(7):1318–1333.
8. Travin MI, Katz MS, Moulton AW, Miele NJ, Sharaf BL, Johnson LL. Accuracy of dipyridamole SPECT imaging in identifying individual coronary stenoses and multivessel disease in women versus men. *J Nucl Cardiol*. 2000;7(3):213–220.
9. Farzaneh-Far A, Phillips HR, Shaw LK, Starr AZ, Fiuzat M, O'Connor CM, et al. Ischemia change in stable coronary artery disease is an independent predictor of death and myocardial infarction. *JACC Cardiovasc Imaging*. 2012;5(7):715–724.
10. Boden WE, O'Rourke RA, Teo KK, et al. Optimal medical therapy with or without PCI for stable coronary disease. *N Engl J Med*. 2007;356(15):1503–1516.
11. Prasad A, Rihal C, Holmes DR, Jr. The COURAGE trial in perspective. *Catheter Cardiovasc Interv*. 2008;72(1):54–59.
12. Shaw LJ, Berman DS, Maron DJ, et al. Optimal medical therapy with or without percutaneous coronary intervention to reduce ischemic burden: Results from the Clinical Outcomes Utilizing Revascularization and Aggressive Drug Evaluation

(COURAGE) trial nuclear substudy. *Circulation*. 2008;117(10): 1283-1291.
13. Shah BR, Cowper PA, O'Brien SM, et al. Patterns of cardiac stress testing after revascularization in community practice. *J Am Coll Cardiol*. 2010;56(16):1328-1334.
14. Wolk MJ, Bailey SR, Doherty JU, et al. ACCF/AHA/ASE/ASNC/HFSA/HRS/SCAI/SCCT/SCMR/STS 2013 multimodality appropriate use criteria for the detection and risk assessment of stable ischemic heart disease: a report of the American College of Cardiology Foundation Appropriate Use Criteria Task Force, American Heart Association, American Society of Echocardiography, American Society of Nuclear Cardiology, Heart Failure Society of America, Heart Rhythm Society, Society for Cardiovascular Angiography and Interventions, Society of Cardiovascular Computed Tomography, Society for Cardiovascular Magnetic Resonance, and Society of Thoracic Surgeons. *J Am Coll Cardiol*. 2014;63(4):380-406.
15. Beller GA. Stress testing after coronary revascularization too much, too soon. *J Am Coll Cardiol*. 2010;56(16):1335-1337.
16. Zellweger MJ, Kaiser C, Jeger R, et al. Coronary artery disease progression late after successful stent implantation. *J Am Coll Cardiol*. 2012;59(9):793-799.
17. Zellweger MJ, Kaiser C, Brunner-La Rocca HP, et al. Value and limitations of target-vessel ischemia in predicting late clinical events after drug-eluting stent implantation. *J Nucl Med*. 2008;49(4):550-556.
18. Beller GA, Zaret BL. Contributions of nuclear cardiology to diagnosis and prognosis of patients with coronary artery disease. *Circulation*. 2000;101(12):1465-1478.
19. Gibbons RS. American Society of Nuclear Cardiology project on myocardial perfusion imaging: measuring outcomes in response to emerging guidelines. *J Nucl Cardiol*. 1996;3(5):436-442.
20. Berman DS, Kang X, Schisterman EF, et al. Serial changes on quantitative myocardial perfusion SPECT in patients undergoing revascularization or conservative therapy. *J Nucl Cardiol*. 2001;8(4):428-437.
21. Zellweger MJ, Lewin HC, Lai S, et al. When to stress patients after coronary artery bypass surgery? Risk stratification in patients early and late post-CABG using stress myocardial perfusion SPECT: Implications of appropriate clinical strategies. *J Am Coll Cardiol*. 2001;37(1):144-152.
22. Acampa W, Petretta M, Evangelista L, et al. Stress cardiac single-photon emission computed tomographic imaging late after coronary artery bypass surgery for risk stratification and estimation of time to cardiac events. *J Thorac Cardiovasc Surg*. 2008;136(1):46-51.
23. Zellweger MJ, Fahrni G, Ritter M, et al. Prognostic value of "routine" cardiac stress imaging 5 years after percutaneous coronary intervention: the prospective long-term observational BASKET (Basel Stent Kosteneffektivitats Trial) LATE IMAGING study. *JACC Cardiovasc Interv*. 2014;7(6):615-621.
24. Hecht HS, Shaw RE, Bruce TR, Ryan C, Stertzer SH, Myler RK. Usefulness of tomographic thallium-201 imaging for detection of restenosis after percutaneous transluminal coronary angioplasty. *Am J Cardiol*. 1990;66(19):1314-1318.
25. Harb SC, Marwick TH. Prognostic value of stress imaging after revascularization: a systematic review of stress echocardiography and stress nuclear imaging. *Am Heart J*. 2014; 167(1):77-85.
26. Manyari DE, Knudtson M, Kloiber R, Roth D. Sequential thallium-201 myocardial perfusion studies after successful percutaneous transluminal coronary artery angioplasty: delayed resolution of exercise-induced scintigraphic abnormalities. *Circulation*. 1988;77(1):86-95.
27. Wilson RF, Johnson MR, Marcus ML, et al. The effect of coronary angioplasty on coronary flow reserve. *Circulation*. 1988;77(4):873-885.
28. Giedd KN, Bergmann SR. Myocardial perfusion imaging following percutaneous coronary intervention: The importance of restenosis, disease progression, and directed reintervention. *J Am Coll Cardiol*. 2004;43(3):328-336.
29. Zellweger MJ, Weinbacher M, Zutter AW, et al. Long-term outcome of patients with silent versus symptomatic ischemia six months after percutaneous coronary intervention and stenting. *J Am Coll Cardiol*. 2003;42(1):33-40.
30. Peterson T, Askew JW, Bell M, Crusan D, Hodge D, Gibbons RJ. Low yield of stress imaging in a population-based study of asymptomatic patients after percutaneous coronary intervention. *Circ Cardiovasc Imaging*. 2014;7(3):438-445.
31. Basu S, Senior R, Dore C, Lahiri A. Value of thallium-201 imaging in detecting adverse cardiac events after myocardial infarction and thrombolysis: A follow up of 100 consecutive patients. *BMJ*. 1996;313(7061):844-848.
32. Dakik HA, Mahmarian JJ, Kimball KT, Koutelou MG, Medrano R, Verani MS. Prognostic value of exercise ^{201}Tl tomography in patients treated with thrombolytic therapy during acute myocardial infarction. *Circulation*. 1996;94(11):2735-2742.
33. Brown KA, Heller GV, Landin RS, et al. Early dipyridamole (99m)Tc-sestamibi single photon emission computed tomographic imaging 2 to 4 days after acute myocardial infarction predicts in-hospital and postdischarge cardiac events: Comparison with submaximal exercise imaging. *Circulation*. 1999;100(20):2060-2066.
34. Brown KA, O'Meara J, Chambers CE, Plante DA. Ability of dipyridamole-thallium-201 imaging one to four days after acute myocardial infarction to predict in-hospital and late recurrent myocardial ischemic events. *Am J Cardiol*. 1990; 65(3):160-167.
35. Mahmarian JJ, Mahmarian AC, Marks GF, Pratt CM, Verani MS. Role of adenosine thallium-201 tomography for defining long-term risk in patients after acute myocardial infarction. *J Am Coll Cardiol*. 1995;25(6):1333-1340.
36. Gimple LW, Hutter AM, Jr., Guiney TE, Boucher CA. Prognostic utility of predischarge dipyridamole-thallium imaging compared to predischarge submaximal exercise electrocardiography and maximal exercise thallium imaging after uncomplicated acute myocardial infarction. *Am J Cardiol*. 1989;64(19):1243-1248.
37. Rai M, Ahlberg AW, Marwell J, et al. Safety of vasodilator stress myocardial perfusion imaging in patients with elevated cardiac biomarkers. *J Nucl Cardiol*. 2016.
38. Mahmarian JJ, Shaw LJ, Filipchuk NG, et al. A multinational study to establish the value of early adenosine technetium-99m sestamibi myocardial perfusion imaging in identifying a low-risk group for early hospital discharge after acute myocardial infarction. *J Am Coll Cardiol*. 2006;48(12):2448-2457.
39. Amsterdam EA, Wenger NK, Brindis RG, et al. 2014 AHA/ACC Guideline for the Management of Patients with Non-ST-Elevation Acute Coronary Syndromes: a report of the

American College of Cardiology/American Heart Association Task Force on Practice Guidelines. *J Am Coll Cardiol.* 2014;64(24):e139-228.
40. Hendel RC, Berman DS, Di Carli MF, et al. ACCF/ASNC/ACR/AHA/ASE/SCCT/SCMR/SNM 2009 Appropriate Use Criteria for Cardiac Radionuclide Imaging: A Report of the American College of Cardiology Foundation Appropriate Use Criteria Task Force, the American Society of Nuclear Cardiology, the American College of Radiology, the American Heart Association, the American Society of Echocardiography, the Society of Cardiovascular Computed Tomography, the Society for Cardiovascular Magnetic Resonance, and the Society of Nuclear Medicine. Endorsed by the American College of Emergency Physicians. *J Am Coll Cardiol.* 2009;53(23):2201-2229.
41. Antman EM, Cohen M, Bernink PJ, et al. The TIMI risk score for unstable angina/non-ST elevation MI: A method for prognostication and therapeutic decision making. *JAMA.* 2000;284(7):835-842.
42. Cannon CP, Weintraub WS, Demopoulos LA, et al. Comparison of early invasive and conservative strategies in patients with unstable coronary syndromes treated with the glycoprotein IIb/IIIa inhibitor tirofiban. *N Engl J Med.* 2001;344(25):1879-1887.
43. Doukky R, Golzar Y. Safety of stress testing in patients with elevated cardiac biomarkers: Are all modalities created equal? *J Nucl Cardiol.* 2016. [Epub ahead of print]
44. Brown KA. Prognostic value of thallium-201 myocardial perfusion imaging in patients with unstable angina who respond to medical treatment. *J Am Coll Cardiol.* 1991;17(5):1053-1057.
45. Freeman MR, Chisholm RJ, Armstrong PW. Usefulness of exercise electrocardiography and thallium scintigraphy in unstable angina pectoris in predicting the extent and severity of coronary artery disease. *Am J Cardiol.* 1988;62(17):1164-1170.
46. Stratmann HG, Williams GA, Wittry MD, Chaitman BR, Miller DD. Exercise technetium-99m sestamibi tomography for cardiac risk stratification of patients with stable chest pain. *Circulation.* 1994;89(2):615-622.
47. Mahmarian JJ, Moye LA, Verani MS, Bloom MF, Pratt CM. High reproducibility of myocardial perfusion defects in patients undergoing serial exercise thallium-201 tomography. *Am J Cardiol.* 1995;75(16):1116-1119.
48. Mahmarian JJ, Cerqueira MD, Iskandrian AE, et al. Regadenoson induces comparable left ventricular perfusion defects as adenosine: a quantitative analysis from the ADVANCE MPI 2 trial. *JACC Cardiovasc Imaging.* 2009;2(8):959-968.
49. Steele P, Sklar J, Kirch D, Vogel R, Rhodes CA. Thallium-201 myocardial imaging during maximal and submaximal exercise: comparison of submaximal exercise with propranolol. *Am Heart J.* 1983;106(6):1353-1357.
50. Shehata AR, Gillam LD, Mascitelli VA, et al. Impact of acute propranolol administration on dobutamine-induced myocardial ischemia as evaluated by myocardial perfusion imaging and echocardiography. *Am J Cardiol.* 1997;80(3):268-272.
51. Marie PY, Danchin N, Branly F, et al. Effects of medical therapy on outcome assessment using exercise thallium-201 single photon emission computed tomography imaging: Evidence of a protective effect of beta-blocking antianginal medications. *J Am Coll Cardiol.* 1999;34(1):113-121.
52. Yamazaki J, Ohsawa H, Uchi T, et al. Study of the efficacy of nicorandil in patients with ischaemic heart disease using Exercise-T1-201 myocardial tomography. *Eur J Clin Pharmacol.* 1993;44(3):211-217.
53. Flaker GC, Warnica JW, Sacks FM, et al. Pravastatin prevents clinical events in revascularized patients with average cholesterol concentrations. Cholesterol and Recurrent Events CARE Investigators. *J Am Coll Cardiol.* 1999;34(1):106-112.
54. Mahmarian JJ, Fenimore NL, Marks GF, et al. Transdermal nitroglycerin patch therapy reduces the extent of exercise-induced myocardial ischemia: Results of a double-blind, placebo-controlled trial using quantitative thallium-201 tomography. *J Am Coll Cardiol.* 1994;24(1):25-32.
55. Taillefer R, Ahlberg AW, Masood Y, et al. Acute beta-blockade reduces the extent and severity of myocardial perfusion defects with dipyridamole Tc-99m sestamibi SPECT imaging. *J Am Coll Cardiol.* 2003;42(8):1475-1483.
56. Cholesterol Treatment Trialists C, Mihaylova B, Emberson J, Blackwell L, et al. The effects of lowering LDL cholesterol with statin therapy in people at low risk of vascular disease: Meta-analysis of individual data from 27 randomised trials. *Lancet.* 2012;380(9841):581-590.
57. Scandinavian Simvastatin Survival Study Group. Randomised trial of cholesterol lowering in 4444 patients with coronary heart disease: the Scandinavian Simvastatin Survival Study (4S). *Lancet.* 1994;344(8934):1383-1389.
58. LaRosa JC, Grundy SM, Waters DD, et al. Intensive lipid lowering with atorvastatin in patients with stable coronary disease. *N Engl J Med.* 2005;352(14):1425-1435.
59. Cannon CP, Braunwald E, McCabe CH, et al. Intensive versus moderate lipid lowering with statins after acute coronary syndromes. *N Engl J Med.* 2004;350(15):1495-1504.
60. Ridker PM, Danielson E, Fonseca FA, et al. Rosuvastatin to prevent vascular events in men and women with elevated C-reactive protein. *N Engl J Med.* 2008;359(21):2195-2207.
61. Gould KL, Martucci JP, Goldberg DI, et al. Short-term cholesterol lowering decreases size and severity of perfusion abnormalities by positron emission tomography after dipyridamole in patients with coronary artery disease. A potential noninvasive marker of healing coronary endothelium. *Circulation.* 1994;89(4):1530-1538.
62. Schwartz RG. Beyond the cholesterol profile: monitoring therapeutic effectiveness of statin therapy. *J Nucl Cardiol.* 2001;8(4):528-532.
63. Schwartz RG, Pearson TA, Kalaria VG, et al. Prospective serial evaluation of myocardial perfusion and lipids during the first six months of pravastatin therapy: Coronary artery disease regression single photon emission computed tomography monitoring trial. *J Am Coll Cardiol.* 2003;42(4):600-610.
64. Zoghbi GJ, Dorfman TA, Iskandrian AE. The effects of medications on myocardial perfusion. *J Am Coll Cardiol.* 2008;52(6):401-416.
65. Rubins HB, Robins SJ, Collins D, et al. Gemfibrozil for the secondary prevention of coronary heart disease in men with low levels of high-density lipoprotein cholesterol. Veterans Affairs High-Density Lipoprotein Cholesterol Intervention Trial Study Group. *N Engl J Med.* 1999;341(6):410-418.

66. Prasad A, Husain S, Quyyumi AA. Abnormal flow-mediated epicardial vasomotion in human coronary arteries is improved by angiotensin-converting enzyme inhibition: A potential role of bradykinin. *J Am Coll Cardiol*. 1999;33(3):796–804.
67. Schlaifer JD, Wargovich TJ, O'Neill B, et al. Effects of quinapril on coronary blood flow in coronary artery disease patients with endothelial dysfunction. TREND Investigators. Trial on Reversing Endothelial Dysfunction. *Am J Cardiol*. 1997;80(12):1594–1597.
68. van den Heuvel AF, Dunselman PH, Kingma T, et al. Reduction of exercise-induced myocardial ischemia during add-on treatment with the angiotensin-converting enzyme inhibitor enalapril in patients with normal left ventricular function and optimal beta blockade. *J Am Coll Cardiol*. 2001;37(2):470–474.
69. Gould KL, Ornish D, Scherwitz L, et al. Changes in myocardial perfusion abnormalities by positron emission tomography after long-term, intense risk factor modification. *JAMA*. 1995;274(11):894–901.

Radionuclide Imaging in Heart Failure

CHAPTER 18

Gautam V. Ramani and Prem Soman

INTRODUCTION

Despite many advances in therapy, chronic heart failure remains a prevalent condition with a high mortality rate.[1] The successful treatment of heart failure patients requires establishing an accurate diagnosis, identifying potentially reversible etiologies, determining the optimal therapy, and reliable risk assessment for stratification of patients at high risk for worsening. Several of these aspects of heart failure care can be gainfully evaluated via radionuclide imaging. This chapter will review established applications of radionuclide imaging in heart failure.

The clinician has several goals when evaluating a heart failure patient. One potential work flow sequence for the evaluation of newly diagnosed heart failure is shown in Figure 18-1. Once a clinical diagnosis of the syndrome of heart failure is made, an initial step is often the determination of left ventricular (LV) systolic function. Approximately one-half of patients will have heart failure with preserved ejection fraction (HFpEF, EF ≥40%), while the remainder will have LV systolic dysfunction (heart failure with reduced ejection fraction HFrEF, EF <40%).[2] Radionuclide imaging methods including single-photon emission computed tomography (SPECT), radionuclide ventriculography (RVG), and positron emission tomography (PET) can all provide highly accurate and repeatable measures of LV systolic and diastolic function (Chapter 11). Despite being as prevalent as HFrRF, the treatment of HFpEF remains largely symptom based and empirical, with very little supportive data from clinical trials. For patients with systolic dysfunction, HFrEF, a critical next step is the determination of etiology. Etiology evaluation can include identifying specific and potentially remediable causes such as valvular disease, coronary artery disease (CAD), specific cardiomyopathies, and pericardial disease. When extensive CAD is found, testing for ischemia and viability is helpful to determine benefit from coronary revascularization. Radionuclide imaging has critical roles in the determination of heart failure etiology (see below), identifying patients for coronary revascularization (Chapter 21), and the evaluation for specific cardiomyopathies such as amyloidosis and sarcoidosis (Chapter 24). For patients with nonischemic cardiomyopathy (NICM), and those with persistent LV systolic dysfunction after specific intervention, a combination of guideline-directed medical therapy (GDMT), and device therapy in selected patients (implantable cardioverter defibrillator [ICD], and cardiac resynchronization therapy [CRT]), form the cornerstone of current recommendations. Evolving applications such as myocardial sympathetic neuronal function (Chapter 23) and dyssynchrony imaging (Chapter 11) may have relevance to the selection of patients for ICD and CRT. Furthermore, PET/CT imaging with F-18 fluorodeoxyglucose (FDG) has established utility in the challenging area of diagnosing device infections (Chapter 24). A minority of patients will receive advanced heart failure therapies, including left and right ventricular assist devices (LVAD and RVAD) and cardiac transplantation. In posttransplant patients,

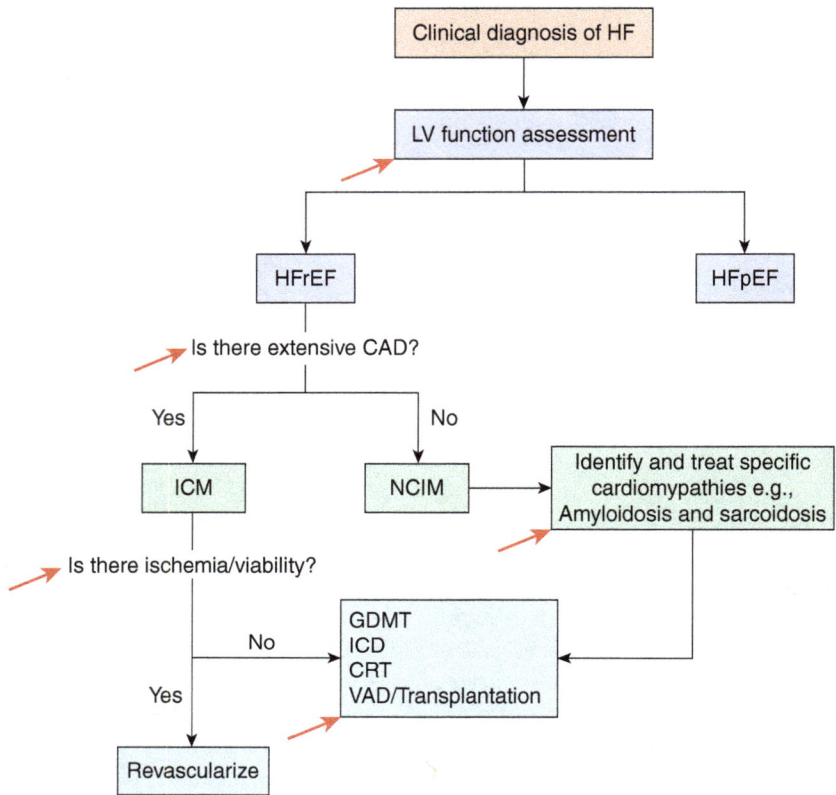

FIGURE 18-1 Scheme for the evaluation of patients with heart failure. Arrows indicate steps where radionuclide imaging has application. HF, heart failure; LV, left Ventricle; HFrEF, heart failure with reduced ejection fraction; HFpEF, heart failure with preserved ejection fraction; CAD, coronary artery disease; ICM, ischemic cardiomyopathy; NICM, nonischemic cardiomyopathy; GDMT, guideline-directed medical therapy; ICD, implantable cardioverter defibrillator; CRT, cardiac resynchronization therapy; VAD, ventricular assist device.

radionuclide imaging has important prognostic value, which may influence therapeutic options in patients with suspected allograft vasculopathy (see below).

▶ Determination of Heart Failure Etiology

The etiology of heart failure varies considerably depending on the population studied.[3] Based on clinical trial data on patients with established heart failure, CAD is the attributed etiology for 60% to 70% of heart failure in the United States.[4] However, the mere presence of CAD in the setting of a cardiomyopathy does not imply an ischemic etiology to the LV dysfunction. What is traditionally referred to as significant CAD in the literature, that is, ≥50% luminal stenosis, may be encountered in 15% to 30% of patients with a dilated cardiomyopathy, and thus may not be sufficiently sensitive for accurate risk stratification of the heart failure population. Felker et al. addressed this question, and tested a more stringent definition of ischemic cardiomyopathy for characterization of heart failure patients.[5] They defined ischemic cardiomyopathy as LV dysfunction with one or more of the following angiographic criteria: significant left main or proximal left anterior descending coronary artery stenosis, at least two-vessel disease with ≥70% stenosis, or single-vessel disease with prior myocardial infarction, or prior coronary revascularization. For example, a patient with LV dysfunction and a 70% stenosis of one major epicardial vessel without antecedent myocardial infarction

Table 18-1

Performance Characteristics of Gated SPECT Tc-99m Sestamibi for CAD Diagnosis in Patients with New-Onset Heart Failure from the IMAGING in Heart Failure Study

CAD Definition	Any CAD: ≥70% Stenosis in Any Coronary Artery	Extensive CAD: Stenosis ≥70% in the LM or Proximal LAD, ≥70% in ≥2 Major Epicardial Coronary Arteries or Any Stenosis ≥70% with a Prior MI or Coronary Revascularization
CAD prevalence by angiography	51% (n = 38)	36% (n = 27)
Sensitivity (95% CI)	82% (66–92)	96% (81–99)
Specificity (95% CI)	57% (40–72)	56% (41–71)
PPV	67%	55%
NPV	75%	96%

CAD, coronary artery disease; LM, left main coronary artery; LAD, left anterior descending coronary artery; NPV, negative predictive value; PPV, positive predictive value. Criteria for positive SPECT was summed stress score >3.
Reproduced with permission from Soman P, Lahiri A, Mieres JH, et al. Etiology and pathophysiology of new-onset heart failure: evaluation by myocardial perfusion imaging. *J Nucl Cardiol.* 2009;16(1):82–91.

or revascularization would be adjudicated to the nonischemic cardiomyopathy group (with coexisting, but not causally related CAD). Using these more restrictive criteria, patients with LV dysfunction and single-vessel CAD had a prognosis comparable to those with nonischemic cardiomyopathy.[5] Patients with true CAD-related heart failure have a worse prognosis than those with nonischemic cardiomyopathy, but the former may improve cardiac function dramatically with revascularization, highlighting the critical importance of an accurate diagnosis. The literature regarding the use of SPECT for the diagnosis of underlying CAD in LV dysfunction has primarily focused upon patients with *chronic* heart failure, with scant data addressing the diagnosis of CAD in new-onset heart failure.

In the setting of newly diagnosed LV systolic dysfunction, the identification of underlying CAD and potential "at risk" dysfunctional myocardium that might recover with coronary revascularization is critical. Although current practice guidelines specifically mandate coronary angiography only in heart failure patients with angina, chest pain is often absent in patients with ischemic cardiomyopathy, even those with significant amounts of viable myocardium.[2,6]

The Investigation of Myocardial Gated SPECT Imaging (IMAGING) in Heart Failure trial specifically addressed the utility of gated SPECT as an initial diagnostic modality in the de novo acute heart failure setting.[7] Two hundred and one patients hospitalized with new-onset heart failure were prospectively enrolled, and underwent exercise or pharmacologic SPECT during the index hospitalization. At the physician's discretion, approximately one-third of the patients underwent coronary angiography. Using a summed stress score (SSS) >3 to define an abnormal study, SPECT had a sensitivity of 96% and a negative predictive value of 96% for the diagnosis of ischemic cardiomyopathy using the criteria proposed by Felker, but was less accurate in detecting limited-extent CAD (Table 18-1). Thus, this study provides proof of concept of the utility of myocardial SPECT for the initial characterization of patients presenting with severe new-onset heart failure. Such patients who have normal stress myocardial SPECT are very unlikely to have underlying extensive CAD that is etiologically related to their heart failure (Fig. 18-2).

Several previous studies have established the utility of myocardial perfusion imaging (MPI) for the diagnosis of CAD in *chronic* heart failure.[8] Although many of these studies predated contemporary MPI, they uniformly demonstrated a very high negative predictive value for excluding CAD. Using more contemporary imaging with gated Tc-99m SPECT, Danias et al. reported an SSS >8 as 87% sensitive for detection of CAD, and that incorporating the SDS with findings of ischemia and regional wall motion abnormalities increased this to 94%.[9] Thus, in the setting of both new-onset and established heart failure, and global dysfunction, a normal stress myocardial

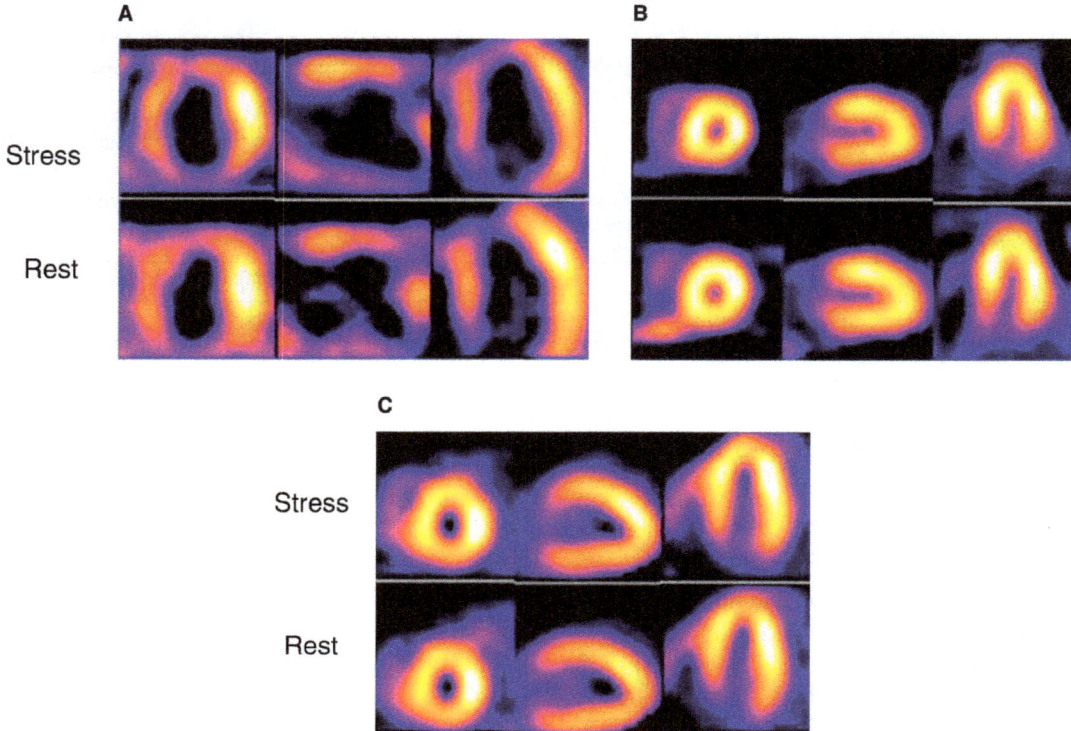

FIGURE 18-2 Categorization of heart failure etiology using technetium-99m sestamibi MPI. **(A)** Left ventricular (LV) dilation (abnormal LV systolic function by gated SPECT not shown) with large, fixed perfusion defects in the septum, anterior wall, apex and inferior wall suggestive of CAD-related ("ischemic") cardiomyopathy. **(B)** Normal stress–rest perfusion and LV size (normal LV EF on gated SPECT not shown) indicative of heart failure likely related to diastolic mechanisms. **(C)** LV dilation (with abnormal LV systolic function on gated SPECT, not shown) and normal perfusion suggestive of non-CAD related ("nonischemic"). (Reproduced with permission from Soman P, Lahiri A, Mieres JH, et al. Etiology and pathophysiology of new-onset heart failure: evaluation by myocardial perfusion imaging. *J Nucl Cardiol.* 2009;16(1):82–91.)

perfusion scan virtually excludes a diagnosis of ischemic LV dysfunction.

One important question remains, and that is whether SPECT MPI can replace coronary angiography as the diagnostic test for important underlying CAD in patients with new-onset heart failure. A major concern is that of balanced ischemia due to extensive CAD which might be missed or underestimated due to the fact that the MPI assessment of regional myocardial perfusion is relative. While it is unlikely that a patient with severe and extensive CAD will have no angina and a normal and rest/stress ECG and MPI, given the critical importance of excluding CAD in this population and the lack of substantive clinical trial data with MPI, patients with new-onset heart failure continue to undergo diagnostic coronary angiography for this purpose. Therefore, although evolving data increasingly suggest that this might be the case, only a large prospective clinical trial can definitively answer this question.

From a practical perspective, new-onset heart failure patients with angina and/or an intermediate to high probability of CAD (based on age, symptoms, and risk factors) should undergo diagnostic coronary angiography. Heart failure patients with a low probability of CAD, with clinical circumstances suggestive of nonischemic LV dysfunction can safely have a rest/stress MPI as the initial diagnostic test. In patients with known CAD being evaluated for new-onset or established heart failure, a rest/stress MPI provides invaluable information on ischemia, viability and quantitative LV function which can be used to drive important management decisions such as the choice between targeted percutaneous or surgical revascularization.

It is important to recognize that mild perfusion defects are common in nonischemic cardiomyopathy, and may reflect true physiological phenomena such as myocardial fibrosis or abnormal coronary vasodilator reserve, and have prognostic significance.[10-12] Inferior defects may also be caused by diaphragmatic attenuation and attenuation from LV dilatation. Attenuation correction is helpful in identifying soft tissue artifacts in SPECT imaging, but its effect on diagnostic accuracy for CAD has not been specifically tested in the heart failure population.

Selecting Patients for Coronary Revascularization

In selected heart failure patients with LV systolic dysfunction, coronary revascularization may offer a unique opportunity for "cure." The selection of patients for coronary revascularization requires a consideration of its potential benefits against perioperative mortality and morbidity. Patients with severe LV systolic dysfunction are at the highest risk, but might also derive the most benefit. While the concept of preserved myocardial viability (Chapter 21) and its impact on prognosis appears physiologically sound, the lack of conclusive evidence from the randomized trials has resulted in uncertainty surrounding it. Two large randomized trials that addressed this issue, STICH and PPAR-2 did not support the selection of patients for revascularization based on the presence of myocardial viability, but could be critiqued for the nonrandomized design (a deviation from the originally intended study design) of the STICH viability substudy, and suboptimal adherence to the protocol-defined treatment arm in PPAR-2. Thus, the major guidelines for the role of viability testing have not been impacted by these trials (revascularization in patients with one- or two-vessel CAD without proximal LAD CAD, but with a large area of viable myocardium and high-risk criteria on noninvasive testing: Class IB).[2] One practical approach might be to revascularize patients with extensive CAD, good coronary target vessels, and average surgical risk without routine prior viability testing. For patients at high surgical risk, the demonstration specifically of hibernating or stunned myocardium establishes the etiology of LV systolic dysfunction and informs the risk–benefit ratio of surgery favorably. A more recent analysis of the STICH cohort revealed better outcomes after coronary artery bypass grafting in patients with preserved functional capacity, multi-vessel CAD, lower ejection fraction, and higher end-systolic volume.[13]

Radionuclide Approaches to Risk Stratification in Heart Failure

The role of myocardial sympathetic neuronal imaging for risk stratification in heart failure patients is discussed in Chapter 23. I-123 metaiodobenzylguanidine (mIBG) is a SPECT agent that was approved by the Food and Drug Administration for this purpose in 2013.[14] C-11 labeled PET agents have also been used for sympathetic neuronal imaging, but the requirement for a cyclotron in close proximity makes clinical use logistically difficult.[15] An F-18 labeled agent, LMI1195 is currently undergoing phase 1 studies.[16]

Other radionuclide approaches have also been proven valuable for risk stratification in heart failure. A preserved myocardial flow reserve on Rb-82 PET MPI is indicative of a more benign prognosis in patients with ischemic and nonischemic cardiomyopathy compared to patients with a low myocardial flow reserve, as demonstrated elegantly in a study of 510 patients followed up for 8 months.[17] The use of PET-derived myocardial flow reserve to identify low-risk patients is a very promising approach to risk stratification, and is addressed again in the section on cardiac transplantation.

The cellular and interstitial changes that underlie the phenomenon of LV remodeling are accompanied by a transformation of the normally ellipsoid LV into a more spherical shape. LV shape indices, such as the sphericity index derived from echocardiography, have established utility in predicting prognosis and response to therapy heart failure patients.[18-20] Analogous measurements derived from gated SPECT have shown similar prognostic value (Fig. 18-3).[21]

Role of Radionuclide Imaging in Device and Advanced Heart Failure Therapies

The potential role of sympathetic neuronal imaging for selecting patients for ICD therapy, and of

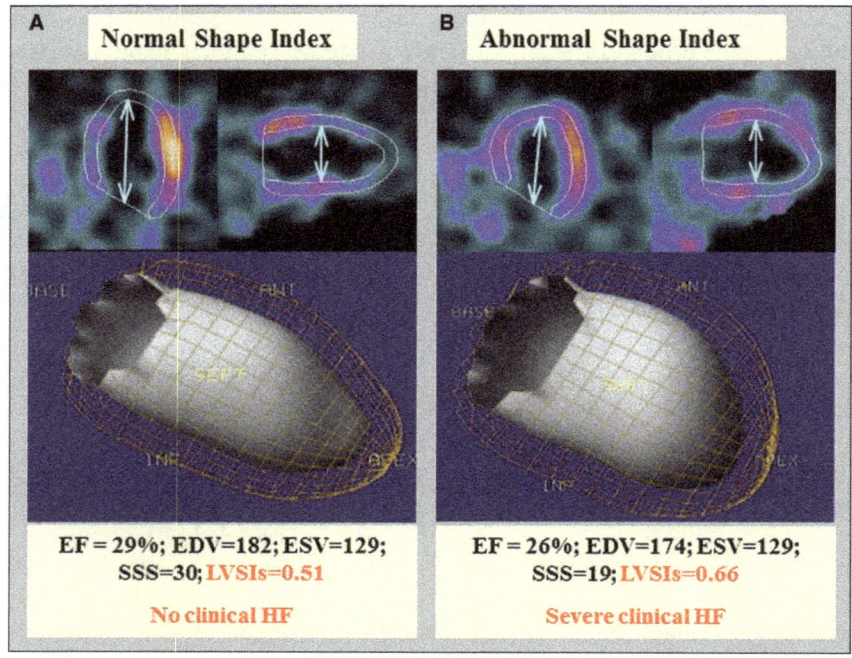

FIGURE 18-3 Illustration of two cases with comparable left ventricular ejection fraction (LVEF) but different left ventricular shape indices (LVSI). The patient with a normal ellipsoid-shaped LV and preserved LVSI **(A)** had no symptoms whereas the patient with a remodeled, spherical LV and abnormal LVSI **(B)** had severe symptoms. (Reproduced with permission from Abidov A, Slomka PJ, Nishina H, et al. Left ventricular shape index assessed by gated stress myocardial perfusion SPECT: initial description of a new variable. *J Nucl Cardiol.* 2006;13(5):652–659.)

dyssynchrony imaging for CRT are discussed in Chapters 23 and 11, respectively. The evolving role of PET/CT for the diagnosis of device infections is discussed in Chapter 24.

Another area of great clinical challenge is the surveillance of patients after orthotopic heart transplantation for the detection of allograft vasculopathy. Currently, posttransplant patients undergo annual surveillance coronary angiography. This disease is characterized by diffuse arterial hyperplasia rather than focal obstruction, and therefore, may be missed by conventional coronary "luminography," particularly in the early stages. Intriguing features include its development in young patients without traditional risk factors for atherosclerosis, and the selective involvement of allograft vessels with sparing of the host's native arterial system.[22] Once developed, there is no therapy proven to definitively reverse the process, and the clinical course is usually one of progressive ischemic LV failure. Survival rates are low (~20% at 1 year) after a clinical ischemic event.[23]

The role of MPI for posttransplant follow-up has been evaluated. Both SPECT perfusion imaging[24] and PET perfusion with myocardial flow reserve estimation[25] have been found to have good prognostic utility for this purpose. Single-center studies indicate that normal perfusion on SPECT or myocardial flow reserve on PET predicts an excellent prognosis in the intermediate term (2–5 years). The ability to risk stratify using noninvasive approaches would be an important clinical advantage for posttransplant patients who are already burdened with a substantial load of testing. Also, these data attest to the fact that, analogous to atherosclerotic CAD, functional testing provides important prognostic information that may not be available from anatomy-based diagnostic approaches.[26]

▶ Molecular Imaging in Heart Failure

Molecular mechanisms of heart failure are operative at the preclinical stage (Stage A of the ACC/AHA classification), and molecular imaging approaches have greatly enhanced our understanding of heart failure pathophysiology. It is hoped that the clinical translation of molecular imaging approaches will identify specific processes that may predominate in individual patients or patient groups, and explain the heterogeneity in response to therapy, for example, beta-blockers, thus facilitating personalized medicine. Such approaches include the imaging cellular mechanisms such as apoptosis (annexin-V)[27,28] and the renin–angiotensin system (F-18 captopril, F-18 lisinopril),[29] myocardial sympathetic innervation (I-123 mIBG, C-11 agents, and F-18 LMI1195), and myocardial metabolism (C-11 palmitate, I-123 BMIPP, F-18 FDG).[30] Molecular imaging techniques have also been applied with success to the monitoring of regenerative cell therapy.[31]

SUMMARY

In summary, several established radionuclide imaging approaches can be used with advantage in the evaluation and management of the heart failure patient. Radionuclide imaging applications in this prevalent and pervasive condition continue to evolve and expand, offering unique insights into pathophysiology. The future clinical translation of molecular imaging approaches may offer opportunities to personalize therapy.

REFERENCES

1. Mozaffarian D, Benjamin EJ, Go AS, et al. Heart disease and stroke statistics—2015 update: A report from the American Heart Association. *Circulation*. 2015;131:e29–322.
2. Yancy CW, Jessup M, Bozkurt B, et al. 2013 ACCF/AHA Guideline for the Management of Heart Failure: A Report of the American College of Cardiology Foundation/American Heart Association Task Force on Practice Guidelines. *Circulation*. 2013;128:e240–e327.
3. Felker GM, Thompson RE, Hare JM, et al. Underlying causes and long-term survival in patients with initially unexplained cardiomyopathy. *N Engl J Med*. 2000;342:1077–1084.
4. Gheorghiade M, Sopko G, De L, et al. Navigating the crossroads of coronary artery disease and heart failure. *Circulation*. 2006;114:1202–1213.
5. Felker GM, Shaw LK, O'Connor CM. A standardized definition of ischemic cardiomyopathy for use in clinical research. *J Am Coll Cardiol*. 2002;39:210–218.
6. Cleland JG, Pennell DJ, Ray SG, et al. Myocardial viability as a determinant of the ejection fraction response to carvedilol in patients with heart failure (CHRISTMAS trial): randomised controlled trial. *Lancet*. 2003;362:14–21.
7. Soman P, Lahiri A, Mieres JH, et al. Etiology and pathophysiology of new-onset heart failure: Evaluation by myocardial perfusion imaging. *J Nucl Cardiol*. 2009;16:82–91.
8. Udelson JE, Shafer CD, Carrio I. Radionuclide imaging in heart failure: Assessing etiology and outcomes and implications for management. *J Nucl Cardiol*. 2002;9:40S–52S.
9. Ahlberg AW, Kazi FA, Azemi T, et al. Usefulness of stress gated technetium-99m single photon emission computed tomographic myocardial perfusion imaging for the prediction of cardiac death in patients with moderate to severe left ventricular systolic dysfunction and suspected coronary artery disease. *Am J Cardiol*. 2012;109:26–30.
10. Doi YL, Chikamori T, Tukata J, et al. Prognostic value of thallium-201 perfusion defects in idiopathic dilated cardiomyopathy. *Am J Cardiol* 1991;67:188–193.
11. Iles L, Pflugger H, Lefkovits L, et al. Myocardial fibrosis predicts appropriate device therapy in patients with implantable cardioverter-defibrillators for primary prevention of sudden cardiac death. *J Am Coll Cardiol*. 2011;57:821–828.
12. van den Heuvel AF, van Veldhuisen DJ, van der Wall EE, et al. Regional myocardial blood flow reserve impairment and metabolic changes suggesting myocardial ischemia in patients with idiopathic dilated cardiomyopathy. *J Am Coll Cardiol*. 2000;35:19–28.
13. Panza JA, Velazquez EJ, She L, et al. Extent of coronary and myocardial disease and benefit from surgical revascularization in ischemic LV dysfunction [Corrected]. *J Am Coll Cardiol*. 2014;64:553–561.
14. Jacobson AF, Senior R, Cerqueira MD, et al. Myocardial iodine-123 meta-iodobenzylguanidine imaging and cardiac events in heart failure. Results of the prospective ADMIRE-HF (AdreView Myocardial Imaging for Risk Evaluation in Heart Failure) study. *J Am Coll Cardiol*. 2010;55:2212–2221.
15. Sasano T, Abraham MR, Chang KC, et al. Abnormal sympathetic innervation of viable myocardium and the substrate of ventricular tachycardia after myocardial infarction. *J Am Coll Cardiol*. 2008;51:2266–2275.
16. Sinusas AJ, Lazewatsky J, Brunetti J, et al. Biodistribution and radiation dosimetry of LMI1195: first-in-human study of a novel 18F-labeled tracer for imaging myocardial innervation. *J Nucl Med*. 2014;55:1445–1451.
17. Majmudar MD, Murthy VL, Shah RV, et al. Quantification of coronary flow reserve in patients with ischaemic and non-ischaemic cardiomyopathy and its association with clinical outcomes. *Eur Heart J Cardiovasc Imaging*. 2015.
18. Douglas PS, Morrow R, Ioli A, Reichek N. Left ventricular shape, afterload and survival in idiopathic dilated cardiomyopathy. *J Am Coll Cardiol*. 1989;13:311–315.
19. Hall SA, Cigarroa CG, Marcoux L, Risser RC, Grayburn PA, Eichhorn EJ. Time course of improvement in left ventricular function, mass and geometry in patients with congestive heart failure treated with beta-adrenergic blockade. *J Am Coll Cardiol*. 1995;25:1154–1161.
20. Lowes BD, Gill EA, Abraham WT, et al. Effects of carvedilol on left ventricular mass, chamber geometry, and mitral regurgitation in chronic heart failure. *Am J Cardiol*. 1999;83:1201–1205.
21. Abidov A, Slomka PJ, Nishina H, et al. Left ventricular shape index assessed by gated stress myocardial perfusion SPECT: Initial description of a new variable. *J Nucl Cardiol*. 2006;13:652–659.

22. Libby P. The vascular biology of atherosclerosis. In: Libby P, Bonow RO, Mann DL, Zipes DP, eds. *Braunwald's Heart Disease*. Philadelphia, PA: Saunders; 2008:985–1002.
23. McCarthy PM. Surgical management of heart failure. In: Libby P, Bonow RO, Mann DL, Zipes DP, eds. *Braunwald's Heart Disease*. Philadelphia, PA: Saunders; 2008:665–683.
24. Manrique A, Bernard M, Hitzel A, et al. Diagnostic and prognostic value of myocardial perfusion gated SPECT in orthotopic heart transplant recipients. *J Nucl Cardiol*. 2010;17:197–206.
25. Mc Ardle BA, Davies RA, Chen L, et al. Prognostic value of rubidium-82 positron emission tomography in patients after heart transplant. *Circulation*. 2014;7:930–937.
26. Soman P, McNamara D. Surveillance for post-transplant coronary artery vasculopathy: Shifting gears from diagnosis to prognosis. *J Nucl Cardiol*. 2010;17:172–174.
27. Thimister PW, Hofstra L, Liem IH, et al. In vivo detection of cell death in the area at risk in acute myocardial infarction. *J Nucl Med*. 2003;44:391–396.
28. Korngold EC, Jaffer FA, Weissleder R, Sosnovik DE. Noninvasive imaging of apoptosis in cardiovascular disease. *Heart Failure Reviews*. 2008;13:163–173.
29. Dilsizian V, Eckelman WC, Loredo ML, Jagoda EM, Shirani J. Evidence for tissue angiotensin-converting enzyme in explanted hearts of ischemic cardiomyopathy using targeted radiotracer technique. *J Nucl Med*. 2007;48:182–187.
30. Dilsizian V. Metabolic adaptation to myocardial ischemia: the role of fatty acid imaging. *J Nucl Cardiol*. 2007;14:S97–S99.
31. Bengel F. Nuclear imaging in cardiac cell therapy. *Heart Failure Reviews*. 2006;11:325–332.

Myocardial Perfusion Imaging in Special Populations

CHAPTER 19

Upamanyu Rampal and Raja C. Pullatt

INTRODUCTION

Previous chapters have demonstrated the important role of myocardial perfusion imaging (MPI) for the diagnosis and risk stratification of coronary artery disease (CAD) in the general population. There is also robust literature validating the use of MPI in different patient cohorts. This chapter will describe the value of MPI for the assessment of CAD and risk stratification in special populations consisting of diabetic patients, women, patients with chronic renal disease, the elderly, and patients with acute chest pain syndromes.

EVALUATION OF DIABETIC PATIENTS

In 2014, the global prevalence of diabetes was estimated to be 9% among adults aged 18+ years by the World Health Organization (WHO).[1] In the United States, the Centers for Disease Control (CDC) estimates those with diabetes is rising, with recently 29 million people (9.3% prevalence) suffering from diabetes.[2] This increase in prevalence of diabetes mirrors the obesity epidemic in the United States with 33% of the population now classified as being obese.[3] The overall prevalence of CAD has been estimated to be as high as 55% in diabetic patients compared with 4% in the general population. In a landmark Finnish observational trial, the authors elegantly demonstrated the similar survival (15.4% vs. 15.9%) and rate of myocardial infarction (MI) (20.2% vs. 18.8%) among diabetic patients without prior MI and nondiabetic patients with prior MI, respectively, leading to the designation of diabetes as CAD equivalent by the Adult Treatment Panel-III (ATP-III) guidelines.[4,5] There are also data demonstrating that these patients have a higher incidence of more severe disease and are at greater risk of developing acute coronary syndromes.[6] From these data it is clear that diabetic patients are at high risk for coronary events. Nuclear cardiology imaging offers potential for early and accurate identification of such patients.

▶ The Role of Stress Myocardial Perfusion Imaging in Symptomatic Diabetic Patients

Stress MPI in symptomatic diabetic patients can be very beneficial in providing the appropriate diagnosis and risk stratification. Several studies demonstrate similar sensitivity (80–86%) and specificity (79–87%) of single-photon emission computed tomography (SPECT) MPI in diabetic patients as compared to nondiabetic patients.[7,8] In the largest study to date, Kang et al.[9] evaluated retrospectively 138 diabetics and 188 nondiabetics with suspected CAD who had SPECT imaging and coronary angiography within 6 months. The diagnostic accuracy was similar between diabetic and nondiabetic patients (p = nonsignificant), respectively. The normalcy rate for low-likelihood patients was 89% in diabetics and 90% in nondiabetics (p = NS). These data indicate a strong diagnostic role for MPI in diabetic patients which is not different from a nondiabetic cohort.

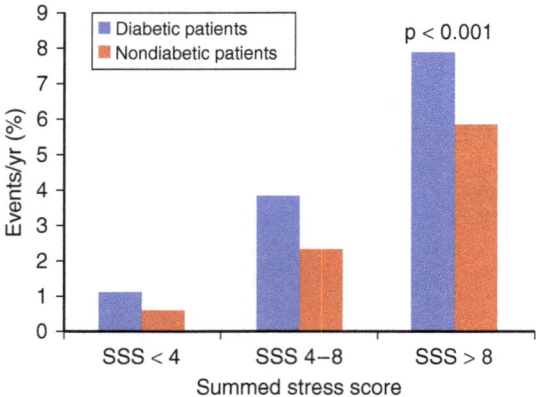

FIGURE 19-1 Cardiac event rates (cardiac death and nonfatal MI) among patients with diabetes and patients without diabetes as a function of stress defect extent and severity. SSS, summed stress score. (Data from Kang X, Berman DS, Lewin H, et al. Comparative ability of myocardial perfusion single-photon emission computed tomography to detect coronary artery disease in patients with and without diabetes mellitus. *Am Heart J.* 1999;137(5):949–957.)

and 5130 nondiabetic patients, Kang et al.[9] evaluated risk stratification according to defect size and extent (Fig. 19-1). As in studies in the general population, they found the greater the defect extent, the greater the risk for coronary events (cardiac death and nonfatal MI). Diabetic patients had more perfusion defects and higher event rates (nonfatal MI, cardiac death, and revascularization) during the follow-up period. The authors' conclusion was that exercise and adenosine stress myocardial perfusion SPECT add incremental prognostic value for patients with diabetes.

Wiersma et al.[10,11] performed a subanalysis of the prematurely terminated MERIDIAN trial (medical therapy vs. invasive therapy in diabetic patients with mild angina and reversible perfusion defects) to examine the prognostic value of SPECT MPI in diabetics with stable angina and documented ischemia on MPI. In multivariate analysis, severe myocardial ischemia (summed difference score >8) ($p = 0.001$) and the use of insulin ($p = 0.02$) were independent predictors of cardiac death/nonfatal MI.

Data from a multicenter analysis also corroborate the above-mentioned findings. Using data from six centers, Giri et al.[12] examined whether the nuclear perfusion study could contribute to risk stratification beyond the presence of diabetes using the incremental chi-square approach (Fig. 19-2). Indeed, for

Risk Stratification in Diabetic Patients with Stress Myocardial Perfusion Imaging

Several studies have reported the value of SPECT MPI for the risk stratification of diabetic patients. In a single-center prospective study of 1080 diabetic

FIGURE 19-2 Abnormal stress MPI result provides the greatest contribution (incremental χ^2) for prediction of either death or death/MI among diabetics. (Reproduced with permission from Giri S, Shaw LJ, Murthy DR, et al. Impact of diabetes on the risk stratification using stress single-photon emission computed tomography myocardial perfusion imaging in patients with symptoms suggestive of coronary artery disease. *Circulation.* 2002;105(1):32–40.)

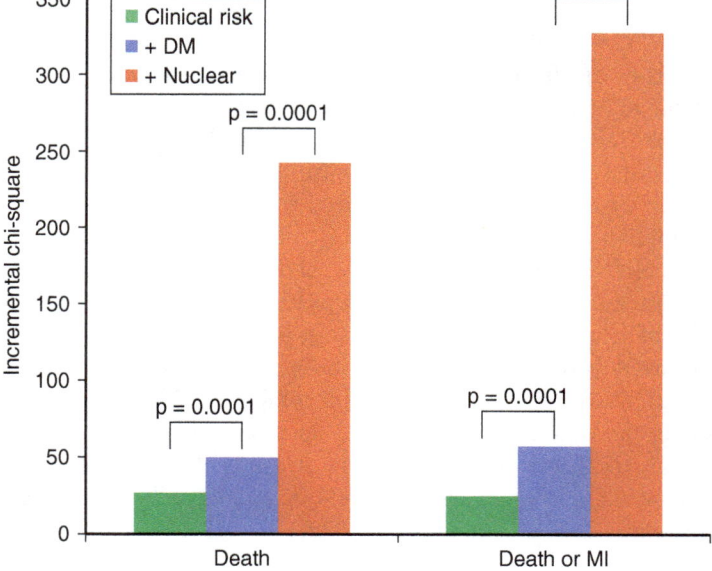

both the prediction of cardiac death alone and as a combined end point with nonfatal MI, the perfusion imaging data were significantly better predictors of cardiac events than the presence of diabetes in combination with clinical risk factors.

Previous studies suggested that diabetic women have a greater risk of adverse outcomes at any level of stress perfusion defects.[13] Recently, Santos et al.[14] reported a large retrospective study of more than 4600 diabetic patients to examine whether the gender differences in cardiovascular event rates persisted in the modern era of aggressive treatment of CAD. This large study demonstrated that size and severity of stress perfusion abnormalities' predicted outcomes equally in both genders. It is also appreciated that patients undergoing pharmacologic as opposed to exercise myocardial perfusion SPECT are at greater risk of cardiac events in diabetic patients.[15] Other aspects of diabetics contributing to cardiac risk were evaluated by Barmpouletos et al.[16] They demonstrated that diabetic patients with moderate to severe perfusion abnormalities are at greater risk for adverse cardiac events with longstanding diabetes (>10 years) and/or receiving insulin therapy.

Various studies have shown a higher rate of cardiac events following a normal MPI in diabetic patients.[9,12] A recent meta-analysis[17] also confirmed these findings revealing an annualized event rate with normal MPI of 1.60%, higher than in the general population (<1%), leading the authors to define diabetic patients with negative stress MPI results as a "relatively low-risk" cohort but not truly at low risk. This study, however, did not account for stress type (pharmacologic or exercise) in either cohort.

Is this higher cardiac risk in diabetic patients inherent to the disease? This question was addressed by a large study ($n > 3000$) by Ghatak et al.[18] to examine how the type of stress SPECT MPI (exercise vs. pharmacologic) impacts outcomes in diabetic patients.[18] They demonstrated that diabetic patients who were able to undergo exercise stress SPECT MPI had significantly lower annualized cardiac event rates compared to diabetic patients undergoing pharmacologic stress SPECT MPI across all perfusion categories. In the normal perfusion category, the subgroup of diabetic patients able to exercise had a low cardiac event rate (<1%) similar to nondiabetic population (Fig. 19-3). This finding suggests that previous studies may have been reflective of a high percentage of pharmacologic stress tests in diabetic patents.

Ventricular function assessment also adds additional prognostic value in diabetic patients. Acampa et al.[19] studied the role of gated SPECT in 520 diabetic and nondiabetic patients with baseline normal MPI and showed that the highest probability of cardiac events and the major risk acceleration was observed in diabetic patients with poststress LVEF <45%. In diabetic patients with poststress LVEF <45%, the time to achieve a risk level of events >3% was earlier at 12 months than nondiabetics (Figs. 19-4 and 19-5).

In summary, MPI provides considerable value in diagnosis and risk stratification of the diabetic patient. The literature suggests that diabetic patients are at greater risk for CAD-related events than nondiabetic patients. The duration of diabetes and insulin use (perhaps an indicator of severity of the disease) are also predictors of greater risk in the same categories of perfusion abnormalities. However, the Ghatak study demonstrates that diabetic patients with good exercise capacity have more favorable outcomes similar to nondiabetic patients. Thus, the form of stress a diabetic patient can perform needs to be considered in management decisions.

▶ Role of Stress Myocardial Perfusion Imaging in Asymptomatic Diabetic Patients

In the last decade, several studies have emerged demonstrating the varying rates of cardiovascular events in asymptomatic diabetics, perhaps reflecting the heterogeneity of risk in this group of patients. The screening of truly asymptomatic patients using MPI remains controversial and is not recommended by professional guidelines. Contemporary evidence regarding this topic is reviewed below.

The Detection of Ischemia in Asymptomatic Diabetics (DIAD) study[20] was a randomized controlled trial that tested the hypothesis that systematic screening would identify higher-risk individuals and beneficially affect their risk of MI or cardiac death. The overall 5-year cardiac event rate was 2.9% (0.6% per year) and use of MPI screening had no discernable effect on subsequent cardiac events in asymptomatic diabetics.[21] More recently, the BARDOT

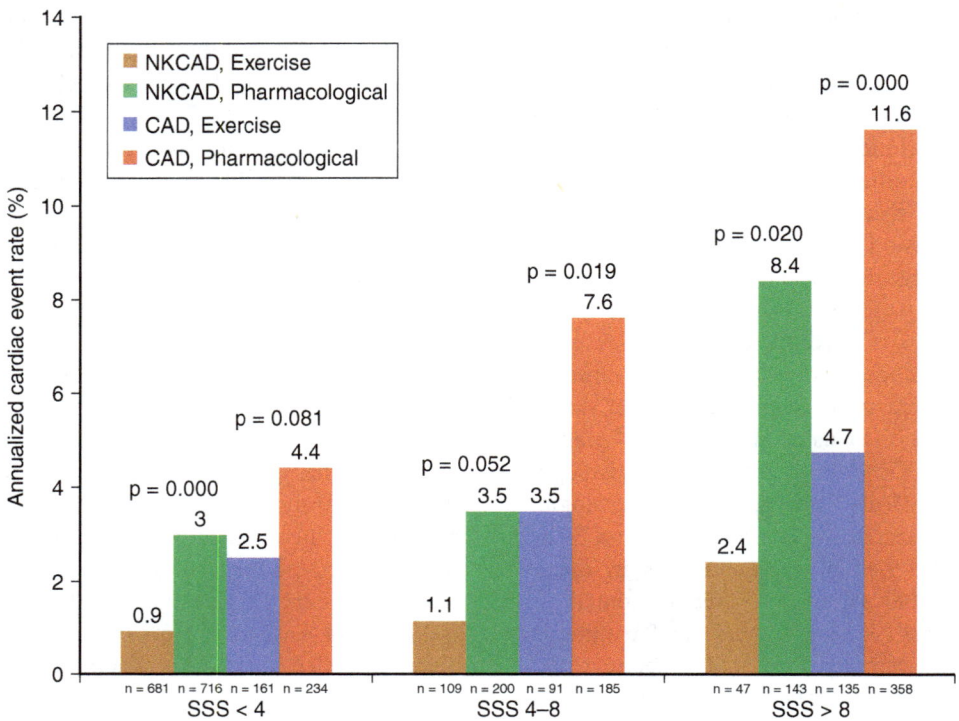

FIGURE 19-3 Annualized cardiac event rates in diabetic patients subcategorized into underlying CAD status and stress modality. NKCAD, no known CAD; SSS, summed stress score; *n*, number of patients in each category as mentioned at the base of data points. (Reproduced with permission from Ghatak A, Padala S, Heller GV. Risk stratification among diabetic patients undergoing stress myocardial perfusion imaging. *J Nucl Cardiol.* 2013;20(4):529–538.)

trial included 400 high-risk asymptomatic diabetic patients. The Patients included had evidence of end-organ damage or composite of age >55 years, diabetes duration >5 years, and at-least two cardiac risk factors of smoking, hypertension, hypercholesterolemia, positive family history of CAD in addition to diabetes. The rate of silent myocardial ischemia (SMI) in this study was 22% and "overt or silent CAD progression" (cardiac events + new ischemia/scar) was seven-fold higher in patients with an abnormal versus

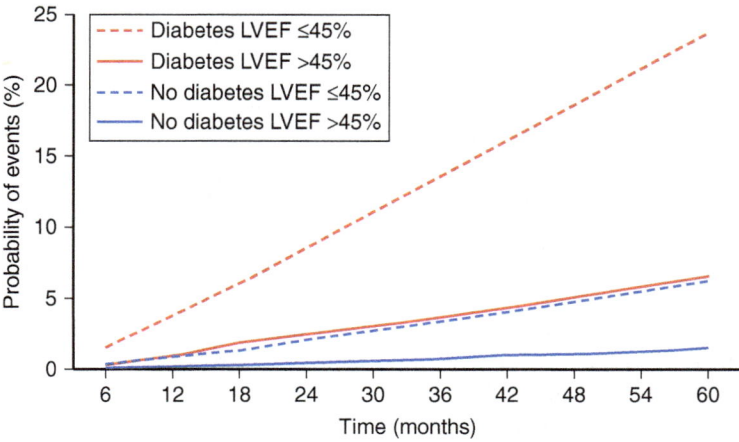

FIGURE 19-4 Probability of cardiac events in diabetic patients and nondiabetic patients with poststress LVEF ≤45% or with preserved LVEF. (Reproduced with permission from Acampa W, Petretta M, Cuocolo R. Warranty period of normal stress myocardial perfusion imaging in diabetic patients: a propensity score analysis. *J Nucl Cardiol.* 2014;21(1):50–56.)

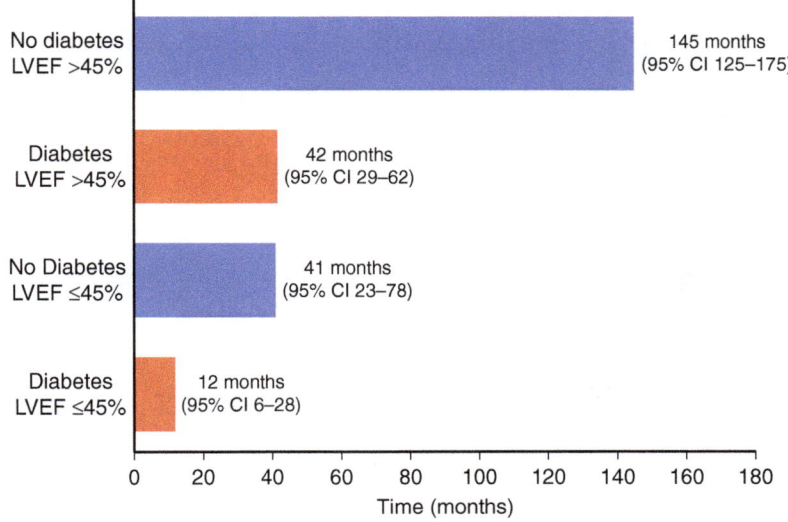

FIGURE 19-5 Time to achieve cumulative cardiac risk level (>3%) in diabetic and nondiabetic patients with reduced poststress LVEF or preserved LVEF. (Reproduced with permission from Acampa W, Petretta M, Cuocolo R. Warranty period of normal stress myocardial perfusion imaging in diabetic patients: a propensity score analysis. *J Nucl Cardiol*. 2014;21(1):50–56.)

a normal MPS (35.6% vs. 4.6%), documenting the screening efficacy of MPS in these patients. Patients randomized to revascularization had similar rates of symptomatic CAD progression, but lower rates of asymptomatic CAD (more ischemia or new scar) progression (54.3% vs. 15.8%; $p < 0.001$).[22] These data in a higher-risk population than the DIAD trial suggest some benefits to screening but this has not been adopted by professional organizations.

A new novel method to identify high-risk asymptomatic diabetics is to estimate coronary microvascular dysfunction (CMD) using coronary flow reserve (CFR) with positron emission tomography (PET). Murthy et al.[23] examined patients with and without diabetes using ^{82}Rb-PET MPI and found that addition of CFR to clinical and imaging risk models improved risk discrimination for both diabetics and nondiabetics. Diabetic patients without known CAD with impaired CFR experienced a rate of cardiac death comparable to that for nondiabetic patients with known CAD (2.8% per year vs. 2.0% per year; $p = 0.33$). Conversely, diabetics without known CAD and preserved CFR had very low annualized cardiac mortality, which was similar to patients without known CAD or diabetes mellitus and normal stress perfusion and systolic function (0.3% per year vs. 0.5% per year; $p = 0.65$) (Fig. 19-6).

These data suggest such a test might be useful in asymptomatic diabetic patients but further prospective studies are necessary.

Conclusions: Diabetic Patients

1. MPI is an effective tool in the diagnosis and risk stratification of diabetic patients.
2. Diabetic patients with longstanding and more severe disease are at greater risk for cardiac events.
3. The ability to perform exercise in diabetic patients conveys a lower risk of cardiac events.
4. Routine stress MPI is not recommended for asymptomatic diabetic patients.
5. The role of cardiac PET with myocardial blood flow (MBF) assessment needs further assessment, but can identify an "at-risk" population.

ASSESSMENT OF WOMEN

While cardiovascular diseases (CVDs), including CAD and stroke, are the leading cause of death in both men and women in the United States, more women die from CVD than men.[24] In 2013, CVDs caused about one death every 80 seconds in women and were responsible for more number of deaths from cancer, chronic lower respiratory disease, and diabetes combined. Younger women (aged 35–45 years) for the first time in the last four decades had higher CAD death rates likely representing the influence of the obesity epidemic in younger women.[25,26] This section will review the data on women and heart disease and the value of MPI in assessment and prognosis.

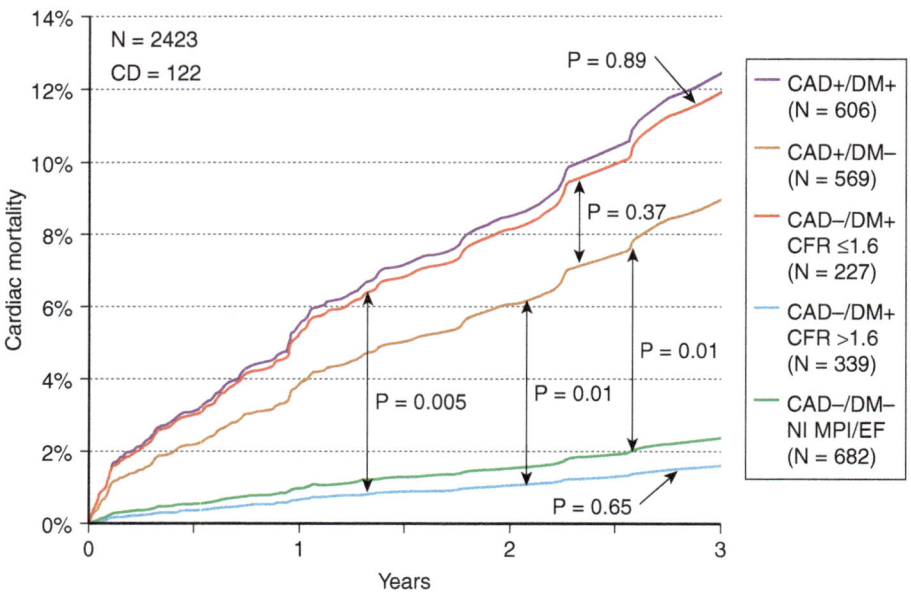

FIGURE 19-6 Annualized cardiac mortality in diabetic and nondiabetic patients with or without coronary artery disease (CAD) and with preserved or reduced coronary flow reserve (CFR). MPI, myocardial perfusion imaging; EF, ejection fraction; NI MPI, normal myocardial perfusion imaging; CD, cardiac death. (Reproduced with permission from Murthy VL, Naya M, Foster CR, et al. Association between coronary vascular dysfunction and cardiac mortality in patients with and without diabetes mellitus. *Circulation*. 2012;126(15):1858–1868.)

▶ Diagnostic Testing in Women

The diagnosis of CAD in women is challenging due to the atypical symptoms often experienced. This leads to less referral for evaluation in women with suspected CAD.[27,28] A recent meta-analysis revealed that women with MI had a lower likelihood of presenting with typical chest pain than men (odds ratio 0.63; 95% CI, 0.59–0.68) and were more likely than men to present with atypical symptoms.[29] Similar findings were also observed in a prospective cohort study which showed that despite chest pain being the most common presentation of acute coronary syndrome in both sexes, women presented more frequently without chest pain than men (19.0% vs. 13.7%; $p = 0.03$).[30]

Adding to the challenge of diagnosing heart disease in women is the high prevalence of nonobstructive disease (40–60%). This finding was confirmed in a more recent analysis by Jespersen et al.,[31] which showed a higher incidence of nonobstructive CAD in women (65% vs. 32%) as compared to men. In this study normal coronary arteries and nonobstructive CAD were associated with a 52% and 85% increased risk of MACE (cardiovascular mortality, hospitalization for MI, heart failure, or stroke) and with 29% and 52% increased risk of all-cause mortality, respectively. Similar findings were demonstrated in the 10-year follow-up of the Women's Ischemia Syndrome Evaluation (WISE) study, which showed that two-thirds (62%) of women with angina had nonobstructive disease. The 10-year adverse outcome rates (cardiovascular death or MI rate) in the women with nonobstructive CAD were almost double (12.8% vs. 6.7%) than that observed in women with angiographically normal coronary arteries.[32] These differences in the presentation and prognosis of CAD in women could be related to the increased incidence of CMD and different characteristics of plaque morphology in women presenting with acute coronary syndrome.[33] However, recent studies using optical coherence tomography (OCT) did not reveal a sex difference in the prevalence of plaque rupture or erosion.[34,35]

Despite the above-mentioned challenges of diagnosing CAD in women, ETT still remains the most

Table 19-1

Women and Heart Disease Exercise Test: Diagnostic Accuracy

Study (Year)	n Women	n Men	Angiographic Endpoint (Degree of Stenosis)	Sensitivity (%)	Specificity (%)
Detry et al.[38]	47	231	≥50	80 in women/87 in men	63 in women/74 in men
Barolsky et al.[37]	92	85	≥75	60 in women/65 in men	68 in women/89 in men
Friedman et al.[39]	60	NA	≥70	32	41
Guiteras et al.[40]	112	NA	≥70	79	66
Hung et al.[36]	92	NA	≥70 or ≥50 left main	73	59
[a]Morise et al.[41]	284	504	≥50	47 ± 5 in women/56 ± 3 in men	73 ± 3 in women/81 ± 3 in men

[a]Subgroup analysis.

common screening test used to detect CAD. However, Table 19-1 summarizes the low sensitivity and specificity of this modality in women.[36–41]

To address the concerns regarding the accuracy of ETT alone in women, the WOMEN (What is the Optimal Method for Ischemia Evaluation in Women) trial was undertaken to examine outcomes rather than diagnoses. In this trial, 824 symptomatic women with intermediate pretest probability of CAD were randomized to one of two diagnostic strategies: exercise tolerance testing (ETT) alone or exercise MPI. At 2 years, there was no difference in major adverse cardiac events (98.0% for ETT and 97.7% for MPI; $p = 0.59$) (Fig. 19-7).

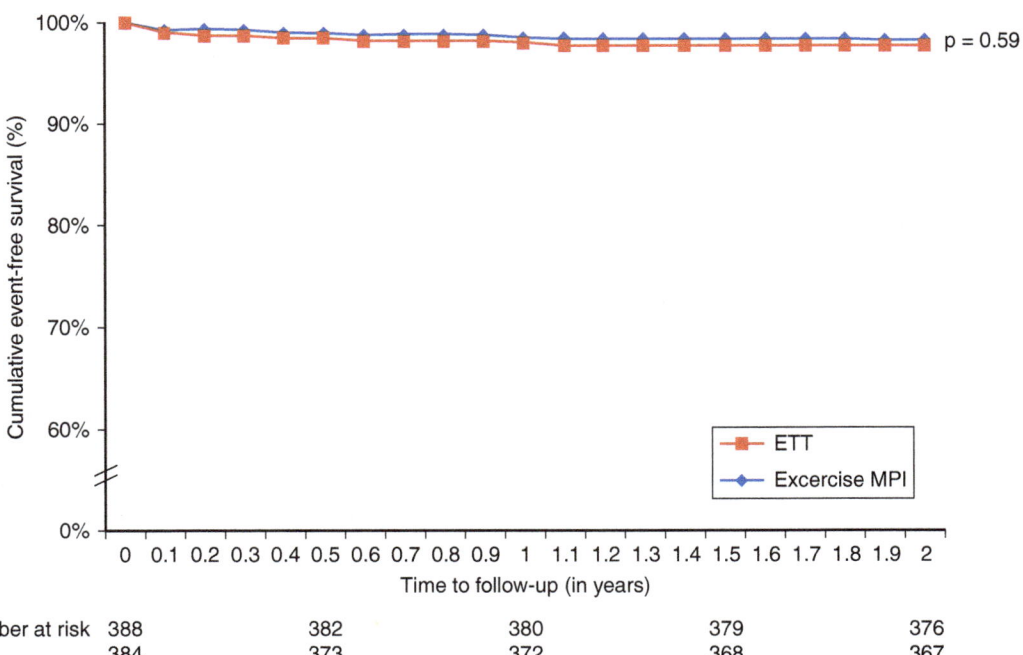

FIGURE 19-7 Comparison of outcomes in a randomized trial between Exercise Tolerance Testing (ETT) versus exercise myocardial perfusion imaging (MPI) strategy in women with chest pain. (Reproduced with permission from Shaw LJ, Mieres JH, Hendel RH, et al. Comparative effectiveness of exercise electrocardiography with or without myocardial perfusion single photon emission computed tomography in women with suspected coronary artery disease: results from the What Is the Optimal Method for Ischemia Evaluation in Women (WOMEN) trial. *Circulation.* 2011;124(11):1239–1249.)

The clinical implications of this trial's results are noteworthy. For low- to intermediate-risk women capable of performing exercise, routine ETT without imaging appears a reasonable first-line test.[42] Women with intermediate–high CAD risk may be referred for stress imaging because of a higher likelihood of CAD. Women at high CAD risk with stable symptoms may be referred for a stress imaging modality for assessment of their ischemic burden and to guide posttest and anti-ischemic therapeutic decision making.[43]

▶ Radionuclide Stress Imaging in Women

Robust data are available for the use of MPI for diagnosis as well as risk stratification of women with known or suspected CAD. The strength of MPI in the diagnostic accuracy of stress testing in women was demonstrated in a contemporary meta-analysis of 14 SPECT studies, which found a sensitivity of 81% and specificity of 78% in women with no known CAD.[44]

The higher specificity of SPECT MPI than ETT alone is particularly useful in identifying the presence of ischemia in women with false-positive exercise tests. In a recent report of >4000 patients of which more than one-third were women, exercise MPI showed a net reclassification improvement of 36% over ETT. Thus, additional ischemic heart disease (IHD) risk information was available by the performance of MPI in one out of every three patients.[45] While radionuclide imaging has a higher sensitivity than exercise stress testing in the detection of single-vessel disease, the highest accuracy has been found in women with multiple-vessel disease compared to those with single-vessel disease.[46,47]

It has also been questioned whether stress MPI is less accurate in women compared to men, similar to ETT. To address this issue, Iskandar et al.[48] performed a bivariate meta-analysis on 26 studies that met criteria. In contrast to ETT, SPECT imaging provided similar and high sensitivity and specificity for both genders, reassuring that SPECT is a reasonable diagnostic modality in women.

Pharmacologic stress is an important alternative for women with limited exercise capacity. Both dipyridamole and adenosine stress have been found to be comparable to exercise imaging in primarily male populations.[49] In a prospective study of 201 women, adenosine SPECT imaging had a 95% sensitivity, 66% specificity, and 85% accuracy in the detection of coronary stenosis greater than 70% regardless of presenting symptoms, prior history of MI, or pretest probability of coronary disease.[50]

Data are also now available for use of SPECT MPI in women of different ethnicity.[51] Cerci et al. studied 2225 Hispanic women in Brazil and showed that women with abnormal SPECT had three times higher event rate (13.1% vs. 4%) as compared to those with normal SPECT studies. Moreover, in the subgroup of patients with abnormal SPECT studies, further risk stratification could be performed using extent of perfusion abnormality and presence or absence of reversible ischemia.

▶ Challenges of Radionuclide Stress Imaging in Women

The accuracy of radionuclide imaging is affected by several factors in women, particularly breast attenuation and small heart size.[52–54] To appreciate breast attenuation artifact, one of the best approaches is to begin with a review of the unprocessed rotating images. On standard display, if a defect correlates with an area of soft tissue on the raw images and the wall motion in the same region is normal with gated SPECT, the finding is consistent with an artifact and not CAD, and the study should be considered normal. The use of technetium-99 imaging agents (higher energy) and ECG gating using this concept has been shown to improve specificity.[55,56] Other techniques to increase specificity of MPI include supine/prone MPI or the use of attenuation correction. In a recent study,[57] the overall correlation between summed stress scores (SSS) for two readers improved with supine/prone imaging in female patients undergoing supine/prone MPI (0.86 vs. 0.75, $p < 0.0001$) as compared to supine-only MPI.

▶ Outcomes and Management of Female Patients Following Stress Imaging

The value of risk stratification in women has been demonstrated in relation to a reversible defect, size, and extent of the defect with MPI in women.[58–60] Patients with both normal and mildly abnormal scans are at low risk of cardiac death (<1% per year of follow-up) and only patients with moderately to severely abnormal scans are at moderate to high risk (>5% per year of follow-up) (Fig. 19-8) for cardiac

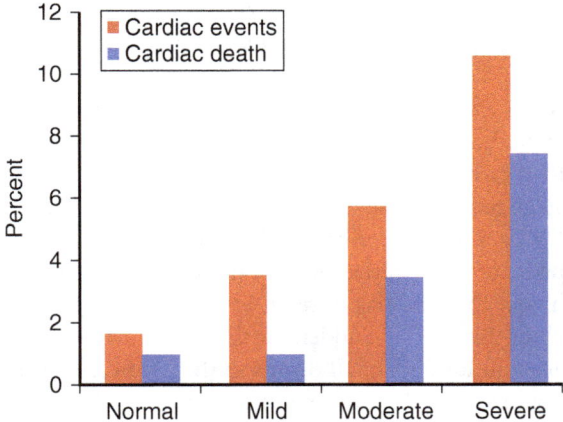

FIGURE 19-8 Risk stratification in women: adenosine Tc-99m sestamibi SPECT. (Data from Hachamovitch R, Berman DS, Kiat H, et al. Incremental prognostic value of adenosine stress myocardial perfusion single-photon emission computed tomography and impact on subsequent management in patients with or suspected of having myocardial ischemia. *Am J Cardiol.* 1997;80(4):426–433.)

death.[61] This can be helpful in management decisions, especially regarding downstream testing. In general, women who have normal studies do not need further testing but medical management is warranted. For those with moderate to severe abnormalities, further testing may be important.

Cardiac PET MPI is another alternative modality, which can be used for diagnosis and cardiovascular risk stratification of women. PET provides higher spatial resolution, significant reduction in attenuation artifact, lower radiation dose (2–4 mSv vs. 13 mSv),[62] ability to measure MBF, and higher diagnostic accuracy as compared to SPECT MPI.[63,64]

Recently, data from the large prospective multicenter PET registry of 6037 men and women who were followed for a mean of 2.2 years were reported. The unadjusted 5-year CAD mortality ranged from 0.9% to 12.9% for women ($p < 0.0001$) and from to 1.5% to 17.4% for men ($p < 0.0001$) for 0% to ≥15% abnormal myocardium at stress[65] (Fig. 19-9). For

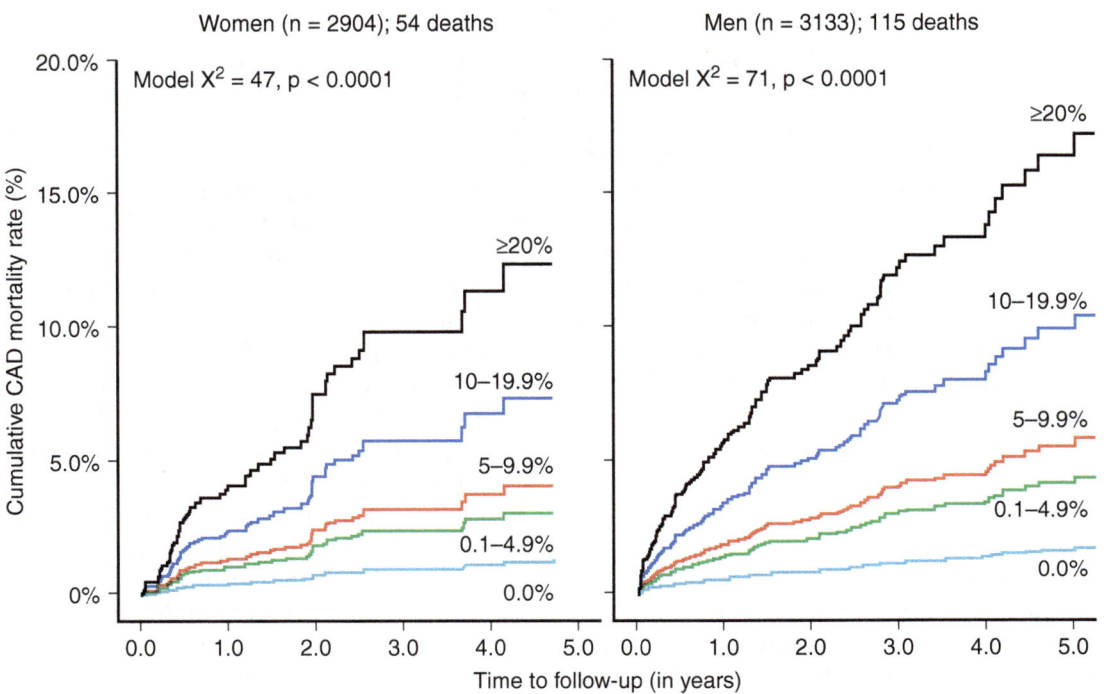

FIGURE 19-9 Comparative CAD mortality estimates from the PET Prognosis Registry in women and men. (Reproduced with permission from Kay J, Dorbala S, Goyal A, et al. Influence of sex on risk stratification with stress myocardial perfusion Rb-82 positron emission tomography: Results from the PET (Positron Emission Tomography) Prognosis Multicenter Registry. *J Am Coll Cardiol.* 2013;62(20):1866–1876.)

women, PET data also improved the detection of high-risk patients (9.3% newly detected), which were more than for men (3.5% newly detected).

A normal cardiac PET study is associated with a very low rate of future cardiac events. In a recent study of 457 women with normal ^{82}Rb-PET MPI, the average risks of death and initial nonfatal cardiac events were 0.72% and 0.47% per year, respectively.[66] This low risk is despite using pharmacologic stress and may be due to the greater diagnostic accuracy of PET.

Historically, testing for the presence of ischemia relied on the demonstration of impaired myocardial perfusion using radiotracers after exercise/pharmacologic stress testing due to obstructive epicardial stenosis. In the past, there was a notion that MPI perfusion imaging in women leads to an increased incidence of "false-positive" results due to the higher prevalence of nonobstructive CAD. However, it is increasingly being recognized that women even with nonobstructive CAD are at higher risk of cardiovascular events, as demonstrated in the WISE study.[33] The identification of the extent and severity of myocardial ischemia that results from coronary CMD and the ensuing elevation of IHD risk is important for risk stratification of women with nonobstructive CAD. Murthy et al.[67] studied the influence of CMD on prognosis in 947 women and 523 men by measuring CFR using ^{82}Rb-PET MPI. The frequency of CFR <2.0, primarily reflecting CMD, was high and similar in men (n = 206; 51%) and women (n = 435; 54%; Fisher exact test p = 0.39 and equivalence p = 0.0002). MACE occurred earlier and more frequently among both men and women with CMD than those without. Thus, detection of abnormal CMD using PET MPI in women may help explain the high cardiac event rates in women with nonobstructive CAD.

CONCLUSION

Based on the results from the WOMEN trial and other data, ETT alone is recommended as the initial test of choice for women at low CAD risk, with MPI reserved for women with intermediate–high risk of CAD. PET MPI, with its higher diagnostic accuracy, lower radiation exposure, and ability to assess CFR holds the potential for improving diagnosis and risk stratification in women.

RISK STRATIFICATION IN PATIENTS WITH CHRONIC KIDNEY DISEASE

More than 26 million adults (13%) in the United States have chronic kidney disease (CKD) and more than half a million Americans are living with end-stage renal disease (ESRD) according to the AHA.[68] CVDs account for more than half the deaths in patients with ESRD. The risk of death from CVD is higher than the risk of requirement of renal replacement therapy.[69,70] Sudden death/cardiac arrhythmias account for 37% of all deaths in the Medicare ESRD population.[71] Patients requiring renal replacement therapy also have worse outcomes following acute coronary syndrome. In an analysis of the Global Registry of Acute Coronary Syndrome (GRACE) registry, patients requiring renal replacement therapy had three-fold greater risk of short- and long-term mortality and had worse actual outcomes (in-hospital mortality) than that predicted by the Grace score (7.8% predicted vs. 12% observed; $p < 0.05$).[72]

The accurate diagnosis and risk stratification of CAD in patients with CKD is challenging.

The Framingham risk score fails to accurately risk stratify patients with renal disease and can underestimate the risk of cardiac events by 50%.[73] Despite the limitations of traditional risk stratification tools in symptomatic patients with renal disease, SPECT MPI has been validated as a powerful prognostic tool in several studies across a wide spectrum of CKD patients.[74–76]

Patients requiring renal replacement have high cardiovascular events equaling patients with known CAD; however, the role of MPI in asymptomatic renal patients is unclear. In a recent study, Kim et al.[77] provided a novel approach for risk stratification of asymptomatic patients (n = 215) with ESRD by using abnormal EKG and echocardiography at the time of initiation of hemodialysis as markers of high risk. Myocardial perfusion defects were identified in 45% of these high-risk patients with a cardiac event rate of 15%, which was significantly higher as compared to high-risk patients without perfusion defects (4.5%). Larger trials are needed to confirm the validity of the above approach for screening ESRD patients.

Despite the robust data (Table 19-2) for SPECT MPI in patients with CKD, several challenges in this high-risk cohort exist. The presence of left ventricular hypertrophy and hypertension decreases the

Table 19-2

Summary of Trials of Myocardial Perfusion Imaging in Patients with Chronic Kidney Disease

No.	Study	Study Participants	Study Description	Key Findings
1	Hakeem et al.[74]	• eGFR <60 • n = 1652	Assess prognostic utility of MPI across varying degrees of CKD	• Both MPS and CKD had incremental power for prediction of cardiac death over baseline risk factors and left ventricular dysfunction • Patients with CKD appear to have a relatively less benign prognosis than those without CKD, even in the presence of a normal scan
2	Hakeem et al.[76]	• eGFR <60 • n = 1747 • 37% diabetics	Evaluate the impact of CKD and diabetes on cardiac death using MPI	In patients with normal scan, annual CD rate was: • 0.9% for those without diabetes and CKD • 0.5% in the DM alone • 2.35% in CKD alone • 2.9% in those with both DM and CKD ($p < 0.001$)
3	Kim et al.[77]	• Asymptomatic ESRD patient at initiation of dialysis • n = 215	Evaluate role of MPI in screening asymptomatic high-risk ESRD patients (abnormal EKG or low EF) for CAD	• High-risk asymptomatic ESRD patients with perfusion defects had threefold increase in relative risk for cardiac events compared with high-risk patients without perfusion defects • Revascularization therapy did not improve the cardiac event-free survival rate as compared to OMT
4	Murthy et al.[78]	• eGFR <60 • n = 0 866	Evaluate if impaired vasodilator function (CFR <1.5) measured using PET MPI plays a role in increased cardiac risk in patients with CKD	• Patients with CFR <1.5 had 3× increase in mortality • 36% of intermediate-risk patients were reclassified into low (21%) or high risk (15%) using abnormal CFR (<1.5)

eGFR, estimated glomerular filtration; ESRD, end-stage renal disease; CFR, coronary flow reserve; CKD, chronic kidney disease; PET, positron emission tomography; MPI, myocardial perfusion imaging; OMT, optimal medical therapy; EF, ejection fraction; CD, cardiac death.

sensitivity of SPECT MPI due to partial volume effect as well as the high prevalence of CMD. Some of these challenges can be overcome by use of cardiac PET MPI's ability to detect CMD by measuring absolute CFR. CMD was evaluated by Murthy et al.[78] in 866 patients with moderate to severe kidney dysfunction using rest and stress PET using ^{82}Rb as perfusion tracer to calculate CFR. In each category of abnormality on PET scanning (combined ischemia and scar extent), an impaired CFR identified higher-risk subgroups, including among those with visually normal scans (Fig. 19-10). Patients with abnormal CFR (<1.5) had a threefold higher rate of cardiac death compared to patients with normal CFR. Using CFR, 36% of patients classified as intermediate risk on MPI could be reclassified to low risk (21%) or high risk (15%) with an annualized cardiac mortality of 0% versus 15%, respectively.

CONCLUSION

SPECT MPI provides incremental information beyond traditional risk estimators in patients with renal disease. However, despite normal MPI, ESRD patients have high cardiac event rates. Cardiac PET MPI by using CFR holds the promise for further risk stratification of this high-risk cohort.

ROLE OF NUCLEAR CARDIOLOGY IN THE ELDERLY PATIENT

Individuals over the age of 65 (elderly) are expected to constitute one-fifth of the U.S. population by 2030 and CVD remains the leading cause of death among both elderly men and women.[79] It is estimated that

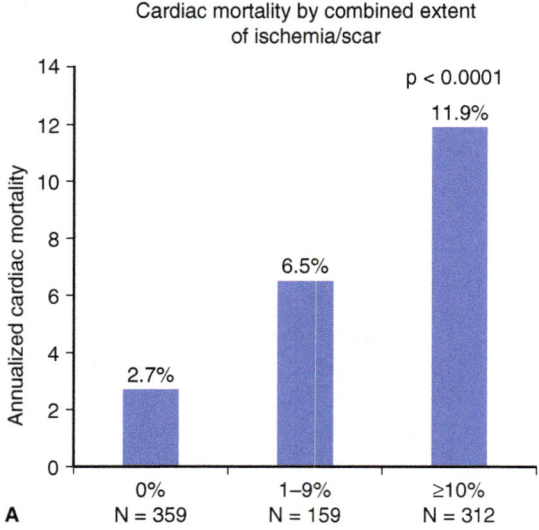

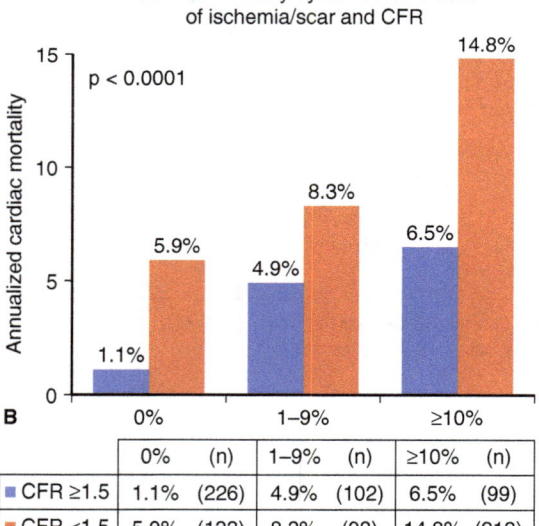

FIGURE 19-10 Annual cardiac mortality in patients with chronic kidney disease (CKD) using combined ischemia/scar on PET imaging **(A)** and identification of high-risk subgroups using CFR **(B)**. (Reproduced with permission from Murthy VL, Naya M, Foster CR, et al. Coronary vascular dysfunction and prognosis in patients with chronic kidney disease. *JACC Cardiovasc Imaging.* 2012;5(10):1025–1034.)

up to 50% of elderly men and 30% of elderly women are living with coronary heart disease.[80]

▶ Diagnosis of CAD in Elderly Patients

In general, ETT is recommended by the ACC/AHA as the initial test for the risk stratification of symptomatic elderly patients with interpretable EKG who are able to exercise.[81,82] However, the overall accuracy of ETT and its ability to risk stratify elderly patients using Duke treadmill score (DTS) for CAD is limited. Moreover, baseline EKG abnormalities have been reported in 40% to 70% of elderly patients, decreasing the utility of ETT in these patients. In a recent study of octogenarians, the use of DTS was found to be a significant predictor of only late revascularization (>3 months) but not of the hard endpoints of cardiac death or MI[83]; in contrast, SSS was a powerful predictor of both soft and hard cardiac endpoints.

To assess the optimal noninvasive strategy of risk stratification of patients over the age of 65, Rai et al.[84] performed a meta-analysis of 17 studies (n = 13,304) comparing ETT to SPECT and stress echocardiography (Fig. 19-11). The results demonstrated effective risk stratification using imaging techniques but no benefit of ETT alone, and SPECT imaging was more successful than stress echocardiography.

Data also support the use of ventricular function assessment for the risk stratification of elderly patients. In a large study (>5000 patients), Hachamovitch et al.[85] reported that MPI and gated ejection fraction provided incremental prognostic value over

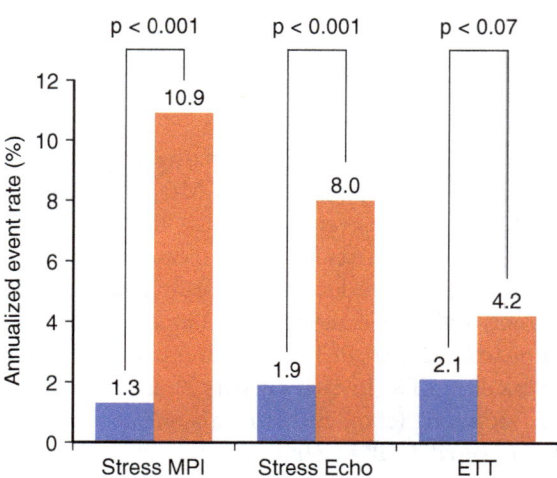

FIGURE 19-11 Comparison of annualized cardiac event rates (percentage) in elderly patients by different techniques depicting abnormal (*red bars*) and normal (*blue bars*) results. Echo, echocardiography. (Reproduced with permission from Rai M, Baker WL, Parker MW, et al. Meta-analysis of optimal risk stratification in patients >65 years of age. *Am J Cardiol.* 2012;110(8):1092–1099.)

Table 19-3
Summary of Trials Supporting Use of Myocardial Perfusion Imaging in Elderly

No.	Study (Year)	Study Participants	Study Description	Key Results
1	Katsikis et al.[83]	• >80 years • n = 137	Evaluate role of DTS in elderly patients undergoing exercise nuclear stress testing	• Duke treadmill score (DTS) unable to predict hard cardiac events
2	Rai et al.[84]	• >65 years • Meta-analysis of 17 studies • n = 13,304	Evaluate the optimal method of noninvasive stress testing in elderly patients	• Stress imaging (nuclear/ECHO) superior to ETT alone
3	Hachamovitch et al.[85]	• Age >75 years • n = 5200	Evaluate role of gated MPI in elderly (age >75, n = 5200)	• MPI and gated EF provide incremental benefit over clinical variables • Early revascularization in elderly patients with small area of ischemia associated with increased cardiac events
4	Nair et al.[86]	• Age >80 years • n = 1093	Investigated the clinical value of MPI in *very elderly patients* with suspected CAD in comparison to younger patients	• Higher events in elderly patients across all SSS categories as compared to younger patients • Low death rate in elderly patients with normal exercise MPI (<0.7%/yr)

ETT, exercise tolerance testing; ECHO, echocardiography; MPI, myocardial perfusion imaging; DTS, Duke treadmill score; SSS, summed stress score; EF, ejection fraction.

traditional scoring systems. The authors also showed significant interaction between the use of early revascularization and percentage of ischemic myocardium. Early revascularization increased cardiovascular risk in the setting of little or no ischemia but decreased the risk in the setting of increasing amounts of ischemia. Recently, Nair et al.[86] demonstrated that very elderly (>80 years) patients with moderate to severely abnormal SSS had a significantly higher annualized cardiac event rate than those with mildly abnormal or normal study (9.6% vs. 3.4% and 2.5%, respectively, $p < 0.001$). Across all categories of SSS, very elderly patients had a significantly higher cardiac event rate as compared to younger patients ($p < 0.001$). Table 19-3 summarizes the key findings of the above-mentioned studies using MPI in elderly patients.

CONCLUSION

SPECT MPI provides improved risk stratification over ETT in the elderly population and can be used to guide decisions regarding medical treatment versus invasive therapy in patients with high-risk scans. ETT alone in this population is of limited value.

ACUTE-REST MYOCARDIAL PERFUSION IMAGING

More than 6 million patients present to the emergency department (ED) with symptoms suggestive of acute coronary syndrome.[87] This cohort of patients presenting to the ED constitutes a diverse group of patients with varying degrees of risk of cardiac events. The initial goal of diagnostic testing includes establishing the correct diagnosis of the patient's symptoms and short-term risk stratification of this cohort. This process is relatively unique in that the goal is to assess whether the patient's symptoms are consistent with CAD, not necessarily whether the patient him/herself has CAD. Thus, the study is performed under resting conditions without performing stress. Low-risk patients, that is, those with normal imaging results should be discharged with outpatient follow-up, while intermediate- to high-risk patients should be admitted for further evaluation and management.

Role of MPI in Diagnosis of Acute Chest Pain Syndromes

In the ischemic cascade chest pain due to increased myocardial demand or decreased supply leads to regional variation in MBF, which occurs prior to development of wall-motion abnormalities, ECG changes, or elevated biomarkers. This regional heterogeneity in blood flow forms the basis of performance of acute-rest myocardial perfusion (ARMP) imaging in patients with chest pain in the acute setting. The use of technetium-based tracers is preferred over thallium due to their higher-energy spectrum (less attenuation) and lack of redistribution.

Data accumulated over several years demonstrate value of the ARMP if tracer is injected during or within 2 hours of an episode of chest pain thought to be consistent with CAD. It is preferable to inject during symptoms and before administration of anti-ischemic regimens. Once the patient is injected with a technetium-based agent, medications can be administered as no clinically significant redistribution occurs and therefore subsequent imaging results are not affected.

Once the patient is injected, imaging should be performed as rapidly as possible to obtain the clinical diagnosis. As this is one study only, attenuation artifact is an issue, best resolved with attenuation correction methods, or with prone imaging if the former is not possible. Since it is one image only, ECG gating is less useful in identifying attenuation artifact from CAD, as normal wall motion may also be possible with an ischemic event.

The accuracy of rest MPI for detection of obstructive CAD or MI in this setting has been validated in a large number of trials with a high sensitivity and negative predictive value (~99%).[88] The specificity is less robust due to attenuation artifact as well as the possibility that the abnormal study might represent ischemia and not infarction. The American Society of Nuclear Cardiology (ASNC)/American College of Cardiology (ACC)/American Heart Association (AHA) recommends the use of acute-rest MPI in the setting of possible ACS in patients with nondiagnostic EKG and gives it a class I recommendation.[89] However, the sensitivity of ARMP imaging is highest when the radiotracer is injected during the episode of chest pain with decreasing accuracy after resolution of symptoms.[90]

Role of MPI in Risk Stratification of Acute Chest Pain Syndromes

The use of acute-rest imaging for prognosis and short-term risk stratification of patients for cardiac events has also been validated in several studies. Normal images carry an extremely low risk of cardiac events as compared to abnormal scans 0% to 1% versus 20% to 70%, respectively.

ARMP imaging also provides superior prognostication as compared to a strategy of using clinical variables and EKG in this diverse cohort (Fig. 19-12).[91]

The use of resting MPI also improves ED triage decisions and leads to appropriate discharge of low-risk patients from the ED. This was demonstrated in the Emergency Room Assessment of Sestamibi for Evaluation (ERASE) of chest pain trial ($n = 2475$), which randomized patients to usual ED care versus receiving acute-rest MPI.[92] The attending physician

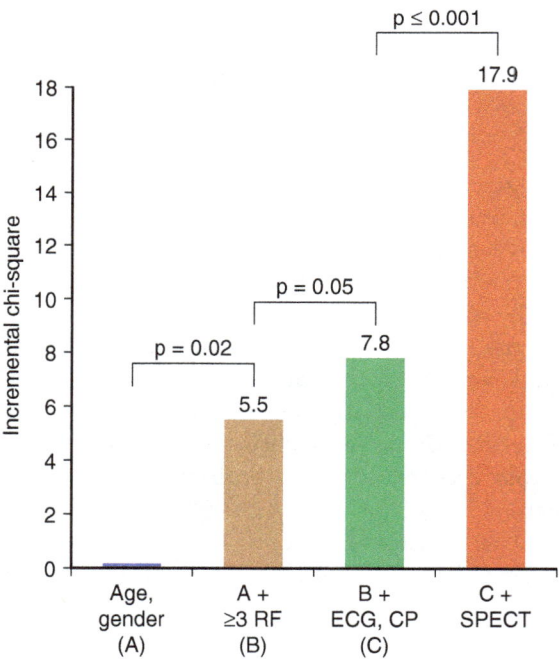

FIGURE 19-12 Incremental prognostic value of rest Tc-99m tetrofosmin SPECT imaging in the ED over clinical variables such as age and gender (base model A), (≥) risk factors (RF) for CAD and a normal admission ECG and chest pain (CP). (Reproduced with permission from Heller GV, Stowers SA, Hendel RC, et al. Clinical value of acute rest technetium-99m tetrofosmin tomographic myocardial perfusion imaging in patients with acute chest pain and nondiagnostic electrocardiograms, *J Am Coll Cardiol*. 1998;31(5):1011–1017.)

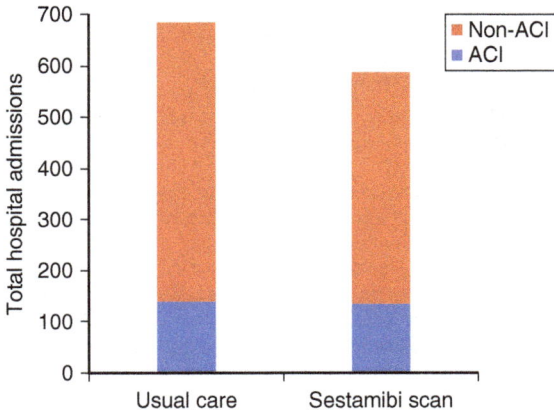

FIGURE 19-13 Effectiveness of acute-rest myocardial perfusion imaging (sestamibi) in risk stratification of emergency department (ED) patients compared with usual ED care. ACI, acute cardiac ischemia. (Data from Udelson JE, Beshansky JR, Ballin DS, et al. Myocardial perfusion imaging for evaluation and triage of patients with suspected acute cardiac ischemia: a randomized controlled trial. *JAMA*. 2002;288(21): 2693–2700.)

was provided imaging results and subsequent management (admission or discharge) was their decision. In this trial Udelson et al. demonstrated a 20% reduction in unnecessary hospitalization with excellent outcomes and a significantly higher event rate and presence of CAD in the admitted patients (Fig. 19-13). The success of triage outcomes in this trial was pivotal to the ACC/AHA class IA indication.[89]

Despite the above-mentioned advantages of using ARMP in patients with chest pain presenting to the ED, its widespread adoption faces several logistical challenges such as 24-hour availability of radiotracer, technologist, and interpreting physicians.

CONCLUSION: ACUTE-REST MPI

Acute-rest MPI can be used for the accurate diagnosis of acute coronary syndromes in the ED if injected during or within 2 hours of symptoms. Negative images during this time frame have a high negative predictive value and can be used to guide triage decisions in the ED, while those with positive studies warrant further evaluation and hospital admission. Under certain conditions such as a patient presenting to a nuclear cardiology laboratory with symptoms, this procedure is also useful.

CONCLUSION

Similar to its role in the general population, SPECT and PET MPI provide accurate diagnosis and prognosis of CAD in the special groups of patients discussed in this chapter, especially diabetic and female patients. These populations also include the elderly, those with renal failure, and patients presenting with chest pain syndromes in which acute-rest MPI is a powerful tool for the risk stratification in the ED setting.

REFERENCES

1. WHO. *Global Status Report on Noncommunicable Diseases 2014*. Geneva: World Health Organization; 2014.
2. Centers for Disease Control and Prevention. *National Diabetes Statistics Report: Estimates of Diabetes and Its Burden in the United States, 2014*. Atlanta, GA: US Department of Health and Human Services; 2014.
3. Roger VL, Go AS, Lloyd-Jones DM, et al.; American Heart Association Statistics Committee and Stroke Statistics Subcommittee. Heart disease and stroke statistics—2012 update: a report from the American Heart Association. *Circulation*. 2012;125(1):e2–e220.
4. Haffner SM, Lehto S, Rönnemaa T. Mortality from coronary heart disease in subjects with type 2 diabetes and in nondiabetic subjects with and without prior myocardial infarction. *N Engl J Med*. 1998;339(4):229–234.
5. National Cholesterol Education Program (NCEP) Expert Panel on Detection, Evaluation, and Treatment of High Blood Cholesterol in Adults (Adult Treatment Panel III). Third Report of the National Cholesterol Education Program (NCEP) Expert Panel on Detection, Evaluation, and Treatment of High Blood Cholesterol in Adults (Adult Treatment Panel III) final report. *Circulation*. 2002;106(25):3143–3421.
6. Zuanetti G, Latini R, Maggioni AP. Influence of diabetes on mortality in acute myocardial infarction: data from the GISSI-2 study. *J Am Coll Cardiol*. 1993;22(7):1788–1794.
7. Boudreau RJ, Strony JT, duCret RP, et al. Perfusion thallium imaging of type I diabetes patients with end stage renal disease: comparison of oral and intravenous dipyridamole administration. *Radiology*. 1990;175:103–105.
8. Bell DS, Yumuk VD. Low incidence of false-positive exercise thallium-201 scintigraphy in a diabetic population. *Diabetes Care*. 1996;19:185–186.
9. Kang X, Berman DS, Lewin H, et al. Comparative ability of myocardial perfusion single-photon emission computed tomography to detect coronary artery disease in patients with and without diabetes mellitus. *Am Heart J*. 1999;137:949–957.
10. Wiersma JJ, Dijksman LE, Ten Holt WL, et al. Cardiac complications in type 2 diabetic patients with mild angina complaints and documented reversible myocardial perfusion defects, results of the MERIDIAN trial. *Neth Heart J*. 2006;14:409–416.
11. Wiersma J, Verberne HJ, Ten Holt WL, et al. Prognostic value of myocardial perfusion scintigraphy in type 2 diabetic

patients with mild, stable angina pectoris. *J Nucl Cardiol.* 2009;16:524–532.
12. Giri S, Shaw LJ, Murthy DR, et al. Impact of diabetes on the risk stratification using stress single-photon emission computed tomography myocardial perfusion imaging in patients with symptoms suggestive of coronary artery disease. *Circulation.* 2002;105:32–40.
13. Berman DS, Kang X, Hayes SW, et al. Adenosine myocardial perfusion single-photon emission computed tomography in women compared with men. Impact of diabetes mellitus on incremental prognostic value and effect on patient management. *JACC.* 2003;41:1125–1133.
14. Santos MT, Parker MW, Heller GV. Evaluating gender differences in prognosis following SPECT myocardial perfusion imaging among patients with diabetes and known or suspected coronary disease in the modern era. *J Nucl Cardiol.* 2013;20(6):1021–1029.
15. Supariwala A, Uretsky S, Depuey EG, et al. Influence of mode of stress and coronary risk factor burden upon long-term mortality following normal stress myocardial perfusion single-photon emission computed tomographic imaging. *Am J Cardiol.* 2013;111(6):846–850.
16. Barmpouletos D, Stavens G, Ahlberg AW, Katten DM, O'sullivan DM, Heller GV. Duration and type of therapy for diabetes: impact on cardiac risk stratification with stress electrocardiographic-gated SPECT myocardial perfusion imaging. *J Nucl Cardiol.* 2010;17(6):1041–1049.
17. Acampa W, Cantoni V, Green R, et al. Prognostic value of normal stress myocardial perfusion imaging in diabetic patients: a meta-analysis. *J Nucl Cardiol.* 2014;21(5):893–902.
18. Ghatak A, Padala S, Heller GV. Risk stratification among diabetic patients undergoing stress myocardial perfusion imaging. *J Nucl Cardiol.* 2013;20(4):529–538.
19. Acampa W, Petretta M, Cuocolo R. Warranty period of normal stress myocardial perfusion imaging in diabetic patients: a propensity score analysis. *J Nucl Cardiol.* 2014;21(1):50–56.
20. Wackers FJT, Young LH, Inzucchi SE, et al. Detection of silent myocardial ischemia in asymptomatic diabetic subjects. The DIAD study. *Diabetes Care.* 2004;27:1954–1961.
21. Young LH, Wackers FJT, Chyun DA, et al. Cardiac outcomes after screening for asymptomatic coronary artery disease in patients with type 2 diabetes. The DIAD study: a randomized controlled trial. *JAMA.* 2009;301:1547–1555.
22. Zellweger MJ, Maraun M, Osterhues HH, et al. Progression to overt or silent CAD in asymptomatic patients with diabetes mellitus at high coronary risk: main findings of the prospective multicenter BARDOT trial with a pilot randomized treatment substudy. *JACC Cardiovasc Imaging.* 2014;7(10):1001–1010.
23. Murthy VL, Naya M, Foster CR, et al. Association between coronary vascular dysfunction and cardiac mortality in patients with and without diabetes mellitus. *Circulation.* 2012;126(15):1858–1868.
24. Rosamond W, Flegal K, Furie K, et al. Heart disease and stroke statistics—2008 update: A report from the American Heart Association Statistics Committee and Stroke Statistics Subcommittee. *Circulation.* 2008;117(4):e25–e146.
25. Roger VL, Go AS, Lloyd-Jones DM, et al. Heart disease and stroke statistics–2011 update: a report from the American Heart Association. *Circulation.* 2011;123(4):e18–e209.
26. Ford ES, Ajani UA, Croft JB, et al. Explaining the decrease in U.S. deaths from coronary disease, 1980–2000. *N Engl J Med.* 2007;356(23):2388–2398.
27. Shaw LJ, Miller DD, Romeis JC, et al. Gender differences in the noninvasive evaluation and management of patients with suspected coronary artery disease. *Ann Intern Med.* 1994;120(7):559–566.
28. Steingart RM, Packer M, Hamm P, et al. Sex differences in the management of coronary artery disease. *N Engl J Med.* 1991;325(4):226–230.
29. Coventry LL, Finn J, Bremner AP. Sex differences in symptom presentation in acute myocardial infarction: a systematic review and meta-analysis. *Heart Lung.* 2011;40(6):477–491.
30. Khan NA, Daskalopoulou SS, Karp I, et al. Sex differences in acute coronary syndrome symptom presentation in young patients. *JAMA Intern Med.* 2013;173(20):1863–1871.
31. Jespersen L, Hvelplund A, Abildstrøm SZ, et al. Stable angina pectoris with no obstructive coronary artery disease is associated with increased risks of major adverse cardiovascular events. *Eur Heart J.* 2012;33(6):734–744.
32. Sharaf B, Wood T, Shaw L, et al. Adverse outcomes among women presenting with signs and symptoms of ischemia and no obstructive coronary artery disease: findings from the National Heart, Lung, and Blood Institute-sponsored Women's Ischemia Syndrome Evaluation (WISE) angiographic core laboratory. *Am Heart J.* 2013;166(1):134–141.
33. Reis SE, Holubkov R, Smith AJC, et al. Coronary microvascular dysfunction is highly prevalent in women with chest pain in the absence of coronary artery disease: results from the NHLBI WISE study. The WISE investigators. *Am Heart J.* 2001;141:735–741.
34. Jia H, Abtahian F, Aguirre AD, et al. In vivo diagnosis of plaque erosion and calcified nodule in patients with acute coronary syndrome by intravascular optical coherence tomography. *J Am Coll Cardiol.* 2013;62(19):1748–1758.
35. Guagliumi G, Capodanno D, Saia F, et al. Mechanisms of atherothrombosis and vascular response to primary percutaneous coronary intervention in women versus men with acute myocardial infarction: results of the OCTAVIA study. *JACC Cardiovasc Interv.* 2014;7(9):958–968.
36. Hung J, Chaitman BR, Lam J, et al. Noninvasive diagnostic test choices for the evaluation of coronary artery disease in women: a multivariate comparison of cardiac fluoroscopy, exercise electrocardiography and exercise thallium myocardial perfusion scintigraphy. *J Am Coll Cardiol.* 1984;4(1):8–16.
37. Barolsky SM, Gilbert CA, Faruqui A, et al. Differences in electrocardiographic response to exercise of women and men: a non-Bayesian factor. *Circulation.* 1979;60(5):1021–1027.
38. Detry JM, Kapita BM, Cosyns J, et al. Diagnostic value of history and maximal exercise electrocardiography in men and women suspected of coronary heart disease. *Circulation.* 1977;56(5):756–761.
39. Friedman TD, Greene AC, Iskandrian AS, et al. Exercise thallium-201 myocardial scintigraphy in women: correlation with coronary arteriography. *Am J Cardiol.* 1982;49:1632–1637.
40. Guiteras P, Chaitman BR, Waters DD, et al. Diagnostic accuracy of exercise ECG lead systems in clinical subsets of women. *Circulation.* 1982;65(7):1465–1474.

41. Morise AP, Dalal JN, Duva RD. Value of a simple measure of estrogen status for improving the diagnosis of coronary artery disease in women. *Am J Med*. 1993;94(5):491–496.
42. Shaw LJ, Mieres JH, Hendel RH, et al. Comparative effectiveness of exercise electrocardiography with or without myocardial perfusion single photon emission computed tomography in women with suspected coronary artery disease: results from the What Is the Optimal Method for Ischemia Evaluation in Women (WOMEN) trial. *Circulation*. 2011;124(11):1239–1249.
43. Mieres JH, Gulati M, Merz NB, et al. Role of noninvasive testing in the clinical evaluation of women with suspected ischemic heart disease: a consensus statement from the American Heart Association. *Circulation*. 2014;130(4):350–379.
44. Dolor RJ, Patel MR, Melloni C, et al. Noninvasive Technologies for the Diagnosis of Coronary Artery Disease in Women [Internet]. Rockville (MD): Agency for Healthcare Research and Quality (US); 2012 Jun. Report No.: 12-EHC034-EF. AHRQ Comparative Effectiveness Reviews.
45. Shaw LJ, Wilson PW, Hachamovitch R. Improved near-term coronary artery disease risk classification with gated stress myocardial perfusion SPECT. *JACC Cardiovasc Imaging*. 2010;3(11):1139–1148.
46. Okada RD, Boucher CA, Strauss HW, et al. Exercise radionuclide imaging approaches to coronary artery disease. *Am J Cardiol*. 1980;46:1188–1204.
47. Amanullah AM, Kiat H, Berman DS. Adenosine technetium-99m sestamibi myocardial perfusion SPECT in women: diagnostic efficacy in detection of coronary artery disease. *J Am Coll Cardiol*. 1996;27(4):803.
48. Iskandar A, Limone B, Parker MW, et al. Gender differences in the diagnostic accuracy of SPECT myocardial perfusion imaging: a bivariate meta-analysis. *J Nucl Cardiol*. 2013;20(1):53–63.
49. Gupta NC, Esterbrooks DJ, Hilleman DE, et al. Comparison of adenosine and exercise thallium-201 single photon emission computed tomography (SPECT) myocardial perfusion imaging. *J Am Coll Cardiol*. 1992;19(2):248–257.
50. Mahmarian JJ, Verani MS. Myocardial perfusion imaging during pharmacologic stress testing. *Cardiol Clin*. 1994;12(2):223–245.
51. Cerci MSJ, Cerci JJ, Cerci RJ, Neto CCP, Trindade E, Delbeke D. Myocardial perfusion imaging is a strong predictor of death in women. *JACC Cardiovasc Imaging*. 2011;4(8):880–888.
52. Wackers FJ. Artifacts in planar SPECT myocardial perfusion imaging. *Am J Cardiac Imaging*. 1992;6(1):42–58.
53. Wackers FJ. Diagnostic pitfalls of myocardial perfusion imaging in women. *J Myocardial Ischemia*. 1992;4(10):23–37.
54. Johnstone DE. Effect of patient positioning on left lateral thallium-201 myocardial images. *J Nucl Med*. 1979;20(3):183–188.
55. DePuey EG, Rozanski A. Using gated technetium-99m-sestamibi SPECT to characterize fixed myocardial defects as infarct or artifact. *J Nucl Med*. 1995;36(6):952–955.
56. Taillefer R, DePuey EG, Udelson JE, et al. Comparative diagnostic accuracy of thallium-201 and Tc-99m sestamibi SPECT imaging (perfusion and ECG-gated SPECT) in detecting coronary artery disease in women. *J Am Coll Cardiol*. 1997;29:69–77.
57. Arsanjani R, Hayes SW, Fish M, et al. Two-position supine/prone myocardial perfusion SPECT (MPS) imaging improves visual inter-observer correlation and agreement. *J Nucl Cardiol*. 2014;21(4):703–711.
58. Roger V, Farkouh M, Weston S, et al. Sex differences in evaluation and outcome of unstable angina. *JAMA*. 2000;283:646–652.
59. Gulati M, Pandy DK, Arnsdorf MF, et al. Exercise capacity and the risk of death in women: the St. James Women Take Heart Project. *Circulation*. 2003;108:1554–1559.
60. Pancholy SB, Fattah AA, Kamal AM, et al. Independent and incremental prognostic value of exercise thallium single-photon emission computed tomographic imaging in women. *J Nucl Cardiol*. 1995;2(2):110–116.
61. Hachamovitch R, Berman DS, Kiat H, et al. Incremental prognostic value of *adenosine* stress myocardial perfusion single-photon emission computed tomography and impact on subsequent management in patients with or suspected of having myocardial ischemia. *Am J Cardiol*. 1997;80:426–432.
62. Einstein AJ, Knuuti J. Cardiac imaging: does radiation matter? *Eur Heart J*. 2012;33(5):573–578.
63. Nandalur KR, Dwamena BA, Choudhri AF. Diagnostic performance of positron emission tomography in the detection of coronary artery disease: a meta-analysis. *Acad Radiol*. 2008;15(4):444–451.
64. Bateman TM, Heller GV, McGhie AI, et al. Diagnostic accuracy of rest/stress ECG-gated Rb-82 myocardial perfusion PET: comparison with ECG-gated Tc-99m sestamibi SPECT. *J Nucl Cardiol*. 2006;13(1):24–33.
65. Kay J, Dorbala S, Goyal A, et al. Influence of sex on risk stratification with stress myocardial perfusion Rb-82 positron emission tomography: Results from the PET (Positron Emission Tomography) Prognosis Multicenter Registry. *J Am Coll Cardiol*. 2013;62(20):1866–1876.
66. Van Tosh A, Supino PG, Nichols KJ, Garza D, Horowitz SF, Reichek N. Prognosis of a normal positron emission tomography 82Rb myocardial perfusion imaging study in women with no history of coronary disease. *Cardiology*. 2010;117(4):301–306.
67. Murthy VL, Naya M, Taqueti VR, et al. Effects of sex on coronary microvascular dysfunction and cardiac outcomes. *Circulation*. 2014;129(24):2518–2527.
68. Mozaffarian D, Benjamin EJ, Go AS, et al. Executive Summary: Heart Disease and Stroke Statistics—2016 Update: A Report From the American Heart Association. *Circulation*. 2016;133(4):447–454.
69. Keith DS, Nichols GA, Gullion CM, Brown JB, Smith DH Longitudinal follow-up and outcomes among a population with chronic kidney disease in a large managed care organization. *Arch Intern Med*. 2004;164(6):659–663.
70. Foley RN, Murray AM, Li S, et al. Chronic kidney disease and the risk for cardiovascular disease, renal replacement, and death in the United States Medicare population, 1998 to 1999. *J Am Soc Nephrol*. 2005;16:489–495.
71. United States Renal Data System. *2015 USRDS Annual Data Report: Epidemiology of Kidney Disease in the United States*. Bethesda, MD: National Institutes of Health, National Institute of Diabetes and Digestive and Kidney Diseases; 2014.
72. Gurm HS, Gore JM, Anderson FA Jr, et al. Comparison of acute coronary syndrome in patients receiving versus not receiving chronic dialysis (from the Global Registry of Acute Coronary Events [GRACE] Registry). *Am J Cardiol*. 2012;109(1):19–25.
73. Weiner DE, Tighiouart H, Elsayed EF, et al. The Framingham predictive instrument in chronic kidney disease. *J Am Coll Cardiol*. 2007;50(3):217–224.

74. Hakeem A, Bhatti S, Dillie KS, et al. Predictive value of myocardial perfusion single-photon emission computed tomography and the impact of renal function on cardiac death. *Circulation*. 2008;118:2540–2549.
75. Al-Mallah MH, Hachamovitch R, Dorbala S, Di Carli MF. Incremental prognostic value of myocardial perfusion imaging in patients referred to stress single-photon emission computed tomography with renal dysfunction. *Circ Cardiovasc Imaging*. 2009;2:429–436.
76. Hakeem A, Bhatti S, Karmali KN, et al. Renal function and risk stratification of diabetic and nondiabetic patients undergoing evaluation for coronary artery disease. *J Am Coll Cardiol Img*. 2010;3:734–745.
77. Kim JK, Kim SG, Kim HJ, Song YR. Cardiac risk assessment by gated single-photon emission computed tomography in asymptomatic end-stage renal disease patients at the start of dialysis. *J Nucl Cardiol*. 2012;19:438–447.
78. Murthy VL, Naya M, Foster CR, et al. Coronary vascular dysfunction and prognosis in patients with chronic kidney disease. *JACC Cardiovasc Imaging*. 2012;5(10):1025–1034.
79. U.S. Bureau of the Census. Current Population Reports, Special Studies, P23-190, 65+ in the United States. Washington, DC: U.S. Government Printing Office; 1996.
80. Steinman MA, Lee SJ, John Boscardin W, et al. Patterns of multimorbidity in elderly veterans. *J Am Geriatr Soc*. 2012; 60(10):1872–1880.
81. Gibbons RJ, Balady GJ, Bricker JT, et al.. ACC/AHA 2002 guideline update for exercise testing: summary article: a report of the American College of Cardiology/American Heart Association Task Force on Practice Guidelines (Committee to Update the 1997 Exercise Testing Guidelines). *Circulation*. 2002;106:1883–1892.
82. Fihn SD, Gardin JM, Abrams J, et al.; 2012 ACCF/AHA/ACP/AATS/PCNA/SCAI/STS guideline for the diagnosis and management of patients with stable ischemic heart disease: a report of the American College of Cardiology Foundation/American Heart Association Task Force on Practice Guidelines, and the American College of Physicians, American Association for Thoracic Surgery, Preventive Cardiovascular Nurses Association, Society for Cardiovascular Angiography and Interventions, and Society of Thoracic Surgeons. *J Am Coll Cardiol*. 2012;60:e44–e164.
83. Katsikis A, Theodorakos A, Kouzoumi A. Prognostic value of the Duke treadmill score in octogenarians undergoing myocardial perfusion imaging. *Atherosclerosis*. 2014;236(2):373–380.
84. Rai M, Baker WL, Parker MW, Heller GV. Meta-analysis of optimal risk stratification in patients >65 years of age. *Am J Cardiol*. 2012;110(8):1092–1099.
85. Hachamovitch R, Kang X, Amanullah AM, et al. Prognostic implications of myocardial perfusion single-photon emission computed tomography in the elderly. *Circulation*. 2009;120(22):2197–2206.
86. Nair SU, Ahlberg AW, Mathur S, Katten DM, Polk DM, Heller GV. The clinical value of single photon emission computed tomography myocardial perfusion imaging in cardiac risk stratification of very elderly patients (≥80 years) with suspected coronary artery disease. *J Nucl Cardiol*. 2012;19(2):244–255.
87. McCaig LF, Burt CW. National Hospital Ambulatory Medical Care Survey: 2002 emergency department summary. *Adv Data*. 2004;340:1–34.
88. Duncan BH, Heller GV. Acute rest myocardial perfusion imaging in the evaluation of patients with chest pain syndromes. *ACC Curr J Rev*. 1999;8:52–56.
89. Klocke FJ, Baird MG, Lorell BH, et al. ACC/AHA/ASNC guidelines for the clinical use of cardiac radionuclide imaging—executive summary: a report of the American College of Cardiology/American Heart Association Task Force on Practice Guidelines (ACC/AHA/ASNC Committee to Revise the 1995 Guidelines for the Clinical Use of Cardiac Radionuclide Imaging). *Circulation*. 2003;108(11):1404–1418.
90. Wackers FJ, Brown KA, Heller GV, et al. American Society of Nuclear Cardiology position statement on radionuclide imaging in patients with suspected acute ischemic syndromes in the emergency department or chest pain center. *J Nucl Cardiol*. 2002;9(2):246–250.
91. Heller GV, Stowers SA, Hendel RC, et al. Clinical value of acute rest technetium-99m tetrofosmin tomographic myocardial perfusion imaging in patients with acute chest pain and nondiagnostic electrocardiograms. *J Am Coll Cardiol*. 1998; 31:1011–1017.
92. Udelson JE, Beshansky JR, Ballin DS, et al. Myocardial perfusion imaging for evaluation and triage of patients with suspected acute cardiac ischemia: a randomized controlled trial. *JAMA*. 2002;288:2693–2700.

Cost-Effectiveness of Nuclear Cardiology

CHAPTER 20

Lawrence M. Phillips, Joe X. Xie, and Leslee J. Shaw

INTRODUCTION

Nuclear cardiology in its over 40 years of use has grown to one of the most utilized and performed medical procedures in the United States, with cardiovascular imaging tests frequently being listed among the top 200 Medicare expenditures.[1-3] As nuclear cardiology has blossomed into an over $1 billion per year industry, increased attention and scrutiny have been given to this testing approach, particularly with cost-effectiveness playing a more central role. This has been seen in several different ways. Appropriate use criteria (AUC) have become mainstream tools in providing decision-making support as to whether or not a test or procedure is indicated based on evidence combined with expert consensus opinion.[4-6] This has contributed to a downtrend in the number of nuclear stress tests performed annually over the last decade (Fig. 20-1).[7] In addition, in an era with continued technological advancements in each of the cardiac

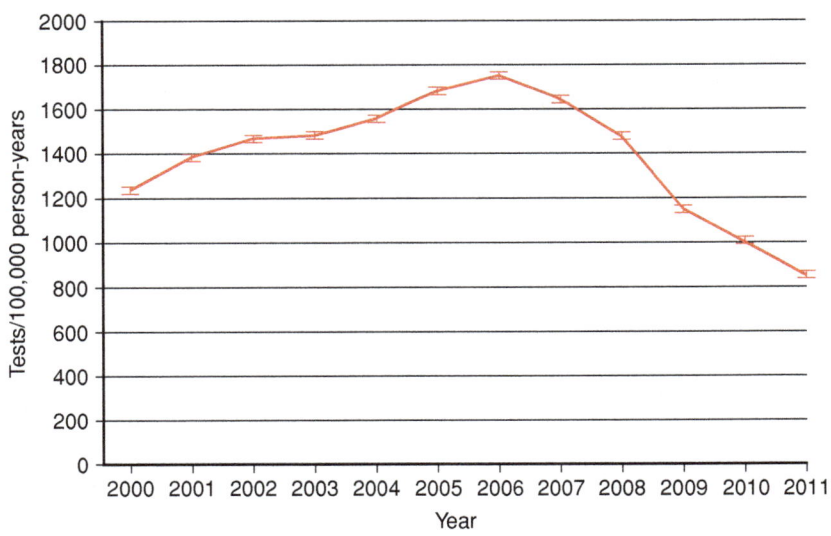

FIGURE 20-1 Age- and sex-adjusted annual rates of nuclear myocardial perfusion imaging tests from 2000 to 2011 showing initial increase in volume up until 2006 followed by a steady decrease in test performance. (Reproduced with permission from McNulty EJ, Hung YY, Almers LM, et al. Population trends from 2000–2011 in nuclear myocardial perfusion imaging use. *JAMA*. 2014;311(12):1248–1249.)

imaging modalities, clinicians often have multiple testing options that can be performed for a particular patient prompting a decision process that necessitates the evaluation of cost-effectiveness.[6,8]

Since 2005, which reflected the peak years of nuclear cardiology reimbursement, there have been increased restrictions on referrals for diagnostic testing including preauthorization and test substitution, as well as reductions in reimbursement for location of testing performed (outpatient vs. hospital based). In addition, the Institute of Medicine in 2009 suggested that 30% or $750 billion per year was spent on unnecessary medical services,[9] which puts all procedures under scrutiny. As the value of an imaging study becomes a pivotal issue, every diagnostic test must now pass individually defined quality and efficiency criteria. The value of the imaging study must balance the cost of the procedure with its impact on changing patient treatment and influencing outcomes. As the Medicare Access and CHIP Reauthorization Act (MACRA) of 2015 is implemented, the net value of the imaging procedure will directly impact on levels of reimbursement.

Thus, as the cost of diagnostic testing now plays a greater role in clinical decision making, clinicians have to be well educated in the science and economics of medicine as it impacts their daily practice. This chapter will discuss approaches to optimize the efficiency and quality of care based on patient selection for testing. This will be followed by a review of the definitions currently used for analysis and determination of cost-effectiveness. Finally, we will discuss sentinel studies that have examined value-based comparative approaches to diagnostic testing using nuclear stress tests as compared to other imaging modalities among patients presenting with stable ischemic heart disease or acute chest pain.

APPROPRIATE USE CRITERIA

The value of a test can be directly correlated to the selection of an appropriate test for a particular patient. In 2005, the AUC were first released by the American College of Cardiology to help guide clinicians in the selection of nuclear stress tests for the most common indications.[4] These were revised in 2009[5] as the initial AUC document was incorporated into payer decisions for test reimbursement. The AUC for stable ischemic heart disease have been updated as part of a new set of multimodality AUC.[6] This latest document also reflects changes in terminology to now include: appropriate, may be appropriate, and rarely appropriate.[6] Refer to Chapter 13 for a more detailed discussion of AUC.

The use of clinical decision support for the selection of appropriate tests is mandatory for most commercial payers and is also a central portion of Medicare health care reform policies. The Protecting Access to Medicare Act of 2014 (PAMA) includes stipulations that require the use of clinical decision support tools as part of the reimbursement process for imaging including nuclear cardiology.[8]

COST-EFFECTIVENESS ANALYSIS IN CARDIAC IMAGING

The passing of the Affordable Care Act of 2010 in the United States brought increased attention to value-based purchasing,[10] which examined health care value and included factors of quality and cost. Value-based purchasing can be mathematically written as:

$$Value = Quality/Cost$$

From this equation, it is clear that value increases as either quality increases or costs decrease. However, how is quality defined? In general, quality has been expressed as efficiency relating the processes incorporated to attain a certain goal. In health care, it is often associated with outcomes, which include survival or quality of life.[11] For cost, the question remains for what period of time the cost is impacted (e.g., episode of care). In value-based imaging, for example, we can compare two test modalities such as an exercise treadmill stress test and a nuclear stress test. For the actual test performed, there is a monetary cost associated with the specific test, which is one portion of the diagnostic evaluation cost.[12] Based on the results of a certain test, additional diagnostic testing, procedures and/or treatments may be required, which result in a higher cost of the diagnostic test approach beyond the index procedure.[13] However, over what timeframe do we allow these additional costs to be attributed to the index imaging procedure? There is as of yet no clear definition to incorporate associated downstream costs, but the length of time must be long enough to see the full benefit of the test and its subsequent results to fruition.[14] Moreover, an episode of care can be quite short for an acute evaluation, but may also be protracted for lower risk, stable patients.

Cost-effectiveness in cardiac imaging may involve two different approaches and compares the costs and outcomes of these testing strategies. It is important to keep in mind that one of the comparators can be no testing at all.[14] Quality-adjusted life-year (QALY) can be used to measure this outcome, which incorporates survival adjusted for quality of life.[14] The incremental cost-effectiveness ratio (ICER) is the summed calculation and allows for comparison of two diagnostic approaches. This can be mathematically written (with 1 and 2 representing the two diagnostic tests) as:

$$ICER = (C_1 - C_2)/(QALY_1 - QALY_2)$$

It is important for the definition of cost-effectiveness to identify both absolute thresholds as well as the impact of selecting one modality over another while incorporating downstream-related expenses. The thresholds of QALY have varied in studies, but have often been designated as $50,000 in previous literature.[14,15] Recently, the World Health Organization has suggested an alternative calculation based on an individual country's gross domestic product (GDP). Using the recommendation of three times the GDP would result in a new threshold in the United States of <$150,000 per life-year saved.[14]

The American College of Cardiology and the American Heart Association Task Force on Performance Measures and Task Force on Practice Guidelines now mandates that in addition to "Level of Evidence" for clinical guideline recommendations, that there also be a category of "Level of Value."[14] This proposal would include four categories: high value (H); intermediate value (I); low value (L); uncertain value (U). The dollar amount associated with these categories is linked with previously defined benchmarks of ICER (Table 20-1).

COST-EFFECTIVENESS IN STABLE ISCHEMIC HEART DISEASE

It has now been almost 20 years since one of the most sentinel papers regarding cost-effectiveness in

Table 20-1

Categorization of the Incremental Cost-Effectiveness Ratio per Quality-Adjusted Life-Year for Determination of Value

Levels of Value	ICER/QALY Gained
High value	ICER < $50,000 per QALY gained
Intermediate value	ICER $50,000 to < $150,000 per QALY gained
Low value	ICER > $150,000 per QALY gained
Uncertain value	Insufficient data to support categorization

ICER, incremental cost-effectiveness ratio; QALY, quality-adjusted life-year.
Reproduced with permission from Anderson JL, Heidenreich PA, Barnett PG, et al. ACC/AHA statement on cost/value methodology in clinical practice guidelines and performance measures: A report of the American College of Cardiology/American Heart Association Task Force on Performance Measures and Task Force on Practice Guidelines. *Circulation*. 2014;129(22):2329–2345.

cardiac imaging was published. The Economics of Noninvasive Diagnosis (END) Multicenter Study Group examined the cost impact of an approach using an initial referral for stress myocardial perfusion tomography versus direct referral for coronary angiography without initial noninvasive testing.[16] In this study, 11,372 patients were prospectively evaluated for costs of care both in their initial diagnostic testing and in composite costs over a 3-year period. The costs of care using radionuclide myocardial perfusion imaging (range, $2,387–$3,010) were lower than for patients undergoing direct angiography (range, $2,878–$4,579) ($p < 0.0001$) despite similar rates of death or myocardial infarction ($p > 0.20$). Part of this increased cost was due to higher rates of revascularization among patients in the invasive arm. Reductions in cost were also seen due to only one-third of patients assigned to the initial imaging strategy undergoing subsequent coronary angiography. Although some interpreted these results as a license to use nuclear stress testing as a "gatekeeper," it should instead be viewed as a precursor to trials such as COURAGE and BARI-2D, in that revascularization based solely on anatomic disease increases cost without a clinical benefit in terms of event-free survival (i.e., death or myocardial infarction-free survival).[17–19]

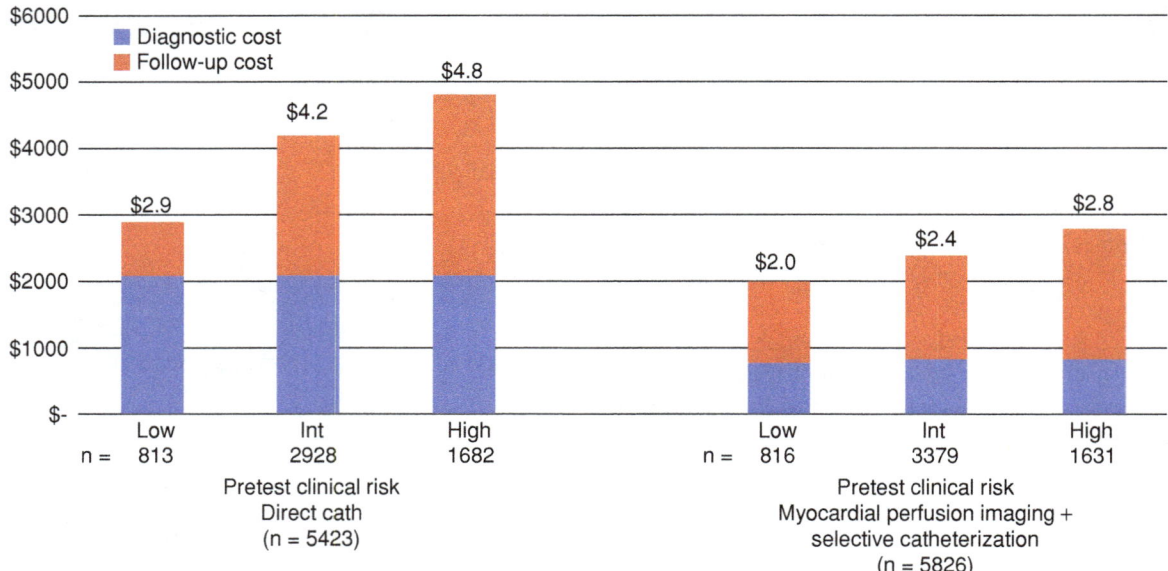

FIGURE 20-2 Diagnostic and follow-up costs for direct catheterization and initial stress perfusion imaging in the END trial based on pretest clinical risk. (Reproduced with permission from Shaw LJ, Hachamovitch R, Berman DS, et al. The economic consequences of available diagnostic and prognostic strategies for the evaluation of stable angina patients: an observational assessment of the value of precatheterization ischemia. Economics of Noninvasive Diagnosis (END) Multicenter Study Group. *J Am Coll Cardiol.* 1999;33(3):661–669.)

Figure 20-2 shows a graph from the END Multicenter Study Group comparing both the diagnostic and follow-up costs for different clinical risk subsets of patients for stress-first versus invasive-first approaches. Upon review of this finding, several factors have to be kept in mind: (1) The dollar amounts in this figure reflect health care costs from 1995 which would clearly underestimate current costs[16]; (2) Both guideline-directed medical therapy and revascularization technologies have improved, which also underestimate the costs to both arms if reproduced at present day; (3) Referral patterns for patients undergoing ischemic heart disease evaluation have changed with recent studies showing lower abnormality rates for single-photon emission computed tomography (SPECT) testing.[20] These factors taken together would suggest a greater cost-effectiveness for a cardiac imaging first approach in stable ischemic heart disease.

In 1999, the Economics of Myocardial Perfusion Imaging in Europe (EMPIRE) study retrospectively examined 396 patients for the cost-effectiveness of several diagnostic strategies, as well as the quality of diagnosis in a patient population undergoing initial evaluation of suspected coronary artery disease.[13] The diagnostic approaches evaluated in this trial were exercise stress testing, nuclear stress testing and coronary angiography with differentiation between institutions using nuclear stress testing routinely and for those who did not. The results from the EMPIRE study revealed that costs associated with both initial diagnostic approaches were reduced for institutions utilizing SPECT stress testing as well as a 32% lower 2-year diagnostic and management costs in these populations among patients without identified obstructive coronary artery disease. In patients where the algorithm was SPECT stress testing followed by coronary angiography versus angiography alone, 2-year costs were reduced 54% and 36% in patients without disease and those with disease, respectively, when using SPECT first (Fig. 20-3).[13]

More recent data presented in the Study of Myocardial Perfusion and Coronary Anatomy Imaging Roles in Coronary Artery Disease (SPARC) registry evaluated 1703 patients who were prospectively monitored after SPECT, positron emission tomography (PET), or 64-slice coronary computed tomography angiography (CCTA) for their 90-day cardiac

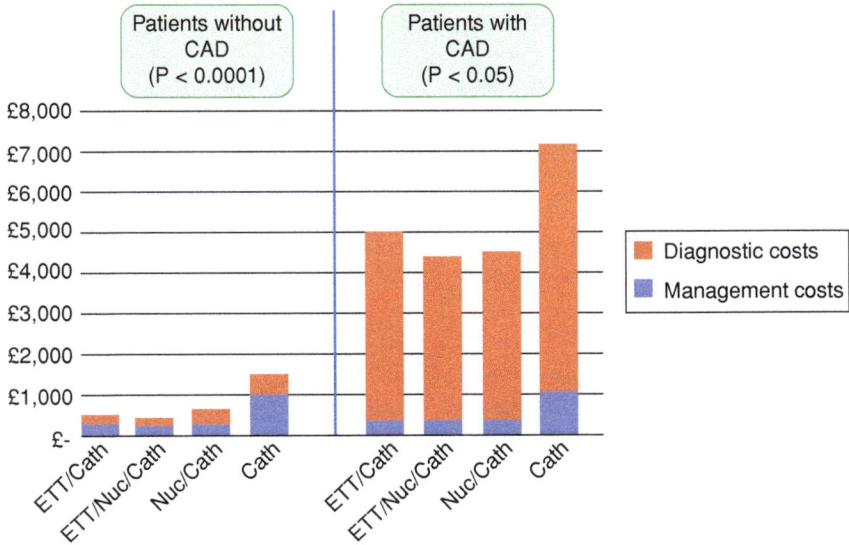

FIGURE 20-3 Mean 2-year diagnostic and management costs for patients with and without coronary artery disease (CAD) based on testing approach utilized in the EMPIRE study. (Data from Underwood SR, Godman B, Salyani S, et al. Economics of myocardial perfusion imaging in Europe—the EMPIRE Study. *Eur Heart J.* 1999;20(2):157–166.)

catheterization rates.[3,21] The results showed that referral to catheterization was relative to the severity of the noninvasive test abnormalities across all modalities, 2.8% catheterization rate in those with normal/nonobstructive results, 20.3% catheterization rate in those with mildly abnormal results, and 48.2% catheterization rate in those with moderate or severe abnormal results ($p < 0.001$). However, the referral rate to catheterization for patients in the CCTA arm (13.2%) was higher when compared to SPECT (4.3%) and PET (11.1%) ($p < 0.001$).[3]

For the purposes of this discussion on cost-effectiveness, subsequent analysis from the SPARC registry was performed to evaluate resource use, medical costs, and clinical outcomes for this cohort, allowing calculation of cost-effectiveness for the varying diagnostic test strategies.[22] These results revealed that 2-year costs were lowest for those who underwent initial SPECT testing compared to CCTA and PET (mean $3,965 vs. $4,909 vs. $6,647, respectively), which persisted after multivariable adjustment for clinical characteristics. Furthermore, patients undergoing CCTA had costs that were 15% higher than those undergoing SPECT. However, after controlling for longer survival, the cost-effectiveness of one modality over another became uncertain.[22] Notably, this registry was based on physician choice for test selection, and not randomization, and thus selection biases and additional confounders may have been present.

In the Cost-Effectiveness of Noninvasive Cardiac Testing (CECat) trial, 898 patients at high risk for obstructive coronary artery disease were randomized to SPECT, stress echocardiography, magnetic resonance perfusion imaging or index coronary angiography.[23] The goal was to compare the index noninvasive test versus direct coronary angiography. Survival was generally similar across the patients randomized to stress echocardiography and radionuclide stress testing when compared to coronary angiography (hazard ratio [HR] 1.0, 95% confidence interval [CI] 0.4–2.9; and HR 1.6, 95% CI 0.6–4.0, respectively). However, magnetic resonance perfusion imaging was noted to have a nearly threefold increased risk of death (HR 2.6, 95% CI 1.1–6.2). In the quality-of-life analysis, no difference was found in any of the four arms, thus revealing a similar pattern across all of the compared patient subsets. Notably, the cost of the index coronary angiography compared to index noninvasive testing was lower, but this was partially attributed to the high rate of subsequent coronary angiography among patients undergoing index noninvasive testing (75–80%). Of note is a key statement made in their report, "Our data clearly demonstrate a limited future role for cost-effective noninvasive imaging if referring physicians are not willing to accept a negative result as ground truth."[23] This underlines the utilization of noninvasive testing results in determining patients who would benefit from coronary angiography.

A different conclusion was reached from the results of the single-center clinical evaluation of magnetic resonance imaging in coronary heart disease (CeMARC). A total of 752 patients with suspected angina and at least one cardiovascular risk factor were recruited to undergo SPECT, CMR, or coronary angiography in order to evaluate the sensitivity, specificity, positive predictive value, and negative predictive value of SPECT versus CMR when using coronary angiography as the gold standard.[24] A subsequent decision analytic model was applied to this data to identify the most cost-effective diagnostic approach in a similar patient population.[25] Two diagnostic approaches using CMR (one with index ETT testing followed by CMR after a positive or inconclusive ETT and the other with index CMR) were concluded to be the most cost-effective with a threshold range cost of £20,000 (index ETT) to £30,000 (index CMR). In the recently published CE-MARC 2 trial, CMR and SPECT both reduced the probability of unnecessary angiography compared with NICE guideline-directed care. There was no statistical significance between the CMR and SPECT arms.[26]

Importantly, one of the least costly of initial noninvasive tests has been the exercise treadmill test (ETT). In the What Is the Optimal Method for Ischemia Evaluation in Women (WOMEN) trial, 824 women with intermediate pretest likelihood of coronary artery disease were randomized to an index diagnostic test of ETT versus exercise SPECT imaging.[12] Of note, all enrolled patients had interpretable EKGs for ischemia and predetermined exercise tolerance >5 METs. Two-year major adverse cardiac event (MACE)-free survival was similar in the two groups with 98.0% in the ETT arm and 97.7% in the MPI arm ($p = 0.59$). The index testing costs for patients undergoing ETT averaged $154.28 compared to exercise MPI of $495.24 ($p \leq 0.001$). This cost benefit was sustained when follow-up testing was also added with the ETT arm averaging $337.80 versus the exercise MPI at $643.24 ($p \leq 0.001$) (Table 20-2). These results support the cost-effectiveness of index diagnostic testing using ETT in lower-risk women who have an ability to exercise and have an interpretable EKG. Although not a cost-effectiveness trial by design, Borque et al. evaluated a similar question of additive benefit of myocardial perfusion imaging among patients who were able to exercise beyond 10 METS without ischemic ECG changes.[27] This study demonstrated that the prevalence of >10% ischemia in this group was very low (0.6%) with an annual cardiac mortality rate of 0.1% per year. Given these low event rates, it appears that there is little incremental value of SPECT MPI for patients who can perform a high-level exercise without ECG evidence for myocardial ischemia.

In 2015, the Prospective Multicenter Imaging Study for Evaluation of Chest Pain (PROMISE) trial published results comparing noninvasive anatomic assessment versus functional testing for patients

Table 20-2

Diagnostic Costs for Women Undergoing Initial ETT Versus Exercise MPI Testing. Results of the WOMEN Trial

Test Strategy	Index Testing Mean (SD)	Follow-Up Testing Mean (SD)	Total Costs
ETT	$1454.28 ($30.42)	$179.97 ($413.64)	$337.80 ($416.26)
Exercise MPI	$495.24 ($8.54)	$144.77 ($407.75)	$643.24 ($411.51)
	$p < 0.001$	$p = 0.0008$	$p < 0.001$

Modified with permission from Shaw LJ, Mieres JH, Hendel RH, et al. Comparative effectiveness of exercise electrocardiography with or without myocardial perfusion single photon emission computed tomography in women with suspected coronary artery disease: Results from the What Is the Optimal Method for Ischemia Evaluation in Women (WOMEN) trial. *Circulation*. 2011;124(11):1239–1249.

presenting with chest pain.[28] A total of 10,003 symptomatic outpatients who required nonurgent, noninvasive cardiac evaluation were randomized to initial evaluation with CCTA versus stress testing (67% stress radionuclide imaging, 23% stress echocardiography, and 10% ETT). The primary endpoint of a composite of death, myocardial infarction, hospitalization for unstable angina, or major procedural complication was similar between the diagnostic arms with an event rate of 3.3% in the CCTA group and 3.0% in the functional-testing group (HR 1.04; 95% CI 0.83–1.29, $p = 0.75$). An economic analysis of 9649 of the enrolled patients was subsequently published.[29] The costs were divided into three sections: First, was the cost of the index testing. The range of mean costs for different modalities ranged from $174 for ETT and up to $1132 for pharmacologic SPECT. The second analysis examined cumulative costs through 90 days. In comparing treatment approaches, the CCTA strategy had mean costs of $2494 compared to the functional strategy costs of $2240. A major component of this cost difference was attributed to coronary angiography and revascularization. In the CCTA group, 12.2% of the patients underwent invasive angiography with 6.2% undergoing revascularization compared to 8.1% of the functional testing group undergoing invasive angiography and 3.2% undergoing revascularization. Through 3 years of follow-up, using bootstrap analysis, the cost differences between anatomic versus functional diagnostic testing were minimal after the first year ($26 in year 2 and $91 in year 3 after removal of an outlier representing a noncardiovascular hospitalization). Figure 20-4 shows the cost differences between the two diagnostic approaches. Similarly, a retrospective analysis of Medicare spending from a sample of 282,830 patients from 2005 to 2008 showed that those undergoing evaluation with CCTA had a higher rate of subsequent invasive angiography compared to patients undergoing SPECT evaluation (22.9% vs. 12.1%, $p < 0.001$),[30] which led to higher total costs for CCTA. Importantly, medication use was not included as part of the cost calculations

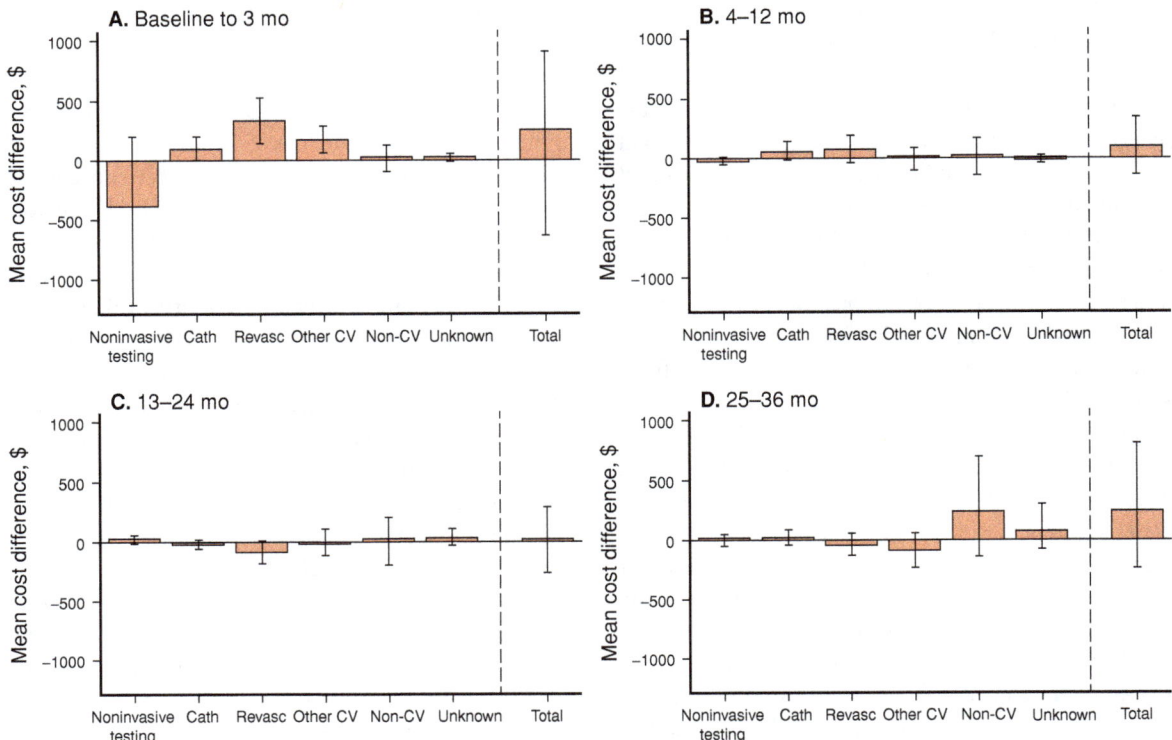

FIGURE 20-4 Mean cost differences between CTA and functional approaches in the PROMISE trial. Values above the baseline show higher cost for CTA compared to below the baseline show higher cost for the functional test. (Reproduced with permission from Mark DB, Federspiel JJ, Cowper PA, et al. Economic outcomes with anatomical versus functional diagnostic testing for coronary artery disease. *Ann Intern Med.* 2016;165(2):94–102.)

in either of these studies. As revealed in a secondary analysis of SPARC, aspirin and statin utilization were greater following an index CCTA as compared to an index SPECT.[3] Whether these changes in medication use could have prevented clinical worsening, additional downstream testing, or coronary hospitalizations are unknown, but are important variables to consider in cost-effectiveness analysis.

COST-EFFECTIVENESS IN THE EVALUATION OF ACUTE CHEST PAIN

A subset of patients where cost-effectiveness of nuclear stress testing is important has been evaluated among those undergoing evaluation in the emergency department (ED) for acute chest pain. Each year, over 8 million patients are evaluated in the ED in the United States for low-risk chest pain with costs in excess of $10 billion per year,[31–34] which has recently gained even more importance as medicine has seen a substantive movement from inpatient to outpatient care. The cost-effectiveness of different diagnostic modalities has additional components in this patient population including: time to diagnosis, hospital length of stay, and need for follow-up testing postdischarge. Thus, within nuclear cardiology, significant attention had been paid to the concept of acute chest pain imaging,[31] which uses an injection of a radiopharmaceutical while the patient is at rest but during or shortly after an episode of chest pain. Using this approach, an injection of radioisotope, in the setting of suspected acute myocardial ischemia, can be used to help differentiate focal-decreased perfusion from ischemia. In a sentinel article looking at early patient hospital discharge, Udelson et al. reported that hospitalizations among patients without evidence of acute ischemia on nuclear testing were reduced by 10% (52% of patients with usual care compared to 42% with sestamibi imaging).[32] Although only modest cost savings per patient ($60–72) were realized due to the added expense of SPECT imaging, the overall impact could be translated into savings of more than $14 million annually. Heller et al. similarly found in a patient sample of 357 patients that normal SPECT findings during the evaluation of acute chest pain resulted in more prompt and higher rates of discharge from the ED, with a mean cost savings of $4258 per patient.[32]

Stowers et al. looked at a sample of 46 patients who were assigned to perfusion imaging-guided diagnostic approach versus conventional evaluation (blinded to the perfusion results) and found a $1843 median reduction in in-hospital costs in the perfusion imaging-guided approach.[34] These results have been replicated in several additional studies.[35]

More commonly, an evaluation to exclude acute coronary syndrome consists of serial cardiac enzymes followed by rest–stress radionuclide imaging. In the Coronary Computed Tomographic Angiography for Systemic Triage of Acute Chest Pain Patients to Treatment (CT-STAT) trial, 699 patients presenting to the ED for evaluation of low-risk chest pain were randomized to index testing with CCTA versus SPECT.[36] Two key findings were relevant to our cost-effectiveness discussion. First, the time to diagnosis was 54% shorter in the arm undergoing index CCTA (median 2.9 hours in the CCTA arm compared to 6.2 hours in the SPECT arm, $p < 0.0001$). However, the amount of time for test completion should be considered given the increased time required for SPECT versus CCTA as well as need for serial biomarker testing. Second, the total ED costs were reduced in the CCTA arm by over 38%. The median CCTA cost was $2137 compared to $3458 for SPECT ($p < 0.0001$) despite no difference in the actual cost of the diagnostic test. Of note, these costs do not take into effect subsequent costs after the initial emergency room discharge and also include the required additional emergency room time needed for serial cardiac enzymes. In the Coronary CT Angiography versus Standard Evaluation in Acute Chest Pain by the ROMICAT-II investigators, early CCTA was compared to standard ED treatment for 1000 patients with suspected acute coronary syndromes.[37] No difference was seen in the cost of the two approaches with the CCTA at $4289 cumulative mean cost and the standard evaluation group at $4060.

The above studies relate times to discharge from the ED. However, new MPI protocols have resulted in reduction in time for testing. One particular protocol using selective stress-only testing can result in significant reduction in time required prior to a negative result. In a retrospective analysis performed by Duvall et al., the utilization of a selective stress-only protocol revealed a lower rate of follow-up testing in the nuclear stress arm as compared to the CCTA arm, which may reduce overall costs associated with

SPECT.[38] In addition, multiple studies have shown that the prognosis associated with a normal stress-only scan is similar to that of a normal rest/stress MPI scan.[39–41]

CONCLUSIONS

In this chapter, we have highlighted the economic evidence and provided clinicians with a clearer understanding of the factors determining varying cost-effectiveness of diagnostic imaging test strategies. Both in patients with suspected stable ischemic heart disease and in those who present to the ED with acute chest pain, radionuclide stress testing has been shown to be a cost-effective approach to the management of these patients. When comparing direct invasive angiography first approaches to radionuclide stress testing, the data have repeatedly shown cost-effectiveness to using a noninvasive testing first approach. In the ED evaluation, studies have shown a more equipoise in the cost-effectiveness among noninvasive tests when comparing radionuclide imaging to coronary CT angiography. As newer technologies become available for clinical use, the comparative cost-effectiveness of these new diagnostic testing modalities will need to be investigated against those which have been our mainstay testing for almost the last half-century.

REFERENCES

1. Zaret BL, Strauss HW, Martin ND, Wells HP, Jr., Flamm MD, Jr. Noninvasive regional myocardial perfusion with radioactive potassium. Study of patients at rest, with exercise and during angina pectoris. *N Engl J Med*. 1973;288(16):809–812.
2. Strauss HW, Harrison K, Langan JK, Lebowitz E, Pitt B. Thallium-201 for myocardial imaging. Relation of thallium-201 to regional myocardial perfusion. *Circulation*. 1975;51(4):641–645.
3. Shaw LJ, Hage FG, Berman DS, Hachamovitch R, Iskandrian A. Prognosis in the era of comparative effectiveness research: Where is nuclear cardiology now and where should it be? *J Nucl Cardiol*. 2012;19(5):1026–1043.
4. Brindis RG, Douglas PS, Hendel RC, et al. ACCF/ASNC appropriateness criteria for single-photon emission computed tomography myocardial perfusion imaging (SPECT MPI): a report of the American College of Cardiology Foundation Quality Strategic Directions Committee Appropriateness Criteria Working Group and the American Society of Nuclear Cardiology endorsed by the American Heart Association. *J Am Coll Cardiol*. 2005;46(8):1587–1605.
5. Hendel RC, Berman DS, Di Carli MF, et al. ACCF/ASNC/ACR/AHA/ASE/SCCT/SCMR/SNM 2009 Appropriate Use Criteria for Cardiac Radionuclide Imaging: A Report of the American College of Cardiology Foundation Appropriate Use Criteria Task Force, the American Society of Nuclear Cardiology, the American College of Radiology, the American Heart Association, the American Society of Echocardiography, the Society of Cardiovascular Computed Tomography, the Society for Cardiovascular Magnetic Resonance, and the Society of Nuclear Medicine. *J Am Coll Cardiol*. 2009;53(23):2201–2229.
6. Ronan G, Wolk MJ, Bailey SR, et al. ACCF/AHA/ASE/ASNC/HFSA/HRS/SCAI/SCCT/SCMR/STS 2013 multimodality appropriate use criteria for the detection and risk assessment of stable ischemic heart disease: a report of the American College of Cardiology Foundation Appropriate Use Criteria Task Force, American Heart Association, American Society of Echocardiography, American Society of Nuclear Cardiology, Heart Failure Society of America, Heart Rhythm Society, Society for Cardiovascular Angiography and Interventions, Society of Cardiovascular Computed Tomography, Society for Cardiovascular Magnetic Resonance, and Society of Thoracic Surgeons. *J Nucl Cardiol*. 2014;21(1):192–220.
7. McNulty EJ, Hung YY, Almers LM, Go AS, Yeh RW. Population trends from 2000–2011 in nuclear myocardial perfusion imaging use. *JAMA*. 2014;311(12):1248–1249.
8. Lin FY, Dunning AM, Narula J, et al. Impact of an automated multimodality point-of-order decision support tool on rates of appropriate testing and clinical decision making for individuals with suspected coronary artery disease: A prospective multicenter study. *J Am Coll Cardiol*. 2013;62(4):308–316.
9. http://www.nationalacademies.org/hmd/~/media/Files/Report%20Files/2012/Best-Care/BestCareReportBrief.pdf. Accessed May 16, 2017.
10. http://archive.ahrq.gov/professionals/quality-patient-safety/quality-resources/value/valuebased/evalvbp1.html#whatisvbp. Accessed May 16, 2017.
11. Porter ME. What is value in health care? *N Engl J Med*. 2010;363(26):2477–2481.
12. Shaw LJ, Mieres JH, Hendel RH, et al. Comparative effectiveness of exercise electrocardiography with or without myocardial perfusion single photon emission computed tomography in women with suspected coronary artery disease: Results from the What Is the Optimal Method for Ischemia Evaluation in Women (WOMEN) trial. *Circulation*. 2011;124(11):1239–1249.
13. Underwood SR, Godman B, Salyani S, Ogle JR, Ell PJ. Economics of myocardial perfusion imaging in Europe–the EMPIRE Study. *Eur Heart J*. 1999;20(2):157–166.
14. Anderson JL, Heidenreich PA, Barnett PG, et al. ACC/AHA statement on cost/value methodology in clinical practice guidelines and performance measures: A report of the American College of Cardiology/American Heart Association Task Force on Performance Measures and Task Force on Practice Guidelines. *Circulation*. 2014;129(22):2329–2345.
15. Owens DK. Interpretation of cost-effectiveness analyses. *J Gen Int Med*. 1998;13(10):716–717.
16. Shaw LJ, Hachamovitch R, Berman DS, et al. The economic consequences of available diagnostic and prognostic strategies for the evaluation of stable angina patients: An observational assessment of the value of precatheterization ischemia.

Economics of Noninvasive Diagnosis (END) Multicenter Study Group. *J Am Coll Cardiol.* 1999;33(3):661–669.
17. Boden WE, O'Rourke RA, Teo KK, et al. Optimal medical therapy with or without PCI for stable coronary disease. *N Engl J Med.* 2007;356(15):1503–1516.
18. Shaw LJ, Berman DS, Maron DJ, et al. Optimal medical therapy with or without percutaneous coronary intervention to reduce ischemic burden: Results from the Clinical Outcomes Utilizing Revascularization and Aggressive Drug Evaluation (COURAGE) trial nuclear substudy. *Circulation.* 2008;117(10):1283–1291.
19. Frye RL, August P, Brooks MM, et al. A randomized trial of therapies for type 2 diabetes and coronary artery disease. *N Engl J Med.* 2009;360(24):2503–2515.
20. Rozanski A, Gransar H, Hayes SW, et al. Temporal trends in the frequency of inducible myocardial ischemia during cardiac stress testing: 1991 to 2009. *J Am Coll Cardiol.* 2013;61(10):1054–1065.
21. Hachamovitch R, Johnson JR, Hlatky MA, et al. The study of myocardial perfusion and coronary anatomy imaging roles in CAD (SPARC): Design, rationale, and baseline patient characteristics of a prospective, multicenter observational registry comparing PET, SPECT, and CTA for resource utilization and clinical outcomes. *J Nucl Cardiol.* 2009;16(6):935–948.
22. Hlatky MA, Shilane D, Hachamovitch R, Dicarli MF. Economic outcomes in the Study of Myocardial Perfusion and Coronary Anatomy Imaging Roles in Coronary Artery Disease registry: The SPARC Study. *Am Coll Cardiol.* 2014;63(10):1002–1008.
23. Thom H, West NE, Hughes V, et al. Cost-effectiveness of initial stress cardiovascular MR, stress SPECT or stress echocardiography as a gate-keeper test, compared with upfront invasive coronary angiography in the investigation and management of patients with stable chest pain: Mid-term outcomes from the CECaT randomised controlled trial. *BMJ open.* 2014;4(2):e003419.
24. Greenwood JP, Maredia N, Younger JF, et al. Cardiovascular magnetic resonance and single-photon emission computed tomography for diagnosis of coronary heart disease (CE-MARC): A prospective trial. *Lancet (London, England).* 2012;379(9814):453–460.
25. Walker S, Girardin F, McKenna C, et al. Cost-effectiveness of cardiovascular magnetic resonance in the diagnosis of coronary heart disease: an economic evaluation using data from the CE-MARC study. *Heart (British Cardiac Society).* 2013;99(12):873–881.
26. Greenwood JP, Ripley DP, Berry C, et al. Effect of Care Guided by Cardiovascular Magnetic Resonance, Myocardial Perfusion Scintigraphy, or NICE Guidelines on Subsequent Unnecessary Angiography Rates: The CE-MARC 2 Randomized Clinical Trial. *JAMA.* 2016;316(10):1051–1060.
27. Bourque JM, Charlton GT, Holland BH, Belyea CM, Watson DD, Beller GA. Prognosis in patients achieving ≥ 10 METS on exercise stress testing: Was SPECT imaging useful? *J Nucl Cardiol.* 2011;18:230–237.
28. Douglas PS, Hoffmann U, Patel MR, et al. Outcomes of anatomical versus functional testing for coronary artery disease. *N Engl J Med.* 2015;372(14):1291–300.
29. Mark DB, Federspiel JJ, Cowper PA, et al. Economic outcomes with anatomical versus functional diagnostic testing for coronary artery disease. *Ann Int Med.* 2016.
30. Shreibati JB, Baker LC, Hlatky MA. Association of coronary CT angiography or stress testing with subsequent utilization and spending among Medicare beneficiaries. *JAMA.* 2011;306(19):2128–2136.
31. Rybicki FJ, Udelson JE, Peacock WF, Goldhaber SZ, Isselbacher EM, Kazerooni E, et al. 2015 ACR/ACC/AHA/AATS/ACEP/ASNC/NASCI/SAEM/SCCT/SCMR/SCPC/SNMMI/STR/STS Appropriate Utilization of Cardiovascular Imaging in Emergency Department Patients With Chest Pain: A Joint Document of the American College of Radiology Appropriateness Criteria Committee and the American College of Cardiology Appropriate Use Criteria Task Force. *J Am Coll Cardiol.* 2016;67(7):853–879.
32. Udelson JE, Beshansky JR, Ballin DS, et al. Myocardial perfusion imaging for evaluation and triage of patients with suspected acute cardiac ischemia: A randomized controlled trial. *JAMA.* 2002;288(21):2693–2700.
33. Heller GV, Stowers SA, Hendel RC, et al. Clinical value of acute rest technetium-99m tetrofosmin tomographic myocardial perfusion imaging in patients with acute chest pain and nondiagnostic electrocardiograms. *J Am Coll Cardiol.* 1998;31(5):1011–1017.
34. Stowers SA, Eisenstein EL, Th Wackers FJ, et al. An economic analysis of an aggressive diagnostic strategy with single photon emission computed tomography myocardial perfusion imaging and early exercise stress testing in emergency department patients who present with chest pain but nondiagnostic electrocardiograms: results from a randomized trial. *Ann Emerg Med.* 2000;35(1):17–25.
35. Wackers FJ, Brown KA, Heller GV, et al. American Society of Nuclear Cardiology position statement on radionuclide imaging in patients with suspected acute ischemic syndromes in the emergency department or chest pain center. *J Nucl Cardiol.* 2002;9(2):246–250.
36. Goldstein JA, Chinnaiyan KM, Abidov A, et al. The CT-STAT (Coronary Computed Tomographic Angiography for Systematic Triage of Acute Chest Pain Patients to Treatment) trial. *J Am Coll Cardiol.* 2011;58(14):1414–1422.
37. Hoffmann U, Truong QA, Schoenfeld DA, et al. Coronary CT angiography versus standard evaluation in acute chest pain. *N Engl J Med.* 2012;367(4):299–308.
38. Duvall WL, Savino JA, Levine EJ, et al. A comparison of coronary CTA and stress testing using high-efficiency SPECT MPI for the evaluation of chest pain in the emergency department. *J Nucl Cardiol.* 2014;21(2):305–318.
39. Chang SM, Nabi F, Xu J, Raza U, Mahmarian JJ. Normal stress-only versus standard stress/rest myocardial perfusion imaging: Similar patient mortality with reduced radiation exposure. *J Am Coll Cardiol.* 2010;55(3):221–230.
40. Duvall WL, Wijetunga MN, Klein TM, et al. The prognosis of a normal stress-only Tc-99m myocardial perfusion imaging study. *J Nucl Cardiol.* 2010;17(3):370–377.
41. Mahmarian JJ. Stress only myocardial perfusion imaging: Is it time for a change? *J Nucl Cardiol.* 2010;17(4):529–535.

SECTION 4

NUCLEAR CARDIOLOGY BEYOND MYOCARDIAL PERFUSION

Nuclear Cardiology Procedures in the Evaluation of Myocardial Viability

CHAPTER 21

Fernanda Erthal, Benjamin Chow, Gary V. Heller, and Rob S.B. Beanlands

INTRODUCTION

It is estimated that 5.7 million Americans adults had heart failure (HF) in 2012 with an associated cost of $30.7 billion in that year alone.[1] The incidence of HF is high, with 870,000 new cases being reported annually and projections suggest a prevalence of >8 million adults in United States by 2030.[1] Mortality attributed to HF in 2011 was 58,309 in the United States, and its mention on death certificates was 284,388 (1 in 9 deaths).[1]

Although survival of patients with diagnosed HF has improved over time, it remains a disease with poor outcome. Approximately 50% of HF patients will be deceased 5 years after diagnosis.[2]

Given the growing prevalence of ischemic HF (IHF) and its high mortality rate, the optimal management strategies for IHF has been the focus of research for the last several decades. Evidence, including randomized controlled trials, have accumulated and support the notion that patients with IHF may benefit from viability imaging to guide therapy and revascularization decisions.[3-9] In some, but not all studies, in patients with IHF, the presence of viability, demonstrated on noninvasive images, is a strong indicator that revascularization may improve survival.[7,8,10-13] This chapter will describe the concepts of viability, nuclear imaging methods of assessing viability, supportive data and finally patients who could benefit from viability assessment.

UNDERSTANDING THE CONCEPTS

Viable, stunning, and hibernating myocardium are important concepts that are often misunderstood. Misconceptions of these three entities sometimes can lead to incorrect clinical decision making.

▶ Viable versus Nonviable Myocardium

Dysfunctional myocardium can be dichotomized into viable or nonviable myocardium. In the latter, the tissue is replaced by irreversible fibrosis and therefore cannot be reversed nor improved with revascularization. Conversely, viable myocardium is that with variable function, metabolism, and blood flow. In cases of dysfunctional but viable myocardium due to repeated episodes or persistent abnormal coronary flow, restoring coronary flow may result in metabolic recovery and recovery of function.[3,14] The main goal of viability imaging is to define the amount of viable myocardium in order to guide decision making to therapies which improve not only LV function but also clinical outcomes.[4-10]

▶ Stunning

Stunned myocardium refers to a post ischemic state where there is mismatch between function and flow. Although resting coronary flow has returned to normal, myocardial function remains impaired. The duration of stunning is dependent on the duration, severity, and size of the ischemic insult.[15-18] In stunned myocardium, metabolic alterations prevail over structural changes. Electron microscopy of stunned myocardium shows normal or just mildly degenerated cells.[14] Observed metabolic derangement includes a decrease in calcium sensitivity of myofilaments.[18] Metabolic changes can be complex and change over time. A GLUT 4 translocation to the sarcolemma and an increase in glucose uptake have been observed[19]; so too has a decrease in glucose uptake on metabolic imaging post-STEMI revascularization.[20] If the injury persists and/or in cases of repetitive stunning, myocardial changes can progress to a hibernation state (viable) or to irreversible fibrosis/scar (nonviable).[3,21,22]

If repeated ischemia is prevented, stunned myocardium is expected to eventually recover. As such, imaging in the post-MI period following large MIs (STEMIs or large non-STEMIs) may be misleading in that viable myocardium may recover spontaneously without needing revascularization. In part because of this (but also because of variable metabolic derangements in the stunned myocardium and potential effects of no reflow-phenomena as well as inflammation, which could each alter tracer uptake and lead to false positive or negative findings regarding viability) performing viability imaging in the post-MI period is challenging. Thus viability imaging is often avoided within 2 to 4 weeks of large myocardial infarctions (MIs).

Hibernation

Hibernating myocardium is thought to occur after repeated episodes of ischemia or stunning[3,23] and by definition, is viable and therefore has the capacity for functional recovery after adequate revascularization.[3,4,24] Myocytes in a hibernating state lose variable amounts of contractile material (sarcomeres) without significant changes in the cell volume. The absence of volume changes is an important characteristic that helps differentiate viable myocardium from atrophic degeneration.[25] Cellular volume, previously occupied by myofilaments, is replaced by glycogen (Fig. 21-1).[25] This adaptive downregulation response is important to

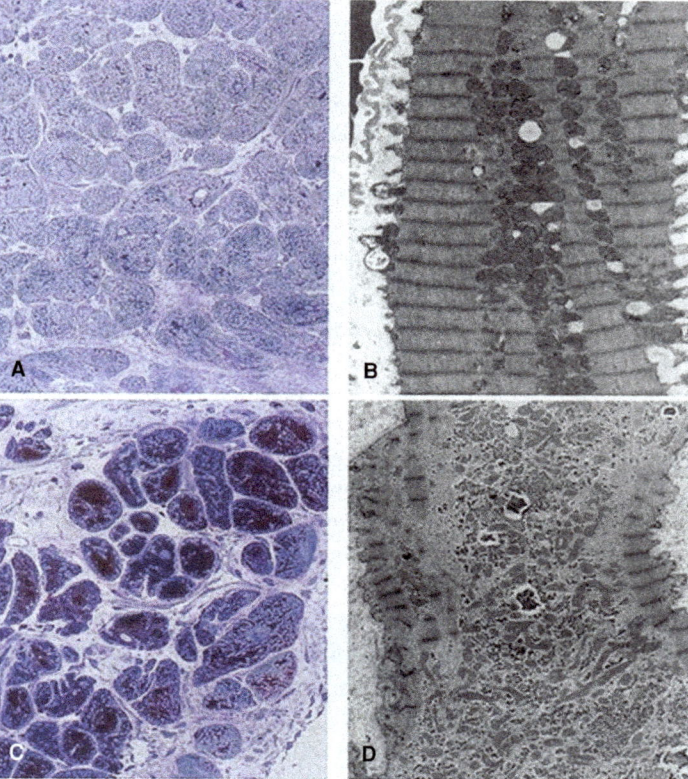

FIGURE 21-1 **(A)** Light micrograph of myocardium showing normal cardiomyocytes with virtually no glycogen (PAS staining in red). **(B)** Transmission electron micrograph of normal cardiac myocyte. **(C)** Representative light micrograph of biopsy sample of human hibernating myocardium. Cardiac myocytes are depleted of their contractile material and filled with glycogen (PAS-positive staining). **(D)** Representative transmission electron micrograph of a hibernating cardiomyocyte. Myolytic cytoplasm is devoid of sarcomeres and filled with glycogen. Magnification: a and c, ×320; b, ×7100; and d, ×7500. (Reproduced with permission from Vanoverschelde JL, Wijns W, Borgers M, et al. Chronic myocardial hibernation in humans from bedside to bench. *Circulation*. 1997;95(7):1961–1971.)

prevent a "supply-demand imbalance" during a period of limited coronary flow reserve.[23] Mitochondria apparatus is preserved. Functionality and oxidative metabolism remain but may be reduced and can be measured by PET with ^{11}C-acetate (acetate is transported into the mitochondria directly via acetyl-CoA and then enters into the tricarboxylic acid cycle to produce energy).[26] Similarly, myocardial glucose metabolism is preserved (via increased glycolysis to offset reduced oxidation) and can be measured by PET with ^{18}fluorodeoxyglucose (^{18}FDG), a glucose analog that is transported into the myocyte and converted to FDG-6-phosphate. This preservation of glucose metabolism is key and makes it possible for cardiac metabolic imaging to distinguish between viable and nonviable myocardium.

Several modalities are available for viability assessment: cardiac PET, single-photon emission computed tomography (SPECT), dobutamine echocardiography (ECHO), dobutamine magnetic resonance imaging (MRI), delayed-enhancement MRI (DE-MRI), delayed-enhancement computed tomography (CT),[4] and myocardial contrast ECHO.[27,28] Metabolic and cellular targets and findings suggestive of viability for each modality are outlined in Table 21-1. The clinically available nuclear imaging methods are summarized below.

NUCLEAR IMAGING METHODS FOR VIABILITY ASSESSMENT

▶ Single-Photon Emission Computed Tomography

Myocardium viability imaging can be performed with 201-thallium (^{201}Tl) or 99m-technetium (^{99m}Tc) and relies on the integrity of the sarcolemma and mitochondria, respectively.[29-31] Comparisons between ^{201}Tl SPECT, ^{99m}Tc SPECT, and ^{18}FDG PET show that scintigraphy with ^{99m}Tc-based imaging may underestimate the amount of viable myocardium,[32-36] while one direct comparison study observed that ^{201}Tl provided comparable information with ^{18}FDG PET.[37] A meta-analysis of 40 studies (1119 patients) using ^{201}Tl SPECT showed a mean sensitivity, specificity, predictive positive value (PPV), and negative predictive value (NPV) of 87%, 54%, 67%, and 79%, respectively.[4] A meta-analysis of 25 studies (721 patients) that used ^{99m}Tc SPECT to assess viability showed sensitivity,

Table 21-1
Imaging Modalities and Mechanisms for Viability Detection

Imaging Modality	Method Target	Indicator of Viability
^{18}FDG PET	Glucose metabolism	Normal perfusion/FDG = viable (not ischemic at rest) Perfusion-Metabolism (a) mismatch = hibernation (b) match = scar
SPECT (Tl-201)	Myocardial perfusion/ Na/K ATPase activity (membrane integrity)	Uptake = viable Redistribution on delayed imaging after stress, rest or reinjection = ischemia or hibernation
SPECT (Tc-99m-based)	Myocardial perfusion/ arterioles vasodilatation Mitochondrial integrity	Uptake = viable Mismatch between rest and post nitro images = hibernating
Dobutamine echocardiography/MRI	Contractile reserve	Improvement in wall motion with low dose dobutamine
Delayed enhancement MRI	Fibrosis tissue	Absence or small amount of scar
Late enhancement CT	Fibrosis tissue	Absence or small amount of scar
Myocardial contrast echocardiography	Microvascular integrity	Homogeneous contrast intensity

^{18}FDG PET, positron emission tomography with ^{18}Fluorodeoxyglucose; SPECT, single-photon emission computed tomography; Tl-201 (Thallium-201); Tc-99m (Technetium-99m); MRI, magnetic resonance imaging; CT, computed tomography.

specificity, PPV, and NPV of 83%, 65%, 74%, and 76%, respectively.[4] Both were not as sensitive as ^{18}FDG PET.[4] However, other studies showed similar values between ^{201}Tl and ^{99m}Tc-based imaging.[38,39] Overall, both approaches are considered reasonable means to assess myocardial viability.[8]

Imaging Protocols for 201-Thallium SPECT

Thallium is a potassium analog and its uptake is both passive and also active via a process requiring the normal function of the sodium-potassium ATPase pump and cellular membrane integrity.[40] Since membrane integrity is a requisite for cell viability, thallium-201 uptake visualized by SPECT images is indicative of myocardium viability.

Different protocols are described to assess viability with ^{201}Tl SPECT. The American Society of Nuclear Cardiology (ASNC) guidelines[41] describe a didactic format (Figs. 21-2 and 21-3). Although the rest-redistribution protocol can be performed (see Fig. 21-2), the most common protocol starts with a stress phase and injection of 2.5 to 3.5 mCi of ^{201}Tl at peak stress (Fig. 21.3). After 10 to 15 minutes, the stress images are acquired with redistribution (rest) imaging acquired 2.5 to 4 hours later. Up to this point, a regular stress/rest ^{201}Tl protocol is described. When a persistent (fixed) defect is present and viability needs to be assessed, a late-redistribution imaging can be performed at 18 to 24 hours. ^{201}Tl redistribution is a continual process that requires blood supply to the viable tissue and thus its uptake is also related to perfusion and the severity of coronary artery stenosis.[42] Studies have shown that in late images (8–72 hours) the viable myocardium segments show thallium redistribution (reversible defects) while truly nonviable myocardium appears as a persistent (fixed) defects on the late perfusion images (no thallium uptake).[42-45] To maximize the protocol, addition 1 to 2 mCi of ^{201}Tl can be reinjected (Fig. 21-3).[41]

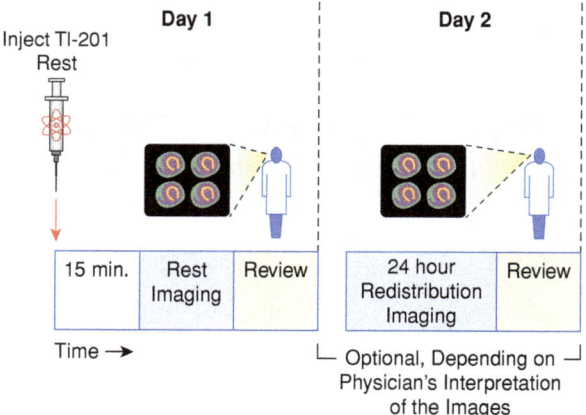

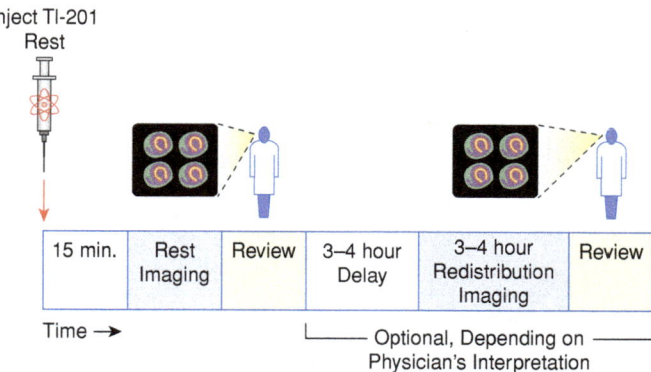

FIGURE 21-2 ^{201}Tl rest-redistribution protocol for viability assessment. (Reproduced with permission from Henzlova MJ, Duvall WL, Einstein AJ, et al. ASNC imaging guidelines for SPECT nuclear cardiology procedures: Stress, protocols, and tracers. J Nucl Cardiol. 2016;23(3):606–639.)

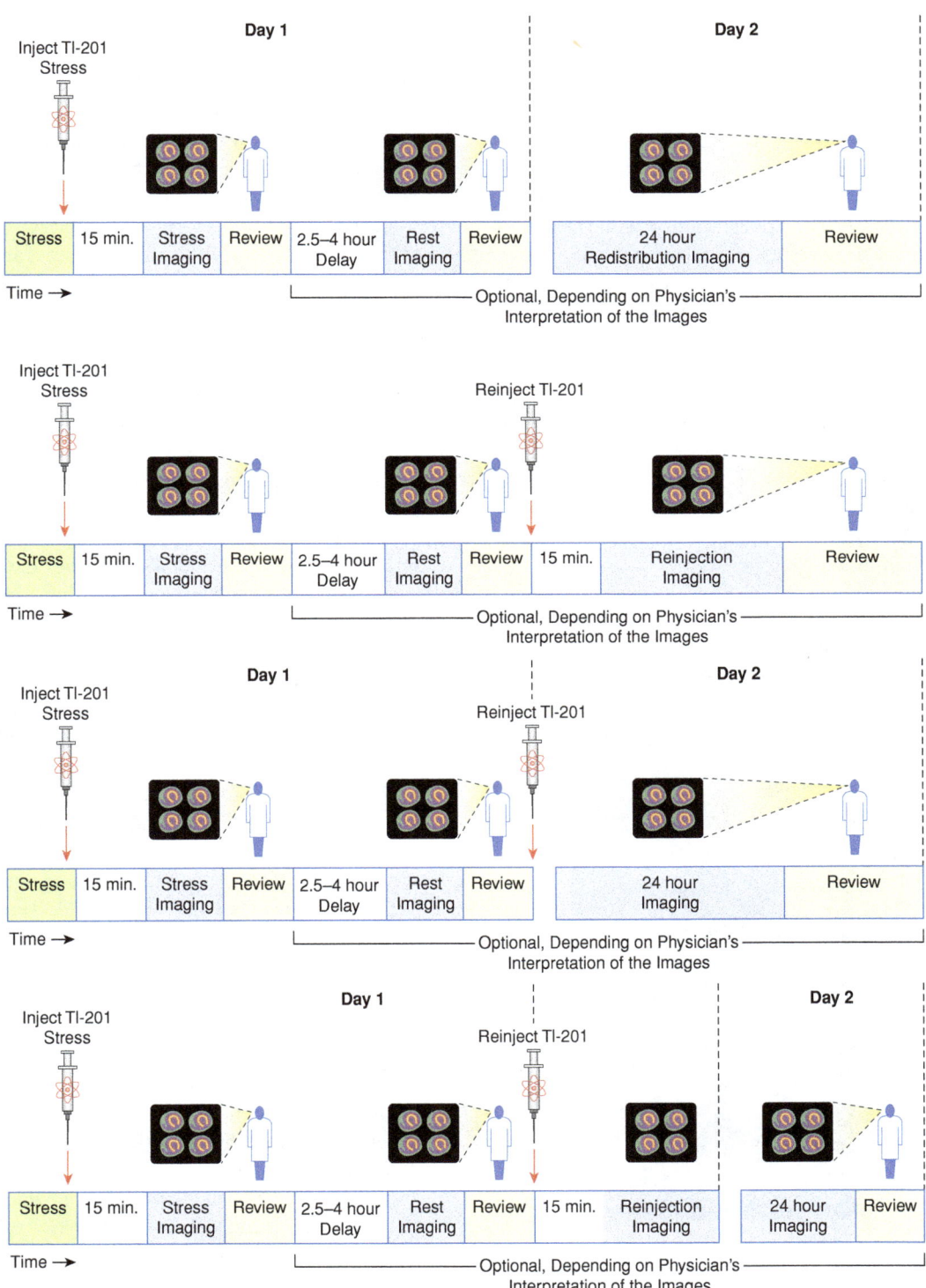

FIGURE 21-3 ^{201}Tl stress–rest imaging protocols. (Reproduced with permission from Henzlova MJ, Duvall WL, Einstein AJ, et al. ASNC imaging guidelines for SPECT nuclear cardiology procedures: Stress, protocols, and tracers. *J Nucl Cardiol.* 2016;23(3):606–639.)

Subanalysis of a pooled meta-analysis compared ^{201}Tl SPECT rest-redistribution to the ^{201}Tl SPECT reinjection protocol and showed comparable sensitivities (87% for both protocols) but with higher specificity and PPV for ^{201}Tl SPECT rest-redistribution (56% vs 50% and 71% vs. 58%, respectively) ($p < 0.05$ for both).[4] On the other hand, head to head comparison between 24-hour redistribution with the reinjection protocol suggested that reinjection may provide better diagnostic information with a significantly greater ability to identify hibernating myocardium.[46] When comparing the reinjection protocol to ^{18}FDG PET, there was very good correlation, although ^{201}Tl may have inferior sensitivity compared to glucose metabolism assessment with PET.[4,37,47,48] The difference in sensitivity may be because perfusion/^{18}FDG PET already considers perfusion. ^{18}FDG then adds metabolic information when there is mismatch. Figure 21-4 shows an example of ^{201}Tl SPECT rest-redistribution imaging.

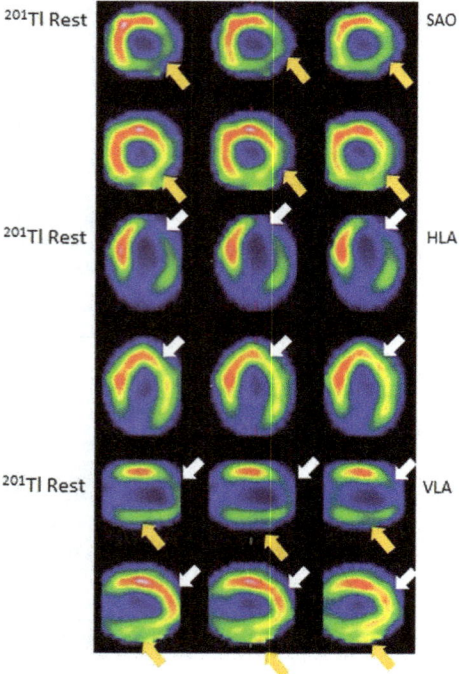

FIGURE 21-4 ^{201}Tl rest-redistribution SPECT in short axis (SAO), horizontal long axis (HLA), and vertical long axis (VLA) showing a mismatch area (viable myocardium) in the mid to distal inferior and inferolateral walls (*yellow arrow*) and distal anterior and lateral walls and apex (*white arrow*).

Imaging Protocols for 99m-Technetium SPECT

^{99m}Technetium-sestamibi and ^{99m}Tc-tetrofosmin have lipophilic proprieties and enter cells passively. However, their retention by the mitochondria is an active process and depends on mitochondrial membrane integrity.[49] ^{99m}Tc-based radiotracers (sestamibi and tetrofosmin) have almost no redistribution when compared to ^{201}Tl,[50] and different approaches are suggested to increase sensitivity for viability detection.

While resting ^{99m}Tc-based perfusion imaging can be used alone to define viability, several studies have shown that the use of nitrates improves viability detection when compared to rest ^{99m}Tc-based imaging and correlates with improvement after revascularization.[39,51-55] Although the exact mechanism is not well understood, it is proposed that it may be related to improvement in blood flow secondary to vasodilation improving blood supply to the hibernating myocardium and therefor tracer uptake.[54] Studies have also demonstrated that abnormal contractility can lead to perfusion defects with SPECT perfusion imaging.[56,57] Incremental value can be achieved by adding electrocardiogram (ECG) gating and dobutamine to ^{99m}Tc-based imaging, enabling the assessment of both perfusion and contractile reserve in a single study.[58]

Dual-isotope imaging with ^{99m}Tc at stress and ^{201}Tl at rest is also possible. The ^{201}Tl rest portion is used for viability interpretation with the addition of late redistribution and reinjection to increase the test sensitivity. However, this protocol is associated with a significantly higher radiation dose and may not be the ideal primary test when other diagnostic options are available.[41]

▶ Imaging Interpretation of SPECT Viability Images

After choosing the image acquisition protocol according to patient characteristics and institutional availability, imaging interpretation should be performed carefully.

While resting ^{99m}Tc-based perfusion imaging can be used alone to define viability, ^{99m}Tc-based SPECT viability imaging interpretation can be enhanced by including both rest and post nitrate images read simultaneously.[50] Persistent (fixed) defects with absence of tracer uptake noticed on both rest and post nitrate images are unlikely to recovery with revascularization,

Table 21-2

Imaging Interpretation of 99m-Technetium SPECT Study. Patterns of Perfusion on Rest and Post Nitrate Images and Clinical Relevance

Interpretation of 99m-Technetium SPECT

Rest Perfusion	Post Nitrate Perfusion	Stress	Category	Clinical Relevance	
Preserved (normal)	Preserved	Not acquired	Normal—viable	Wall motion	Normal—Normal / Abnormal—Stunning
Preserved[a 50,61]	Not acquired	Not acquired	viable	May benefit with revascularization[50,61]	
Preserved	Not acquired	Reduced	Ischemia	Ischemia—may benefit from revascularization[b]	
Reduced	Preserved (50–55% of peak activity)[50,61]	Not acquired	Hibernating myocardium—viable	Likely to recover with adequate revascularization[51–55,59,60]; may be observed after post-MI revascularization[112]	
Reduced	Reduced	Not acquired	Scar—nonviable	Unlikely to recover with adequate revascularization[4]	

[a]Preserved meaning 50–55% of peak activity.
[b]Refer to chapters on Ischemia—also evidence for the benefit of revascularization in patients with moderate to severe ischemia without severe LV dysfunction is being assessed in the ISCHEMIA trial.
Data from Hesse B, Tägil K, Cuocolo A, et al. EANM/ESC procedural guidelines for myocardial perfusion imaging in nuclear cardiology. *Eur J Nucl Med Mol Imaging*. 2005;32(7):855–897; Acampa W, Cuocolo A, Petretta M, et al. Tetrofosmin imaging in the detection of myocardial viability in patients with previous myocardial infarction: Comparison with sestamibi and Tl-201 scintigraphy. *J Nucl Cardiol Off Publ Am Soc Nucl Cardiol*. 2002;9(1):33–40.

and represent the so-called nonviable myocardium (scar). Dysfunctional segments with tracer uptake similar to other segments with normal wall thickening may recover, and segments that improve tracer uptake with nitroglycerin administration are likely to recover (viable hibernating myocardium).[50,59,60] For ^{99m}Tc-based SPECT, 50% to 55% of peak activity is usually defined as the cutoff to predict functional recovery and, therefore, to determine viability[61] (Table 21-2). It is important to remember that ^{99m}Tc-based SPECT can also be performed to assess ischemia. In this case, images would be acquired in rest and post stress (exercise or pharmacological stress). A moderate to severe reversible defect in this case represents ischemia and may benefit from revascularization—viability imaging would not be needed. (Stress perfusion imaging is considered in a separate chapter.) In general, viability testing should be reserved for patients where there are persistent defects on stress perfusion imaging with mild or no ischemia or in patients where stress imaging may be considered to have increased risk such as severe multivessel disease or very severe LV dysfunction.

Similar approaches may be used when ^{201}Tl SPECT imaging is performed. In the first step of the ^{201}Tl protocol, images are acquired at stress and after rest and then, a third optional delayed image (redistribution) is acquired if a persistent defect is present on stress and rest images.[50] After acquisition of the first set of images (stress/rest), images should be reviewed. If the defect is reversible, the interpretation is that myocardium is ischemic and therefore viable (and thus may benefit from revascularization). If the defect is persistent (fixed), then a redistribution image is acquired and interpreted.[50] A persistent (fixed) severe defect (<50% of peak tracer uptake) present in all three images suggests a myocardium which is unlikely to recovery after revascularization (nonviable). A reversible defect on the third set of images (late redistribution) or delayed images of a rest-redistribution protocol, with tracer uptake 55% to 60% of peak activity,[50,61] indicates the presence of viable hibernating myocardium which is likely to benefit from revascularization (Table 21-3).

Positron Emission Tomography

The rationale for ^{18}FDG PET use in viability assessment is based on the fundamentals of myocardial metabolism. The cardiomyocytes can use free fatty acid (FFA), glucose, lactate, pyruvate, and ketone as

Table 21-3

Imaging Interpretation of 201-Thallium SPECT Study. Patterns of Perfusion on Stress, Rest, and Redistribution Images and Clinical Relevance

Interpretation of 201-Thallium SPECT

Stress Perfusion	Rest (Redistribution) Perfusion	Late Redistribution Perfusion (or Post-Reinjection)	Category	Clinical Relevance
Preserved-normal	Preserved	Not acquired	Normal—viable	Wall motion { Normal—Normal / Abnormal—Stunning[b]
Preserved[a]	Preserved[a]	Not acquired	viable	May benefit with revascularization
Reduced	Preserved	Not acquired	Ischemia	Ischemia—may benefit from revascularization[c]
Reduced	Reduced	Preserved (55–60% of peak activity) / Increased activity from rest	Viable (Hibernating myocardium)	Likely to recover with adequate revascularization[56–59]
Reduced	Reduced	Reduced	Scar—nonviable	Unlikely to recover with adequate revascularization[4]

[a]Preserved meaning 50–55% of peak activity.
[b]Could also be due to remodeled myocardium.
[c]Refer to chapters on Ischemia—also evidence for the benefit of revascularization in patients with moderate to severe ischemia without severe LV dysfunction is being assessed in the ISCHEMIA trial.
Data from Hesse B, Tägil K, Cuocolo A, et al. EANM/ESC procedural guidelines for myocardial perfusion imaging in nuclear cardiology. *Eur J Nucl Med Mol Imaging.* 2005;32(7):855–897; Acampa W, Cuocolo A, Petretta M, et al. Tetrofosmin imaging in the detection of myocardial viability in patients with previous myocardial infarction: Comparison with sestamibi and Tl-201 scintigraphy. *J Nucl Cardiol Off Publ Am Soc Nucl Cardiol.* 2002;9(1):33–40.

energy substrates, with the first two being the most important sources of energy.[62–65] Fasting, adrenergic stimulation, ischemia, or insulin can shift the preferred energy substrate toward either FFA (in the case of fasting) or glucose.[66–69]

During fasting, FFAs are the preferred energy substrate. FFA plasma levels are increased as a consequence of low insulin levels and increased peripheral lipolysis in adipose tissue.[65,69] However, during hyperglycemic states (postprandial), the higher insulin plasma level suppresses lipolysis[70] and stimulates myocardial glucose uptake, with glucose becoming the primary substrate.[71] This process is primarily mediated by the glucose transporters 1 and 4 (GLUT 1 and 4). During ischemia and high insulin metabolic state, GLUT 1 and GLUT 4 are transported from intracellular storages to the plasma membrane to increase glucose uptake by the myocyte.[72,73] Similarly, under adrenergic stimulation and ischemic conditions (myocardial ischemia), the FFA oxidation process decreases or may cease and glycolysis (anaerobic glycolysis) facilitates the use of glucose as the main source of myocardial energy.[66,68,71] Glucose is the primary substrate in hibernating myocardium and is the basis for the utility of ^{18}FDG PET for viability imaging.

^{18}FDG is a glucose analog and is used clinically to assess and quantify glucose utilization. Although ^{18}FDG is thought of as a marker of glucose metabolism, technically speaking, it is more specifically a direct measure of exogenous glucose uptake. After ^{18}FDG is transported across cellular membranes, it is converted to FDG-6-phosphate and becomes trapped in the myocyte where it is trapped and does not continue down the metabolic pathway.[74]

▶ Imaging Protocols for FDG

Viability imaging protocols using PET are usually composed of two portions: rest perfusion imaging with 13-ammonia (^{13}N) or 82-rubidium (^{82}Rb) and metabolic imaging with ^{18}FDG. However, ^{99m}Tc-based SPECT and ^{201}Tl SPECT rest perfusion images can also be used to compare with metabolic ^{18}FDG PET images in cases where PET perfusion with ^{13}N or ^{82}Rb are not available (preferably with attenuation correction of the SPECT MPI).[75]

Patient preparation is an important component of the ^{18}FDG PET viability protocol. In a region of reduced perfusion, areas of ^{18}FDG uptake indicate viable myocardium, while the absence of uptake indicates nonviable myocardium.[50,76–79] Thus patient preparation is very important for the success of the viability study. Options include:

1. Fasting: Fasting is a simple approach but can lead to inferior image quality when compared to glucose loaded.[80] The rationale behind this approach is that the normal myocardium will consume FFA while ischemic myocardium (viable) will preferentially use ^{18}FDG and appear as a "hot spot." This approach is generally not recommended as an isolated technique.[50,76] However, fasting is routinely needed as a part of the preparation before administration of glucose +/− insulin used in the three current methods (Fig. 21-5).

    a. Glucose loading: Following a fasting period of at least 6 hours (preferable 12 hours), a glucose load is administered intravenously or orally.[76] Due to its simplicity, this protocol is commonly used at many centers. By increasing glucose plasma levels, insulin release is stimulated which decreases FFA plasma levels and shifts the myocytes toward glucose (and therefore ^{18}FDG) utilization. However, 20% to 25% of the patients with CAD may have poor image quality.[50] This is most commonly problematic in diabetics who have impaired insulin release or insulin resistance. In such cases, intravenous (IV) insulin may need to be administered according to a sliding scale[81] (45–60 minutes after glucose loading) repeating every 15 minutes targeting a glucose serum level between 100 and 140 mg/dL.[76] FDG is administered approximately 1 hour after glucose load.

    b. Hyperinsulinemic/euglycemic clamp: The hyperinsulinemic/euglycemic clamp protocol uses the intravenous infusion of both glucose and insulin. Blood glucose levels need to be monitored and the amount of glucose/insulin is tailored to each individual patient.[50,76] Although this is a more time-consuming protocol and requires an experienced team, the image quality is superior to the standard glucose loading protocol.[78,82] Some centers use this method routinely in all patients; others reserve it for all patients with diabetes.

    c. Acipimox: Acipimox is a nicotinic acid derivative that inhibits peripheral lipolysis thus reducing FFA availability. This process indirectly forces myocardial utilization of glucose as preferable substrate by reducing circulating FFAs. Acipimox administration provides comparable image quality as the hyperinsulinemic/euglycemic IV clamp[77,79] although nicotinic acid itself (i.e., Niacin) does not.[78,82]

After adequate patient preparation, ^{18}FDG (5–10 mCi/185–370 MBq) is administered and image

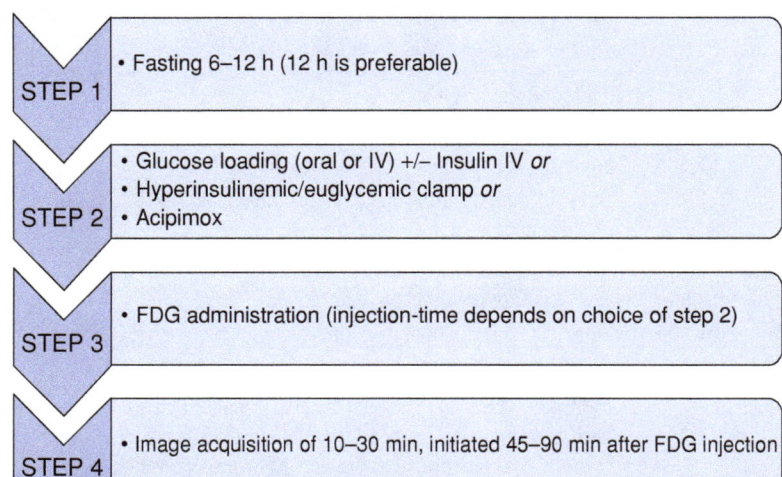

FIGURE 21-5 ^{18}FDG PET imaging protocol adapted from ASNC/SNMMI PET guidelines. (Data from Dilsizian V, Bacharach SL, Beanlands RS, et al. ASNC imaging guidelines/SNMMI procedure standard for positron emission tomography (PET) nuclear cardiology procedures. *J Nucl Cardiol.* 2016;23(5):1187–1226.)

acquisition begins 40 to 60 minutes after ^{18}FDG injection. Imaging can be performed using 2D or 3D scanners, in static, ECG-gated or list-mode and lasts 10 to 30 minutes. Attenuation correction should be applied and images reconstructed using an iterative statistical method. Preferable reconstructed pixel size is 2 to 3 mm but 3 to 4 mm is also acceptable.[50,76]

It is important to carefully review and align CT used for attenuation correction and emission images in all views (transaxial, coronal, and sagittal). Misaligned images can cause artifacts and misinterpretation. As for SPECT, ^{18}FDG images are reoriented and displayed in short-axis (SAO), horizontal long-axis (HLA) and vertical long-axis (VLA) and metabolism images are normalized according to rest perfusion images. For interpretation, a combined assessment is performed and ^{18}FDG scan metabolism images are compared with rest perfusion images in the same way we compare SPECT rest/stress images.[76]

Imaging Interpretation of FDG

^{18}FDG and rest (^{13}N or ^{82}Rb) myocardial PET perfusion images are reviewed simultaneously. ^{18}FDG PET images can be also interpreted in conjunction with resting SPECT MPI.[83] Care is needed with the later approach, especially when comparing a non–attenuation-corrected SPECT myocardial perfusion images with attenuation-corrected ^{18}FDG PET images.[74]

Four patterns of flow/metabolism can be observed (Table 21-4)[84]: (1) normal myocardial perfusion and glucose metabolism (viable, not ischemic myocardium at rest), (2) mismatch with reduced perfusion and preserved (or partly preserved) metabolism (hibernating [viable] myocardium), (3) matched reduction in perfusion and metabolism (nonviable myocardium = scar), and (4) normal perfusion with reduced metabolism (reverse mismatch). Figures 21-6 and 21-7 show examples of clinical cases and their interpretation. Further details are also noted in the next section below.

Reverse mismatch is described in patients with left bundle branch block (LBBB) with altered septal metabolism in ischemic and nonischemic cardiomyopathy, in patients with diabetes where glucose uptake is impaired in nonischemic tissue,[85] in repetitive stunning and early postrevascularization following acute MI.[3,20,86]

Evidence for the Clinical Role of Viability Imaging in Ischemic Heart Disease

Nuclear, dobutamine echo and MRI viability imaging modalities have demonstrated ability to predict LV function recovery and outcome benefit in observational trials. In a previous comparative systematic review meta-analysis, ^{18}FDG PET emerged as the most sensitive imaging technique to predict function recovery after revascularization,[4] with a pooled analysis of

Table 21-4

Imaging Interpretation of FDG PET Study. Patterns of Flow–Glucose Metabolism and Clinical Relevance

Perfusion	FDG Uptake	Category	Clinical Relevance
Preserved	Preserved	Normal—viable	Normal Stunning Ischemia (normal perfusion at rest and abnormal during stress—would benefit from revascularization)
Reduced	Preserved	Mismatch perfusion metabolism (hibernation myocardium)—viable	Likely to recover with adequate revascularization[4]; may be observed after post-MI revascularization[112]
Reduced	Reduced	Scar (match)—nonviable	Unlikely to recover with adequate revascularization[4]
Preserved	Reduced	Reverse mismatch	LBBB with altered septal metabolism in ischemic and nonischemic cardiomyopathy (may respond to CRT),[86,113] diabetes,[85] repetitive stunning, may be observed after post-MI revascularization[20]

Reproduced with permission from Erthal F, Aleksova N, Chong AY, et al. Microvascular function, is there a link to myocardial viability: Is this another piece to the puzzle? *J Nucl Cardiol.* 2016;1–6.

Chapter 21 Nuclear Cardiology Procedures in the Evaluation of Myocardial Viability 319

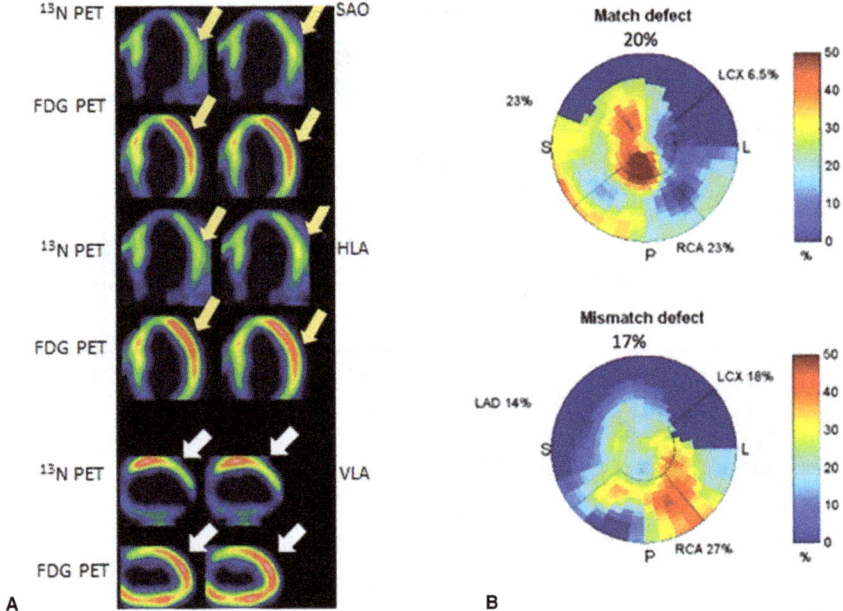

FIGURE 21-6 **(A)** ¹³N PET perfusion PET and ¹⁸FDG metabolism PET in short axis (SAO), horizontal long axis (HLA), and vertical long axis (VLA) showing extensive area of mismatch in the mid to distal anterior wall and apex (*white arrow*) and inferolateral wall (*yellow arrow*). **(B)** Polar map with quantitative analysis of the amount of scar (match defect) (top) and hibernating myocardium (mismatch) (bottom). The patient was referred for CABG.

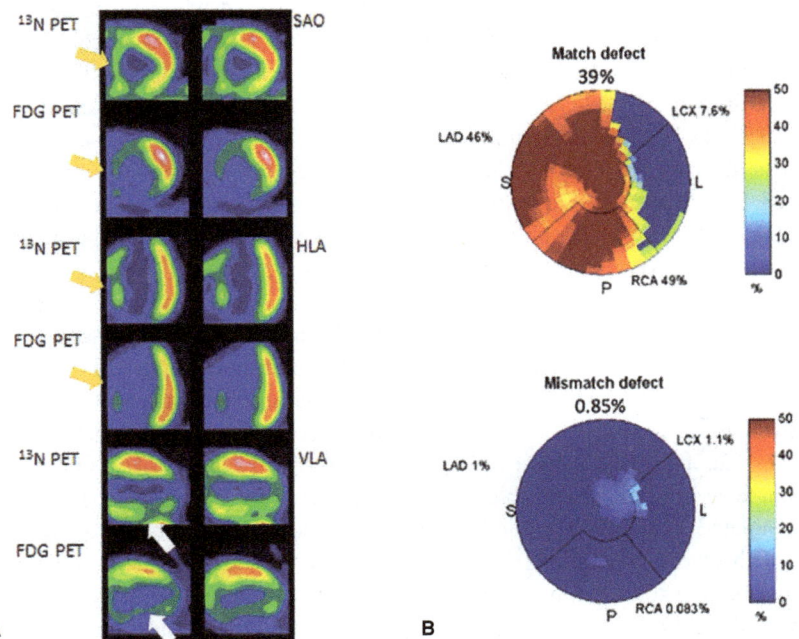

FIGURE 21-7 **(A)** ¹³N PET perfusion PET and ¹⁸FDG metabolism PET in short axis (SAO), horizontal long axis (HLA), and vertical long axis (VLA) showing no significant mismatch (scar) in the entire septal wall and apex (*yellow arrow*) and inferior wall (*white arrow*)—39% of scar and <1% of hibernated myocardium. **(B)** Polar map with quantitative analysis of the amount of scar (match defect) (top) and hibernating myocardium (mismatch) (bottom).

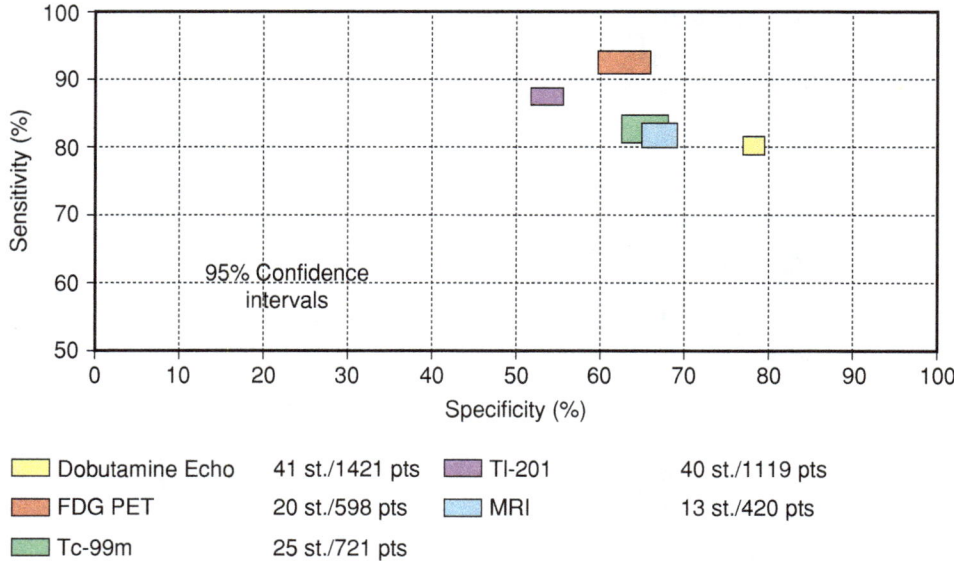

FIGURE 21-8 Comparison of sensitivities and specificities with 95% confidence intervals of the various techniques for the prediction of recovery of regional function after revascularization. (Reproduced with permission from Schinkel AF, Bax JJ, Poldermans D, et al. Hibernating myocardium: Diagnosis and patient outcomes. *Curr Probl Cardiol.* 2007;32(7):375–410.)

24 studies (756 patients) showing a mean sensitivity of 92%, specificity of 63%, and positive and negative predictive values of 74% and 87%, respectively.[4] Differences in sensitivity and specificity between ^{18}FDG PET, dobutamine echocardiography, SPECT with thallium (^{201}Tl-SPECT) and SPECT with technetium (^{99m}Tc SPECT) are illustrated in Figure 21-8. While ^{18}FDG PET is recognized as a sensitivity modality, dobutamine ECHO was the most specific for predicting the recovery of function.[4] However, cardiac MRI was underrepresented in this prior analysis. More recent meta-analysis that considered cardiac MRI alone, showed delayed-enhancement (DE-MRI) to also be highly sensitive while low-dose dobutamine cardiac MRI was more specific.[87]

Providing prospective data for viability assessment is very important, but fewer studies are available. One randomized trial evaluated ^{18}FDG PET-guided management in patients with severe LV dysfunction. In the PARR-2 (Positron emission tomography And Recovery following Revascularization Phase 2), 430 patients from 9 centers were randomized to undergo ^{18}FDG PET or standard care before revascularization decisions.[5] Patients were followed for cardiac death, MI and cardiac hospitalization at 1 year. A trend of benefit was noticed when using PET to assist with management decisions.[5] The composite event was 30% in the PET arm and 36% in the standard care arm (relative risk 0.82; $p = 0.16$ and hazard ratio (HR) 0.78; $p = 0.15$).[5] However, it was observed that clinicians did not uniformly adhere to the advice from imaging results. Therefore, a post-hoc analysis was performed in patients whose revascularization decisions were based on imaging results. In this analysis, a significant reduction in adverse outcome was observed in the ^{18}FDG PET arm (HR 0.62; $p = 0.019$).[5]

Further post-hoc sub-group analyses of PARR-2 showed that not only is adherence important, but also the amount of hibernating myocardium.[6] Among 182 patients in the PET arm, increasing amounts of mismatch (hibernating myocardium) was associated with increasing likelihood of benefit from revascularization. A threshold of 7% LV mismatch appeared to differentiate between those who benefit from revascularization versus optimal medical therapy (Fig. 21-9).[6] A subsequent PARR-2 substudy focusing on an experienced cardiac PET center (the Ottawa-FIVE study) included 111 patients from a center with experience,

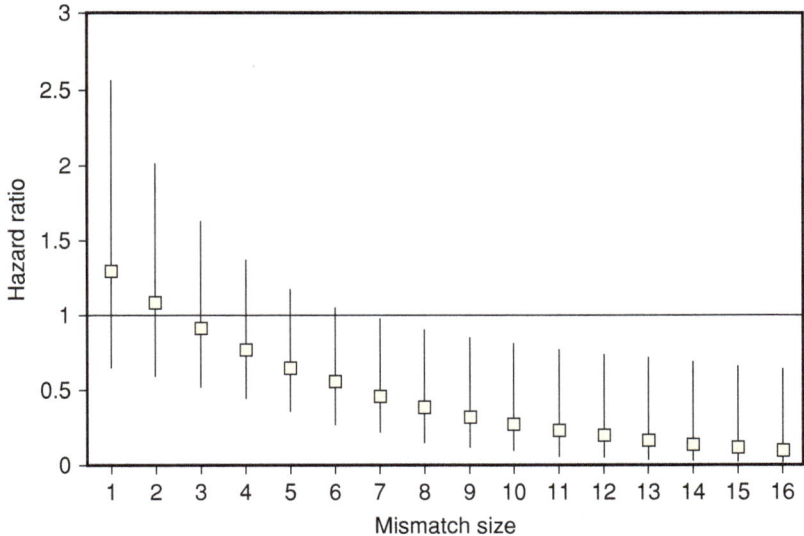

FIGURE 21-9 Hazard ratios and 95% confidence interval at various levels of mismatch measured as a continuous variable. The figure is a derivation from the multivariable model. For those with mismatch of <7% there is no significant difference in the risk of the primary outcome if revascularization is done compared with not done. As mismatch increases (i.e., ≥7%), there is a decreased risk of the primary outcome for those who undergo revascularization. For those with mismatch of 7%, there is a 0.46 times lower risk for the primary outcome if revascularization is done. (Reproduced with permission from D'Egidio G, Nichol G, Williams KA, et al. Increasing benefit from revascularization is associated with increasing amounts of myocardial hibernation: A substudy of the PARR-2 trial. *JACC Cardiovasc Imaging.* 2009;2(9):1060–1068.)

ready access to [18]FDG PET and integration between imaging, HF and revascularization teams, supporting that PET-assisted management improved outcome.[7] The cumulative proportion of events in the standard care group was 41% versus 19% in the PET-assisted management group.[7] In a multivariable Cox proportional hazards regression, the [18]FDG PET–assisted strategy showed benefit (HR 0.34; confidence interval, 0.16–0.72; $p = 0.005$). The 5-year follow-up of PARR-2, demonstrated similar findings as the 1-year study regarding the use of FDG PET to direct clinical management (revascularization vs. medical therapy). When PET recommendations were followed, primary outcome (cardiac death, MI, or cardiac hospitalization) improved, with an HR of 0.73 (95% confidence interval 0.54–0.99; $p = 0.042$).[10]

Revascularization decisions based on the amount of hibernating myocardium found by PARR-2 were similar to the findings of previous work by Di Carli et al. (5%)[12] and Lee et al. (7.6%).[13] Ling et al. also described the relationship between increasing amounts of hibernating myocardium and increasing likelihood of revascularization benefit for reducing all-cause death and found that the threshold was approximately 10% (Fig. 21-10).[11]

Despite all the current supporting literature regarding the benefit of viability imaging-guided revascularization[5-8,88-91] and its ability to cost-effectively select patients who would likely improve HF symptoms,[9,92,93] the STICH trial suggested the opposite.[94] Among the 1212 patients enrolled in the main STICH trial[94] to compare optimal medical therapy (OMT) with revascularization plus OMT, 601 underwent myocardial viability assessment with either SPECT or dobutamine echocardiography.[94] Viability imaging was not part of the randomization. Of this group, 303 received optimal medical therapy alone and 298 received optimal medical therapy plus

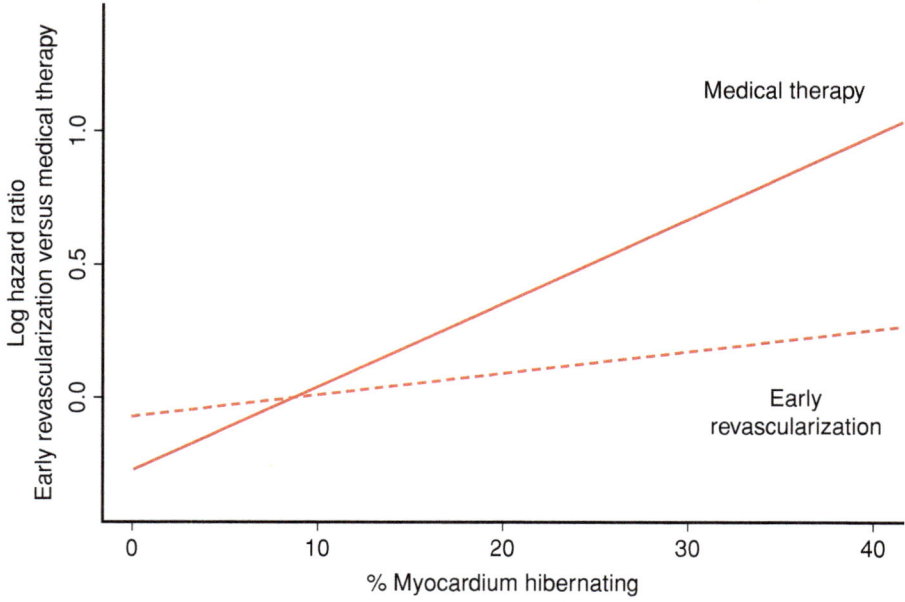

FIGURE 21-10 Relationship between percent myocardium hibernation and adjusted hazard ratio for (all cause of death in) patients treated with early revascularization versus medical therapy. Risk increases as a function of percent myocardium hibernation in medically treated patients. In patients referred to early revascularization risk seems to be relatively unchanged across the range of values. Percent myocardium hibernation–treatment interaction; $p = 0.0009$. (Reproduced with permission from Ling LF, Marwick TH, Flores DR, et al. Identification of therapeutic benefit from revascularization in patients with left ventricular systolic dysfunction: Inducible ischemia versus hibernating myocardium. *Circ Cardiovasc Imaging.* 2013;6(3):363–372.)

coronary artery bypass graft (CABG). Although HR for death in the group with viable myocardium was 0.64 ($p = 0.003$), after adjustment for patients' baseline variables this association was no longer significant ($p = 0.21$), suggesting no benefit of myocardial viability assessment in this population.[94]

PARR-2 and STICH trials appear to yield conflicting interpretation, but their results should be interpreted with caution.[90] The trial design and populations differed between the two studies. PARR-2 was a randomized trial that enrolled subjects with uncertain revascularization plans, and therefore viability assessment was clinically needed.[5] Conversely, in the STICH study, the allocation of patients for viability assessment was not randomized and all subjects were already accepted for revascularization (and thus had suitable coronary anatomy). There were also differences in comorbidities (specifically renal dysfunction and prior CABG).[90,94]

A smaller randomized trial by Siebelink et al.[95] compared ^{13}N-ammonia/^{18}FDG PET with ^{99m}Tc-sestamibi SPECT viability to guide therapy. They enrolled a total of 112 patients and observed no difference in cardiac event-free survival (cardiac death, MI, and revascularization) between the PET versus SPECT (11 vs. 13, p = NS, respectively).[95] However, this study also suffered from patient selection bias since only 35% of the population had severe LV dysfunction. Since there was a low rate of total events, the study was likely underpowered to detect a difference between groups.[96]

Although currently the literature has these mixed results, current recommendations support the use of viability imaging assessment prior to revascularization in patients with CAD and LV dysfunction.[97–99] The level of evidence, class of recommendation, and appropriate use criteria for radionuclide imaging are outlined in Table 21-5.

Despite the recognition of the importance of viability assessment, updated practical guidelines are needed. A multicenter trial[100] and registry[101] are currently being conducted and will hopefully

Table 21-5
Recommendations for Myocardial Viability Assessment According to Published Guidelines, Position Statements, and Appropriate Use Criteria

Recommendation	Grade	Level	Organization
Noninvasive imaging to detect myocardial ischemia and viability is reasonable in HF and CAD	IIa	C	ACCF/AHA Heart Failure Guideline 2013[114]
Viability assessment is reasonable before revascularization in HF patients with CAD	IIa	B	ACCF/AHA Heart Failure Guideline 2013[114]
Myocardial perfusion/ischemia imaging (echocardiography, CMR, SPECT, or PET) should be considered in patients through to have CAD, and who are considered suitable for coronary revascularization, to determine whether there is reversible ischemia and viable myocardium	IIa	C	ESC Heart Failure Guideline 2012[115]
Cardiac PET and CMR should be used in the evaluation and prognostication of *patients with ICM and LV dysfunction*	I	B	CCS/CAR/CANM/CNCS/CanSCMR Advanced Imaging 2007[106]
Surgical revascularization may be considered in HF patients with appropriate anatomy and demonstrable areas of reversible ischemia or viability	IIb	C	CCS Heart Failure Guideline 2006[116]
Nuclear imaging for assessment of *myocardial viability* for consideration of *revascularization* in patients with CAD and *LV dysfunction who do not have angina*	I	B	ACC/AHA/ASNC Radionuclide Imaging 2003[97]
Myocardial viability testing should be considered in patients with ischemic CM and reduced LVEF eligible for revascularization	Appropriate Use Score: 9		AACF/ASNC/ACR/ASE/SCCT/SCMR/SNM 2009 Appropriate Use Criteria[98]

HF, heart failure; CAD, coronary artery disease; ICM, ischemic cardiomyopathy; CMR, cardiac magnetic resonance; PET, positron emission tomography; SPECT, single-photon emission computed tomography; LV, left ventricle; LVEF, left ventricle ejection fraction; CM, cardiomyopathy.

address many unanswered questions that still exist. Alternative Imaging Modalities Ischemic Heart Failure (AIMI-HF) IMAGE HF includes centers from North America, Europe, and Latin America and is a large trial comparing standard investigations with SPECT to advanced imaging modalities (PET and cardiac magnetic resonance [CMR]).[100] Currently, most centers rely on their local experience to guide therapy which may be subjective and biased by limited personal experiences of the imaging physician, cardiologist, and cardiac surgeon. The standardized algorithm for reporting and guiding recommendations being used in the AIMI-HF trial of the IMAGE HF program is shown in Figure 21-11.

Recently published, the STICH Extension Study (STICHES),[102] a 10-year follow-up of the original trial,[94] showed benefit of revascularization for all cause of death, cardiovascular death, and cardiovascular hospitalization. The STICHE study did not assess the impact of viability imaging but the knowledge of greater benefit of revascularization against medical treatment in a long-term follow-up highlights the importance of proper assessment of each patient with ischemic cardiomyopathy weighing long-term benefit versus procedural risk. Viability assessment may have value in helping to define the extent of hibernating myocardium, and thus may be an important parameter to consider with other factors in decision making for revascularization.[6,11,99]

When Should Viability Imaging Be Used?

Although the importance of viability imaging is recognized, in clinical practice it can be difficult to determine the best approach according to each clinical scenario. The first step is to understand

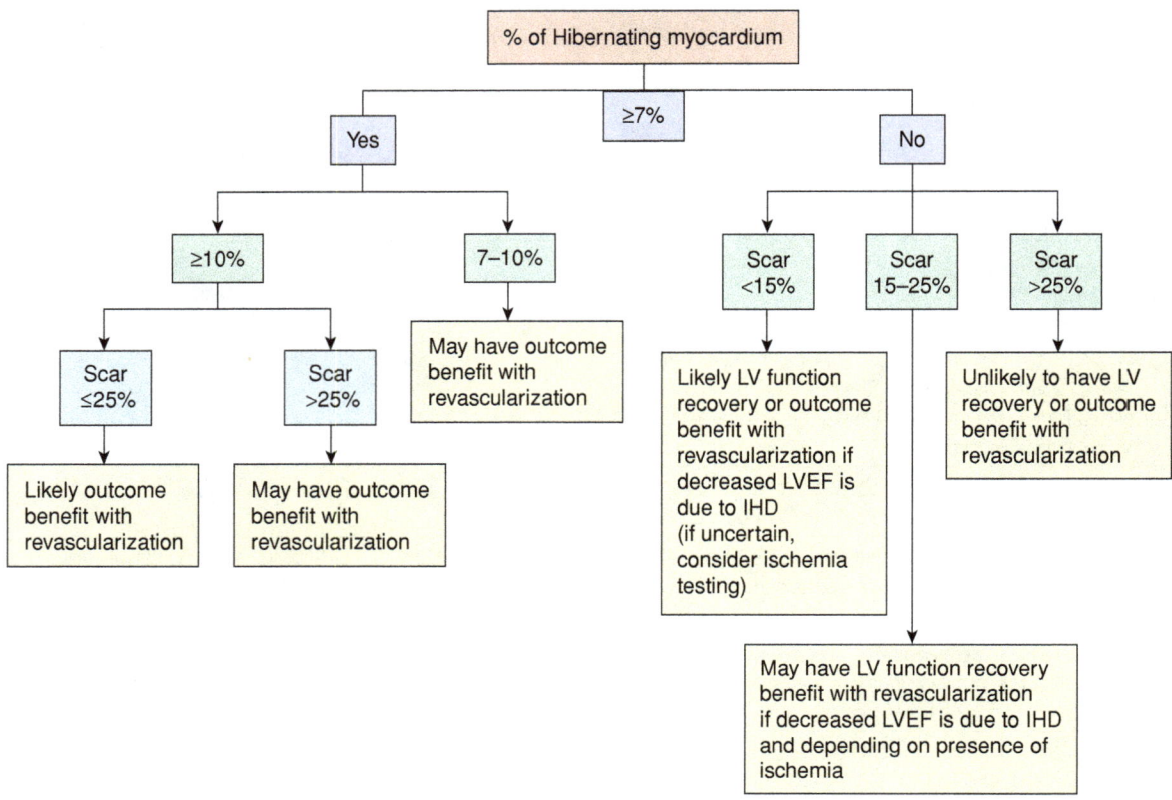

FIGURE 21-11 Algorithm to guide ^{18}FDG PET viability imaging reporting and therapy recommendations. IHD (ischemic heart disease), LVEF (left ventricular ejection fraction), LV (left ventricular). (Data from Hall AB, Ziadi MC, Guo A, et al. 516 Cardiac fdg pet results impact decisions and identify patients likely to benefit from revascularization in a multi-center provincial registry (CADRE). *Can J Cardiol.* 2011;27(5):S249–S250.)

patient symptoms, clinical history, and other imaging results.

As exemplified in a previous review by Di Carli et al.,[103] defining treatment strategy may be challenging for some patients. Consider the contrast, for example, whereby in (i) a 50-year-old patient with ischemic cardiomyopathy, three-vessel CAD, LV ejection fraction of 30%, angina class III, no other comorbidities, and good target vessels, the decision to revascularization would generally be straightforward for most physicians. As opposed to a clinical scenario whereby (ii) an elderly patient with NYHA class III, no angina, multiple comorbidities (including renal impairment, diabetes and COPD), severe LV dysfunction, LV dilatation, history of previous CABG, and mediocre target vessels; the risks versus benefit of revascularization may be less clear.[103] Viability assessment is a great tool to assist the decision making in such patients.[90] Figure 21-12 suggests an algorithm for use of viability imaging adapted from prior work.[104,105] A pragmatic approach at least for FDG PET imaging is considered below.[106]

In our hands we consider FDG PET imaging for patients with:

a. Known or strongly suspected IHD*
b. NYHA II*
c. Moderate–severe LV dysfunction (LVEF <40%)*
d. Moderate-to-large persistent perfusion defects– no significant ischemia*
e. +/− Significant comorbidities +/or poor distal targets
f. +/or Equivocal viability results on another test

*Note that (a–d) are required for insurance reimbursement for FDG PET in the province of Ontario in Canada.

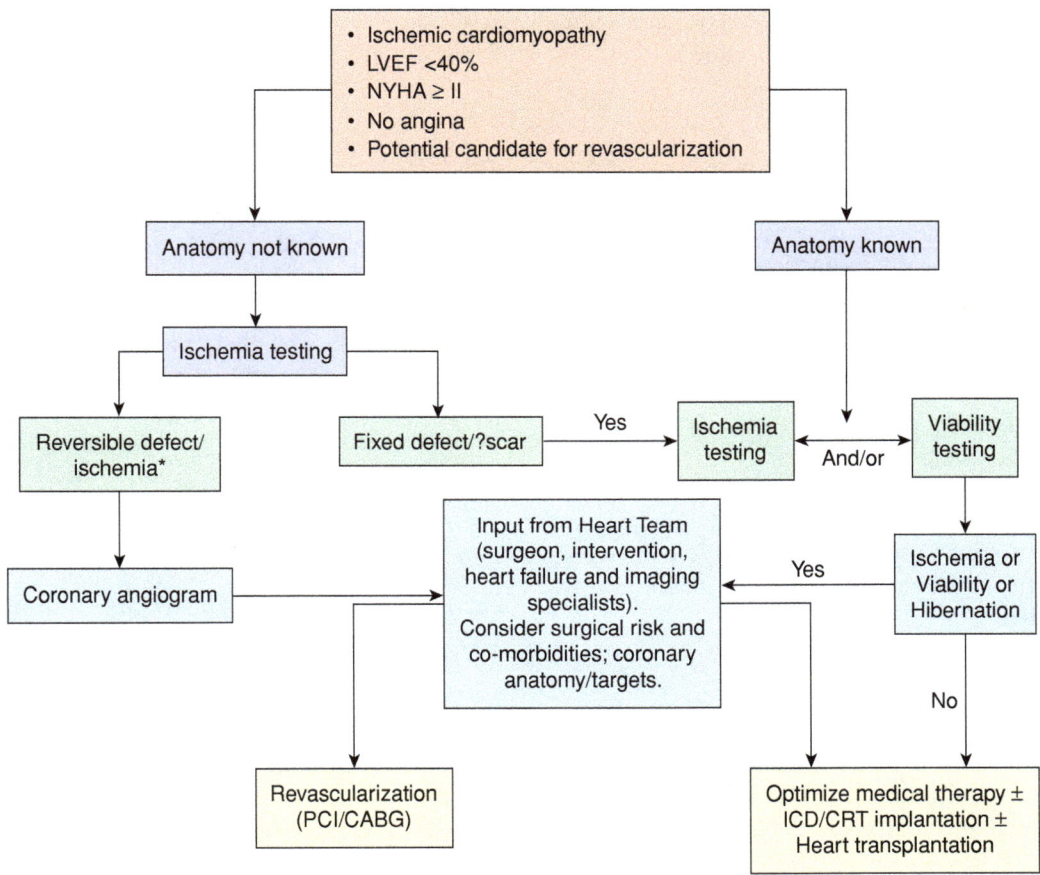

FIGURE 21-12 Flow algorithm for viability imaging approach for patients with ischemic heart failure. LVEF (Left ventricle ejection fraction), NYHA (New York Heart Association), ICD (Implantable cardiac defibrillator), CRT (cardiac resynchronization therapy), PCI (percutaneous coronary intervention), CABG (coronary artery bypass grafting). *ISCHEMIA trial is randomizing patients with EF >35% and ischemia >10% to revascularization versus optimal medical therapy. Patients with low ischemia and low scar may have other causes contributing to cardiomyopathy. (Data from McArdle BA, Beanlands RS. Myocardial viability: Whom, what, why, which, and how? *Can J Cardiol*. 2013;29(3): 399–402; Shah BN, Khattar RS, Senior R. The hibernating myocardium: Current concepts, diagnostic dilemmas, and clinical challenges in the post-STICH era. *Eur Heart J*. 2013;34(18):1323–1336.)

In our hands, FDG PET viability imaging is often not considered in patients with:

a. Predominantly Angina CCS >II
b. Normal or mild LV dysfunction
c. Critical LMCA (left main coronary artery) disease
d. Good targets
e. Documented moderate or severe ischemia
f. Minimal or no comorbidities

After deciding on the need for viability imaging, it is necessary to choose the most appropriate test for each patient. Although some studies report superior sensitivity for ^{18}FDG PET[4] and specificity for dobutamine echocardiogram and MRI,[4,87] there is lack of head-to-head study to help us decide the "right test for the right patient." All techniques (^{18}FDG PET, dobutamine echocardiography, ^{201}Tl-SPECT, ^{99m}Tc-SPECT, and cardiac MRI) can be used for viability assessment and guidance in decision making. Contraindications for modalities (e.g., pacemakers and implantable cardiac defibrillators for MRI), technique availability, and center expertise are key factors to take into account when deciding about the right test for the right patient. A practical approach to consider regarding which test to use in which patient circumstances (used by the author) is as follows:

a. Normal or mild LV dysfunction—viability imaging is rarely needed.
b. Moderate LV dysfunction—any method can be considered depending on availability and local expertise.
c. Very severe LV dysfunction, consider nuclear methods (SPECT, FDG PET) or MRI which is more sensitive than contractile reserve.[4,87,107]
d. Renal failure (GFR <30) or implanted devices—avoid MRI.
e. LMCA disease or severe proximal three-vessel disease—avoid dobutamine.
f. Equivocal results on another viability test or negative results on another viability test where certainty is needed to completely rule of viability—consider FDG PET or MRI as they are highly sensitive methods.[4,87,107]

FUTURE DIRECTIONS

PET/MRI scanners may permit advances in viability assessment. MRI and ^{18}FDG PET indicators of viability are different. While in the first the target is the fibrotic tissue and/or myocardium contractile reserve, PET assessment is based on metabolic and perfusion evaluation. PET/MRI fused scans may integrate information from both on a per patient basis. The additional benefit of this strategy is still unknown.

Previous studies have shown that hibernating myocardium is a substrate that increases patient's risk of sudden cardiac death.[108] Recent data suggest that this may be due to inhomogeneity of sympathetic innervation,[109] as measured by PET with ^{11}C-hydroxyephedrine (HED), a specific tracer for sympathetic presynaptic nerve function. The PAREPET study demonstrated that in ischemic cardiomyopathy, HED PET done in conjunction with perfusion and FDG PET for viability, was able to assess myocardium denervation and predict risk for sudden cardiac arrest.[110] Future studies are needed to consider the role of neurohormonal imaging in conjunction with viability imaging to assist in decision making.

Preliminary data with biomarkers in AIMI-HF[100] raise the consideration for their use in the future as an additional tool to assist imaging-based viability assessment in guiding revascularization recommendations.[111]

CONCLUSION

IHF is an important cause of patient morbidity and mortality, and significantly impacts patient quality of life and health care costs. Management decisions for patients with IHF continue to be a challenge and are compounded by their multiple comorbidities and their high risk with revascularization. Viability assessment with nuclear imaging enables individualized tailoring of therapies, serving to guide the choice between revascularization versus medical therapy alone.

ACKNOWLEDGMENTS AND DISCLOSURES

RSB is a career investigator supported by the Heart and Stroke Foundation of Ontario, a Tier 1 Research Chair supported by the University of Ottawa, and the University of Ottawa Heart Institute Vered Chair in Cardiology. He receives research support and honoraria from Lantheus Medical Imaging, Jubilant Drax-Image, and GE.

GVH is Research Officer, Intersocietal Accreditation Commission (IAC), Ellicott City, MD, and Consultant, Gagnon Cardiovascular Institute, Morristown Medical Center, Morristown, NJ.

BJC holds the Saul and Edna Goldfarb Chair in Cardiac Imaging Research. He receives research support from GE Healthcare and educational support from TeraRecon.

FE is a Cardiac Imaging Fellow at the University of Ottawa Heart Institute supported by the UOHI Associates in Cardiology.

REFERENCES

1. Mozaffarian D, Benjamin EJ, Go AS, et al. Heart disease and stroke statistics–2015 update: A report from the American Heart Association. *Circulation*. 2015;131(4):e29–e322.
2. Levy D, Kenchaiah S, Larson MG, et al. Long-term trends in the incidence of and survival with heart failure. *N Engl J Med*. 2002;347(18):1397–1402.

3. Ghosh N, Rimoldi OE, Beanlands RS, et al. Assessment of myocardial ischaemia and viability: Role of positron emission tomography. *Eur Heart J*. 2010;31(24):2984–2995.
4. Schinkel AF, Bax JJ, Poldermans D, et al. Hibernating myocardium: Diagnosis and patient outcomes. *Curr Probl Cardiol*. 2007;32(7):375–410.
5. Beanlands RS, Nichol G, Huszti E, et al. F-18-Fluorodeoxyglucose positron emission tomography imaging-assisted management of patients with severe left ventricular dysfunction and suspected coronary disease: A randomized, controlled trial (PARR-2). *J Am Coll Cardiol*. 2007;50(20):2002–2012.
6. D'Egidio G, Nichol G, Williams KA, et al. Increasing benefit from revascularization is associated with increasing amounts of myocardial hibernation: A substudy of the PARR-2 trial. *JACC Cardiovasc Imaging*. 2009;2(9):1060–1068.
7. Abraham A, Nichol G, Williams KA, et al. 18F-FDG PET imaging of myocardial viability in an experienced center with access to 18F-FDG and integration with clinical management teams: The Ottawa-FIVE substudy of the PARR 2 trial. *J Nucl Med Off Publ Soc Nucl Med*. 2010;51(4):567–574.
8. Allman KC, Shaw LJ, Hachamovitch R, et al. Myocardial viability testing and impact of revascularization on prognosis in patients with coronary artery disease and left ventricular dysfunction: A meta-analysis. *J Am Coll Cardiol*. 2002; 39(7):1151–1158.
9. Di Carli MF, Asgarzadie F, Schelbert HR, et al. Quantitative relation between myocardial viability and improvement in heart failure symptoms after revascularization in patients with ischemic cardiomyopathy. *Circulation*. 1995;92(12):3436–3444.
10. McArdle B, Shukla T, Nichol G, et al. Long-term follow-up of outcomes with F-18-Fluorodeoxyglucose positron emission tomography imaging–assisted management of patients with severe left ventricular dysfunction secondary to coronary disease. *Circ Cardiovasc Imaging*. 2016;9(9):e004331.
11. Ling LF, Marwick TH, Flores DR, et al. Identification of therapeutic benefit from revascularization in patients with left ventricular systolic dysfunction: Inducible ischemia versus hibernating myocardium. *Circ Cardiovasc Imaging*. 2013; 6(3):363–372.
12. Di Carli MF, Davidson M, Little R, et al. Value of metabolic imaging with positron emission tomography for evaluating prognosis in patients with coronary artery disease and left ventricular dysfunction. *Am J Cardiol*. 1994;73(8):527–533.
13. Lee KS, Marwick TH, Cook SA, et al. Prognosis of patients with left ventricular dysfunction, with and without viable myocardium after myocardial infarction. Relative efficacy of medical therapy and revascularization. *Circulation*. 1994; 90(6):2687–2694.
14. Lim SP, McArdle BA, Beanlands RS, et al. Myocardial viability: It is still alive. *Semin Nucl Med*. 2014;44(5):358–374.
15. Braunwald E, Kloner RA. The stunned myocardium: Prolonged, postischemic ventricular dysfunction. *Circulation*. 1982;66(6):1146–1149.
16. Ambrosio G, Betocchi S, Pace L, et al. Prolonged impairment of regional contractile function after resolution of exercise-induced angina evidence of myocardial stunning in patients with coronary artery disease. *Circulation*. 1996;94(10):2455–2464.
17. Barnes E, Hall RJC, Dutka DP, et al. Absolute blood flow and oxygen consumption in stunned myocardium in patients with coronary artery disease. *J Am Coll Cardiol*. 2002; 39(3):420–427.
18. Kloner RA, Bolli R, Marban E, et al. Medical and cellular implications of stunning, hibernation, and preconditioning: An NHLBI workshop. *Circulation*. 1998;97(18):1848–1867.
19. Hashimoto K, Nishimura T, Ishikawa M, et al. Enhancement of glucose uptake in stunned myocardium: Role of glucose transporter. *Am J Physiol—Heart Circ Physiol*. 1997; 272(3):H1122–H1130.
20. Anselm DD, Anselm AH, Renaud J, et al. Altered myocardial glucose utilization and the reverse mismatch pattern on rubidium-82 perfusion/F-18-FDG PET during the subacute phase following reperfusion of acute anterior myocardial infarction. *J Nucl Cardiol Off Publ Am Soc Nucl Cardiol*. 2011;18(4):657–667.
21. Canty JM, Fallavollita JA. Hibernating myocardium. *J Nucl Cardiol Off Publ Am Soc Nucl Cardiol*. 2005;12(1):104–119.
22. Camici PG, Dutka DP. Repetitive stunning, hibernation, and heart failure: Contribution of PET to establishing a link. *Am J Physiol Heart Circ Physiol*. 2001;280(3):H929–H936.
23. Fallavollita JA, Malm BJ, Canty JM. Hibernating myocardium retains metabolic and contractile reserve despite regional reductions in flow, function, and oxygen consumption at rest. *Circ Res*. 2003;92(1):48–55.
24. Tillisch J, Brunken R, Marshall R, et al. Reversibility of cardiac wall-motion abnormalities predicted by positron tomography. *N Engl J Med*. 1986;314(14):884–888.
25. Vanoverschelde J-LJ, Wijns W, Borgers M, et al. Chronic myocardial hibernation in humans from bedside to bench. *Circulation*. 1997;95(7):1961–1971.
26. Grassi I, Nanni C, Allegri V, et al. The clinical use of PET with 11C-acetate. *Am J Nucl Med Mol Imaging*. 2011;2(1):33–47.
27. Kaul S. Myocardial contrast echocardiography: A 25-year retrospective. *Circulation*. 2008;118(3):291–308.
28. Camici PG, Prasad SK, Rimoldi OE. Stunning, hibernation, and assessment of myocardial viability. *Circulation*. 2008; 117(1):103–114.
29. Sinusas AJ, Watson DD, Cannon JM, et al. Effect of ischemia and postischemic dysfunction on myocardial uptake of technetium-99m-labeled methoxyisobutyl isonitrile and thallium-201. *J Am Coll Cardiol*. 1989;14(7):1785–1793.
30. Freeman I, Grunwald AM, Hoory S, et al. Effect of coronary occlusion and myocardial viability on myocardial activity of technetium-99m-sestamibi. *J Nucl Med Off Publ Soc Nucl Med*. 1991;32(2):292–298.
31. Beanlands RS, Dawood F, Wen WH, et al. Are the kinetics of technetium-99m methoxyisobutyl isonitrile affected by cell metabolism and viability? *Circulation*. 1990;82(5): 1802–1814.
32. Sawada SG, Allman KC, Muzik O, et al. Positron emission tomography detects evidence of viability in rest technetium-99m sestamibi defects. *J Am Coll Cardiol*. 1994;23(1):92–98.
33. Marzullo P, Sambuceti G, Parodi O. The role of sestamibi scintigraphy in the radioisotopic assessment of myocardial viability. *J Nucl Med Off Publ Soc Nucl Med*. 1992;33(11):1925–1930.
34. Marzullo P, Parodi O, Reisenhofer B, et al. Value of rest thallium-201/technetium-99m sestamibi scans and dobutamine echocardiography for detecting myocardial viability. *Am J Cardiol*. 1993;71(2):166–172.

35. Cuocolo A, Pace L, Ricciardelli B, et al. Identification of viable myocardium in patients with chronic coronary artery disease: Comparison of thallium-201 scintigraphy with reinjection and technetium-99m-methoxyisobutyl isonitrile. *J Nucl Med Off Publ Soc Nucl Med*. 1992;33(4):505–511.
36. Dilsizian V, Arrighi JA, Diodati JG, et al. Myocardial viability in patients with chronic coronary artery disease. Comparison of 99mTc-sestamibi with thallium reinjection and [18F] fluorodeoxyglucose. *Circulation*. 1994;89(2):578–587.
37. Bonow RO, Dilsizian V, Cuocolo A, et al. Identification of viable myocardium in patients with chronic coronary artery disease and left ventricular dysfunction. Comparison of thallium scintigraphy with reinjection and PET imaging with 18F-fluorodeoxyglucose. *Circulation*. 1991;83(1):26–37.
38. Kauffman GJ, Boyne TS, Watson DD, et al. Comparison of rest thallium-201 imaging and rest technetium-99m sestamibi imaging for assessment of myocardial viability in patients with coronary artery disease and severe left ventricular dysfunction. *J Am Coll Cardiol*. 1996;27(7):1592–1597.
39. Sciagrà R, Bisi G, Santoro GM, et al. Comparison of baseline-nitrate technetium-99m sestamibi with rest-redistribution thallium-201 tomography in detecting viable hibernating myocardium and predicting postvascularization recovery. *J Am Coll Cardiol*. 1997;30(2):384–391.
40. Grunwald AM, Watson DD, Holzgrefe HH, et al. Myocardial thallium-201 kinetics in normal and ischemic myocardium. *Circulation*. 1981;64(3):610–618.
41. Henzlova MJ, Duvall WL, Einstein AJ, et al. ASNC imaging guidelines for SPECT nuclear cardiology procedures: Stress, protocols, and tracers. *J Nucl Cardiol Off Publ Am Soc Nucl Cardiol*. 2016;23(3):606–639.
42. Gutman J, Berman DS, Freeman M, et al. Time to completed redistribution of thallium-201 in exercise myocardial scintigraphy: Relationship to the degree of coronary artery stenosis. *Am Heart J*. 1983;106(5 Pt 1):989–995.
43. Kiat H, Berman DS, Maddahi J, et al. Late reversibility of tomographic myocardial thallium-201 defects: An accurate marker of myocardial viability. *J Am Coll Cardiol*. 1988;12(6):1456–1463.
44. Cloninger KG, DePuey EG, Garcia EV, et al. Incomplete redistribution in delayed thallium-201 single photon emission computed tomographic (SPECT) images: An overestimation of myocardial scarring. *J Am Coll Cardiol*. 1988;12(4):955–963.
45. Yang LD, Berman DS, Kiat H, et al. The frequency of late reversibility in SPECT thallium-201 stress-redistribution studies. *J Am Coll Cardiol*. 1990;15(2):334–340.
46. Kayden DS, Sigal S, Soufer R, et al. Thallium-201 for assessment of myocardial viability: Quantitative comparison of 24-hour redistribution imaging with imaging after reinjection at rest. *J Am Coll Cardiol*. 1991;18(6):1480–1486.
47. Tamaki N, Ohtani H, Yamashita K, et al. Metabolic activity in the areas of new fill-in after thallium-201 reinjection: Comparison with positron emission tomography using fluorine-18-deoxyglucose. *J Nucl Med Off Publ Soc Nucl Med*. 1991;32(4):673–678.
48. Perrone Filardi P, Bacharach SL, Bonow RO. [Identification of viable myocardium in patients with chronic ischemic disease and left ventricular dysfunction: Correlations between blood flow, metabolic activity and regional function]. *Cardiol Rome Italy*. 1991;36(4):299–307.
49. Li QS, Solot G, Frank TL, et al. Myocardial redistribution of technetium-99m-methoxyisobutyl isonitrile (SESTAMIBI). *J Nucl Med Off Publ Soc Nucl Med*. 1990;31(6):1069–1076.
50. Hesse B, Tägil K, Cuocolo A, et al. EANM/ESC procedural guidelines for myocardial perfusion imaging in nuclear cardiology. *Eur J Nucl Med Mol Imaging*. 2005;32(7):855–897.
51. Schneider CA, Voth E, Gawlich S, et al. Significance of rest technetium-99m sestamibi imaging for the prediction of improvement of left ventricular dysfunction after Q wave myocardial infarction: Importance of infarct location adjusted thresholds. *J Am Coll Cardiol*. 1998;32(3):648–654.
52. Bisi G, Sciagrà R, Santoro GM et al. Rest technetium-99m sestamibi tomography in combination with short-term administration of nitrates: Feasibility and reliability for prediction of postvascularization outcome of asynergic territories. *J Am Coll Cardiol*. 1994;24(5):1282–1289.
53. Bisi G, Sciagrà R, Santoro GM. Technetium-99m-sestamibi imaging with nitrate infusion to detect viable hibernating myocardium and predict postvascularization recovery. *J Nucl Med Off Publ Soc Nucl Med*. 1995;36(11):1994–2000.
54. Galli M, Marcassa C, Imparato A, et al. Effects of nitroglycerin by technetium-99m sestamibi tomoscintigraphy on resting regional myocardial hypoperfusion in stable patients with healed myocardial infarction. *Am J Cardiol*. 1994;74(9):843–848.
55. Maurea S, Cuocolo A, Soricelli A, et al. Enhanced detection of viable myocardium by technetium-99m-MIBI imaging after nitrate administration in chronic coronary artery disease. *J Nucl Med Off Publ Soc Nucl Med*. 1995;36(11):1945–1952.
56. Sinusas AJ, Shi Q, Vitols PJ, et al. Impact of regional ventricular function, geometry, and dobutamine stress on quantitative 99mTc-sestamibi defect size. *Circulation*. 1993;88(5 Pt 1):2224–2234.
57. Eisner RL, Schmarkey LS, Martin SE, et al. Defects on SPECT "perfusion" images can occur due to abnormal segmental contraction. *J Nucl Med Off Publ Soc Nucl Med*. 1994;35(4):638–643.
58. Leoncini M, Marcucci G, Sciagrà R, et al. Prediction of functional recovery in patients with chronic coronary artery disease and left ventricular dysfunction combining the evaluation of myocardial perfusion and of contractile reserve using nitrate-enhanced technetium-99m sestamibi gated single-photon emission computed tomography and dobutamine stress. *Am J Cardiol*. 2001;87(12):1346–1350.
59. Peix A, López A, Ponce F, et al. Enhanced detection of reversible myocardial hypoperfusion by technetium 99m-tetrofosmin imaging and first-pass radionuclide angiography after nitroglycerin administration. *J Nucl Cardiol Off Publ Am Soc Nucl Cardiol*. 1998;5(5):469–476.
60. Greco C, Ciavolella M, Tanzilli G, et al. Preoperative identification of viable myocardium: Effectiveness of nitroglycerine-induced changes in myocardial sestamibi uptake. *Cardiovasc Surg Lond Engl*. 1998;6(2):149–155.
61. Acampa W, Cuocolo A, Petretta M, et al. Tetrofosmin imaging in the detection of myocardial viability in patients with previous myocardial infarction: Comparison with sestamibi and Tl-201 scintigraphy. *J Nucl Cardiol Off Publ Am Soc Nucl Cardiol*. 2002;9(1):33–40.
62. Bing RJ, Siegel A, Vitale A, et al. Metabolic studies on the human heart in vivo. I. Studies on carbohydrate metabolism of the human heart. *Am J Med*. 1953;15(3):284–296.

63. Camici P, Ferrannini E, Opie LH. Myocardial metabolism in ischemic heart disease: Basic principles and application to imaging by positron emission tomography. *Prog Cardiovasc Dis.* 1989;32(3):217–238.
64. Depre C, Vanoverschelde JL, Taegtmeyer H. Glucose for the heart. *Circulation.* 1999;99(4):578–588.
65. Neely JR, Morgan HE. Relationship between carbohydrate and lipid metabolism and the energy balance of heart muscle. *Annu Rev Physiol.* 1974;36:413–459.
66. Liedtke AJ Alterations of carbohydrate and lipid metabolism in the acutely ischemic heart. *Prog Cardiovasc Dis.* 1981;23(5):321–336.
67. Stanley WC, Lopaschuk GD, Hall JL, et al. Regulation of myocardial carbohydrate metabolism under normal and ischaemic conditions. Potential for pharmacological interventions. *Cardiovasc Res.* 1997;33(2):243–257.
68. Goodwin GW, Ahmad F, Doenst T, et al. Energy provision from glycogen, glucose, and fatty acids on adrenergic stimulation of isolated working rat hearts. *Am J Physiol.* 1998;274(4 Pt 2):H1239–H1247.
69. Barger PM, Kelly DP. PPAR signaling in the control of cardiac energy metabolism. *Trends Cardiovasc Med.* 2000;10(6):238–245.
70. Choi SM, Tucker DF, Gross DN, et al. Insulin Regulates Adipocyte Lipolysis via an Akt-Independent Signaling Pathway. *Mol Cell Biol.* 2010;30(21):5009–5020.
71. Di Carli MF, Lipton MJ. *Cardiac PET and PET/CT Imaging.* Springer; 2007.
72. Mueckler M. Facilitative glucose transporters. *Eur J Biochem.* 1994;219(3):713–725.
73. Egert S, Nguyen N, Schwaiger M. Myocardial glucose transporter GLUT1: Translocation induced by insulin and ischemia. *J Mol Cell Cardiol.* 1999;31(7):1337–1344.
74. Zaret BL, Beller GA. *Clinical Nuclear Cardiology: State of the Art and Future Directions.* 4th ed. Philadelphia, PA: Elsevier Mosby; 2010.
75. Beanlands RSB, Ruddy TD, deKemp RA, et al. Positron emission tomography and recovery following revascularization (PARR-1): The importance of scar and the development of a prediction rule for the degree of recovery of left ventricular function. *J Am Coll Cardiol.* 2002;40(10):1735–1743.
76. Bacharach SL, Bax JJ, Case J, et al. PET myocardial glucose metabolism and perfusion imaging: Part 1—Guidelines for data acquisition and patient preparation. *J Nucl Cardiol Off Publ Am Soc Nucl Cardiol.* 2003;10(5):543–556.
77. Bax JJ, Veening MA, Visser FC, et al. Optimal metabolic conditions during fluorine-18 fluorodeoxyglucose imaging; a comparative study using different protocols. *Eur J Nucl Med.* 1997;24(1):35–41.
78. Knuuti MJ, Nuutila P, Ruotsalainen U, et al. Euglycemic hyperinsulinemic clamp and oral glucose load in stimulating myocardial glucose utilization during positron emission tomography. *J Nucl Med Off Publ Soc Nucl Med.* 1992;33(7):1255–1262.
79. Knuuti MJ, Yki-Järvinen H, Voipio-Pulkki LM, et al. Enhancement of myocardial [fluorine-18]fluorodeoxyglucose uptake by a nicotinic acid derivative. *J Nucl Med Off Publ Soc Nucl Med.* 1994;35(6):989–998.
80. Berry JJ, Baker JA, Pieper KS, et al. The effect of metabolic milieu on cardiac PET imaging using fluorine-18-deoxyglucose and nitrogen-13-ammonia in normal volunteers. *J Nucl Med Off Publ Soc Nucl Med.* 1991;32(8):1518–1525.
81. Dilsizian V, Bacharach SL, Beanlands RS, et al. ASNC imaging guidelines/SNMMI procedure standard for positron emission tomography (PET) nuclear cardiology procedures. *J Nucl Cardiol Off Publ Am Soc Nucl Cardiol.* 2016;23(5):1187–1226.
82. Vitale GD, deKemp RA, Ruddy TD, et al. Myocardial glucose utilization and optimization of (18)F-FDG PET imaging in patients with non-insulin-dependent diabetes mellitus, coronary artery disease, and left ventricular dysfunction. *J Nucl Med Off Publ Soc Nucl Med.* 2001;42(12):1730–1736.
83. Schelbert HR, Beanlands R, Bengel F, et al. PET myocardial perfusion and glucose metabolism imaging: Part 2—Guidelines for interpretation and reporting. *J Nucl Cardiol Off Publ Am Soc Nucl Cardiol.* 2003;10(5):557–571.
84. Erthal F, Aleksova N, Chong AY, et al. Microvascular function, is there a link to myocardial viability: Is this another piece to the puzzle? *J Nucl Cardiol Off Publ Am Soc Nucl Cardiol.* 2016.
85. Paternostro G, Camici PG, Lammerstma AA, et al. Cardiac and skeletal muscle insulin resistance in patients with coronary heart disease. A study with positron emission tomography. *J Clin Invest.* 1996;98(9):2094–2099.
86. Thompson K, Saab G, Birnie D, et al. Is septal glucose metabolism altered in patients with left bundle branch block and ischemic cardiomyopathy? *J Nucl Med Off Publ Soc Nucl Med.* 2006;47(11):1763–1768.
87. Romero J, Xue X, Gonzalez W, et al. CMR imaging assessing viability in patients with chronic ventricular dysfunction due to coronary artery disease: A meta-analysis of prospective trials. *JACC Cardiovasc Imaging.* 2012;5(5):494–508.
88. Haas F, Haehnel CJ, Picker W, et al. Preoperative positron emission tomographic viability assessment and perioperative and postoperative risk in patients with advanced ischemic heart disease. *J Am Coll Cardiol.* 1997;30(7):1693–1700.
89. Mule JD, Bax JJ, Zingone B, et al. The beneficial effect of revascularization on jeopardized myocardium: Reverse remodeling and improved long-term prognosis. *Eur J Cardio-Thorac Surg Off J Eur Assoc Cardio-Thorac Surg.* 2002;22(3):426–430.
90. Mielniczuk LM, Beanlands RS. Does imaging-guided selection of patients with ischemic heart failure for high risk revascularization improve identification of those with the highest clinical benefit?: Imaging-guided selection of patients with ischemic heart failure for high-risk revascularization improves identification of those with the highest clinical benefit. *Circ Cardiovasc Imaging.* 2012;5(2):262–270.
91. Tamaki N, Yonekura Y, Yamashita K, et al. Positron emission tomography using fluorine-18 deoxyglucose in evaluation of coronary artery bypass grafting. *Am J Cardiol.* 1989;64(14):860–865.
92. Shukla T, Nichol G, Wells G, et al. Does FDG PET-assisted management of patients with left ventricular dysfunction improve quality of life? A substudy of the PARR-2 trial. *Can J Cardiol.* 2012;28(1):54–61.
93. Jacklin PB, Barrington SF, Roxburgh JC, et al. Cost-effectiveness of preoperative positron emission tomography in ischemic heart disease. *Ann Thorac Surg.* 2002;73(5):1403–1409; discussion 1410.

94. Bonow RO, Maurer G, Lee KL, et al. Myocardial viability and survival in ischemic left ventricular dysfunction. *N Engl J Med*. 2011;364(17):1617–1625.
95. Siebelink HM, Blanksma PK, Crijns HJ, et al. No difference in cardiac event-free survival between positron emission tomography-guided and single-photon emission computed tomography-guided patient management: A prospective, randomized comparison of patients with suspicion of jeopardized myocardium. *J Am Coll Cardiol*. 2001;37(1):81–88.
96. Beanlands RS, Ruddy TD, Freeman M, et al. Patient management guided by viability imaging. *J Am Coll Cardiol*. 2001;38(4):1271–1273.
97. Members C, Klocke FJ, Baird MG, et al. ACC/AHA/ASNC Guidelines for the Clinical Use of Cardiac Radionuclide Imaging—Executive Summary A Report of the American College of Cardiology/American Heart Association Task Force on Practice Guidelines (ACC/AHA/ASNC Committee to Revise the 1995 Guidelines for the Clinical Use of Cardiac Radionuclide Imaging). *Circulation*. 2003;108(11):1404–1418.
98. Hendel RC, Berman DS, Di Carli MF, et al. ACCF/ASNC/ACR/AHA/ASE/SCCT/SCMR/SNM 2009 appropriate use criteria for cardiac radionuclide imaging: A report of the American College of Cardiology Foundation Appropriate Use Criteria Task Force, the American Society of Nuclear Cardiology, the American College of Radiology, the American Heart Association, the American Society of Echocardiography, the Society of Cardiovascular Computed Tomography, the Society for Cardiovascular Magnetic Resonance, and the Society of Nuclear Medicine. *Circulation*. 2009;119(22):e561–e587.
99. Anavekar NS, Chareonthaitawee P, Narula J, et al. Revascularization in patients with severe left ventricular dysfunction: Is the assessment of viability still viable? *J Am Coll Cardiol*. 2016;67(24):2874–2887.
100. O'Meara E, Mielniczuk LM, Wells GA, et al. Alternative imaging modalities in ischemic heart failure (AIMI-HF) IMAGE HF Project I-A: Study protocol for a randomized controlled trial. *Trials*. 2013;14(1):218.
101. Hall AB, Ziadi MC, Guo A, et al. 516 Cardiac FDG PET results impact decisions and identify patients likely to benefit from revascularization in a multi-center provincial registry (CADRE). *Can J Cardiol*. 2011;27(5):S249–S250.
102. Velazquez EJ, Lee KL, Jones RH, et al. Coronary-artery bypass surgery in patients with ischemic cardiomyopathy. *N Engl J Med*. 2016;374(16):1511–1520.
103. Di Carli MF, Hachamovitch R. New Technology for noninvasive evaluation of coronary artery disease. *Circulation*. 2007;115(11):1464–1480.
104. Mc Ardle BA, Beanlands RS. Myocardial viability: Whom, what, why, which, and how? *Can J Cardiol*. 2013;29(3):399–402.
105. Shah BN, Khattar RS, Senior R. The hibernating myocardium: Current concepts, diagnostic dilemmas, and clinical challenges in the post-STICH era. *Eur Heart J*. 2013;34(18):1323–1336.
106. Beanlands R, Chow B, Dick A, et al. CCS/CAR/CANM/CNCS/CanSCMR joint position statement on advanced noninvasive cardiac imaging using positron emission tomography, magnetic resonance imaging and multidetector computed tomographic angiography in the diagnosis and evaluation of ischemic heart disease—executive summary. *Can J Cardiol*. 2007;23(2):107–119.
107. Pagano D, Bonser RS, Townend JN, et al. Predictive value of dobutamine echocardiography and positron emission tomography in identifying hibernating myocardium in patients with postischaemic heart failure. *Heart Br Card Soc*. 1998;79(3):281–288.
108. Canty JM, Suzuki G, Banas MD, et al. Hibernating myocardium: Chronically adapted to ischemia but vulnerable to sudden death. *Circ Res*. 2004;94(8):1142–1149.
109. Luisi AJ, Suzuki G, Dekemp R, et al. Regional 11C-hydroxyephedrine retention in hibernating myocardium: Chronic inhomogeneity of sympathetic innervation in the absence of infarction. *J Nucl Med Off Publ Soc Nucl Med*. 2005;46(8):1368–1374.
110. Fallavollita JA, Heavey BM, Luisi AJ, et al. Regional myocardial sympathetic denervation predicts the risk of sudden cardiac arrest in ischemic cardiomyopathy. *J Am Coll Cardiol*. 2014;63(2):141–149.
111. Zelt JG, Liu PP, Erthal F, et al. Brain natriuretic peptide and high sensitivity Troponin T levels are related to the extent of global and regional hibernating myocardium in patients with ischemic heart failure. *Can J Cardiol*. 2017. In press.
112. Fukuoka Y, Nakano A, Tama N, et al. Impaired myocardial microcirculation in the flow–glucose metabolism mismatch regions in revascularized acute myocardial infarction. *J Nucl Cardiol*. 2016:1–10. doi: 10.1007/s12350-016-0526-z.
113. Birnie D, de Kemp RA, Tang AS, et al. Reduced septal glucose metabolism predicts response to cardiac resynchronization therapy. *J Nucl Cardiol Off Publ Am Soc Nucl Cardiol*. 2012;19(1):73–83.
114. Yancy CW, Jessup M, Bozkurt B, et al. 2013 ACCF/AHA guideline for the management of heart failure. *Circulation*. 2013;128(16):e240–327.
115. McMurray JJ, Adamopoulos S, Anker SD, et al. ESC Guidelines for the diagnosis and treatment of acute and chronic heart failure 2012: The Task Force for the Diagnosis and Treatment of Acute and Chronic Heart Failure 2012 of the European Society of Cardiology. Developed in collaboration with the Heart Failure Association (HFA) of the ESC. *Eur Heart J*. 2012;33(14):1787–1847.
116. Arnold JM, Liu P, Demers C, et al. Canadian cardiovascular society consensus conference recommendations on heart failure 2006: Diagnosis and management. *Can J Cardiol*. 2006;22(1):23–45.

Radionuclide Angiography: Equilibrium and First Pass

CHAPTER 22

Rupa M. Sanghani and Kim A. Williams

INTRODUCTION

The noninvasive assessment of resting left ventricular (LV) performance is an integral part of the evaluation of patients with known or suspected cardiac disease, having important diagnostic, therapeutic, and prognostic significance.[1-11] Although scintigraphic measures of cardiac function historically included measurement of ejection fraction (EF), estimation of cardiac output, valvular regurgitant fraction, and detection of intracardiac shunts have also been successfully performed. Other than EF, these potential applications for nuclear cardiology techniques have been largely supplanted by echocardiography, cardiac computed tomography, and magnetic resonance imaging (MRI) techniques over the past two decades.

Gated equilibrium radionuclide angiography (ERNA, often called multiple-gated acquisition [MUGA] and equilibrium radionuclide ventriculography [RNV]) were introduced nearly 30 years ago. These techniques were routinely utilized in the evaluation of patients with known or suspected LV dysfunction, postmyocardial infarction (MI), and valvular disease, and for monitoring the cardiotoxic effects of chemotherapeutic drugs. Exercise radionuclide angiography (RNA), particularly with the first-pass radionuclide angiographic (FPRNA) technique, was widely used to diagnose or evaluate known coronary artery disease (CAD),[5-9] competing favorably with and often complementing planar myocardial perfusion imaging (MPI). However, since its introduction, RNA has evolved little, while other noninvasive methods, such as gated single-photon emission computed tomography (SPECT) MPI, echocardiography, and cardiac magnetic resonance, have been introduced and become increasingly sophisticated and cost effective.

TECHNICAL ASPECTS

▶ Red Blood Cell Labeling

For FPRNA alone, Tc-99m DTPA is often used if no equilibrium images are required. For ERNA, red blood cell labeling can be performed via multiple methods. The in vitro method, usually using a commercial kit, is preferred, and offers the highest level of labeling efficiency (>97%). Blood is withdrawn from the patient, mixed into a "reaction vial" containing stannous pyrophosphate. After 5 minutes it is mixed with sodium hypochlorite to destroy extracellular stannous ion, and then with citrate buffer. After shaking lightly, 25mCi Tc-99m is added, incubated for 20 minutes and then reinjected back into the patient. The in vivo method, although simple, cheap and fast, is no longer recommended as it provides the lowest labeling efficiency (80–85%). It involves giving stannous pyrophosphate directly to the patient, followed by Tc-99m 15 to 20 minutes later (which can be given as a rapid bolus if for FPRNA). Finally, a modified in vivo/in vitro method can be used with labeling efficiency of 92% to 95%. Perfusion imaging can also be performed if desired.[12-14]

First-Pass Radionuclide Angiography

FPRNA images are usually obtained using a single- or multicrystal high-count rate gamma camera fitted with a high-sensitivity parallel hole collimator (e.g., SIM 400, Scinticor, Milwaukee, WI; or ElGems CardiaL [formerly Elscint], Haifa, Israel). Images are acquired in the anterior or the right anterior oblique (RAO) projection using 25 (±4) frames per cardiac cycle. Preliminary work suggests that FPRNA can also be performed with positron emission tomography (PET) using images acquired during a bolus of radiolabeled water ($H_2^{15}O$), but this has not yet achieved widespread utilization or validation.[15]

FPRNA data are analyzed using the frame method for LVEF using commercially available computer software,[16-18] as shown in Figures 22-1 to 22-3. This software creates a representative LV volume curve

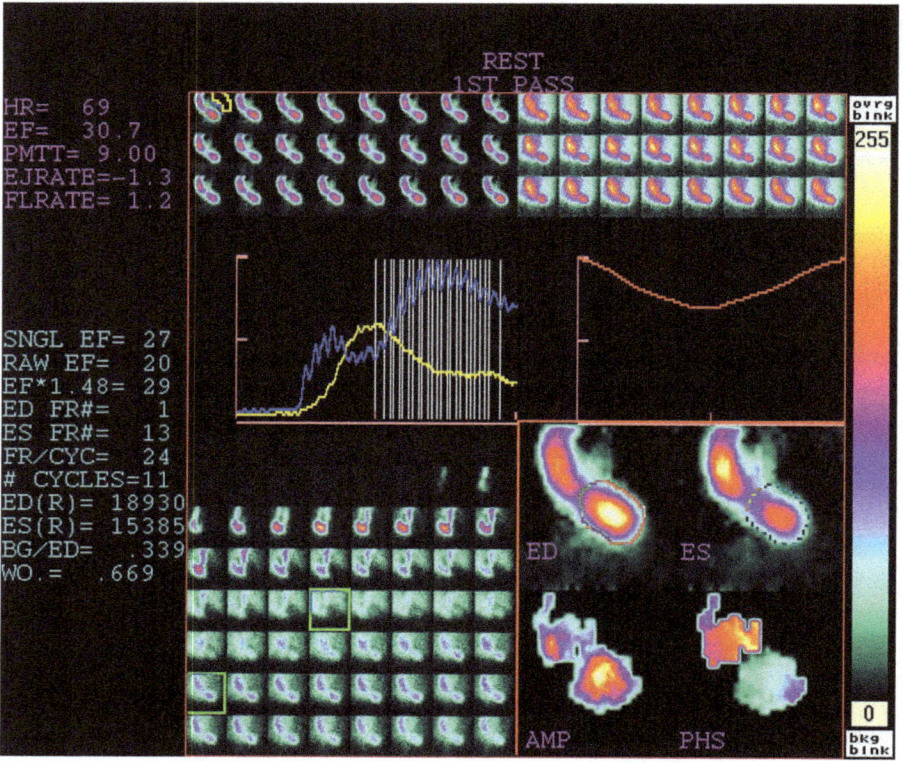

FIGURE 22-1 FPRNA (anterior projection) images are shown, with the serial images at the lower left, demonstrating tracer transit from the superior vena cava, to the right atrium, to the right ventricle to the pulmonary phase, left heart phase, and systemic circulation. Using regions of interest (ROIs) drawn over the LV and left lung (far upper left image), histograms are obtained (shown above serial images), which show overlapping RV counts with systoles (curve valleys) and diastoles (curve peaks) from which the cardiac cycles (CYC) are derived that comprise the representative cycle. Each cardiac cycle is marked. The pulmonary curve is used to compute the pulmonary mean transit time (PMTT). The length of the representative cycle in frames (FR) is used to derive the heart rate (HR). The images of the raw representative cycle are shown at upper right. This is subjected to the frame method of background subtraction (i.e., using the background to end-diastolic image ratio [BG/ED] and the washout factor [WO] needed to set the pulmonary area to zero counts), in order to derive the corrected representative cycle (upper left images) from which single ROI ejection fraction (SNGL EF), which is higher than the raw EF, but lower than the dual ROI-derived EF, which is used to account for valve plane motion. The Fourier amplitude (AMP) and phase (PHS) images at the lower right demonstrate reduced apical amplitude and delayed contraction of the apex, respectively.

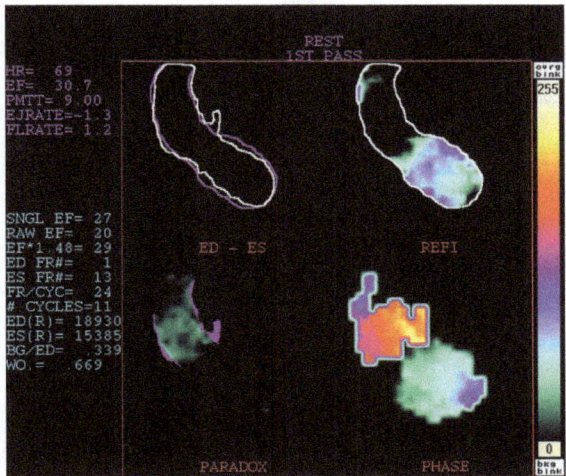
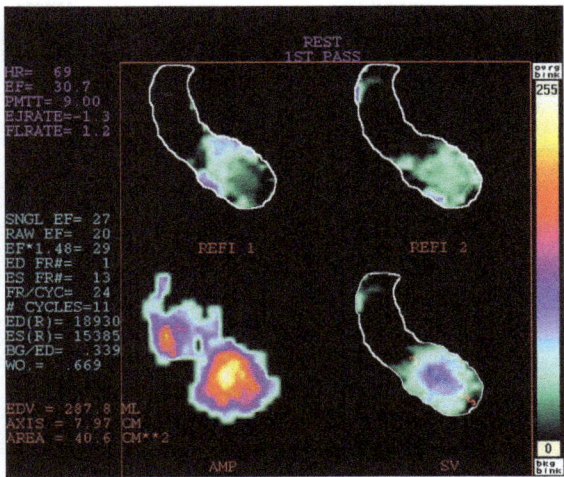

FIGURE 22-2 FPRNA (anterior projection) functional images are shown, with end-diastolic and end-systolic perimeter images at the upper left (ED – ES), a paradox image (lower left), regional ejection fraction index (REFI, upper right), and Fourier phase images (lower right) shown. The Fourier phase image demonstrates delayed contraction of the majority of the apex, with a small area of paradoxical movement (aneurysmal) evident at the apex on the paradox (ES counts – ED counts) image. These functional images allow assessment of regional function without the need for visual interpretation of cine images.

FIGURE 22-3 Additional FPRNA (anterior projection) functional images are shown, with regional ejection fraction index for the first and second halves of systole (REFI 1 and REFI 2, upper frames), an alternative method of determining the presence of delayed contraction. Note that the apical region has more ejection fraction in the latter half of systole, compared with the inferobasal wall. Fourier amplitude (AMP, lower left) and stroke volume (SV, ED – ES, lower right) images are shown. The graphic extending from the valve plane to the apex on the SV image is used to compute the LV volume using the Sandler and Dodge equation for the anterior projection.

by summing frames of several (usually 5–10) cardiac cycles, which are aligned by matching their end diastoles (histogram peaks) and end systoles (histogram valleys) during the operator-defined levophase of radioactive tracer transit. The pulmonary-frame background-corrected representative cycle is then examined with a fixed region of interest (ROI) in order to obtain the final first-pass LV time–activity curve. This ROI is drawn over the LV as defined by a first harmonic Fourier transformation phase image, which distinguishes clearly the LV from the aortic counts. End diastole is taken as the first frame of the representative cycle, and end systole is defined as the frame with the minimum counts in the histogram. Historically, the LVEF was taken as the end-diastolic counts minus the end-systolic counts, divided by the background-subtracted end-diastolic counts.

A second ROI (end diastolic) can be derived from a Fourier transformation amplitude image with masking of the lower 10% of image intensity, which extends the ROI in a basal direction, usually one to four pixels, depending on the vigor of ventricular contraction, up to the amplitude signal of the aortic root. The remainder of this ROI is drawn to match the first ROI (end systolic). The dual ROI LVEF is determined as the end-diastolic ROI counts minus the end-systolic ROI counts, divided by the background-subtracted end-diastolic ROI counts. This results in an accounting for valve plane motion during the cardiac cycle, using Fourier-guided dual ROI analysis of FPRNA, giving EFs that are highly reproducible and similar in value to ERNA.[18]

Gated Planar Equilibrium Blood Pool Imaging

Electrocardiogram (ECG)-gated planar equilibrium blood pool images (Fig. 22-4) can be performed with any of the several blood pool agents, such as Tc-99m–labeled red blood cells (described above and the standard) and Tc-99m–labeled human serum albumin. These images are best when acquired using high-resolution collimation. Images for planar LVEF calculation are obtained in the best septal (shallow) left anterior oblique (LAO) view. For regional

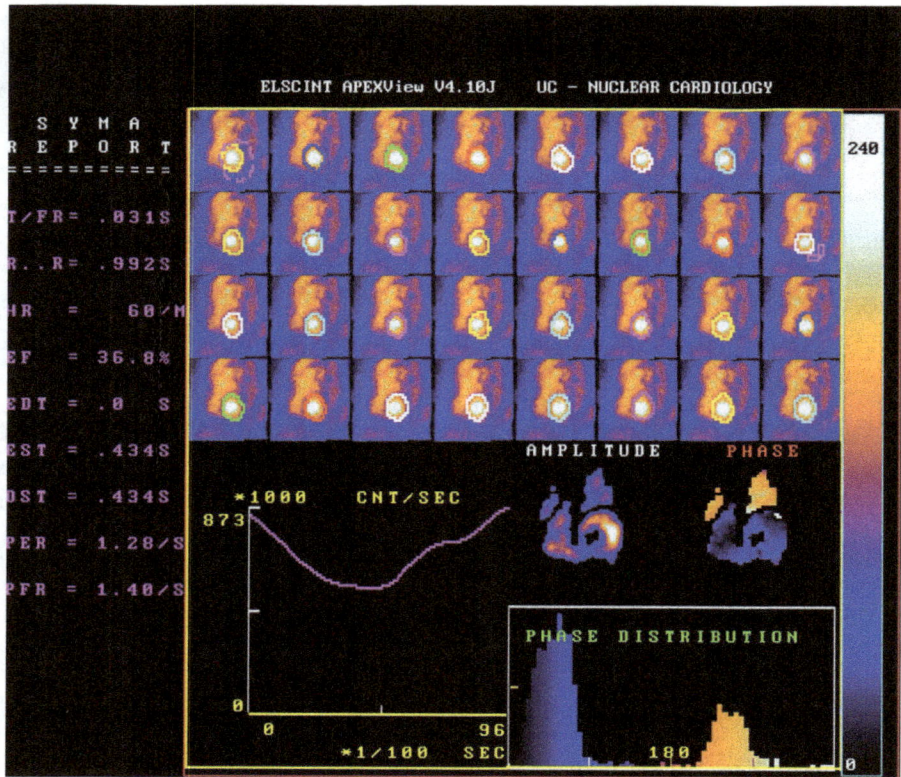

FIGURE 22-4 ERNA analysis is shown for images obtained in the LAO 45-degree projection. The 32 ECG-gated frames are analyzed using a guiding ROI (frame 1) obtained either manually or using Fourier phase and amplitude images to automatically locate and outline the LV. Automated LV edge detection is performed using a combination of first and second derivatives of count profiles inside the guiding or master ROI. Background correction is performed based on the counts per pixel within a small periventricular ROI (frame 16) drawn carefully to avoid the ventricle or the spleen. The counts within the 32 ROIs are shown after background correction in the lower left histogram. The first derivative of this ventricular volume curve is used to compute the peak filling and emptying rates (PFR and PER). The Fourier phase and amplitude functional images demonstrate inferoapical and septal hypokinesis with late contraction, when compared with the RV and the basal lateral portion of the LV.

wall motion assessment, the best septal view ±45 degrees should be obtained (approximately "anterior" and "lateral" views). Each of these planar-gated images should be acquired for 6- to 10-minute duration, dividing each cardiac cycle into a minimum of 32 frames. A smaller number of frames (e.g., 16) are adequate for assessment of EF due to the usual length of the isovolumic ejection period (at end diastole) and relaxation period (at end systole). However, more frames are desirable if quantitative assessment of diastolic performance is needed.

For LVEF, automated regions of interest are generated on the planar-gated equilibrium blood pool data throughout the cardiac cycle using the commercially available software. An automated periventricular background ROI must be adjusted routinely in order to avoid inclusion of high-count structures (e.g., spleen and descending aorta), which would artifactually increase the LVEF if included.

▶ Gated Tomographic Equilibrium Blood Pool Imaging

ECG-gated projections for SPECT reconstruction are usually obtained using high-resolution collimation in a fashion similar to gated SPECT perfusion imaging

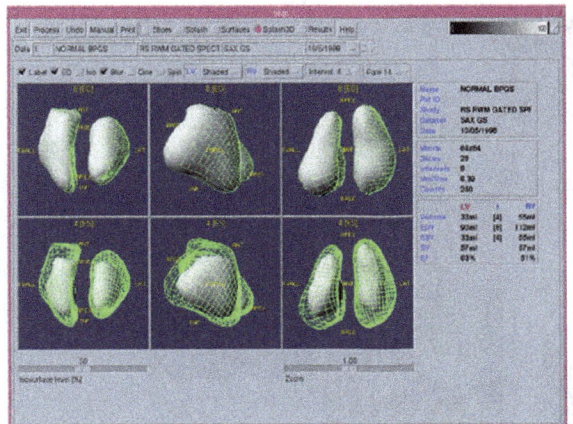

FIGURE 22-5 Gated tomographic ERNA analysis is shown after three-dimensional reconstruction of the left and right ventricles and surface rendering. This display (BPQS, Cedars-Sinai, Los Angeles) is termed *Splash3D*. All three synchronized pairs of 3D views are displayed. The lower views can be gated, and each of these views can be rotated interactively. It is also possible to superimpose an isosurface in this mode for rapid display of regional wall motion.

(Fig. 22-5), scanning from RAO 45 degrees to left posterior oblique (LPO) 45 degrees projections. A total of 45 to 60 projections of 20- to 30-second duration, at 4-degree or 3-degree steps, respectively, should give adequate count density. At each projection, either 8 or 16 frames per cardiac cycle should be acquired. After collimator sensitivity and center of rotation correction, projections are reconstructed into transaxial slices of the blood pool for each of the 8 or 16 frames of the cardiac cycle. The transaxial slice sets can then be reoriented in cardiac planes (i.e., short axis, horizontal long axis, and vertical long axis) for each of the eight frames of the cardiac cycle.

Multiple methods of quantifying blood pool SPECT images have been published using either three-dimensional images or midventricular horizontal and vertical long-axis slices, which can be analyzed for wall motion or EF.[19-25] The LVEF and RVEF can be calculated for each long axis as the end-diastolic counts minus the end-systolic counts, divided by the end-diastolic counts, combining them for a biplane EF.

The three-dimensional techniques are useful for blood pool volume rendering, which is used for delineation of myocardial (actually endocardial) topography. This technique is limited by the accuracy of automated valve plane definition since there is often little count density change at the mitral or tricuspid valve planes. However, this method has been validated against standard approaches, such as cardiac magnetic resonance.[25] Due to the uniformly high contrast and lack of overlap between cardiac blood pool and extracardiac structures, no background subtraction algorithm should be employed for these analyses.

▶ Gated SPECT Myocardial Perfusion Imaging

Gated SPECT MPI (Fig. 22-6) has become one of the most powerful tools available in nuclear cardiology and is discussed in detail in Chapter 11. Acquisition of SPECT data, synchronized with the electrocardiographic R wave, is generally performed using 8 or 16 gating intervals and allows evaluation of both global (EF) and regional (myocardial wall motion and wall thickening) cardiac function. Gated SPECT acquisition is now recommended for all perfusion studies whenever possible. It is estimated that over 90% of all SPECT studies in the United States are currently performed using the gated acquisition technique.[26] Gated SPECT MPI is most often performed with poststress ECG gating. Ungated SPECT perfusion imaging is usually reserved for resting images in some institutions or for patients with cardiac arrhythmias.

Two- and three-dimensional techniques for display of gated perfusion SPECT have been well validated for EF.[26-31] Gated SPECT has been utilized extensively for determination of EF and wall motion, adding incremental diagnostic and prognostic information. The addition of wall motion has improved the specificity of myocardial perfusion SPECT by distinguishing myocardial scarring from attenuation artifacts, both of which may result in "fixed" defects.[32]

The exponential increase in the use of gated SPECT perfusion has been fueled by the increased availability of automatic and semiautomatic algorithms for the quantification of cardiac function. DePuey et al.[29] described a method based on the automated detection of endocardial borders. Williams and Taillon[28] developed a method based on digitally subtracting and inverting the perfusion images and analyzing the change in counts occurring in the ventricular chamber, using an edge-detection method identical to that commonly used in gated ERNA. Germano et al.[27,30] developed a totally automated method of fitting geometric shapes to the endocardial borders to obtain

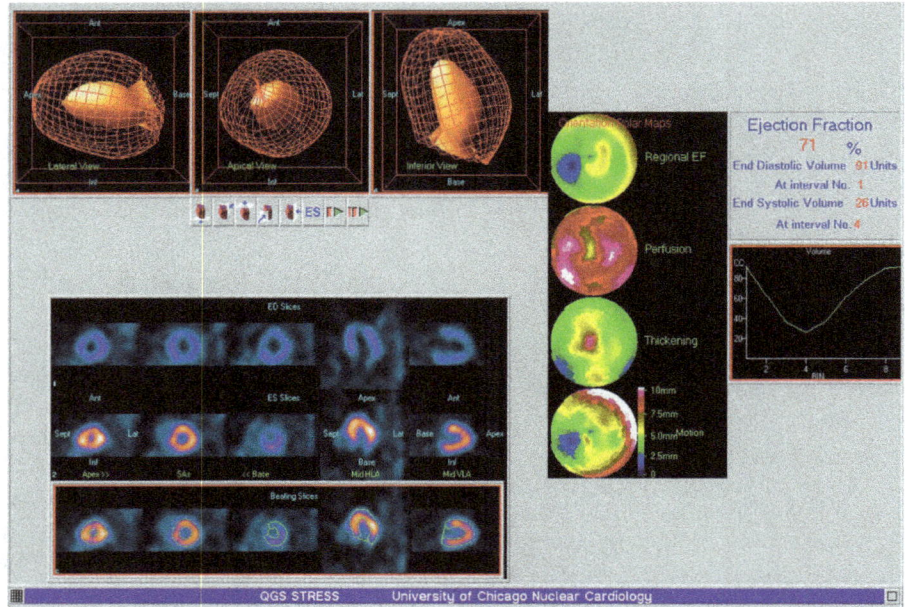

FIGURE 22-6 Gated SPECT myocardial perfusion images are shown analyzed with the commercially available QGS program (Cedars-Sinai) used for display and automated calculation of ejection fraction and volume. Changes in volume are tracked from ED to ES, for calculation of wall motion and regional thickening, displayed in polar map format. Three-dimensional surface-rendered diagrams (above) and actual SPECT slices with fitted edges (below) are also shown. These images were obtained with Tl-201 in a normal patient.

systolic and diastolic volumes and EFs. Smith et al.[31] have used partial volume effect to quantitate regional thickening and estimate LVEF, without need for any edge-detection algorithm. Each of these techniques has been well "correlated" with standard methods of performing EF, but each demonstrating varying degrees of "substitutability."[28]

For these reasons, the gated SPECT policy statement of the American Society of Nuclear Cardiology encourages the use of gated SPECT with every perfusion study in which gating is feasible. This reflects the improved quality control and diagnostic accuracy of interpreting perfusion images in light of regional and global LV performance, as well as the incremental value of gated SPECT over perfusion imaging alone for prognosis.[32-35]

Functional Images

Each of the scintigraphic modalities described above, whether planar or gated SPECT ERNA, FPRNA, or gated SPECT MPI, consists of a series of digital images. These series can be evaluated by computer techniques, which allow automated analyses and aid image interpretation, particularly for the assessment of regional function. The resultant images are the so-called functional images.

Functional images may be as simple as a subtraction (e.g., end-diastole image – end-systole image = stroke volume image) or more complex computer calculations (e.g., Fourier transformation phase and amplitude images).[36-39] The Fourier transformation process fits the changes that occur in each pixel (picture element) to a cosine wave, which is characterized by the height of change throughout the cycle (amplitude) and the relative timing of the wave (phase).

The amplitude images may be used to detect regions of decreased wall motion (hypokinesis) on blood pool or FPRNA images or to quantitate myocardial wall thickening on gated SPECT perfusion images. The presence of amplitude on Fourier transformation of perfusion polar maps has been shown to correlate with perfusion residual myocardial perfusion defect reversibility.[36]

The phase images are used to detect alterations in regional timing, such as the dyskinesis (outward wall motion) of an aneurysmal myocardial segment, or the often subtle degrees of late contraction (tardokinesis), typical of myocardial ischemia or prior infarction. They have also been utilized to detect the location of ventricular tachycardia or insertion of an accessory conduction bypass tract in Wolff–Parkinson–White syndrome.[36,37] In fact, a delay in segmental right ventricular (RV) activation compared with the LV detected on Fourier phase images of gated blood pool RNA is consistent with arrhythmogenic RV dysplasia and has been correlated with a poor prognosis.[37–39]

CLINICAL APPLICATIONS

The assessment of LV size, systolic function, diastolic function, regional wall motion, and timing of mechanical activation remain diagnostically and prognostically important uses of radionuclide imaging. The exercise FPRNA LVEF has particularly greater prognostic value in patients with ischemic heart disease than many other clinical, noninvasive, and invasively derived variables.[5–9] An exercise LVEF of 0.50 (50%) has been identified as the inflection point below which patients with CAD demonstrate a probability of cardiac death, which increases as the EF decreases.[7] However, the direct applicability of these numerical data when the EF is obtained with other protocols or techniques, such as the more widely utilized ERNA technique, is uncertain.

The evaluation of LV systolic function has become one of the most common applications of nuclear imaging, using FPRNA, planar ERNA, and, more recently, gated SPECT perfusion and SPECT ERNA. Each noninvasive imaging technique has unique strengths and limitations. Detection of regional global ventricular dysfunction can be performed with many noninvasive methods, but the nuclear imaging techniques are inherently quantitative, rather than relying on visual estimation of ventricular size and function. Factors to consider upon test selection include local expertise, local access, cost, and the need for reproducible quantitative measurements. The ability to distinguish systolic from diastolic dysfunction should also be considered. The RNA techniques can be used to compute quantitative estimates of LV, as well as RV EFs, and absolute volumes with geometric or count-based methods.

FPRNA has some distinct advantages over ERNA. These include (1) the acquisition of data in <30 seconds; (2) the evaluation of RV function with less overlap of the activity from other chambers[40]; (3) the use of multiple radiopharmaceuticals, including bone, renal, and myocardial scintigraphic agents[13]; (4) a proven robust measurement of stress ventricular function at the true point of peak exercise[5,7,9]; and (5) the presence of a wealth of prognostic information available for management of patients with ischemic heart disease based on stratification by FPRNA exercise LVEFs.[5,7,9] Despite these advantages, widespread use of FPRNA has been limited by the need for large-bore intravenous access, absence of significant tricuspid regurgitation,[40] impeccable bolus technique,[28] and a high-count rate-capable, often dedicated, gamma camera.[16–18] Currently, ERNA use is far more widespread than FPRNA and allows for multiple views of imaging.

In terms of feasibility, quantitation of LV chamber volume and EFs are obtainable in essentially 100% of patients. If venous access is poor, FPRNA cannot be performed, but ERNA requires no bolus, and therefore can be performed with a minimally sized intravenous catheter or direct venous punctures. If ERNA is difficult due to poor tagging of red cells (e.g., with heparin infusion), a Tc-99m–labeled perfusion agent may be employed for gated SPECT perfusion imaging. As noted earlier, the latter test has become the most commonly performed scintigraphic ejection EF, as a diagnostically and prognostically important addition to myocardial perfusion SPECT. The high degree of reproducibility in the EF makes RNA an ideal choice for the assessment of medical interventions on LV function, such as in oncology patients receiving chemotherapy. In particular, this is an ideal choice for serial imaging to assess for cardiotoxicity in patients receiving anthracycline-based drugs such as daunorubicin, discussed further below.

▶ Assessment of Systolic Function

Left Ventricle

The assessment of systolic function is an important component of the initial evaluation of all patients with the clinical symptoms of right- or left-sided congestive heart failure (CHF), ischemic heart disease, and in patients who are undergoing potentially cardiotoxic treatments, such as doxorubicin. Systolic dysfunction is usually defined by the presence of an LVEF <50%, while a normal RVEF is 10 to 15 units lower than that of the LV. However, it should be recalled that the EF is an ejection phase index, which is dependent on loading conditions of the ventricle. Preload (i.e., fiber stretch) deficiency or inappropriate afterload (e.g., severe hypertension) may result in lowering of the EF in the absence of any real decrease in inotropic state or contractile reserve. Compensatory dilatation of the ventricle is present in most patients with systolic dysfunction. Assessment of ventricular volume indices has both diagnostic and therapeutic implications. The presence of ventricular enlargement in the absence of systolic dysfunction in the patient with clinical symptoms of heart failure raises the possibility of heart failure secondary to high-output states, such as anemia or valvular heart disease. For example, when systolic function deteriorates in the RV or LV, this is an indicator of the need to proceed with mitral or aortic (respectively) valvular replacement surgery.[11,41] In the absence of dilatation or systolic dysfunction, heart failure symptoms suggest the presence of pulmonary disease (RV dysfunction), pericardial disease (biventricular dysfunction), or predominant diastolic dysfunction.

Right Ventricle

Right ventricular function is less commonly assessed than LV function but can have diagnostic and prognostic implications in assessment of lung disease and lung transplantation patients, congestive heart failure, and assessment of arrhythmogenic RV dysplasia.[39,42–45] FPRNA offers the most accurate scintigraphic assessment of RVEF, but again, is rarely performed these days.

Assessment of Diastolic Function

The presence and severity of diastolic dysfunction should be assessed in every patient presenting with evidence for heart failure, since it is the predominant abnormality in as many as 30% to 40% of such patients.[46] Most often, this sways both the diagnostic considerations (e.g., hypertension, diabetes mellitus, hypertrophic myopathies, or myocardial infiltration) and the therapeutic options (e.g., antihypertensives and tight glucose control). This may indicate the need for further procedures, such as myocardial biopsy.

In RNA studies, the rate of change (first derivative) of counts in diastole can be analyzed to calculate indices of diastolic filling, including the peak LV filling rate, time to peak filling, and atrial contribution to filling.[47] In practice, Doppler blood flow velocity indices of transmitral flow are used much more commonly to assess LV diastolic filling parameters. For RNA, a peak diastolic filling rate of >2.5 end-diastolic volumes per second (EDV/s) is considered normal.[47,48] Age- and gender-specific criteria for diagnosing LV diastolic dysfunction using Doppler blood flow velocity from transmitral flow based on large population studies have been defined that are applicable to clinical practice.[49,50] However, large population-based criteria, adjusted for age and gender, for abnormal diastolic function have not yet been established for RNA.

Assessment of Ventricular Dyssynchrony

Recent advancements in the management of CHF include prevention of sudden death with implanted defibrillators and improvement of mechanical efficiency by synchronizing the timing of ventricular contraction. Ventricular dyssynchrony is typified by a wide QRS complex on electrocardiography, often with a left bundle branch block morphology,[51] and is associated with a higher risk of sudden cardiac death.[52] Various parameters have been looked at to help delineate which patients would be optimal candidates for cardiac resynchronization therapy, including LV dyssynchrony, scar burden, and site of late activation for placement of the LV lead.[53]

Echocardiography has been highly touted as the method of choice for evaluation of ventricular dyssynchrony, but suffers from its two-dimensional nature, and lack of reproducibility.[54] Recent data have indicated that gated SPECT perfusion[55,56] and SPECT blood pool[57] imaging can be utilized as three-dimensional methods that easily evaluate regional timing of myocardial contraction in an automated operator-independent fashion (Fig. 22-7). SPECT phase analysis has been shown to be reproducible,

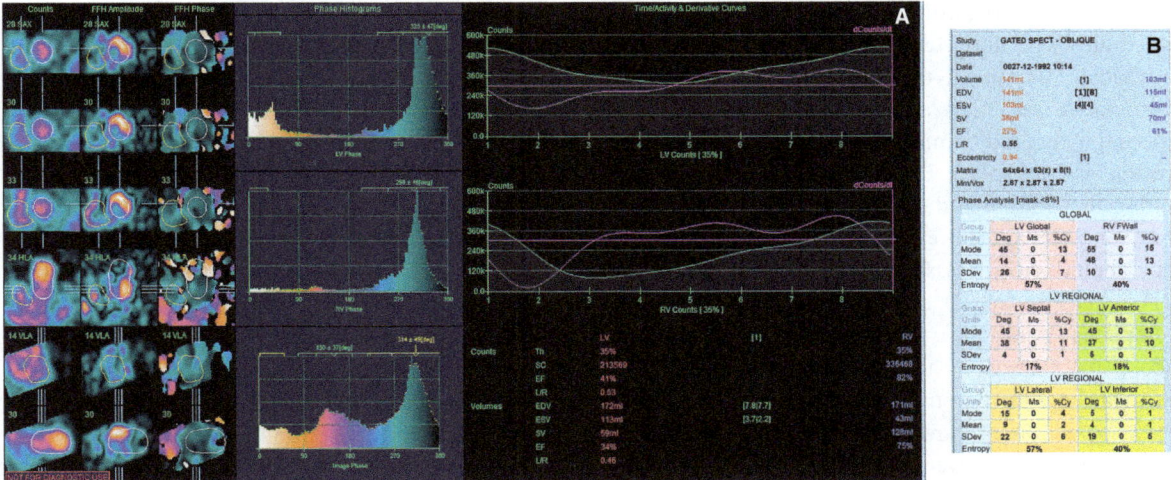

FIGURE 22-7 Gated SPECT blood pool imaging with phase and amplitude analysis is shown in the same patient depicted with planar imaging in Figure 22-4. **(A)** Time–activity curves of LV and RV volume and flow (first derivative of volume) are shown on the right. Tomographic slices at ED and ES are shown for three short and two short-axis images on the left. The middle panel depicts the LV, RV, and total image phase histogram. The presence of many apical pixels with phases that are opposite (180 degrees out of synchrony with the base) is consistent with aneurysm formation. **(B)** Degree of dyssynchrony can be quantitated in terms of mean phase angle, the standard deviation of the angles, and "entropy" or histogram bandwidth.

validated using commercially available software and has been validated again dyssynchrony parameters measured by tissue Doppler imaging and speckle tracking echocardiography.[58–61] Phase analysis holds promise for improving the evaluation and selection of patients with CHF and QRS widening, but further randomized clinical trials are needed.

▶ Monitoring the Effects of Chemotherapy

Monitoring for cardiotoxicity from chemotherapy is an important use of radionuclide angiography. The two main classes of chemotherapy that cause cardiac toxicity include anthracyclines and the newer tyrosine kinase inhibitors (TKIs).

Anthracyclines include daunorubicin (the most commonly used) and various analogs of anthracyclines (including doxorubicin, epirubicin, idarubicin, mitoxantrone, and others).[62] They cause myocardial necrosis due to free radical formation, characterized by myocellular vacuolization. Risk factors for the development of more rapid deterioration in LV function with anthracyclines include cumulative anthracycline dose, extremes of age, female gender, cardiovascular comorbidities, adjuvant chemotherapies, and adjuvant thoracic radiation therapy.[63]

Anthracyclines cause what is traditionally called type I cardiotoxicity, with irreversible injury from cardiomyocyte death.[64] This results in progressive lowering of the LVEF as the cumulative dose of the agent increases and is clearly dose related.

The tyrosine kinase inhibitors include trastuzumab, lapatinib, imatinib, sorafenib, and sunitinib, among others.[65] They cause type 2 cardiotoxicity which is characterized by cardiomyocyte dysfunction, rather than cell death, which is felt to be reversible. For TKIs, the toxicity is not dose related and usually responds to standard medical treatment or discontinuation of drug.[66] Risk factors for the development of trastuzumab-induced cardiotoxicity include previous or concurrent anthracycline use and older age.

Noninvasive monitoring of LVEF during chemotherapy with anthracyclines or TKIs is recommended for the early assessment of cardiotoxicity; however there is no clear consensus on how to monitor. Both ECHO and ERNA techniques have been evaluated for chemotherapy monitoring. FPRNA has been found to be more sensitive than echocardiography for the detection of anthracycline-induced LV dysfunction,[67] but is no longer readily available. ERNA is well established and is still commonly used. It has extensive data regarding its accuracy and reproducibility with long-term follow-up and is widely available.[68] However, there are concerns about its cumulative radiation exposure. As such, echocardiography is used commonly these days, and certain protocols intersperse ECHO with RNA to provide reduced radiation and still have the improved accuracy of RNA. ECHO evaluation during chemotherapy should include assessment of LVEF (ideally by 3D echo, else by 2D echo using modified biplane Simpson's technique), assessment of wall motion score index, and global longitudinal strain.[69] Other echocardiogram parameters being assessed for the early detection of cardiotoxicity include fractional shortening, and newer tissue Doppler and speckle tracking indices (strain).[67] Although ECHO is used commonly these days, concerns do exist regarding the reproducibility of LVEF by ECHO. Regardless of which imaging technique is used, the LVEFs are likely not interchangeable, and it is recommended that a single technique be used in an individual patient for serial monitoring of LVEF.

There are no definitive guidelines on the optimal timing and duration of cardiac monitoring for patients receiving anthracycline-based chemotherapy. All patients that are at high risk for cardiotoxicity should receive a baseline evaluation of LVEF. The newest guidelines by the European Society of Medical Oncology and the American Society of Echocardiography recommend: a baseline evaluation of LV function with ECHO and Troponin levels.[69,70] For asymptomatic patients, serial evaluation should be considered at 6 months after completion of treatment, annually for 2 to 3 years thereafter, and then at 3- to 5-year intervals for life. High-risk patients may be monitored more frequently. Assessment of subclinical LV dysfunction should be considered with evaluation of global longitudinal strain on ECHO. American Society of Clinical Oncology (ASCO) guidelines include: (1) an evaluation of EF prior to each planned course of doxorubicin (per the labeling guidelines of the drug), (2) monitoring after a cumulative dose of 400 mg/m^2 is reached, (3) repeated after 500 mg/m^2 cumulative dose, and (4) thereafter after every 50 mg/m^2 dose.[71] Traditional ERNA assessment has included EF assessment at baseline, measurement at 250 to 300 mg/m^2, at 450 mg/m^2 and measurement before each dose above 450 mg/m^2. If the baseline EF is >50%, then therapy should be discontinued once it decreases by >10% from baseline and LVEF is <50%. If EF is <50% at baseline, serial measurements should be obtained before each dose, with discontinuation of therapy once LVEF <30% or drops by >10%.[72] It has been advocated that keeping a table of RNA/EF results along with cumulative doses may be helpful for proper monitoring.

In general, if test results indicate deterioration in cardiac function associated with an anthracycline, the benefit of continued therapy must be carefully evaluated against the risk of producing irreversible cardiac damage.

For tyrosine kinase inhibitors, especially trastuzumab, baseline cardiac function and troponin should be assessed prior to treatment.[69,70] Optimal surveillance with these agents has also not been established, but higher-risk patients should be followed more closely. Both ERNA and ECHO are being used for monitoring of LV function. Serial assessment in an individual patient should be performed by a consistent method.

CONCLUSION

This chapter details the technical aspects and the wide range of clinical diagnostic possibilities available by dynamic imaging of myocardial function using scintigraphic techniques. These principles are now finding new applications in the realm of myocardial timing and mechanics and for the monitoring of chemotherapy-induced cardiomyopathy.

REFERENCES

1. Greenberg H, McMaster P, Dwyer EM; The Multicenter Postinfarction Research Group. Left ventricular dysfunction after acute myocardial infarction: The results of a prospective multicenter study. *J Am Coll Cardiol*. 1984;4:867–874.
2. Nesto RW, Cohn LH, Collins JJ Jr, et al. Inotropic contractile reserve: A useful predictor of increased 5 year survival and improved post-operative left ventricular function in patients with coronary artery disease and reduced ejection fraction. *Am J Cardiol*. 1982;50:39–44.
3. Ritchie JL, Hallstrom AP, Troubaugh GB, et al. Out-of-hospital sudden coronary death: Rest and exercise left ventricular function in survivors. *Am J Cardiol*. 1985;55:645–651.
4. Williams KA, Sherwood DF, Fisher KM. The frequency of asymptomatic and electrically silent exercise-induced regional myocardial ischemia during first-pass radionuclide

angiography with upright bicycle ergometry. *J Nucl Med.* 1992;33:359–364.
5. Lee KL, Pryor DB, Pieper KS. Prognostic value of radionuclide angiography in medically treated patients with coronary artery disease: A comparison with clinical and catheterization variables. *Circulation.* 1990;82:1705–1717.
6. Muhlbaier LH, Pryor DB, Rankin JS, et al. Observational comparison of event-free survival with medical and surgical therapy in patients with coronary artery disease: 20 years of follow-up. *Circulation.* 1992;86(5 suppl):II198–II204.
7. Jones RH, Johnson SH, Bigelow C, et al. Exercise radionuclide angiocardiography predicts cardiac death in patients with coronary artery disease. *Circulation.* 1991;84(3 suppl): 152–158.
8. Johnson SH, Bigelow C, Lee KL, et al. Prediction of death and myocardial infarction by radionuclide angiocardiography in patients with suspected coronary artery disease. *Am J Cardiol.* 1991;67(11):919–926.
9. Pryor DB, Harrell FE Jr, Lee KL, et al. Prognostic indicators from radionuclide angiography in medically treated patients with coronary artery disease. *Am J Cardiol.* 1984;53(1):18–22.
10. Zhu WX, Gibbons RJ, Bailey KR, Gersh BJ. Predischarge exercise radionuclide angiography in predicting multivessel coronary artery disease and subsequent cardiac events after thrombolytic therapy for acute myocardial infarction. *Am J Cardiol.* 1994;74:554–559.
11. Borer JS, Hochreiter C, Herrold EM, et al. Prediction of indications for valve replacement among asymptomatic or minimally symptomatic patients with chronic aortic regurgitation and normal left ventricular performance. *Circulation.* 1998;97:525–534.
12. Berman DS, Kiat H, Maddahi J. The new ^{99m}Tc myocardial perfusion imaging agents: ^{99m}Tc-sestamibi and ^{99m}Tc-teboroxime. *Circulation.* 1991;84(3 suppl):I7–I21.
13. Williams KA, Taillon LA, Draho JM, Foisy MF. First-pass radionuclide angiographic studies of left ventricular function with Tc-99m-teboroxime, Tc-99m-sestamibi and Tc-99m-DTPA. *J Nucl Med.* 1993;35:394–399.
14. Jones RH, Borges-Neto S, Potts JM. Simultaneous measurement of myocardial perfusion and ventricular function during exercise from a single injection of Tc-99m sestamibi in coronary artery disease. *Am J Cardiol.* 1990;66:68E–71E.
15. Knaapen P, Lubberink M, Rijzewijk LJ, et al. Stroke volume measurements with first-pass dynamic positron emission tomography: Comparison with cardiovascular magnetic resonance. *J Nucl Cardiol.* 2008;15(2):218–224.
16. Gal R, Grenier RP, Carpenter J, et al. High count rate first-pass radionuclide angiography using a digital gamma camera. *J Nucl Med.* 1986;27:198–206.
17. Gal R, Grenier RP, Schmidt DH, Port SC. Background correction in first-pass radionuclide angiography: Comparison of several approaches. *J Nucl Med.* 1986;27:1480–1486.
18. Williams KA, Bryant TA, Taillon LA. First-pass radionuclide angiographic analysis with two regions of interest: Improved "substitutability" for gated equilibrium ejection fractions. *J Nucl Med.* 1998;39(11):1857–1861.
19. Faber TL, Stokely EM, Templeton GH, et al. Quantification of three-dimensional left ventricular segmental wall motion and volumes from gated tomographic radionuclide ventriculograms. *J Nucl Med.* 1989;30:638–649.
20. Bartlett ML, Srinivasan G, Barker WC, et al. Left ventricular ejection fraction: Comparison of results from planar and SPECT gated blood-pool studies. *J Nucl Med.* 1996;37:1795–1799.
21. Chin BB, Bloomgarden DC, Xia W, et al. Right and left ventricular volume and ejection fraction by tomographic gated blood-pool scintigraphy. *J Nucl Med.* 1997;38:942–948.
22. Groch MW, Marshall RC, Erwin WD, et al. Quantitative gated blood pool SPECT for the assessment of coronary artery disease at rest. *J Nucl Cardiol.* 1998;5:567–573.
23. Van Kriekinge SD, Berman DS, Germano G. Automatic quantification of left ventricular ejection fraction from gated blood pool SPECT. *J Nucl Cardiol.* 1999;6:498–506.
24. Vanhove C, Franken PR, Defrise M, et al. Automatic determination of left ventricular ejection fraction from gated blood-pool tomography. *J Nucl Med.* 2001;42:401–407.
25. Nichols K, Saouaf R, Ababneh AA, et al. Validation of SPECT equilibrium radionuclide angiographic right ventricular parameters by cardiac magnetic resonance imaging. *J Nucl Cardiol.* 2002;9:153–160.
26. Beller GA, Zaret BL. Wintergreen summary: Panel on instrumentation and quantification. *J Nucl Cardiol.* 1999;6(1):94–103.
27. Germano G, Erel J, Kiat H, et al. Quantitative LVEF and qualitative regional function from gated thallium-201 perfusion SPECT. *J Nucl Med.* 1997;38(5):749–754.
28. Williams KA, Taillon LA. Left ventricular function in patients with coronary artery disease using gated tomographic myocardial perfusion images: Comparison with contrast ventriculography and first-pass radionuclide angiography. *J Am Coll Cardiol.* 1996;27:173–181.
29. DePuey EG, Nichols K, Dobrinsky C. Left ventricular ejection fraction assessed from gated technetium-99m-sestamibi SPECT. *J Nucl Med.* 1993;34(11):1871–1876.
30. Germano G, Kiat H, Kavanagh PB, et al. Automatic quantification of ejection fraction from gated myocardial perfusion SPECT. *J Nucl Med.* 1995;36(11):2138–2147.
31. Smith WH, Kastner RJ, Calnon DA, et al. Quantitative gated single photon emission computed tomography imaging: A counts-based method for display and measurement of regional and global ventricular systolic function. *J Nucl Cardiol.* 1997; 4(6):451–463.
32. DePuey EG, Rozanski AR. Using gated technetium-99m sestamibi SPECT to characterize fixed myocardial defects as infarct or artifact. *J Nucl Med.* 1995;36:952–955.
33. Taillefer R, DePuey EG, Udelson JE, et al. Comparative diagnostic accuracy of Tl-201 and Tc-99m sestamibi SPECT imaging (perfusion and ECG-gated SPECT) in detecting coronary artery disease in women. *J Am Coll Cardiol.* 1997;29: 69–77.
34. Smanio PE, Watson DD, Segalla DL, et al. Value of gating of technetium 99m sestamibi single-photon emission computed tomographic imaging. *J Am Coll Cardiol.* 1997;30: 1687–1692.
35. Chua T, Kiat H, Germano G, et al. Gated technetium 99m sestamibi for simultaneous assessment of stress myocardial perfusion, post-exercise regional ventricular function and myocardial viability. *J Am Coll Cardiol.* 1994;23:1107–1114.
36. Le Guludec D, Bourguignon M, Sebag C, et al. Phase mapping of radionuclide gated biventriculograms in patients with sustained ventricular tachycardia or Wolff–Parkinson–White syndrome. *Int J Card Imaging.* 1987;2:117–126.

37. Casset-Senon D, Babuty D, Alison D, et al. Delayed contraction area responsible for sustained ventricular tachycardia in an arrhythmogenic right ventricular cardiomyopathy: Demonstration by Fourier analysis of SPECT equilibrium radionuclide angiography. *J Nucl Cardiol*. 2000;7:539–542.
38. Casset-Senon D, Philippe L, Babuty D, et al. Diagnosis of arrhythmogenic right ventricular cardiomyopathy by Fourier analysis of gated blood pool single-photon emission tomography. *J Cardiol*. 1998;82:1399–1404.
39. Le Guludec D, Gauthier H, Porcher R, et al. Prognostic value of radionuclide angiography in patients with right ventricular arrhythmias. *Circulation*. 2001;103:1972–1976.
40. Williams KA, Walley PE, Ryan JW. Detection and assessment of severity of tricuspid regurgitation using first-pass radionuclide angiography and comparison with pulsed Doppler echocardiography. *Am J Cardiol*. 1990;66:333–339.
41. Wencker D, Borer JS, Hochreiter C, et al. Preoperative predictors of late postoperative outcome among patients with nonischemic mitral regurgitation with "high risk" descriptors and comparison with unoperated patients. *Cardiology*. 2000;93:37–42.
42. Van der Maas N, Braam RL, Van der Zaag-Loonen HJ, et al. Right ventricular ejection fraction measured by multigated planar equilibrium radionuclide ventriculography is an independent prognostic factor in patients with ischemic heart disease. *J Nucl Cardiol*. 2012;19:1162–1169.
43. Sciurba FC, Rogers RM, Keenan RJ, et al. Improvement in pulmonary function and elastic recoil after lung-reduction surgery for diffuse emphysema. *N Engl J Med*. 1996; 334: 1095–1099.
44. Di Salvo TG, Mathier M, Semigran MJ, Dec GW. Preserved right ventricular ejection fraction predicts exercise capacity and survival in advanced heart failure. *J Am Coll Cardiol*. 1995;25:1143–1153.
45. Baker BJ, Wilen MM, Boyd CM, et al. Relation of right ventricular ejection fraction to exercise capacity in chronic left ventricular failure. *Am J Cardiol*. 1984;54:596–599.
46. Ruzumna P, Gheorghiade M, Bonow RO. Mechanisms and management of heart failure due to diastolic dysfunction. *Curr Opin Cardiol*. 1996;11:269–275.
47. Muntinga HJ, van den BF, Knol HR, et al. Normal values and reproducibility of left ventricular filling parameters by radionuclide angiography. *Int J Card Imaging*. 1997;13:165–171.
48. Bonow RO. Radionuclide angiographic evaluation of left ventricular function. *Circulation*. 1991;84:I208–1215.
49. Schirmer H, Lunde P, Rasmussen K. Mitral flow derived Doppler indices of left ventricular diastolic function in a general population: the Tromso study. *Eur Heart J*. 2000;21:1376–1386.
50. Nagueh SF, Smiseth OA, Appleton CP, et al. Recommendations for the evaluation of left ventricular diastolic function by echocardiography: An update from the American Society of Echocardiography and the European Association of Cardiovascular Imaging. *J Am Soc Echocardiogr*. 2016;29:277–314.
51. Tavazzi L. Ventricular pacing: A promising new therapeutic strategy in heart failure. For whom? Editorial. *Eur Heart J*. 2000;21:1211–1214.
52. Iuliano S, Fisher SG, Karasik PE, Fletcher RD, Singh SN; Department of Veterans Affairs Survival Trial of Antiarrhythmic Therapy in Congestive Heart Failure. QRS duration and mortality in patients with congestive heart failure. *Am Heart J*. 2002;143:1085–1091.
53. Chen J, Boogers MJ, Bax JJ, et al. The use of nuclear imaging for cardiac resynchronization therapy. *Current Cardiol Reports*. 2010;12:185–191.
54. Chung ES, Leon AR, Tavazzi L, et al. Results of the Predictors of Response to CRT (PROSPECT) trial. *Circulation*. 2008;117(20):2608–2616.
55. Chen J, Garcia EV, Lerakis S, et al. Left ventricular mechanical dyssynchrony as assessed by phase analysis of ECG-gated SPECT myocardial perfusion imaging. *Echocardiography*. 2008;25(10):1186–1194.
56. Boogers MM, Van Kriekinge SD, Henneman MM, et al. Quantitative gated SPECT-derived phase analysis on gated myocardial perfusion SPECT detects left ventricular dyssynchrony and predicts response to cardiac resynchronization therapy. *J Nucl Med*. 2009;50(5):718–725.
57. Nichols KJ, Van Tosh A, De Bondt P, Bergmann R, Palestro CJ, Reichek NR. Normal limits of gated blood-pool SPECT count-based regional cardiac function parameters. *Int J Card Imaging*. 2008;24(7):717–725.
58. Singh H, Singhal A, Sharma P, et al. Quantitative assessment of cardiac mechanical synchrony using equilibrium radionuclide angiography. *J Nuc Cardiol*. 2013;20:415–425.
59. Henneman MM, Chen J, Ypenburg C, et al. Phase analysis of gated myocardial perfusion SPECT compared to tissue Doppler imaging for the assessment of left ventricular dyssynchrony. *J Am Coll Cardiol*. 2007; 49:1708–1714.
60. Marsan NA. Henneman MM, Chen J, et al. Left ventricular dyssynchrony assessed by two 3-dimensional imaging modalities: Phase analysis of gated myocardial perfusion SPECT and tri-plane tissue Doppler imaging. *Eur J Nucl Med Mol Imaging*. 2008;35:166–173.
61. Hsu TH, Huang WS, Chen CC, et al. Left ventricular systolic and diastolic dyssynchrony assessed by phase analysis of gated SPECT myocardial perfusion imaging: A comparison with speckle tracking echocardiography. *Ann Nucl Med*. 2013;27:764–771.
62. Singal PK, Iliskovic N. Doxorubicin-induced cardiomyopathy. *N Engl J Med*. 1998;339:900–905.
63. Groarke J, Norhia A. Anthracycline cardiotoxicity: A new paradigm for an old classic. *Circulation*. 2015;131:1946–1949.
64. Volkova M, Russell R 3rd. Anthracycline cardiotoxicity: Prevalence, pathogenesis and treatment. *Curr Cardiol Rev*. 2011;7:214–220.
65. Meller HR, Bell AR, Valentin JP, Roberts RR. Cardiotoxicity associated with targeting kinase pathways in cancer. *Tox Sci*. 2011;120:14–32.
66. Decara JM. Early detection of chemotherapy-related left ventricular dysfunction. *Current Cardiol Reports*. 2012;14: 334–341.
67. Lahtinen R, Uusitupa M, Kuikka J, Lanseimies E. Noninvasive evaluation of anthracycline-induced cardiotoxicity in man. *Acta Med Scand*. 1982;212:201–206.
68. Bellenger, NG, Burgess MI, Ray SG, et al. Comparison of left ventricular ejection fraction and volumes in heart failure by echocardiography, radionuclide ventriculography and cardiovascular magnetic resonance; are they interchangeable? *Eur Heart J*. 2000;21:1387–1396.

69. Plana, J, Galderisi M, Barac A, et al. Expert Consensus for multimodality imaging evaluation of adult patient during and after cancer therapy: A report from the American society of echocardiography and the European association of cardiovascular imaging. *J Am Soc Echo*. 2014;27:911–939.
70. Curigliano G, Cardinale D, Suter T, et al. Cardiovascular toxicity induced by chemotherapy targeted agents and radiotherapy: ESMO clinical practice guidelines. *Ann Oncol*. 2010;21(Suppl 5):v277–v282.
71. Hensely ML, Hagerty KL, Kewaltamani T, et al. American Society of Clinical Oncology 2008 clinical practice guideline update: Use of chemotherapy and radiation therapy protectants. *J Clin Oncol*. 2009;27:127–145.
72. Schwartz RG, McKenzie WB, Alexander J, et al. Congestive heart failure and left ventricular dysfunction complicating doxorubicin therapy. Seven year experience using radionuclide angiocardiography. *Am J Med*. 1987;82:1109–1118.

Radionuclide Imaging of Cardiac Innervation

CHAPTER 23

Mark I. Travin

INTRODUCTION

It is recognized by many in the field of nuclear cardiology that in order to thrive and advance, the discipline needs to go beyond myocardial perfusion imaging (MPI). The high diagnostic and risk stratification utilities of radionuclide single-photon emission computed tomography (SPECT) and positron emission tomography (PET) MPI are well established,[1-4] with observational studies[5-7] strongly suggesting that performing and properly acting upon the results of MPI can lead to improved patient outcome, with a study in progress designed to firmly establish this.[8] Nevertheless, there is an increased focus on developing radionuclide techniques that rely on a unique strength of the modality, that is, the ability to image the underlying molecular processes of cardiac disease.[9] Among such nonperfusion radionuclide imaging methods of current interest is assessment of cardiac autonomic innervation.[10,11]

Neurohormonal regulation of the cardiovascular system is crucial for maintaining body function. One major component is circulating hormones that include epinephrine, norepinephrine (NE), arginine vasopressin, B-type natriuretic peptide (BNP), and substances of the renin-angiotensin aldosterone system (RAAS).[12] Another component, working in conjunction with the hormonal mediators, is direct innervation via the sympathetic and parasympathetic autonomic nervous system. Together, these neurohormonal (sometimes also referred to as "neurohumoral") processes control cardiac output (CO), vascular tone, and blood volume, serving to maintain proper perfusion to body organs as needed for normal conditions and activities. In response to stressors or insults, such as volume depletion or diminished CO from cardiac dysfunction, neurohormonal mechanisms compensate with vasoconstriction, augmentation of myocardial contractility, increased heart rate, and expansion of extracellular volume.[13] In many situations, such adaptations are necessary and beneficial, but in other circumstances neurohormonal activation can be excessive and persist beyond what is needed, thus maladaptive and potentially harmful.[14] The ability to directly visualize these mechanisms via radionuclide imaging provides important insights into the pathophysiology of various cardiac diseases. Much recent work shows a robust ability of cardiac autonomic innervation imaging to effectively assess a patient's condition beyond other commonly used methods. There is much promise that such imaging will lead to improved disease management, thus a reduction of adverse events and improved patient outcome and well-being.

CARDIAC AUTONOMIC INNERVATION

The heart is richly innervated by sympathetic and parasympathetic fibers which are controlled by regulatory centers in the brain that integrate input signals from other parts of the brain and from receptors throughout the body. Efferent sympathetic signals from the regulatory centers follow descending pathways in the spinal cord, and synapse with preganglionic fibers that leave the spinal cord at levels T1–L3, subsequently synapsing with paravertebral stellate ganglia, and eventually innervating the right ventricle, and the anterior and lateral left ventricle. In the heart sympathetic nerves follow the coronary arteries in the subepicardium, and then penetrate the myocardium. Adrenergic output from this sympathetic innervation increases HR (chronotropic effect), augments contractility (inotropic effect), and enhances atrioventricular (AV) conduction (dromotropic effect). The major chemical mediator of sympathetic innervation is NE.[15,16]

Parasympathetic fibers, scarce in comparison with sympathetic fibers, originate in the medulla and travel alongside the vagus nerves. In the heart, these fibers start epicardially, cross the AV groove, and penetrate the myocardium, thereby becoming located in the subendocardium. Parasympathetic fibers predominantly innervate the atria, but are scarce in the ventricle (densest in the inferior wall). The parasympathetic system modulates output of the sinoatrial (SA) and AV nodes to control HR and conduction. The chemical mediator of parasympathetic function is acetylcholine.

Most published literature and impending clinical applicability of autonomic radionuclide imaging is of the sympathetic system, with parasympathetic imaging limited mostly to animals. The ensuing discussion will focus on cardiac sympathetic imaging.

RADIONUCLIDE IMAGING OF CARDIAC SYMPATHETIC INNERVATION

Cardiac sympathetic innervation imaging visualizes processes at the synaptic junction, illustrated in Figure 23-1.[17] To date, most autonomic tracers investigated image presynaptic anatomy and function, though tracers designed to specifically assess postsynaptic α- and β-receptors have also been studied.

NE is synthesized in presynaptic sympathetic terminals from tyrosine, and stored in presynaptic vesicles. In response to stimuli, the vesicles are released into the synaptic space, freeing the NE which interacts with postsynaptic α, β1, and β2 receptors on the myocyte membrane, leading to adrenergic effect(s).[18,19] To control and terminate these effects, NE is actively taken back into the presynaptic terminal mostly via norepinephrine transporter-1 (NET1),

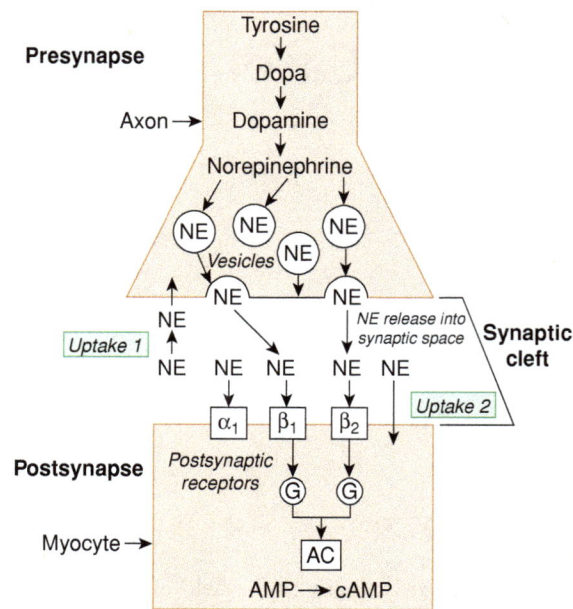

FIGURE 23-1 Schematic representation of the sympathetic neuron synapse. In response to a stimulus, vesicles containing NE are released into the synaptic space and interact with postsynaptic receptors. Sympathetic response is controlled by reuptake of norepinephrine into the presynaptic terminal via the "uptake-1" norepinephrine transporter. AC, adenylyl cyclase; AMP, adenosine monophosphate; cAMP, cyclic adenosine monophosphate; G, G proteins; NE, norepinephrine. (Reproduced with permission from Travin MI. Cardiac neuronal imaging at the edge of clinical application. *Cardiol Clin.* 2009;27(2):311–327.)

a protein-mediated, sodium-, energy-, and temperature-dependent "uptake-1" process, for storage or catabolic disposal by monoamine oxidase (MAO) or catechol-o-methyltransferase.[20] A smaller amount of NE is also taken up by postsynaptic, nonneuronal cells, probably by sodium-independent passive diffusion, referred to as the "uptake-2" process.[21,22]

In the 1970s, while investigating adrenal imaging using modifications of the adrenergic blocking antiarrhythmic drug bretylium, Wieland et al. focused on a similar false neurotransmitter analogue of NE, guanethidine, and discovered that synthesizing a compound with iodine in the meta position, that is, *meta*-iodobenzylguanidine (*m*IBG) could satisfactorily image both the adrenal medulla and the heart.[23–25] However, unlike NE, this false neurotransmitter is not catabolized after NET1 uptake, thus localizing to high concentrations in the presynaptic adrenergic

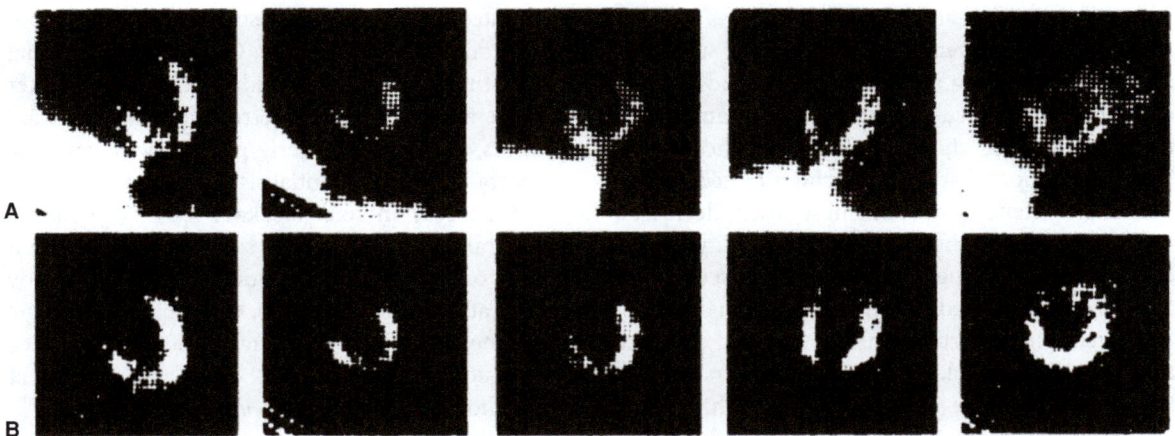

FIGURE 23-2 The first images showing cardiac uptake of ^{123}I-*m*IBG in humans. ^{123}I-*m*IBG images of myocardium in five normal volunteers, acquired over 15 minutes in the 40-degree angle LAO projection. **(A)** Unprocessed digital images. **(B)** Images after interpolated background subtraction. LAO, left anterior oblique; *m*IBG, metaiodobenzylguanidine. (Reproduced with permission from Kline RC, Swanson DP, Wieland DM, et al. Myocardial imaging in man with I-123 meta-iodobenzylguanidine. *J Nucl Med.* 1981;22(2):129–132.)

terminals. Following IV injection of iodine-labeled radiotracer that diffuses into cardiac synaptic clefts and is taken via NET1 into cardiac presympathetic terminals, the heart can be visualized, with the measured counts reflecting the physical integrity and physiologic health of cardiac adrenergic innervation.[26,27] The first cardiac *m*IBG images in humans are shown in Figure 23-2. As opposed to ^{201}Tl- or ^{99m}Tc-based perfusion tracers that image the "plumbing of the heart," *m*IBG has been characterized as providing "clinicians with insight into 'wiring' of the heart."[23]

Initial clinical work that focused on adrenal tumor imaging used iodine-131 for labeling, but as this isotope gives off relatively high-energy (365 keV) γ emissions, emits β particles, and has a relatively long half-life of about 8.02 days, ^{123}I labeling has been developed and is preferred. ^{123}I emits predominantly γ photons with energies of 159 keV and has a half-life of 13.2 hours, therefore easily imaged and well tolerated. Thus, ^{123}I *meta*-iodobenzylguanidine (^{123}I-*m*IBG) is currently the preferred compound for clinical use, and was approved by the Food and Drug Administration (FDA) for cardiac use in 2013.

Various PET adrenergic radiotracers have also been developed, but are currently under investigation and not approved for clinical use.[22] Compared with ^{123}I-*m*IBG, PET tracers not only have superior physical properties for imaging, but also potential biologic advantages. ^{11}C-meta-hydroxyephedrine (HED) has been most widely studied, with its higher NET1 selectivity resulting in better differentiation between innervated and denervated myocardium, reportedly better for evaluating neuronal heterogeneity in hibernating myocardium.[28] Other less well-studied PET tracers include ^{11}C-epinephrine and ^{11}C-phenylephrine. However, as the need for a nearby cyclotron makes ^{11}C-tracers impractical for most potential users, ^{18}F compounds, such as ^{18}F-LMI-1195 (fluorobenzylguanidine) are in development.[29]

CLINICAL IMAGING WITH ^{123}I-*m*IBG

▶ Patient Preparation

^{123}I-*m*IBG is performed at rest and requires only minimal preparation, with details described in published guidelines.[30,31] The patient is customarily kept NPO after midnight on the day of imaging. Standard guidelines directed HF medications, such as β blockers, angiotensin-converting enzyme inhibitors (ACE-I), and/or angiotensin receptor blockers (ARBs), need not be withheld. Published guidelines list and recommend holding medications and substances known to interfere directly with the mechanisms of NE uptake and granule storage, such as opioids, cocaine, tramadol, tricyclic antidepressants, sympathomimetics and antipsychotics, as well as foods containing vanillin (an artificial substance added as a flavoring agent to various foods, beverages, and pharmaceuticals) and catecholamine-like compounds (e.g., chocolate and blue cheese).[30-33] There is a report that neuropsychiatric medications with high potency can result in a falsely decreased tracer uptake in the heart and thus overestimate cardiac risk.[34] Regarding standard cardiovascular and antihypertensive medications, other than labetalol and rarely used reserpine, there is no solid evidence that β blockers or calcium channel blockers directly affect cardiac uptake. Investigations into this matter are hampered by the fact that cardiovascular medicines can alter cardiac ^{123}I-mIBG uptake by improving a patient's cardiac condition as opposed to having a direct effect on cellular mechanisms.[35]

Recommendations regarding medication holding prior to an ^{123}I-mIBG study remain under investigation. At the time of this writing, the specific wording in the package insert from a commercially available preparation is to "consider the withdrawal of the following categories of medications if the withdrawal can be accomplished safely: antihypertensives that deplete NE stores or inhibit reuptake (e.g., reserpine, labetalol), antidepressants that inhibit NE transporter function (e.g., amitriptyline and derivatives, imipramine and derivatives, selective serotonin reuptake inhibitors), and sympathomimetic amines (e.g., phenylephrine, phenylpropanolamine, pseudoephedrine, and ephedrine). The period of time necessary to discontinue any specific medication prior to ^{123}I-mIBG dosing has not been established."[36]

Iodine Prophylaxis

Opinions differ with respect to the need for prophylactic administration of iodine to block thyroid uptake of unbound radioactive ^{123}I. While some people advocate routine pretreatment to prevent thyroid radiation exposure from the unbound impurities, others feel that the risk of iodine allergy outweighs the danger from the minimal amount of unbound tracer present after modern production methods. Nevertheless, one study showed that even with an ^{123}I-mIBG preparation of 98% radiochemical purity, unblocked patients have a 50% higher 4-hour thyroid accumulation of unbound ^{123}I compared with pretreated patients, with an estimated 70-mGy exposure from a 10-mCi dose.[37] One approach is that pretreatment can be individualized, with greater consideration given to pretreatment for younger patients, but less for elderly patients with multiple comorbidities and potential risk of iodine allergy.[38]

If chosen, thyroid blockade can be achieved with oral administration of solutions of potassium iodide or Lugol's (100-mg iodide for adults, body weight adjusted for children), or for patients allergic to iodine, potassium perchlorate (400 mg for adults, weight adjusted for children), orally administered at least 1 hour, minutes prior to mIBG injection.[36]

At the time of this writing, the specific wording in the package insert from a commercially available preparation is that thyroid blockade should be done in "patients at risk for thyroid accumulation of the drug," but can be individualized in that "blockade may not be necessary for patients who have undergone thyroidectomy or those with a very limited life expectancy." The package insert also states that "failure to block thyroid uptake of ^{123}I may result in an increased long-term risk for thyroid neoplasia."[36]

Radiotracer Administration

Regarding tracer dosage, older studies in the literature used 3 to 5 mCi (111–185 MBq). However, as these dosages frequently result in unsatisfactory SPECT images, particularly in patients with severe cardiac dysfunction, recent investigations have used up to 10 mCi (370 MBq)[18] including a phase III study[39,40] that helped lead to FDA approval. A 10-mCi dosage results in a radiation exposure of ~5 mSv, with the highest exposure to the bladder, liver, spleen, gall bladder, heart, and adrenals; the absorbed dose may be higher in patients with severe renal impairment.[30] Recent work suggests that with a solid-state camera, satisfactory planar and tomographic images can be obtained with a reduced tracer dosage of 2 to 3 mCi (74–111 MBq).[41]

It has been recommended that patients lie quietly in a supine position for about 5 to 15 minutes before administration. As initial images are acquired a few minutes after injection, the patient should be lying under the camera or in close proximity. Tracer is then administered slowly over 1 to 2 minutes, followed by a saline flush. Adverse reactions are extremely rare.

Protocol

While acquisition and processing of planar and SPECT ^{123}I-*m*IBG images are customarily performed in a manner typical for perfusion imaging, special issues need to be considered, and there will likely be methodological changes in the future. The current key parameters for ^{123}I-*m*IBG image interpretation—heart-to-mediastinum ratio (HMR) and washout—require accurate and robust quantitative analysis of counts in the heart and adjacent background regions, and thus could vary in relation to differences in the acquisition field of view, the type of collimator used, and how the multiple energy emissions of ^{123}I are considered during acquisition and processing. Current literature data are based on images obtained without attenuation correction, Compton scatter, or depth-dependent loss of spatial resolution, with use of such techniques expected to produce different values. Finally, increased use of solid-state cameras results in quantitative ^{123}I-*m*IBG results from what has been reported for standard Anger cameras.

Figure 23-3 shows a guidelines-recommended protocol for performing cardiac ^{123}I-*m*IBG imaging.[31] Anterior planar ^{123}I-*m*IBG images are acquired for 10 minutes with the patient supine at ~15 minutes (early) and beginning ~3 hours, 50 minutes (late) after tracer administration, with the images stored in a 128 × 128 or 256 × 256 matrix.[30,38] The field of view should include as much of the heart and upper chest as possible, avoiding having the heart be too close to the edge of the field or too close to the center. Positioning should be the same for the early and late planar images.

A large field-of-view camera has customarily been used for acquiring the anterior planar image that is important for deriving global cardiac uptake as measured by the HMR. The technique for obtaining suitable images from a small-field-of-view SPECT camera is unclear. In a pilot study of 67 subjects, HMRs calculated from SPECT images, using mean counts between heart and mediastinum volumes of interest drawn on transaxial images, were equivalent to those obtained by planar techniques for differentiating subjects with normal versus abnormal *m*IBG uptake.[42] More investigations are required to validate this further. Investigations are also ongoing to determine proper techniques for acquiring and interpreting images with solid-state cameras.[43]

Although the utility of SPECT imaging assessment of regional defects is currently uncertain, and thus considered in guidelines as an option,[30] based on theoretic consideration[44] and reports showing utility for arrhythmias,[45–47] tomographic acquisitions are commonly performed immediately following both the early and late planar images. SPECT images are obtained using a standard 180-degree angle circular acquisition from 45-degree angle right anterior oblique to 45-degree angle left posterior oblique, with a total of 60 stops (30 stops per head if done

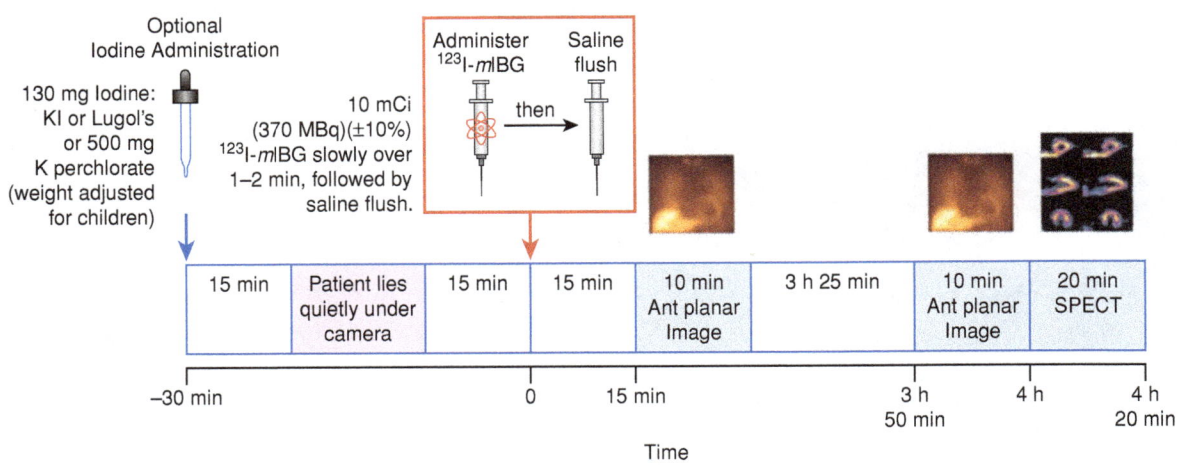

FIGURE 23-3 A recommended protocol for performing cardiac ^{123}I-*m*IBG imaging. Ant, anterior; KI, potassium iodide; MBq, megabecquerel; mCi, millicurie; *m*IBG, meta-iodobenzylguanidine; SPECT, single-photon emission computed tomography. (Reproduced with permission from Henzlova MJ, Duvall WL, Einstein AJ, et al. ASNC imaging guidelines for SPECT nuclear cardiology procedures: stress, protocols, and tracers. *J Nucl Cardiol*. 2016;23(3):606–639.)

with a dual-headed camera) at 30 seconds per stop, and are stored in a 64 × 64 matrix.

Extensive literature describes data derived from image acquisition using low-energy high-resolution (LEHR) collimators, with a symmetrically centered energy window of 20% around the main 159-keV isotope photopeak. However, HMR values vary depending on the collimator used, differing for low-energy versus medium-energy collimators, but also among different collimator brands.[48–50] Contributing to these differences are multiple higher-energy photon emissions (e.g., 529 keV) that penetrate the septa and degrade image quality.[51] Methods to compensate for this effect and improve quantitative accuracy are under investigation, including employing a calibration phantom to derive a conversion coefficient for each camera-collimation system.[52–54]

Protocols for acquiring and processing ^{123}I-*m*IBG images will evolve with increased clinical use and further investigations. Ultimately, the standard will depend on the technique that provides the best clinical value in relation to the lowest radiation exposure, and to the highest efficiency and patient comfort.

^{123}I-*m*IBG Image Interpretation

Most published studies of ^{123}I-*m*IBG have focused on planar imaging. The standard measure of global tracer uptake is the HMR, derived from regions of interest (ROIs) over the heart and upper mediastinum in an anterior planar image. Uptake in late ^{123}I-*m*IBG images is considered more representative of tracer retention, and is better predictive of patient outcome than that in early images.[40] While various methods have been used to create ROIs,[55–57] the currently recommended method is dividing counts per pixel in an irregular ROI defining the epicardial border of the heart by counts per pixel in a square 7 × 7 pixel ROI in the upper mediastinum.[30,31] While there are attempts to automate the process,[58] at present the standard is manual drawing of ROIs that has been shown to be robust,[59] with Veltman et al.[60] reporting extremely high intraclass correlation coefficients 0.98 and 0.96 for intra- and interobserver analyses, respectively. Normal HMRs (for Anger cameras) range from 1.9 to 2.8, a mean of 2.2 ± 0.3 with ≥1.6 (within 2 standard deviations) on the late image indicating lower risk.[26,39,40] Recent work suggests that because of differences in scatter, HMRs derived from solid-state camera-acquired images are higher.[43] Figure 23-4 shows representative planar images with HMRs from patients in different stages of heart failure (HF).[61]

The utility of performing both early and late planar images has been questioned given that the latter provides stronger prognostic utility,[40] with an ongoing multicenter prospective study[62] requiring only

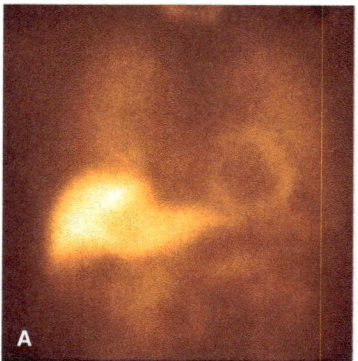
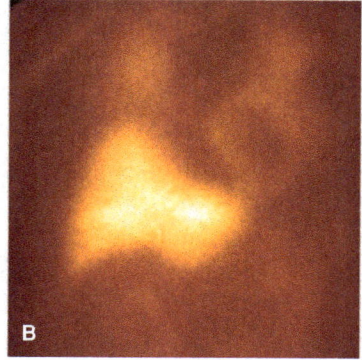
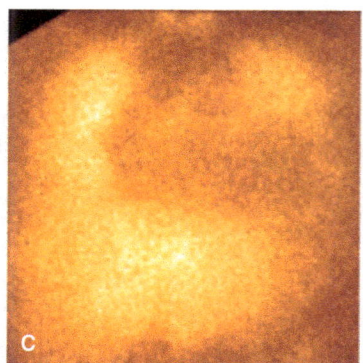

FIGURE 23-4 Examples of planar ^{123}I-*m*IBG images in patients with heart failure, with HMRs and patient outcomes described. **(A)** A 79-year-old male with nonischemic NYHA II HF and LVEF of 35%. HMR = 2.02. No cardiac event over 5-year follow-up. **(B)** A 64-year-old female with nonischemic NYHA III HF and LVEF 25% to 30%. HMR = 1.38. Experienced numerous arrhythmic events/ICD discharges over the next 2 years, requiring VT ablation. **(C)** A 28-year-old male with nonischemic NYHA II HF and LVEF = 20%. HMR = 1.17 (cardiac uptake is barely above background). Progressed within 1 year from NYHA II to NYHA III. HF, heart failure; HMR, heart-to-mediastinum ratio; ICD, implantable cardioverter defibrillator; LVEF, left ventricular ejection fraction; NYHA, New York Heart Association; VT, ventricular tachycardia. (Used with permission from the American College of Cardiology. http://www.acc.org/latest-in-cardiology/articles/2015/04/08/09/45/radionuclide-molecular-imaging-in-heart-failure.)

the late images. To improve image efficiency, use of a single 2-hour postinjection planar image has been investigated,[63] but the clinical utility of this approach has not been established.

At the same time, a frequently measured planar image parameter that requires both an early and late planar image is ^{123}I-*m*IBG washout[64] which relates to integrity and function of the neuron, but also reflects competition from circulating NE.[65] As with HMR, various methods for determining washout have been explored,[60] although guideline recommendations exist.[30] A normal washout value in control subjects is reported as 10 ± 9%.[66] While higher values are associated with worsened prognosis,[64,67] the washout variable often drops out in multivariate analyses.[40]

With regard to SPECT, although most studies examine images processed with filtered back projection, phantom studies suggest that higher image quality is obtained using ordered subsets expectation maximization (OSEM) iterative reconstruction along with deconvolution of septal penetration (DSP) to correct for image contamination from high-energy ^{123}I photons.[51] Tomographic ^{123}I-*m*IBG slices are customarily displayed in a manner similar to that done for MPI,[68] and can be shown alongside ^{99m}Tc-sestamibi or ^{99m}Tc-tetrofosmin perfusion image slices acquired at a separate time in an attempt to detect regions of innervation/perfusion mismatch that may indicate predisposition to ventricular arrhythmias.[44,69] Visual image interpretation can be done using scoring methods similar to perfusion SPECT, but quantitation has unique considerations in that while for perfusion images there are usually regions with normal perfusion that can serve as a reference to which count profiles are normalized, with ^{123}I-*m*IBG, globally reduced tracer uptake is often present. One report used a "mixed reference" method in which classifying a region as "abnormal" varied in relation to global tracer uptake measured by the HMR.[70] Another challenge is that unlike for MPI in which validity and accuracy of a methodology is customarily assessed in reference to "gold standard" coronary anatomy findings, there is no such standard upon which to validate adrenergic image-quantitative findings.[71] In addition, lung and liver tracer uptake overlying myocardial walls can make SPECT images difficult to interpret fully. Finally, one must also consider that adrenergic imaging assesses a physiologic phenomenon different from perfusion, and thus while more extensive and severe defect(s) on MPI predict poorer outcome, this may not hold for ^{123}I-*m*IBG imaging in which a more intermediate degree of abnormality that could reflect more electrical heterogeneity may increase predisposition to lethal arrhythmias.[72,73]

One final issue is that ideally cardiac ^{123}I-*m*IBG uptake would be homogeneous in normal patients, but some variability occurs in relation to age and gender, as well as from body conditioning, and may be different for SPECT versus PET tracers. Such discussion is beyond the scope of this review, and described in various references.[66,74–76] These variations need to be investigated further.

CLINICAL APPLICATIONS OF IMAGING WITH ^{123}I-*m*IBG AND OTHER ADRENERGIC TRACERS

Myocardial innervation imaging has demonstrated the potential benefits in numerous clinical situations, summarized in Table 23-1. While given its widespread prevalence, high mortality, and close association with neurohormonal and sympathetic perturbations, HF with reduced ejection fraction (HFrEF) and associated arrhythmias have been most studied, ^{123}I-*m*IBG imaging also has demonstrated utility in evaluating patients postcardiac transplant, those with primary arrhythmic diseases, myocardial ischemia and diabetes mellitus (DM), and in monitoring toxic effects of chemotherapy.

▶ ^{123}I-*m*IBG Imaging to Assess Heart Failure

HF affects more than 5 million Americans and is expected to increase to >8 million by 2030.[77] Annual mortality is 40% to 60%, with a cost >$30 billion. While older approaches to HF focused on hemodynamic pathophysiology, the contemporary emphasis is on the neurohormonal model.[78] As a result of decreased cardiac function, the sympathetic adrenergic system (SAS) and the renin–angiotensin aldosterone system (RAAS) are activated, that is, at-first beneficially compensatory. However, the processes often become excessive and maladaptive, with deleterious downregulation of β receptors, decreasing myocardial catecholamine levels, and increased

Table 23-1

Demonstrated and Potential Clinical Uses of Cardiac Adrenergic Imaging

- Heart failure
  - Investigated predominantly in patients with HFrEF
  - Demonstrated robust risk stratification utility in terms of cardiac events—HF progression, ventricular arrhythmic events, cardiac death, and all-cause mortality—that are independent of other commonly used parameters. Indicated to patients with lower risk of 1- to 2-year mortality.
  - Can monitor cardiac improvement after guidelines-directed medical therapy
    - Potential utility for directing advanced therapies—CRT, LVAD, transplant—particularly in patients not adequately responsive to medical therapy.
- Ventricular arrhythmias associated with heart failure
  - Demonstrated arrhythmic risk stratification utility
  - Can enhance identification of patients at extremely low risk for lethal ventricular arrhythmias.
    - Potential utility in identifying patients unlikely to benefit from an ICD, at least in the short term (about 2 years).
    - Potential to help decision making for ICD end-of-life battery replacement, and in the setting of device infection.
- Other potential uses
  - Evaluation of patients with primary ventricular arrhythmias and Chagas cardiomyopathy
  - Direct ventricular tachycardia ablation therapy
  - Evaluation of patients with ischemic heart disease
    - Demonstrated ability to risk stratify high-risk patients with hibernating myocardium
    - Quantify myocardial territory at risk during an acute ischemic event
  - Monitor reinnervation of the transplanted heart
  - Detection of cardiac innervation abnormalities in diabetes mellitus that worsen prognosis
  - Monitor innervation abnormalities after cardiotoxic chemotherapy

CRT, cardiac resynchronization therapy; HF, heart failure; HFrEF, heart failure with reduced ejection fraction; ICD, implantable cardioverter defibrillator; LVAD, left ventricular assist device.

plasma NE, with development of anatomic structural changes such as hypertrophy, remodeling, and apoptosis. Continuation of these processes, along with further insults and injury, increase susceptibility to lethal arrhythmias and can lead to a downward clinical spiral toward end-stage HF and death.[79]

At the sympathetic cellular level, there is an initial increase of NE release into the synaptic cleft, promoting an increase in the NET1 process. Eventually, the system is overwhelmed, with a reduction in carrier density leading to increased spillover of NE into plasma that may account for the increased washout seen with ^{123}I-mIBG imaging in HF patients. As disease becomes advanced, there is diminished presynaptic function from loss of neurons and downregulation of NET1, with decreased global radiotracer uptake and thus a lower HMR.[65] HF pathophysiologic processes, as well as insults leading to it such as ischemia and infarction, can cause temporary sympathetic dysfunction that has been referred to as "dysinnervation" (or sympathetic nerve "dysfunction") that has recovery potential, or "denervation" in which there is anatomic loss of the nerve fibers.[80]

Potential utility of ^{123}I-mIBG imaging in HF was first reported by Schofer et al.[81] who found decreasing tracer uptake as disease worsened. In a key study by Merlet et al.[82] in patients with moderate to severe HF and LVEF <45%, an HMR <1.2 was associated with 6- and 12-month survivals of 60% and 40%, respectively, compared with a 100% 12-month survival for patients with an HMR ≥1.2. By multivariate analysis, HMR was better than LVEF for mortality prediction. A study by Nakata et al.[83] showed progressively worsened survival as HMR decreased. In a multicenter European 290-patient study pooling previously collected data of patients with HF, Agostini reported that the only significant predictors of 2-year major cardiac events (cardiac death, transplant, and potentially fatal arrhythmias) were LVEF and HMR. Particularly striking was the ability of HMR to risk stratify patients with LVEF ≤35%, with event rates ranging from <5% for those with HMR ≥2.18 to over

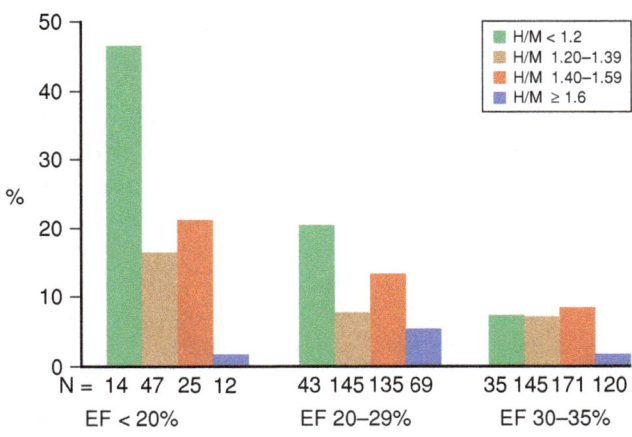

FIGURE 23-5 Relationship of left ventricular ejection fraction (EF) and heart-to-mediastinum ratio (H/M) to 2-year cardiac mortality in the ADMIRE-HF study. ADMIRE-HF, AdreView Myocardial Imaging for Risk Evaluation in Heart Failure. (Reproduced with permission from Chirumamilla A, Travin MI. Cardiac applications of 123I-mIBG imaging. Semin Nucl Med. 2011;41(5):374–387.)

50% for those with HMR ≤1.45.[84] A 1755-patient meta-analysis by Verberne et al.[85] reported that an abnormal WR had a pooled hazard ratio (HR) of 1.72 ($p = 0.006$) for cardiac death, and 1.08 ($p < 0.001$) for cardiac events (cardiac death, myocardial infarction [MI], transplant, HF hospitalization), with the best studies yielding an HR for late HMR of 1.82 ($p = 0.015$) for cardiac death and 1.98 ($p < 0.001$) for cardiac events.

To date, the landmark prospective international multicenter "AdreView Myocardial Imaging for Risk Evaluation in Heart Failure (ADMIRE-HF)" phase III study of 961 patients with New York Heart Association (NYHA) class II to III HF and LVEF ≤35% found, over a 17-month median follow-up, an event-free survival of 85% in patients with HMR ≥1.60 versus 63% for those with HMR <1.60 ($p < 0.0001$).[40] The ability of HMR to predict cardiac events was independent of conventional HF variables such as LVEF and BNP. Figure 23-4 shows representative images from the ADMIRE-HF study. Most striking was that for the approximately 20% of patients with HMR ≥1.6, the negative predictive value for freedom from cardiac death was extremely high (>98%) (Fig. 23-5).[86]

In a later subanalysis of ADMIRE-HF data, Ketchum et al.[87] found that HMR provided incremental risk stratification power beyond the comprehensive Seattle Heart Failure Model algorithm of demographic, imaging, laboratory, and therapeutic parameters. 14.9% of patients who died were correctly reclassified by the HMR as higher risk, while 7.9% of those who survived were correctly reclassified as lower risk, an overall 22.7% improvement.

An analysis by Nakata et al.[88] of 1322 HF patients, who had previously collected ^{123}I-mIBG data available at 6 Japanese medical centers, found that over ~6½ years of follow-up, late HMR (threshold 1.68) and WR (threshold 43%) effectively separated patients in relation to all-cause mortality. By multivariate analysis, the predictive ability of HMR was independent of NYHA class, BNP, LVEF, and age. Of note, this study from Japan also found that ^{123}I-mIBG could effectively risk stratify HF patients with LVEFs more than 35%. A subanalysis of ADMIRE-HF data also suggested utility of ^{123}I-mIBG imaging for patients with higher LVEFs.[89]

Based on the ADMIRE HF phase III study, the study from Japan, and a large accumulation of other work, in March 2013 ^{123}I-mIBG was FDA approved for "scintigraphic assessment of sympathetic innervation of the myocardium by measurement of the heart-to-mediastinum (H/M) ratio of radioactivity uptake in patients with NYHA class II or class III HF and left ventricular ejection fraction (LVEF) ≤35%. Among these patients, ^{123}I-mIBG may be used to help identify patients with lower 1- and 2-year mortality risks, as indicated by an H/M ratio ≥1.6."[36]

^{123}I-mIBG Imaging to Follow and Potentially Guide Therapy in Patients with Heart Failure

To become of widespread clinical use, ^{123}I-mIBG imaging must help guide therapy in ways that other less expensive and more customarily used techniques do not. Test value is limited if it does not improve outcome, especially if testing costs are high.[90] Studies consistently show that cardiac ^{123}I-*m*IBG imaging can help monitor response to various pharmacologic treatments.[91] These include β-blockers,[55,56,92–93] medications that impact on the RAAS system such as ACE-I, angiotensin receptor blocking agents (ARBs), and spironolactone,[94–96] as well as amiodarone,[97] which have been associated with improvements in ^{123}I-*m*IBG image parameters that are in some cases linked to decreased ventricular volumes and increased LVEF. At the same time, ^{123}I-*m*IBG imaging has been shown to identify patients responding to therapy who would not be identified by customary means.[98] Some have considered how cardiac ^{123}I-*m*IBG imaging could specifically direct medical therapies,[99,100] but given the high benefit-to-risk ratio of these, ^{123}I-*m*IBG study results are unlikely to preclude their use.[79]

Thus, a potential of ^{123}I-*m*IBG imaging is to assess if a particular patient's medical therapy is adequate. A study by Matsui et al.[101] of subjects with dilated cardiomyopathy and LVEF <45% showed that among 19 clinical, serum, and image variables, a worsening HMR after 6 months of optimized medical therapy had, with BNP, the highest predictive value for cardiac death, with a sensitivity of 92% and a specificity of 73%. It is possible that additional and/or alternate therapies in the patients with worsening HMR would have improved outcome. Thus, serial ^{123}I-*m*IBG imaging of patients on guideline-directed medical therapies could potentially help guide use of higher-risk, usually more expensive, invasive device therapies and heart transplant.

Invasive devices work to prevent or forestall the two major catastrophic outcomes of HF—progressive debilitating and life-threatening pump failure, and sudden cardiac death (SCD) from ventricular arrhythmias. The likelihood of each particular outcome varies over time in relation to the etiology of the HF.[102] Thus, the promise of using ^{123}I-*m*IBG to direct advanced therapies must take into account the adverse outcome more likely to occur in a particular patient as determined by the clinical scenario, as well as specific image findings in that while the planar derived global uptake, that is, the HMR effectively predicts pump failure-related outcomes such as the need for transplant, arrhythmic outcomes may be better predicted by regional abnormalities seen on tomographic imaging.[73,103,104]

Current device therapies that address pump failure are cardiac resynchronization therapy (CRT) and the left ventricular assist device (LVAD). CRT can improve outcome in patients with chronic HF,[105] but not all patients who meet recommended criteria benefit.[106,107] There is evidence that ^{123}I-*m*IBG imaging could potentially improve CRT patient selection. D'Orio Nishioka et al.[108] showed that in relation to clinical variables, echocardiographic volumes, and LVEF, an HMR >1.36 was the only independent predictor of HF functional class improvement (sensitivity 75%, specificity 71%). Tanaka et al.[109] found that advanced HF patients with HMR ≥1.6 had a higher frequency of response (improvement in echocardiographic speckle-tracking radial strain) to CRT and a more favorable event-free survival compared with HMR <1.6. ^{123}I-*m*IBG imaging can help monitor clinical improvement with CRT,[110] paralleling improved LV dimensions and ejection fraction (EF),[111] and improved exercise capacity.[112]

For guidance of LVAD therapy, in a small study of 27 patients with advanced HF showed that a pre-implant ^{123}I-*m*IBG washout rate ≤39% increased the likelihood of a 6-month decrease in end-diastolic dimension and an increase in LVEF, indicative of reverse remodeling.[113] Several small studies have shown that HMR improvement while on LVAD therapy could potentially help direct patients to successful explant rather than permanent LVAD use or referral for cardiac transplant.[114,115]

Some small studies show potential benefit of using ^{123}I-*m*IBG imaging to prioritize patients for heart transplant.[116,117] A larger 636-patient meta-analysis by Verschure et al.[103] found that late HMR is an independent predictor of need for cardiac transplantation. For sure, larger prospective studies are needed in this regard. For posttransplant patient evaluation, there are much data showing utility of adrenergic imaging with ^{123}I-*m*IBG and related PET tracers.[118] In particular, adrenergic imaging helps assess posttransplant cardiac reinnervation that can be imaged, lack of which may indicate complications such as vasculopathy.[119–121]

In summary, at the present time the established use of ^{123}I-*m*IBG imaging in advanced HF patients is improved risk stratification, and there is consistent evidence that the technique can monitor how these patients are progressing. However, the key to effective clinical utility would appear to be guidance of advanced therapies in ways that improve patient outcomes.

Guiding Use of an Implantable Cardioverter Defibrillator in Heart Failure Patients

In patients with advanced HF, up to 50% of deaths are sudden, most often from ventricular tachycardia progressing to ventricular fibrillation (VT/VF).[122] Based on large prospective randomized trials, implantable cardioverter defibrillator (ICD) implantation is a class IA indication for "primary prevention of SCD to reduce total mortality in selected patients with nonischemic (dilated cardiomyopathy) or ischemic heart disease at least 40 days post-MI with LVEF of 35% or less and NYHA class II or III symptoms on guideline-directed medical therapy, who have a reasonable expectation of meaningful survival for more than 1 year."[123] Nevertheless, this approach is widely considered to be deficient[124,125] as most patients with an ICD do not have therapeutic discharges,[126] the device implantation and management are costly,[127] and there can be serious complications.[128] Clinicians often do not follow guidelines indicating that better patient selection methods are needed.[129] As cardiac autonomic innervation more closely relates to the underlying mechanisms of ventricular arrhythmias than LVEF, imaging with ^{123}I-mIBG or an analogous PET tracer would be expected to better guide ICD use.[19,130,131]

Early animal work showed that artificial creation of focal cardiac denervation produced regional ^{123}I-mIBG defects, and associated with production of supersensitive action potential refractory periods.[44] Early clinical work in the post-MI setting showed an association between focal ^{123}I-mIBG defects and ventricular arrhythmias on Holter monitoring.[132,133] Arora et al.[134] were among the first to report on the potential use of ^{123}I-mIBG to guide ICD therapy in a pilot study of 17 patients in which a reduced late HMR (<1.54) was associated with increased occurrence of an ICD shock. A subsequent 54-patient study by Nagahara et al.[135] showed that late HMR correlated with SCD or an ICD discharge (HR = 0.141, p = 0.008) independent of other variables including LVEF. One study reported an association of high ^{123}I-mIBG washout with SCD that was independent of numerous ventricular and ECG variables.[67] In ADMIRE HF, arrhythmic events (ArEs) occurred less often in patients with an HMR ≥1.6 (3.5% vs. 10.4%, p < 0.01) with only one fatal arrhythmic event over the 17-month median follow-up that was in a patient with an HMR at exactly 1.60.[40] In the ADMIRE-HFX study that extended the median follow-up from 17 to 24 months, fatal or potentially fatal ArEs (SCD, resuscitated cardiopulmonary arrest, and appropriate ICD defibrillation) occurred in 6% to 10% of patients with an HMR <1.6, but there were none in patients with an HMR ≥1.8.[72] Interestingly, as in Figure 23-6, the largest proportion of ArEs occurred with a moderately reduced HMR (1.30–1.59), perhaps reflecting that a

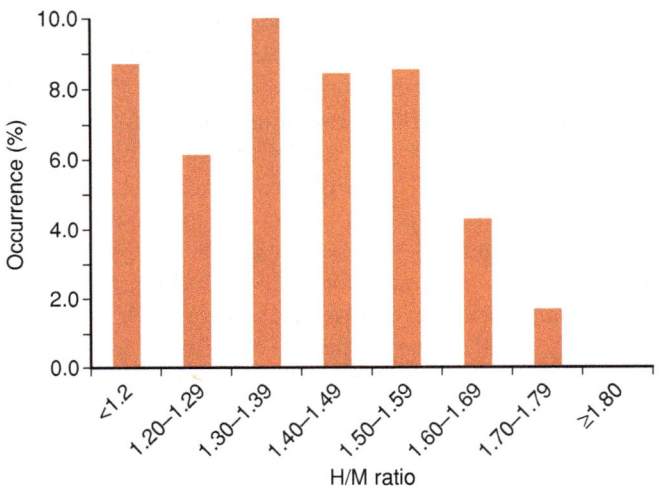

FIGURE 23-6 Occurrence of fatal and potentially fatal arrhythmic events (sudden death, resuscitated arrest, ICD defibrillation) (n = 70) in relation to H/M. Peak occurrence was in 1.30 to 1.39 range, with progressive decline for higher H/Ms. There were no fatal or potentially fatal arrhythmic events among subjects with H/M ≥1.80. H/M, heart-to-mediastinum ratio; ICD, implantable cardioverter defibrillator. (Reproduced with permission from Narula J, Gerson M, Thomas GS, et al. ^{123}I-MIBG Imaging for Prediction of Mortality and Potentially Fatal Events in Heart Failure: The ADMIRE-HFX Study. *J Nucl Med.* 2015;56(7):1011–1018.)

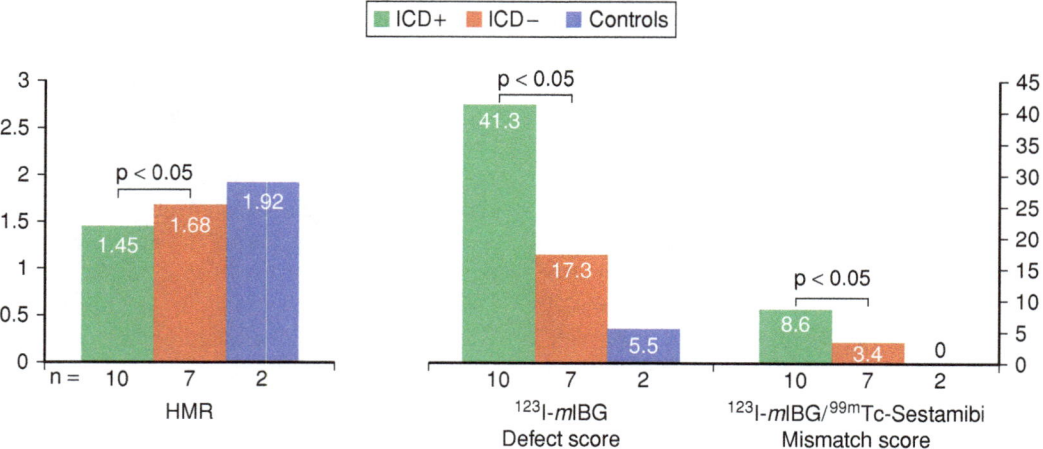

FIGURE 23-7 ^{123}I-*m*IBG results in relation to the occurrence of implantable cardioverter defibrillator (ICD) discharges in 17 patients with ICDs and 2 control patients without heart disease. Compared with patients who have not had ICD discharge (ICD–), patients with a discharge (ICD+) had a lower mean heart-to-mediastinum ratio (HMR), a higher mean neuronal tracer defect score, and a higher mean neuronal tracer uptake/perfusion tracer mismatch score. (Data from Arora R, Ferrick KJ, Nakata T, et al. ^{123}I-MIBG imaging and heart rate variability analysis to predict the need for an implantable cardioverter defibrillator. *J Nucl Cardiol.* 2003;10:121–131.)

very low lower HMR increases the likelihood of dying from pump failure, while an intermediate degree of cardiac denervation leads to greater electrical heterogeneity that predisposes to higher arrhythmic risk.

Despite robust planar imaging data, many investigators feel that tomographic imaging should be superior for prediction ArEs given its ability to detect regional innervation abnormalities that reflect action potential and impulse conduction heterogeneity. A previously cited 636-patient meta-analysis study by Verschure et al.[103] found that arrhythmic risk assessment with planar imaging was limited. Several small studies demonstrated potential strength of SPECT for identifying arrhythmic risk. Arora et al.[134] reported that patients with ICD discharges had more extensive tomographic ^{123}I-*m*IBG defects, as well as more extensive autonomic/perfusion mismatches (Fig. 23-7). In 50 post-MI patients with a reduced LVEF, Bax et al.[136] found an association between electrophysiological (EP) inducibility of a sustained ventricular arrhythmia and the ^{123}I-*m*IBG summed segmental dysinnervation defect score (SSDyS). For 116 HF patients referred for ICD therapy, Boogers et al.[104] found that an ^{123}I-*m*IBG SPECT SSDyS above the median of 26 was independently predictive of ICD discharges ($p < 0.001$). A 27-patient study by Marshall et al.[137] found that both summed innervation and innervation/perfusion mismatch scores predicted ArEs.

With regard to ADMIRE-HF, although SPECT image interpretation was part of the data analysis, findings did not show value for primary study endpoints that were dominated by HF progression events. To address potential limitations of ADMIRE-HF SPECT methodology, SPECT images from the study were rigorously reinterpreted, focusing on 471 patients with ischemic HF whose images were reprocessed by iterative reconstruction with application of DSP.[73] By multivariate proportional hazards analysis, the ^{123}I-*m*IBG SPECT summed dysinnervation score was independently predictive of ArEs ($p = 0.042$). Surprisingly, an HR <1 was found as patients with intermediately abnormal studies, perhaps indicative of more electrical heterogeneity, had a higher likelihood of ArEs than patients with more extensive abnormalities. Figure 23-8 shows an example of a patient with SPECT dysinnervation defects, including areas of mismatch, who experienced subsequent ArEs.

Further support of the benefit of tomographic adrenergic imaging to better assess arrhythmic risk was provided by Fallavollita et al.[138] using the PET tracer ^{11}C-HED. Their Prediction of Arrhythmic Events with Positron Emission Tomography

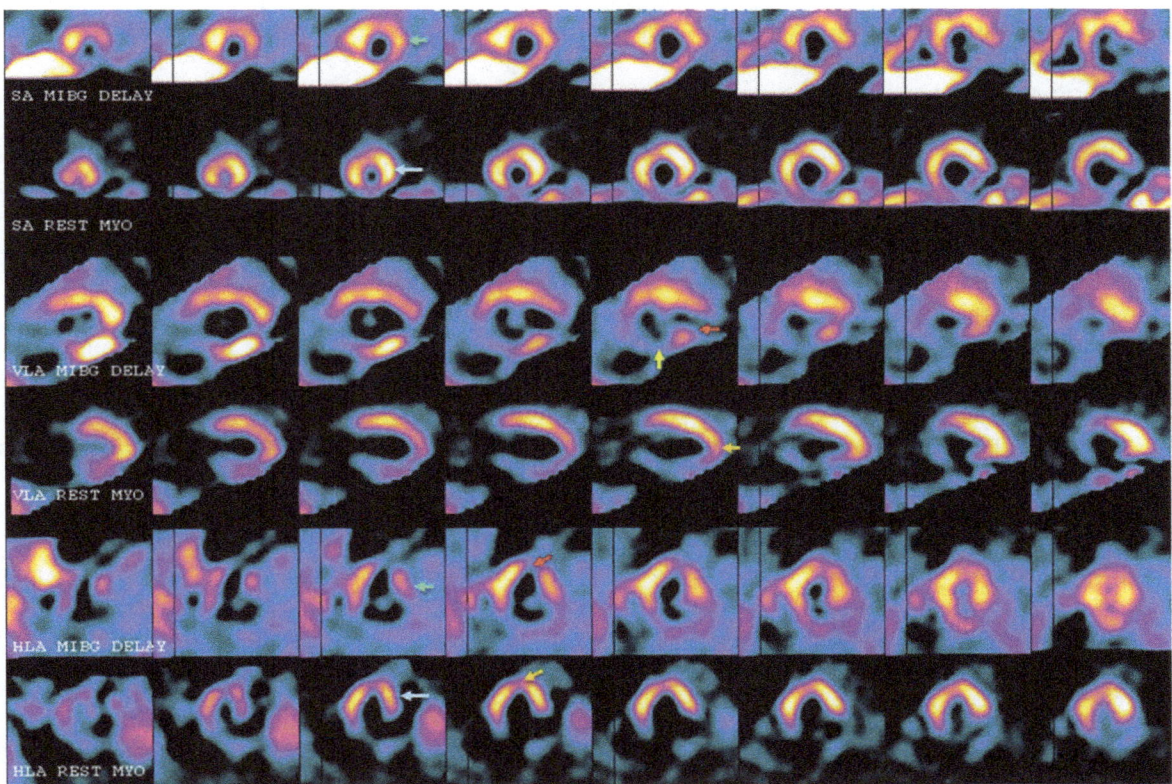

FIGURE 23-8 Adrenergic (MIBG) and perfusion (MYO) tomographic images of a 79-year-old man with nonischemic cardiomyopathy, NYHA II heart failure, EF = 35%. Had HMR of 1.6, but moderate degree of ^{123}I-mIBG defects involving the inferior wall (*yellow arrow* in MIBG slices), anterolateral wall (*green arrow* in MIBG slices) and apex (*red arrow* in MIBG slices). There are innervation perfusion mismatches at the apex (*orange arrow* in MYO slices) and anterolateral wall (*light blue arrow* in MYO slices). In follow-up, the patient had multiple VT episodes requiring ICD shocks and burst pacing. EF, ejection fraction; HLA, horizontal long axis; HMR, heart-to-mediastinum ratio; MIBG, meta-iodobenzylguanidine; NYHA, New York Heart Association; ICD, implantable cardioverter defibrillator; MYO, myoview (tetrofosmin); SA, short axis; VLA, vertical long axis; VT, ventricular tachycardia.

(PAREPET) study showed that in patients with ischemic cardiomyopathy followed over 4 years, sudden cardiac arrest (arrhythmic death, or ICD discharge for VF or VT >240 beats/min) increased in relation to ^{11}C-HED tomographic abnormalities independent of BNP, clinical symptoms, or LVEF.

Thus, there is robust data showing the ability of ^{123}I-mIBG and analogous PET adrenergic imaging to stratify arrhythmic risk in HF patients, with imaging parameters consistently independent of other commonly used variables, especially LVEF. However, as the data are all from observational trials, most investigators and clinicians agree that large prospective randomized trials are essential before adrenergic imaging can be included in guidelines for ICD use.

At the time of this writing, the ongoing corporate-sponsored prospective "International Study to Determine if AdreView Heart Function Scan Can be Used to Identify Patients With Mild or Moderate Heart Failure (HF) That Benefit From Implanted Medical Device (ADMIRE-ICD)" seeks conclusively to demonstrate utility in NYHA Class II to II HF patients who have an LVEF between 30% and 35%, inclusive.[62] The trial plans to randomize 2216 subjects to ^{123}I-mIBG HMR-guided ICD implantation versus the guidelines-directed standard approach, and will compare the occurrence over a mean of 2.75 to 3 years of a primary outcome of all-cause mortality, and various secondary outcomes that include ventricular arrhythmias.

▶ Further Potential Utility of ^{123}I-mIBG Imaging for Assessing and Managing Arrhythmias

Adrenergic imaging can also provide insight into patients with primary ventricular arrhythmic conditions. Wichter et al.[47] reported that patients with Brugada syndrome frequently have inferior and inferoseptal wall adrenergic defects, indicating that local dominance of parasympathetic tone there may contribute to arrhythmogenesis. In patients with arrhythmogenic right ventricular dysplasia (ARVD), Paul et al.[46] reported that focal SPECT ^{123}I-mIBG defects were present in over half of patients with life-threatening ventricular tachyarrhythmias, and led to worsened survival independent of RV dysfunction. Finally, in patients with chronic Chagas cardiomyopathy, Miranda et al.[45] found that the presence of tomographic ^{123}I-mIBG defects increased the occurrence of spontaneous or electrophysiologic-induced sustained VT. These data from primary arrhythmic conditions further support the likely utility of ^{123}I-mIBG in the HF setting in terms of guiding ICD use.

Recent work also shows potential for adrenergic image guiding of electrophysiologic studies. An area of interest is "border zone" myocardial regions adjacent to infarcted or fibrosed tissue containing mixtures of scar and viable tissue that have increased arrhythmic susceptibility.[139] These border zones can become fully or partially denervated as sympathetic fibers are damaged more easily and remain dysfunctional longer than cardiomyocytes. In a study of post-MI patients with LVEF ≤40%, Zhou et al.[140] reported that an ^{123}I-mIBG border zone to mediastinum ratio below 2.2 was better predictive of electrophysiologic inducibility than either scar or border zone size.

Adrenergic imaging can also potentially guide VT ablation therapy. In a study of 15 patients with ischemic cardiomyopathy in which 3D renditions of tomographic ^{123}I-mIBG findings were registered with electroanatomic high-density voltage maps, Klein et al.[141] found that successful ablation sites were often located in ^{123}I-mIBG denervation border areas outside of voltage mapped scar, illustrated in Figure 23-9.

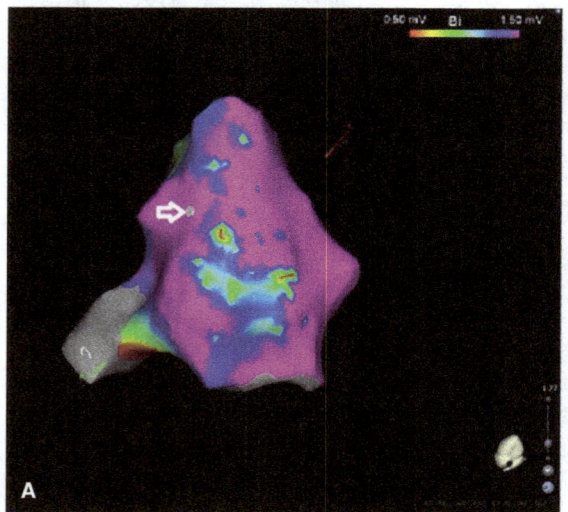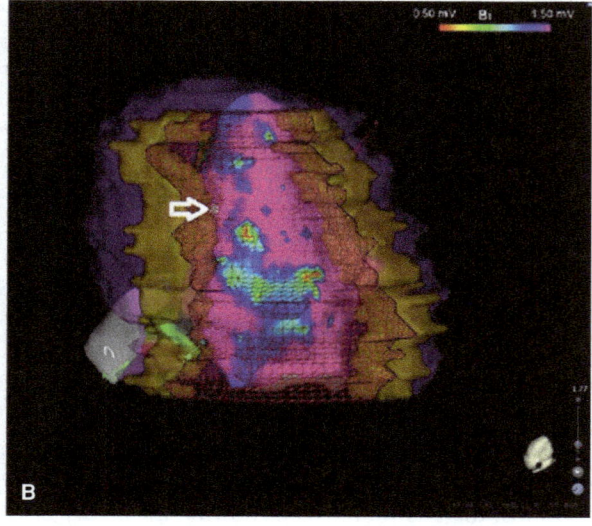

FIGURE 23-9 Comparison of 3D innervation map and electroanatomic map: discordant preserved voltage-denervation location and successful ablation site. **(A)** Bipolar electroanatomic map, inferior view, demonstrating inferior scar with ablation site (*yellow dot; white arrow*) at inferior septal location within area of preserved bipolar voltage (>1.5 mV). **(B)** Coregistration of electroanatomic bipolar map and innervation map demonstrating significantly larger area of denervation than bipolar voltage scar or border zone. Successful ablation point (*yellow dot; white arrow*) is located within the area of denervation (red transparent mesh) close to the denervation/neuronal transition zone interface despite preserved bipolar voltage (^{123}I-mIBG transition zone in overlying transparent yellow, and normal innervated myocardium in overlying transparent purple). (Reproduced with permission from Klein T, Abdulghani M, Smith M, et al. Three-dimensional ^{123}I-meta-iodobenzylguanidine cardiac innervation maps to assess substrate and successful ablation sites for ventricular tachycardia: A feasibility study for a novel paradigm of innervation imaging. *Circ Arrhythm Electrophysiol.* 2015;8(3):583–591.)

▶ Potential Utility of ¹²³I-*m*IBG Imaging in Other Clinical Situations

While the major focus of ¹²³I-*m*IBG and adrenergic PET imaging has been on HF and ventricular arrhythmias, there is much potential use in other clinical entities. These include patients with myocardial ischemia, DM, and monitoring cardiac damage from cancer chemotherapy, as well as cardiac involvement from systemic conditions such as Parkinson disease.

Neuronal imaging has much potential for assessing patients with known or suspected ischemic heart disease.[142] Adrenergic neurons are more sensitive to oxygen deprivation than cardiac myocytes, resulting in areas of denervation supersensitivity that have increased susceptibility to arrhythmias.[143,144] Following an ischemic insult, cardiac sympathetic injury lasts longer than perfusion abnormalities,[145] and thus ¹²³I-*m*IBG imaging can serve as an effective tracer for ischemic memory.[146] ¹²³I-*m*IBG imaging can also assess the area threatened during acute myocardial infarction, able to depict area at-risk similar-to-simple coronary anatomic models[147] but likely superior in terms of accounting for factors such as residual flow through the culprit artery, metabolic factors, and collateral flow. ¹²³I-*m*IBG imaging performed several days after patient presentation has been shown to depict the original area at risk better than standard perfusion techniques.[69,148] ¹²³I-*m*IBG imaging has also shown ability to detect of subclinical CAD,[149] perhaps because silent endothelial dysfunction causes episodes of vasoconstriction, activating neurohormonal events that affect local sympathetic output.

In patients with DM, imaging with ¹²³I-*m*IBG or similar PET tracers can detect cardiac autonomic abnormalities prior to clinical manifestations.[150] Adrenergic defects have been found in 80% of type II DM patients,[151] correlate with subclinical diastolic abnormalities on tissue Doppler echocardiography,[152] may increase risk of life-threatening arrhythmias,[153] are associated with more rapid progression of HF,[154] predict more frequent future occurrence of cardiac events and increased all-cause mortality over 7 years.[155]

Finally, given the enhanced sensitivity of sympathetic nerves to myocardial insults, ¹²³I-*m*IBG imaging has been investigated as a potential method of assessing cardiac damage from chemotherapeutic agents. Cardiac uptake of ¹²³I-*m*IBG decreases as the cumulative dose of doxorubicin increased, with subsequent deterioration in LVEF.[156] After a cumulative doxorubicin dose of 240 to 300 mg/m^2, cardiac ¹²³I-*m*IBG abnormalities have been shown to correlate with cardiac uptake of ¹¹¹In-antimyosin antibody.[157] Most recently, in breast cancer survivors 1 year after anthracycline treatment, an abnormally delayed HMR has been associated with abnormal echocardiographic global radial strain.[158]

FINAL THOUGHTS

Nuclear cardiology is poised to move beyond MPI. The ability of nuclear tracers to depict underlying molecular aspects of disease make them ideal and unique for assessing conditions such as HF and arrhythmias in ways that clinical methods and alternate imaging techniques cannot. Much data demonstrate the robust risk stratification power of cardiac adrenergic innervation imaging using ¹²³I-*m*IBG and related PET tracers. The key to clinical acceptance will be demonstrating management guiding utility that improves event-free survival and patient well-being.

REFERENCES

1. Klocke FJ, Baird MG, Bateman TM, et al.; American College of Cardiology; American Heart Association; American Society for Nuclear Cardiology. ACC/AHA/ASNC guidelines for the clinical use of cardiac radionuclide imaging–executive summary: a report of the American College of Cardiology/American Heart Association Task Force on Practice Guidelines (ACC/AHA/ASNC Committee to Revise the 1995 Guidelines for the Clinical Use of Radionuclide Imaging). *J Am Coll Cardiol.* 2003;42:1318–1333.
2. Shaw LJ, Iskandrian AE. Prognostic value of gated myocardial perfusion SPECT. *J Nucl Cardiol.* 2004;11:171–185.
3. McArdle BA, Dowsley TF, deKemp RA, Wells GA, Beanlands RS. Does rubidium-82 PET have superior accuracy to SPECT perfusion imaging for the diagnosis of obstructive coronary disease?: A systematic review and meta-analysis. *J Am Coll Cardiol.* 2012;60:1828–1837.
4. Dorbala S, Di Carli MF, Beanlands RS, et al. Prognostic value of stress myocardial perfusion positron emission tomography. Results from a multicenter observational registry. *J Am Coll Cardiol.* 2013;61:176–184.
5. Hachamovitch R, Hayes S, Friedman JD, et al. Determinants of risk and its temporal variation in patients with normal stress myocardial perfusion scans: what is the warranty period of a normal scan? *J Am Coll Cardiol.* 2003;41:1329–1340.

6. Hachamovitch R, Rozanski A, Hayes SW, et al. Predicting therapeutic benefit from myocardial revascularization procedures: are measurements of both resting left ventricular ejection fraction and stress-induced myocardial ischemia necessary? *J Nucl Cardiol.* 2006;13:768–778.
7. Shaw LJ, Berman DS, Maron DJ, et al. Optimal medical therapy with or without percutaneous coronary intervention to reduce ischemic burden. Results from the clinical outcomes utilizing revascularization and aggressive drug evaluation (COURAGE) trial nuclear substudy. *Circulation.* 2008;117:1283–1291.
8. Shaw LJ, Berman DS, Picard MH, et al. Comparative definitions for moderate-severe ischemia in stress nuclear, echocardiography and magnetic resonance imaging. *J Am Coll Cardiol Img.* 2014;7:593–604.
9. Sinusas AJ, Thomas JD, Mills G. The future of molecular imaging. *J Am Coll Cardiol Img.* 2011;7:799–806.
10. Travin MI. Application of cardiac neurohormonal imaging to heart failure, transplantation, and diabetes. *Curr Cardiovasc Imaging Rep.* 2015;8:8.
11. Travin MI. Clinical applications of myocardial innervation imaging. *Cardiol Clin.* 2016;34:133–147.
12. Bell DR. Control mechanisms in circulatory function. In: Rhoades RA, Bell DR, eds. *Medical Physiology: Principles of Clinical Medicine.* 4th ed. Philadelphia, PA: Lippincott Williams & Wilkins; 2013:317–320.
13. Colucci WS. Pathophysiology of heart failure: Neurohumoral adaptations. http://www.uptodate.com/contents/pathophysiology-of-heart-failure-neurohumoral-adaptations. Topic last updated August 11, 2015. Accessed April 27, 2016.
14. Francis GS. Neurohormonal control of heart failure. *Cleve Clin J Med.* 2011;78:S75–S79.
15. Carrió I. Cardiac neurotransmission imaging. *J Nucl Med.* 2001;42:1062–1076.
16. Zipes DP. Autonomic modulation of cardiac arrhythmias. In: Zipes DP, Jalife J, eds. *Cardiac Electrophysiology: From Cell to Bedside.* 2nd ed. Philadelphia, PA: WB Saunders Company; 1995:441–442.
17. Travin MI. Cardiac neuronal imaging at the edge of clinical application. *Cardiol Clin.* 2009;27:311–327.
18. Flotats A, Carrió I. Cardiac neurotransmission SPECT imaging. *J Nucl Cardiol.* 2004;11:587–602.
19. Verrier RL, Antzelevich C. Autonomic aspects of arrhythmogenesis: the enduring and the new. *Curr Opin Cardiol.* 2004;19:2–11.
20. Haider N, Baliga RR, Chandrashekhar Y, Narula J. Adrenergic excess, hNET1 down-regulation, and compromised mIBG uptake in heart failure poverty in the presence of plenty. *JACC Cardiovasc Imaging.* 2010;3:71–75.
21. Sisson JC, Wieland DM. Radiolabelled *meta*-iodobenzylguanidine pharmacology: pharmacology and clinical studies. *Am J Physiol Imaging.* 1986;1:96–103.
22. Bengel FM, Schwaiger M. Assessment of cardiac sympathetic neuronal function using PET imaging. *J Nucl Cardiol.* 2004;11:603–616.
23. Raffel DM, Wieland DM. Development of mIBG as a cardiac innervation imaging agent. *JACC Cardiovasc Imaging.* 2010;3:111–116.
24. Counsell RE, Yu T, Ranade VV, et al. Radioiodinated bretylium analogs for myocardial scanning. *J Nucl Med.* 1974;15:991–996.
25. Wieland DM, Mangner TJ, Inbasekaran MN, et al. Adrenal medulla imaging agents: a structure-distribution relationship study of radiolabeled aralkylguanidines. *J Med Chem.* 1984;27:149–155.
26. Hattori N, Schwaiger M. Metaiodobenzylguanidine scintigraphy of the heart. What have we learned clinically? *Eur J Nucl Med.* 2000;27:1–6.
27. Kline RC, Swanson DP, Wieland DM, et al. Myocardial imaging in man with I-123 meta-iodobenzylguanidine. *J Nucl Med.* 1981;22:129–132.
28. Luisi AJ, Suzuki G, deKemp R, et al. Regional ^{11}C-hydroxyephedrine retention in hibernating myocardium: chronic inhomogeneity of sympathetic innervation in the absence of infarction. *J Nucl Med.* 2005;46:1368–1374.
29. Sinusas AJ, Lazewatsky J, Brunetti J, et al. Biodistribution and radiation dosimetry of LMI1195: first-in-human study of a novel 18F-labeled tracer for imaging myocardial innervation. *J Nucl Med.* 2014;55:1–7.
30. Flotats A, Carrió I, Agostini D, et al. Proposal for standardization of ^{123}I-metaiodobenzylguanidine (MIBG) cardiac sympathetic imaging by the EANM Cardiovascular Committee and the European Council of Nuclear Cardiology. *Eur J Nucl Med Mol Imaging.* 2010;37:1802–1812.
31. Henzlova MJ, Duvall WL, Einstein AJ, Travin MI, Verberne HJ. ASNC imaging guidelines for SPECT nuclear cardiology procedures: stress, protocols, and tracers. *J Nucl Cardiol.* 2016;23:606–639.
32. Solanki KK, Bomanji J, Moyes J, Mather SJ, Trainer PJ, Britton KE. A pharmacological guide to medicines which interfere with the biodistribution of radiolabelled meta-iodobenzylguanidine (MIBG). *Nucl Med Commun.* 1992;13:513–521.
33. Wafelman AR, Hoefnagel CA, Maes RA, Beijnen JH. Radioiodinated metaiodobenzylguanidine: a review of its biodistribution and pharmacokinetics, drug interactions, cytotoxicity and dosimetry. *Eur J Nucl Med.* 1994; 21:545–559.
34. Jacobson A, Travin M. Impact of neuropsychiatric medications on cardiac uptake of i123 mIBG in heart failure subjects. *J Nucl Med.* 2013;54:1708.
35. Jacobson AF, Travin MI. Impact of medications on mIBG uptake, with specific attention to the heart: comprehensive review of the literature. *J Nucl Cardiol.* 2015;22 980–993.
36. FDA package insert. http://medlibrary.org/lib/rx/meds/adreview-1/, Accessed July 26, 2016.
37. Friedman NC, Hassan A, Grady E, Matsuoka DT, Jacobson AF. Efficacy of thyroid blockade on thyroid radioiodine uptake in ^{123}I-mIBG imaging. *J Nucl Med.* 2014;55:211–215.
38. Jacobson AF. Thyroid blockade in 123I-mIBG cardiac imaging: A common sense approach. *J Nucl Cardiol.* 2016;23(6):1340–1342.
39. Jacobson AF, Lombard J, Banerjee G, Camici PG. ^{123}I-mIBG scintigraphy to predict risk for adverse cardiac outcomes in heart failure patients: design of two prospective multicenter international trials. *J Nucl Cardiol.* 2009;16:113–121.
40. Jacobson AF, Senior R, Cerqueira MD. Myocardial iodine 123 meta-iodobenzylguanidine imaging and cardiac events in heart failure: results of the prospective ADMIRE-HF (Adreview myocardial imaging for risk evaluation in heart failure). *J Am Coll Cardiol.* 2010;55:2212–2221.
41. Gimelli A, Liga R, Giorgetti A, et al. Assessment of myocardial adrenergic innervation with a solid-state dedicated

cardiac cadmium-zinc-telluride camera: First clinical experience. *Eur Heart Journal-CV Imaging.* 2014;15:575-585.
42. Chen J, Folks RD, Verdes L, Manatunga DN, Jacobson AF, Garcia EV. Quantitative I-123 mIBG SPECT in differentiating abnormal and normal mIBG myocardial uptake. *J Nucl Cardiol.* 2012;19:92-99.
43. Bellevre D, Manrique A, Legallois D, et al. First determination of the heart-to-mediastinum ratio using cardiac dual isotope (^{123}I-MIBG/^{99m}Tc-tetrofosmin) CZT imaging in patients with heart failure: the ADRECARD study. *Eur J Nucl Med Mol Imaging.* 2015;42:1912-1919.
44. Minardo JD, Tuli MM, Mock BH, et al. Scintigraphic and electrophysiological evidence of canine myocardial sympathetic denervation and reinnervation produced by myocardial infarction or phenol application. *Circulation.* 1988;78: 1008-1019.
45. Miranda CH, Figueiredo AB, Maciel BC, Marin-Neto JA, Simoes MV. Sustained ventricular tachycardia is associated with regional myocardial sympathetic denervation assessed with 123I-metaiodobenzylguanidine in chronic Chagas cardiomyopathy. *J Nucl Med.* 2011;52:504-510.
46. Paul M, Wichter T, Kies P, et al. Cardiac sympathetic dysfunction in genotyped patients with arrhythmogenic right ventricular cardiomyopathy and risk of recurrent ventricular tachyarrhythmias. *J Nucl Med.* 2011;52:1559-1565.
47. Wichter T, Matheja P, Eckardt L, et al. Cardiac autonomic dysfunction in Brugada syndrome. *Circulation.* 2002;105: 702-706.
48. Dobbeleir AA, Hambye AS, Franken PR. Influence of high-energy photons on the spectrum of iodine-123 with low- and medium-energy collimators: Consequences for imaging with ^{123}I-labelled compounds in clinical practice. *Eur J Nucl Med.* 1999;26:655-658.
49. Inoue Y, Suzuki A, Shirouzu I, et al. Effect of collimator choice on quantitative assessment of cardiac iodine-123 mIBG uptake. *J Nucl Cardiol.* 2003;10:623-632.
50. Verberne HJ, Feenstra C, de Jong WM, Somsen GA, van Eck-Smit BL, Busemann Sokole E. Influence of collimator choice and simulated clinical conditions on ^{123}I-mIBG heart/mediastinum ratios: A phantom study. *Eur J Nucl Med.* 2005;32:1100-1107.
51. Chen J, Garcia EV, Galt JR, Folks RD, Carrio I. Optimized acquisition and processing protocols for I-123 cardiac SPECT imaging. *J Nucl Cardiol.* 2006;13:251-260.
52. Matsuo S, Nakajima K, Okuda K, et al. Standardization of the heart-to-mediastinum ratio of ^{123}I-labelled-metaiodobenzylguanidine uptake using the dual energy window method: feasibility of correction with different camera-collimator combinations. *Eur J Nucl Med.* 2009;36:560-566.
53. Nakajima K, Okuda K, Matsuo S, et al. Standardization of metaiodobenzylguanidine heart to mediastinum ratio using a calibration phantom: Effects of correction on normal databases and a multicentre study. *Eur J Nucl Med.* 2012;39: 113-119.
54. Nakajima K, Okuda K, Yoshimura M, et al. Multicenter cross-calibration of I-123 metaiodobenzylguanidine heart-to-mediastinum ratios to overcome camera-collimator variations. *J Nucl Cardiol.* 2014;21:970-978.
55. Agostini D, Belin A, Amar MH, et al. Improvement of cardiac neuronal function after carvedilol treatment in dilated cardiomyopathy: a ^{123}I-MIBG scintigraphic study. *J Nucl Med.* 2000;41:845-851.
56. Gerson MC, Craft LL, McGuire N, et al. Carvedilol improves left ventricular function in heart failure patients with idiopathic dilated cardiomyopathy and a wide range of sympathetic nervous system function as measured by iodine 123 metaiodobenzylguanidine. *J Nucl Cardiol.* 2002;9:608-615.
57. Yamada T, Shimonagata T, Fukunami M, et al. Comparison of the prognostic value of cardiac iodine-123 metaiodobenzylguanidine imaging and heart rate variability in patients with chronic heart failure. *J Am Coll Cardiol.* 2003;41:231-238.
58. Okuda K, Nakajima K, Hosoya T, et al. Semi-automated algorithm for calculating heart-to-mediastinum ratio in cardiac iodine-123 mIBG imaging. *J Nucl Cardiol.* 2011;18:82-89.
59. Jacobson AF, Matsuoka DT. Influence of myocardial region of interest definition on quantitative analysis of planar 123I-mIBG images. *Eur J Nucl Med Mol Imaging.* 2013;40: 558-564.
60. Veltman CE, Boogers MJ, Meinardi JE, et al. Reproducibility of planar 123I-meta-iodobenzylguanidine (MIBG) myocardial scintigraphy in patients with heart failure. *Eur J Nucl Med Mol Imaging.* 2012;39:1599-1608.
61. Travin MI, Polk DM. Radionuclide molecular imaging in heart failure. http://www.acc.org/latest-in-cardiology/articles/2015/04/08/09/45/radionuclide-molecular-imaging-in-heart-failure. Published April 9, 2015.
62. ClinicalTrials.gov. https://www.clinicaltrials.gov/ct2/show/NCT02656329. Accessed July 26, 2016.
63. Dimitriu-Leen AC, Gimelli A, Younis I, et al. The impact of acquisition time of planar cardiac ^{123}I-MIBG imaging on the late heart to mediastinum ratio. *Eur J Nucl Med Mol Imaging.* 2016:43:326-332.
64. Ogita H, Shimonagata T, Fukunami M, et al. Prognostic significance of cardiac ^{123}I metaiodobenzylguanidine imaging for mortality and morbidity in patients with chronic heart failure: a prospective study. *Heart.* 2001;86:656-660.
65. Chen GP, Tabibiazar R, Branch KR, et al. Cardiac receptor physiology and imaging: an update. *J Nucl Cardiol.* 2005;12: 714-730.
66. Morozumi T, Kusuoka H, Fukuchi K, et al. Myocardial iodine-123-metaiodobenzylguanidine images and autonomic nerve activity in normal subjects. *J Nucl Med.* 1997;38:49-52.
67. Tamaki S, Yamada T, Okuyama Y, et al. Cardiac iodine-123 metaiodobenzylguanidine imaging predicts sudden cardiac death independently of left ventricular ejection fraction in patients with chronic heart failure and left ventricular systolic dysfunction: results from a comparative study with signal-averaged electrocardiogram, heart rate variability, and QT dispersion. *J Am Coll Cardiol.* 2009;53:426-435.
68. Holly TA, Abbott BG, Al-Mallah M, et al.; American Society of Nuclear Cardiology. Single photon-emission computed tomography. *J Nucl Cardiol.* 2010;17:941-973.
69. Simões MV, Barthel P, Matsunari I, et al. Presence of sympathetically denervated but viable myocardium and its electrophysiologic correlates after early revascularised, acute myocardial infarction. *Eur Heart J.* 2004;25:551-557.
70. Clements IP, Garcia EV, Chen J, Folks RD, Butler J, Jacobson AF. Quantitative iodine-123-metaiodobenzylguanidine (MIBG) SPECT imaging in heart failure with left ventricular systolic dysfunction: Development and validation of

70. automated procedures in conjunction with technetium-99m tetrofosmin myocardial perfusion SPECT. *J Nucl Cardiol.* 2016;23:425–435.
71. Travin MI. It's not all in the numbers. *J Nucl Cardiol.* 2016; 23:436–441.
72. Narula J, Gerson M, Thomas GS, Cerqueira MD, Jacobson AF. ^{123}I-MIBG imaging for prediction of mortality and potentially fatal events in heart failure: The ADMIRE-HFX Study. *J Nucl Med.* 2015;56:1011–1018.
73. Travin MI, Henzlova MJ, van Eck-Smit BLF, et al. Assessment of ^{123}I-mIBG and ^{99m}Tc-tetrofosmin single-photon emission computed tomographic images for the prediction of arrhythmic events in patients with ischemic heart failure. Intermediate severity innervation defects are associated with higher arrhythmic risk. *J Nucl Cardiol.* 2017;24:377–391.
74. Gill JS, Hunter GJ, Gane G, Camm AJ. Heterogeneity of the human myocardial sympathetic innervation: in vivo demonstration by iodine 123-labeled *meta*-iodobenzylguanidine scintigraphy. *Am Heart J.* 1993;126:390–398.
75. Tsuchimochi S, Tamaki N, Tadamura E, et al. Age and gender differences in normal myocardial adrenergic neuronal function evaluated by iodine-123-MIBG imaging. *J Nucl Med.* 1995;36:969–974.
76. Estorch M, Serra-Grima R, Flotats A, et al. Myocardial sympathetic innervation in the athlete's sinus bradycardia: is there selective inferior myocardial wall denervation? *J Nucl Cardiol.* 2000;7:354–358.
77. Mozaffarian D, Benjamin EJ, Go AS, et al.; Writing Group Members; American Heart Association Statistics Committee; Stroke Statistics Subcommittee. Heart Disease and Stroke Statistics—2016 Update: A Report from the American Heart Association. *Circulation.* 2016;133(4):e38–e360.
78. Braunwald E. Heart failure. *JACC Heart Fail.* 2013;1:1–20.
79. Udelson JE, Shafer CD, Carrió I. Radionuclide imaging in heart failure: assessing etiology and outcomes and implications for management. *J Nucl Cardiol.* 2002;9:S40–S52.
80. Fallavollita JA, Canty JM. Dysinnervated but viable myocardium in ischemic heart disease. *J Nucl Cardiol.* 2010;17:1107–1115.
81. Schofer J, Spielmann R, Schuchert A, et al. Iodine-123 meta-iodobenzylguanidine scintigraphy: a noninvasive method to demonstrate myocardial adrenergic nervous system disintegrity in patients with idiopathic dilated cardiomyopathy. *J Am Coll Cardiol.* 1988;12:1252–1258.
82. Merlet P, Valette H, Dubois-Randé J, et al. Prognostic value of cardiac metaiodobenzylguanidine in patients with heart failure. *J Nucl Med.* 1992;33:471–477.
83. Nakata T, Miyamoto K, Doi A, et al. Cardiac death prediction and impaired cardiac sympathetic innervation assessed by MIBG in patients with failing and nonfailing hearts. *J Nucl Cardiol.* 1998;5:579–590.
84. Agostini D, Verberne HJ, Burchert W, et al. I-123-*m*IBG myocardial imaging for assessment of risk for a major cardiac event in heart failure patients: insights from a retrospective European multicenter study. *Eur J Nucl Med Mol Imaging.* 2008;35:535–546.
85. Verberne HJ, Brewster LM, Somsen GA, van Eck-Smit BL. Prognostic value of myocardial 123I-metaiodobenzylguanidine (MIBG) parameters in patients with heart failure: a systematic review. *Eur Heart J.* 2008;29:1147–1159.
86. Chirumamilla A, Travin MI. Cardiac applications of ^{123}I-mIBG imaging. *Semin Nucl Med.* 2011;41:374–387.
87. Ketchum ES, Jacobson AF, Caldwell JH, et al. Selective improvement in Seattle heart failure model risk stratification using iodine-123 meta-iodobenzylguanidine imaging. *J Nucl Cardiol.* 2012;19:1007–1016.
88. Nakata T, Nakajima K, Yamashina S, et al. A pooled analysis of multicenter cohort studies of I-123-mIBG cardiac sympathetic innervation imaging for assessment of long-term prognosis in chronic heart failure. *JACC Cardiovasc Imaging.* 2013;6:772–784.
89. Shah AM, Bourgoun M, Narula J, Jacobson AF, Solomon SD. Influence of ejection fraction on the prognostic value of sympathetic innervation imaging with iodine-123 MIBG in Heart Failure. *JACC Cardiovasc Imaging.* 2012;5:1139–1146.
90. Shaw LJ, Min JK, Hachamovitch R, et al. Cardiovascular imaging research at the crossroads. *JACC Cardiovasc Imaging.* 2010;3:316–324.
91. Treglia G, Stefanelli I, Giordano BA. Clinical usefulness of myocardial innervation imaging using Iodine-123-meta-iodobenzylguanidine scintigraphy in evaluating the effectiveness of pharmacological treatments in patients with heart failure: an overview. *Eur Rev Med Pharmacol Sci.* 2013;17:56–58.
92. Cohen-Solal A, Rouzet F, Berdeaux A, et al. Effects of carvedilol on myocardial sympathetic innervation in patients with chronic heart failure. *J Nucl Med.* 2005;46:1796–1803.
93. Merlet P, Pouillart F, Dubois-Randé J, et al. Sympathetic nerve alterations assessed with ^{123}I-MIBG in the failing human heart. *J Nucl Med.* 1999;40:224–231.
94. Takeishi Y, Atsumi H, Fujiwara S, et al. ACE inhibition reduces cardiac iodine-123-MIBG release in heart failure. *J Nucl Med.* 1997;38:1085–1089.
95. Toyama T, Aihara Y, Iwasaki T, et al. Cardiac sympathetic activity estimated by ^{123}I-MIBG myocardial imaging in patients with dilated cardiomyopathy after β-blocker or angiotensin-converting enzyme inhibitor therapy. *J Nucl Med.* 1999;40:217–223.
96. Kasama S, Toyama T, Kumakura H, et al. Spironolactone improves cardiac sympathetic nerve activity and symptoms in patients with congestive heart failure. *J Nucl Med.* 2002;43:1279–1285.
97. Toyama T, Hoshizaki H, Seki R, et al. Efficacy of amiodarone treatment on cardiac symptom, function, and sympathetic nerve activity in patients with dilated cardiomyopathy: comparison with beta-blocker therapy. *J Nucl Cardiol.* 2004;11:134–141.
98. Lotze U, Kaepplinger S, Kober A, et al. Recovery of the cardiac adrenergic nervous system after long-term beta-blocker therapy in idiopathic dilated cardiomyopathy: assessment by increase in myocardial ^{123}I-metaiodobenzylguanidine uptake. *J Nucl Med.* 2001;42:49–54.
99. Suwa M, Otake Y, Moriguchi A, et al. Iodine-123 metaiodobenzylguanidine myocardial scintigraphy for prediction of response to beta-blocker therapy in patients with dilated cardiomyopathy. *Am Heart J.* 1997;133:353–358.
100. Choi JY, Lee KH, Hong KP, et al. Iodine-123 MIBG imaging before treatment of heart failure with carvedilol to predict improvement of left ventricular function and exercise capacity. *J Nucl Cardiol.* 2001;8:4–9.

101. Matsui T, Tsutamoto T, Maeda K, Kusukawa J, Kinoshita M. Prognostic value of repeated ^{123}I-metaiodobenzylguanidine imaging in patients with dilated cardiomyopathy with congestive heart failure before and after optimized treatments—comparison with neurohumoral factors. *Circ J.* 2002;66:537–543.
102. Nakajima K, Nakata T, Matsuo S, Jacobson AF. Creation of mortality risk charts using ^{123}I meta-iodobenzylguanidine heart-to-mediastinum ratio in patients with heart failure: 2- and 5-year risk models. *Eur Heart J Cardiovasc Imaging.* 2016;17:1138–1145.
103. Verschure DO, Veltman CE, Manrique A, et al. For what endpoint does myocardial ^{123}I-MIBG scintigraphy have the greatest prognostic value in patients with chronic heart failure? Results of a pooled individual patient data meta-analysis. *Eur Heart J Cardiovasc Imaging.* 2014;15:996–1003.
104. Boogers MJ, Borleffs CJ, Henneman MM, et al. Cardiac sympathetic denervation assessed with 123-Iodine metaiodobenzylguanidine imaging predicts ventricular arrhythmias in implantable cardioverter-defibrillator patients. *J Am Coll Cardiol.* 2010;55:2769–2777.
105. Cleland JG, Daubert JC, Erdmann E, et al. The effect of cardiac resynchronization on morbidity and mortality in heart failure. *N Engl J Med.* 2005;352:1539–1549.
106. Swedberg K, Cleland J, Dargie H, et al. Guidelines for the diagnosis and treatment of chronic failure: executive summary (update 2005): the Task Force for the Diagnosis and Treatment of Chronic Heart Failure of the European Society of Cardiology. *Eur Heart J.* 2005;26:1115–1140.
107. Yu CM, Zhang Q, Fung JW, et al. A novel tool to assess systolic asynchrony and identify responders of cardiac resynchronization therapy by tissue synchronization imaging. *J Am Coll Cardiol.* 2005;45:677–684.
108. D'Orio Nishioka SA, Filho MM, Soares Brandão SC, et al. Cardiac sympathetic activity pre and post resynchronization therapy evaluated by ^{123}I-MIBG myocardial scintigraphy. *J Nucl Cardiol.* 2007;14:852–859.
109. Tanaka H, Tatsumi K, Fujiwara S, et al. Effect of left ventricular dyssynchrony on cardiac sympathetic activity in heart failure patients with wide QRS duration. *Circ J.* 2012;76:382–389.
110. Scholtens AM, Braat AJ, Tuinenburg A, Meine M, Verberne HJ. Cardiac sympathetic innervation and cardiac resynchronization therapy. *Heart Fail Rev.* 2014;19:567–573.
111. Erol-Yilmaz A, Verberne HJ, Schrama TA, et al. Cardiac resynchronization induces favorable neurohumoral changes. *Pacing Clin Electrophysiol.* 2005;28:304–310.
112. Gould PA, Kong G, Kalff V, et al. Improvement in cardiac adrenergic function post biventricular pacing for heart failure. *Europace.* 2007;9:751–756.
113. Imamura T, Kinugawa K, Nitta D, Kinoshita O, Nawata K, Ono M. Preoperative iodine-123 meta-iodobenzylguanidine imaging is a novel predictor of left ventricular reverse remodeling during treatment with a left ventricular assist device. *J Artif Organs.* 2016;19:29–36.
114. Drakos SG, Athanasoulis T, Malliaras KG, et al. Myocardial sympathetic innervation and long-term left ventricular mechanical unloading. *J Am Coll Cardiol Imaging.* 2010;3:64–70.
115. George RS, Birks EJ, Cheetham A, et al. The effect of long-term left ventricular assist device support on myocardial sympathetic activity in patients with non-ischaemic dilated cardiomyopathy. *Eur J Heart Fail.* 2013;15:1035–1043.
116. Cohen-Solal A, Esanu Y, Logeart D, et al. Cardiac metaiodobenzylguanidine uptake in patients with moderate chronic heart failure: relationship with peak oxygen uptake and prognosis. *J Am Coll Cardiol.* 1999;33:759–660.
117. Gerson MC, McGuire N, Wagoner LE. Sympathetic nervous system function as measured by I-123 metaiodobenzylguanidine predicts transplant-free survival in heart failure patients with idiopathic dilated cardiomyopathy. *J Card Fail.* 2003;9:384–391.
118. Flotats A, Carrió I. Value of radionuclide studies in cardiac transplantation. *Ann Nucl Med.* 2006;20:13–21.
119. Di Carli MF, Tobes MC, Mangner T, et al. Effects of cardiac sympathetic innervation on coronary blood flow. *N Engl J Med.* 1997;336:1208–1215.
120. Estorch M, Campreciós M, Flotats A, et al. Sympathetic reinnervation of cardiac allografts evaluated by ^{123}I-MIBG imaging. *J Nucl Med.* 1999;40:911–916.
121. Bengel FM, Ueberfuhr P, Schiepel N, et al. Effect of sympathetic reinnervation on cardiac performance after heart transplantation. *N Engl J Med.* 2001;345:731–738.
122. Zipes DP, Camm AJ, Borggrefe M, et al. ACC/AHA/ESC 2006 guidelines for management of patients with ventricular arrhythmias and the prevention of sudden cardiac death—executive summary: a report of the American College of Cardiology/American Heart Association Task Force and the European Society of Cardiology Committee for Practice Guidelines (Writing Committee to Develop Guidelines for Management of Patients with Ventricular Arrhythmias and the Prevention of Sudden Cardiac Death). *J Am Coll Cardiol.* 2006;48:1064–1108.
123. Yancy CW, Jessup M, Bozkurt B, et al. 2013 ACCF/AHA guideline for the management of heart failure: a report of the American College of Cardiology Foundation/American Heart Association Task Force on Practice Guidelines. *Circulation.* 2013;128:e240–e327.
124. Buxton AE, Lee KL, Hafley GE, et al. Limitations of ejection fraction for prediction of sudden death risk in patients with coronary artery disease: lessons from the MUSTT study. *J Am Coll Cardiol.* 2007;50:1150–1157.
125. Myerburg RJ. Implantable cardioverter-defibrillators after myocardial infarction. *N Engl J Med.* 2008;359:2245–2253.
126. Kremers MS, Hammill SC, Berul CI, et al. The National ICD Registry Report: Version 2.1 including leads and pediatrics for years 2010 and 2011. *Heart Rhythm.* 2013;10:e59–e65.
127. Sanders GD, Hlatky MA, Owens DK. Cost-effectiveness of implantable cardioverter-defibrillators. *N Engl J Med.* 2005;353:1471–1480.
128. Lee DS, Krahn AD, Healey JS, et al. Evaluation of early complications related to de novo cardioverter defibrillator implantation: Insights from the Ontario ICD database. *J Am Coll Cardiol.* 2010;55:774–782.
129. Al-Khatib SM, Hellkamp A, Curtis J, et al. Non-evidence-based ICD implantations in the United States. *JAMA.* 2011;305:43–49.
130. Barron HV, Lesh MD. Autonomic nervous system and sudden cardiac death. *J Am Coll Cardiol.* 1996;27:1053–1060.
131. Tomaselli GF, Zipes DP. What causes sudden death in heart failure? *Circ Res.* 2004;95:754–763.
132. Stanton MS, Tuli MM, Radtke NL, et al. Regional sympathetic denervation after MI in humans detected noninvasively using I-123-MIBG. *J Am Coll Cardiol.* 1989;14:1519–1526.

133. McGhie AI, Corbett JR, Aks MS, et al. Regional cardiac adrenergic function using I-123 MIBG SPECT imaging after acute myocardial infarction. *Am J Cardiol.* 1991;67:236–242.
134. Arora R, Ferrick KJ, Nakata T, et al. I-123 MIBG imaging and heart rate variability analysis to predict the need for an implantable cardioverter defibrillator. *J Nucl Cardiol.* 2003;10:121–131.
135. Nagahara D, Nakata T, Hashimoto A, et al. Predicting the need for an implantable cardioverter defibrillator using cardiac metaiodobenzylguanidine activity together with plasma natriuretic peptide concentration or left ventricular function. *J Nucl Med.* 2008;49:225–233.
136. Bax JJ, Kraft O, Buxton AE, et al. ^{123}I-mIBG scintigraphy to predict inducibility of ventricular arrhythmias on cardiac electrophysiology testing: a prospective multicenter pilot study. *Circ Cardiovasc Imaging.* 2008;1:131–140.
137. Marshall A, Cheetham A, George RS, et al. Cardiac iodine-123 metaiodobenzylguanidine imaging predicts ventricular arrhythmia in heart failure patients receiving an implantable cardioverter-defibrillator for primary prevention. *Heart.* 2012;98:1359–1365.
138. Fallavollita JA, Heavey BM, Luisi AJ Jr, et al. Regional myocardial sympathetic denervation predicts the risk of sudden cardiac arrest in ischemic cardiomyopathy. *J Am Coll Cardiol.* 2014;63:141–149.
139. Roes SD, Borleffs XJ, van der Geest RJ, et al. Infract tissue heterogeneity assessed with contrast-enhanced MRI predicts spontaneous ventricular arrhythmia in patients with ischemic cardiomyopathy and implantable cardioverter-defibrillator. *Circ Cardiovasc Imaging.* 2009;2:183–190.
140. Zhou Y, Zhou W, Folks RD, et al. I-123 mIBG and Tc-99m myocardial SPECT imaging to predict inducibility of ventricular arrhythmia on electrophysiology testing: A retrospective analysis. *J Nucl Cardiol.* 2014;21:913–920.
141. Klein T, Abdulghani M, Smith M, et al. Three-dimensional 123I-meta-iodobenzylguanidine cardiac innervation maps to assess substrate and successful ablation sites for ventricular tachycardia: A feasibility study for a novel paradigm of innervation imaging. *Circ Arrhythm Electrophysiol.* 2015;8:583–591.
142. Henneman MM, Bengel FM, van der Wall EE, Knuuti J, Bax JJ. Cardiac neuronal imaging: Application in the evaluation of cardiac disease. *J Nucl Cardiol.* 2008;3:442–455.
143. Inoue H, Zipes DP. Results of sympathetic denervation in the canine heart: supersensitivity that may be arrhythmogenic. *Circulation.* 1987;75:877–887.
144. Sasano T, Abraham R, Chang KC, et al. Abnormal sympathetic innervation of viable myocardium and the substrate of ventricular tachycardia after myocardial infarction. *J Am Coll Cardiol.* 2008;51:2266–2275.
145. Zipes DP. Influence of myocardial ischemia and infarction on autonomic innervation of heart. *Circulation.* 1990;82:1095–1105.
146. Inobe Y, Kugiyama K, Miyagi H, et al. Long-lasting abnormalities in cardiac sympathetic nervous system in patients with coronary spastic angina: Quantitative analysis with iodine 123 metaiodobenzylguanidine myocardial scintigraphy. *Am Heart J.* 1997;134:112–118.
147. D'estanque E, Hedon C, Lattuca B, et al. Optimization of a simultaneous dual isotope Tl/123IMIBG myocardial SPECT imaging protocol with a CZT camera for trigger zone assessment after myocardial infarction for routine clinical settings: are delayed acquisition and scatter correction necessary? *J Nucl Cardiol.* 2016 May 25, doi: 10.1007/s12350-016-0524-1 [Epub ahead of print].
148. Matsunari I, Schricke U, Bengel FM, et al. Extent of cardiac sympathetic neuronal damage is determined by the area of ischemia in patients with acute coronary syndromes. *Circulation.* 2000;101:2579–2585.
149. Simula S, Vanninen E, Viitanen L, et al. Cardiac adrenergic innervation is affected in asymptomatic subjects with very early stage of coronary disease. *J Nucl Med.* 2002;43:1–7.
150. Langer A, Freeman MR, Josse RG, et al. Metaiodobenzylguanidine imaging in diabetes mellitus: Assessment of cardiac sympathetic denervation and its relation to autonomic dysfunction and silent myocardial ischemia. *J Am Coll Cardiol.* 1995;25:610–618.
151. Hattori N, Tamaki N, Hayashi T, et al. Regional abnormality of iodine-123-MIBG in diabetic hearts. *J Nucl Med.* 1996;37:1985–1990.
152. Sacre JW, Franjic B, Jellis CL, et al. Association of cardiac autonomic neuropathy with subclinical myocardial dysfunction in type 2 diabetes. *JACC Cardiovasc Imaging.* 2010;3:1207–1215.
153. Stevens MJ, Raffel DM, Allman KC, et al. Cardiac sympathetic dysinnervation in diabetes: Implications for enhanced cardiovascular risk. *Circulation.* 1998;98:961–968.
154. Gerson MC, Caldwell JH, Ananthasubramaniam K, et al. Influence of diabetes mellitus on prognostic utility of imaging of myocardial sympathetic innervation in heart failure patients. *Circ Cardiovasc Imaging.* 2011;4:87–93.
155. Nagamachi S, Fujita S, Nishii R, et al. Prognostic value of cardiac I-123 metaiodobenzylguanidine imaging in patients with non-insulin-dependent diabetes mellitus. *J Nucl Cardiol.* 2006;13:34–42.
156. Olmos RAV, ten Bokkel Huinink WW, ten Hoeve RFA, et al. Assessment of anthracycline-related myocardial adrenergic derangement by [^{123}I]metaiodobenzylguanidine scintigraphy. *Eur J Cancer.* 1995;31:26–31.
157. Carrió I, Estorch M, Berná L, et al. Indium-111-antimyosin and iodine-123-MIBG studies in early assessment of doxorubicin cardiotoxicity. *J Nucl Med.* 1995;36:2024–2049.
158. Bulten BF, Verberne HJ, Bellersen L, et al. Relationship of promising methods in the detection of anthracycline-induced cardiotoxicity in breast cancer patients. *Cancer Chemother Pharmacol.* 2015;76:957–967.

Cardiac Amyloid Imaging and ^{18}F-FDG PET/CT for Imaging Sarcoidosis and Cardiovascular Infection

CHAPTER 24

Dillenia Rosica and Sharmila Dorbala

INTRODUCTION

Cardiac amyloidosis, sarcoidosis, and cardiovascular infections are major causes of morbidity and mortality. Early diagnosis and timely application of specific therapy are critical to improve clinical outcomes.[1,2] Echocardiography, cardiac magnetic resonance imaging (CMR), and cardiac CT can detect increased wall thickness, expanded extracellular volume, diffuse late gadolinium enhancement, wall motion abnormalities, fibrosis, vegetations, and abscesses resulting from cardiac amyloidosis, sarcoidosis, or infection. However, by the time the above cardiac structural changes are evident, the disease is at a fairly advanced stage. Moreover, some of these changes are nonspecific and may represent sequelae of other forms of heart diseases and are not disease specific. Radionuclide imaging methods are evolving as specific disease markers in amyloidosis, sarcoidosis, and infection imaging.

RADIONUCLIDE IMAGING OF CARDIAC AMYLOIDOSIS

▶ Introduction

Cardiac amyloidosis is a subset of systemic amyloidosis, which is caused by deposition of insoluble nonbranching protein aggregates of amyloid fibrils in the extracellular space of the myocardium. This results in left ventricular thickening and heart failure. Heart failure is a frequent cause of death in these patients. Two major forms of systemic amyloidosis have cardiac involvement[3,4]: (1) Light chain amyloidosis (AL) where amyloid fibrils are formed from immunoglobulin light chains produced by clonal population of plasma cells and (2) Transthyretin amyloidosis (ATTR) where misfolded monomers or dimers from either mutant or wild type TTR deposit as fibrils in the myocardium. The mutant type (ATTRm) is an autosomal dominant disorder while the wild type disease (ATTRwt) is associated with aging (senile systemic amyloidosis). Some of the ATTRm diseases have predominant cardiomyopathic manifestations while others have coexistent or predominant neuropathy, including carpal tunnel syndrome and/or autonomic neuropathy along with cardiomyopathy. ATTRwt may be significantly underdiagnosed clinically, as a recent autopsy study showed a prevalence of up to 30% of myocardial amyloid deposits in individuals over 75 years with heart failure and preserved ejection fraction.[5]

Distinction between the two types of cardiac amyloidosis is critical as the treatment and prognosis are vastly different. For AL amyloidosis, chemotherapy is used to inhibit the plasma cell dyscrasia which results in the abnormal light-chain production. Overall mortality as well as treatment-related mortality for AL patients is markedly increased in individuals with cardiac involvement, therefore demonstrating cardiac involvement can guide treatment in these patients. AL cardiac amyloidosis can be rapidly progressive (median survival, if untreated, is <12 months after heart failure onset).[3] On the other hand, median survival after heart failure onset is better for ATTR patients (median survival 75 months)[4] and within this subset, individuals with ATTRwt do better than those with ATTRm. In recent years, new therapies for ATTR have emerged including drugs that inhibit TTR synthesis, stabilize TTR, or degrade proteins.[6] Hence, there is an urgent need to image and quantify myocardial amyloid burden for early diagnosis and for assessment of response to therapy with these new therapies.

Imaging with echocardiography and CMR typically raises the suspicion of cardiac amyloidosis in individuals with heart failure.[7] However, imaging features on structural imaging, though highly suggestive, may not be definitively diagnostic for cardiac amyloidosis. Importantly, no specific imaging feature on echocardiography or CMR can distinguish AL from ATTR amyloidosis.[7] Several radiotracers have been used for imaging cardiac amyloidosis including bone imaging compounds, ^{123}I metaiodobenzylguanidine (*m*IBG, to image myocardial denervation in familial amyloidosis), and amyloid binding agents (^{123}I-serum amyloid p-component SAP, ^{18}F-florbetapir, flutemetamol, florbetaben, ^{11}C-Pittsburgh B compound).[7] In this chapter, we will focus on ^{99m}Tc bone imaging compounds, which are widely used clinically and are highly sensitive and specific for imaging cardiac ATTR amyloidosis.

▶ Indications

Diagnosis

Radionuclide imaging plays an important role in noninvasive diagnosis of cardiac ATTR amyloidosis. ^{99m}Tc-pyrophosphate (PYP) and ^{99m}Tc-3,3-diphosphono-1,2-propranodicarboxylic acid (DPD) are two radiopharmaceuticals that are used for imaging cardiac amyloidosis. In a recent multicenter study, ^{99m}Tc-PYP has been shown to identify ATTR amyloidosis with 97% sensitivity and 100% specificity.[8-10] ^{99m}Tc-DPD, available in Europe but not approved for clinical use in the United States, has a specificity of 88% and a sensitivity of 100%.[10-12]

Several other amyloid binding radiotracers, in particular PET agents that have been used for beta-amyloid imaging in the brain (^{11}C Pittsburgh B-compound,[13,14] ^{18}F-florbetapir,[15,16] ^{18}F-flutemetamol, and ^{18}F-florbetaben[17]) are being investigated for cardiac amyloid imaging.

^{123}I-MIBG had been used for the diagnosis of early myocardial denervation in ATTRm.[18-21] *m*IBG imaging is discussed in Chapter 23.

Echocardiography and CMR have well-established roles in the diagnosis and follow-up of cardiac amyloidosis and a proposed algorithm incorporating radionuclide imaging is shown in Figure 24-1.

In patients with CHF and unexplained left ventricular thickening with suspected cardiac amyloidosis who either have echo findings that are classic for cardiac amyloid and no evidence of plasma cell dyscrasia or patients with suggestive but not classical echo findings and a negative cardiac MRI (or cannot get an MRI) without plasma cell dyscrasia, ^{99m}TcPYP/DPD scan can be performed to assess for ATTR amyloidosis. Patients with familial ATTR and suspected cardiac amyloidosis can also be evaluated with ^{99m}TcPYP/DPD scan. Patients with a typical echocardiographic appearance and strongly positive (grade 2 or 3 myocardial radiotracer uptake ≥ rib uptake) ^{99m}TcPYP/DPD scan can be considered to have ATTR amyloidosis (Fig. 24-2). In these patients, biopsy is not necessary, but may be performed for typing of amyloid. A negative scan, however, does not exclude AL amyloidosis and further evaluation is necessary.[7] In these patients, bone marrow, fat pad, or endomyocardial biopsy can be performed to confirm the diagnosis of AL. Early studies of cardiac PET imaging for amyloidosis such as with ^{18}F-florbetapir show potential for detection of AL cardiac amyloidosis. However, this is not yet currently in routine clinical use.

Response to Therapy

Currently, response to therapy for cardiac ATTR is mainly monitored using echocardiography and CMR. However, they are limited due to the temporal delay in detection of change in myocardial wall thickness. Extracellular volume fraction on CMR is emerging as a novel and quantitative marker to diagnose changes in cardiac amyloidosis burden. SPECT/CT with ^{99m}TcPYP/DPD has the potential to provide quantitative imaging for monitoring response. Results to date, with planar imaging, however, have been disappointing.[22] However, it is unclear whether the therapy was not successful or the imaging technique was limited at detecting changes. Amyloid imaging using PET amyloid tracers is inherently quantitative and offers the promise to detect changes in amyloid burden following response to therapy.[23]

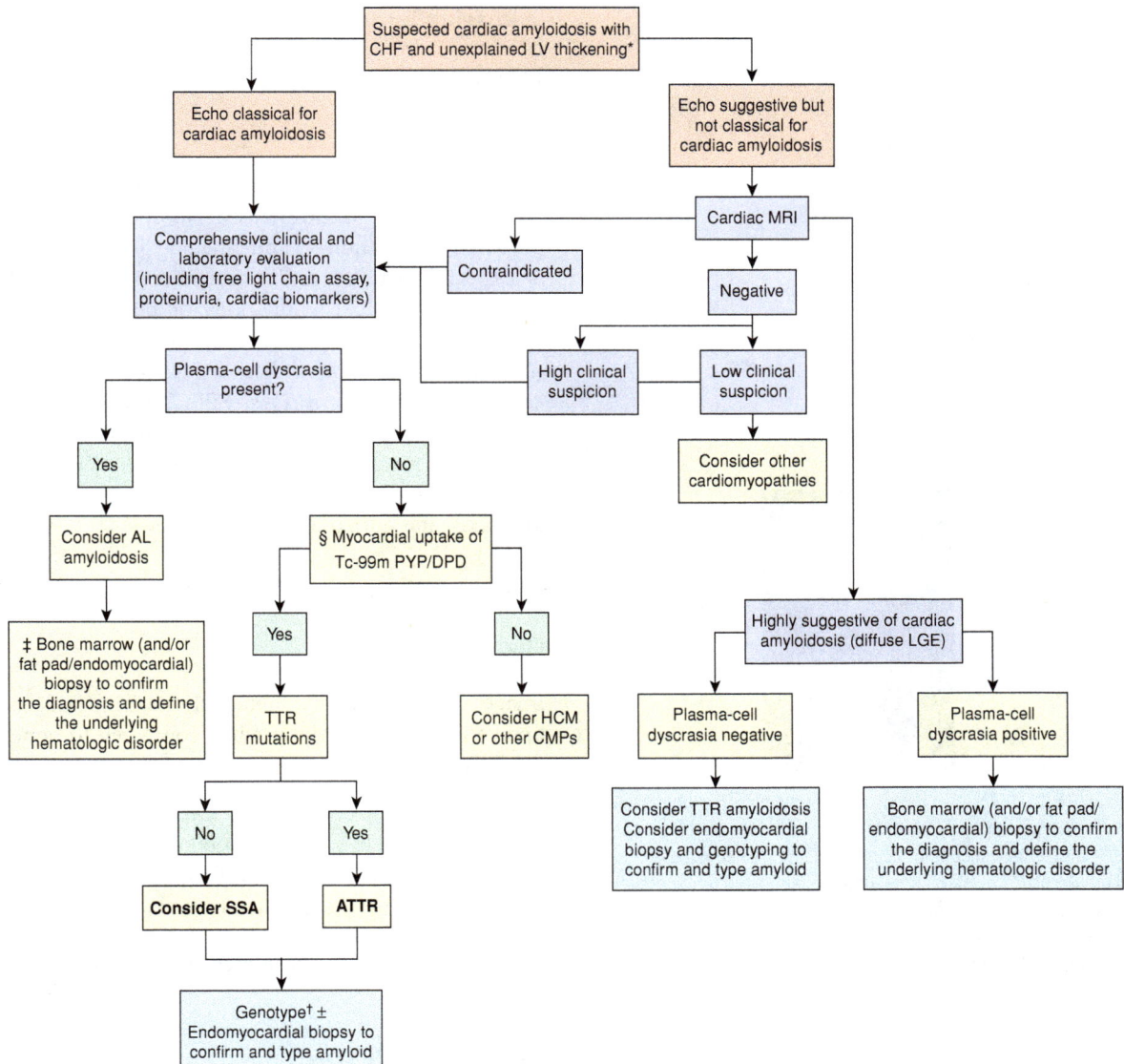

FIGURE 24-1 A proposed algorithm for the evaluation of patients with suspected cardiac amyloidosis. (Reproduced with permission from Falk RH, Quarta CC, Dorbala S. How to image cardiac amyloidosis. *Circ Cardiovasc Imaging*. 2014;7(3):552–562.)
*unexplained symmetric LVH with nondilated LV on echocardiogram, absence of ECG QRS voltage for LVH.
†if genotype positive, probably no need for biopsy?
‡consider the potential of misdiagnosis of ATTR amyloidosis as AL in the presence of monoclonal gammopathy of uncertain significance (MGUS).
§may be an initial test (instead of MRI) in patients with suspected ATTR.
LV, left ventricular; LVH, left ventricular hypertrophy; CHF, congestive heart failure; LGE, late gadolinium enhancement; PYP, pyrophosphate; DPD, 3, 3-diphosphono-1,2-propanodicarboxylic acid; HCM, hypertrophic cardiomyopathy; CMP, cardiomyopathy; SSA, senile systemic amyloidosis; ATTR, transthyretin amyloidosis.

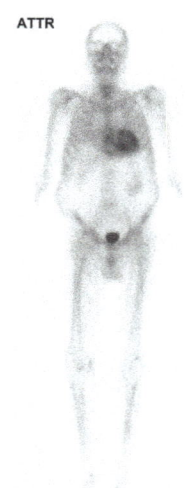

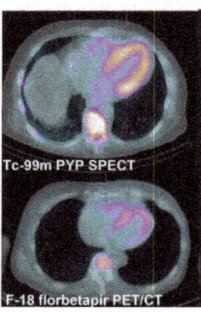

FIGURE 24-2 ^{99m}Tc-PYP and ^{18}F-florbetapir PET/CT images in a 78-year-old man with heart failure. SPECT images obtained 2.5 hours after injection of 20 mCi of ^{99m}Tc-PYP showed grade 3 uptake of ^{99m}Tc-PYP (cardiac radiotracer uptake > rib uptake). Research protocol ^{18}F-florbetapir PET/CT images show diffuse biventricular uptake of radiotracer. Endomyocardial biopsy confirmed ATTR cardiac amyloidosis.

Prognosis

For patients with ATTRm, it has been shown that the heart-to-whole body ratio (>7.5) combined with LV wall thickness (>12 mm) was associated with the highest rate of major adverse cardiovascular events (defined as cardiovascular death, hospitalization or stroke).[12] A heart-to-contralateral lung ratio of ≥1.6 on planar ^{99m}Tc-PYP scan is associated with worse survival.[9] Among individuals with V30M mutation ATTRm a heart to mediastinal (H/M) ratio of <1.6 on late ^{123}I-*m*IBG imaging was associated with a significantly worse 5-year mortality (42% vs. 7% for H/M ratio of <1.6 and ≥1.6, respectively, $p < 0.001$).

Imaging Technique

Protocol

^{99m}Tc-PYP/DPD

The standard dose for ^{99m}Tc-PYP/DPD is 20 to 25 mCi injected intravenously. No special patient preparation is required and imaging is performed at 1 to 2.5 hours after radiotracer injection. Protocol options include: (1) whole-body or planar cardiac with chest/cardiac SPECT if planar is abnormal and (2) planar and chest/cardiac SPECT or (3) chest/cardiac SPECT-only images. SPECT-only imaging is adequate and provides quickest imaging times. Images are reconstructed with standard ^{99m}Tc protocols and displayed in standard short-axis, vertical long-axis, and horizontal long-axis views.

Image Interpretation ^{99m}Tc-PYP

Qualitative

Images are evaluated qualitatively with regard to uptake in the myocardium when compared to bone (ribs) as follows:

- Negative/grade 0: no uptake
- Mild/grade 1: less than rib uptake
- Moderate/grade 2: equal to rib uptake
- Severe/grade 3: greater than rib uptake

Grade 2 or greater is considered positive for ATTR amyloidosis.[24]

Quantitative Analysis

Regions of interest over the heart and in the contralateral lung can be used to assess heart-to-contralateral-lung ratio.[6] The heart-to-contralateral-lung ratio is derived by drawing a region of interest (ROI) over the heart and copying it over to the right chest. Visual uptake in the heart is compared to visual radiotracer uptake in the ribs on planar images and preferably on SPECT images.

Other Findings

Normal physiologic distribution of ^{99m}Tc-PYP/DPD is similar to a standard nuclear medicine bone scan with uptake in the osseous structures and excretion in the genitourinary system.

Pitfalls

A potential pitfall is myocardial blood pool uptake in early images or in individuals with renal dysfunction. Myocardial radiotracer uptake in ATTR amyloidosis is usually clear-cut with excellent contrast between myocardium and blood pool, if there is any question on early images, more delayed images can be obtained to increase the contrast between the myocardium and the blood pool.

Reporting

Report should contain the presence and degree of myocardial uptake, as well as other incidental findings on whole-body imaging and SPECT/CT, if performed. If qualitative analysis is requested, the heart-to-contralateral-lung ratio on planar imaging can be reported as well. Readers are referred to American Society of Nuclear Cardiology (ASNC) practice points on ^{99m}Tc-PYP imaging for more details.[25]

Conclusion/Future Directions

Radionuclide imaging of cardiac ATTR amyloidosis with ^{99m}Tc-PYP/DPD is easy to perform with essentially no contraindications. Image analysis is relatively straightforward and nuclear imaging can provide important adjunct diagnostic and prognostic information to echocardiography and CMR. ^{123}I-mIBG imaging can be useful to identify myocardial denervation and stratify risk of adverse clinical outcomes in individuals with ATTRm. Amyloid-binding PET radiotracers that are approved for beta-amyloid brain imaging are currently under investigation and show promise, particularly for quantitation and for characterization of the AL subtype of amyloidosis.

CARDIAC PET RADIONUCLIDE IMAGING OF CARDIAC SARCOIDOSIS AND CARDIOVASCULAR INFECTION

Positron emission tomography (PET) with ^{18}F-2-fluoro-2-deoxy glucose (^{18}F-FDG) is emerging as a robust technique for early diagnosis of focal myocardial inflammation and infection, particularly prosthetic material infection. ^{18}F-FDG is a cyclotron-produced glucose analog with a half-life of 110 minutes. Due to its long half-life, ^{18}F-FDG can be shipped as unit doses to sites without a cyclotron on-site. ^{18}F-FDG is a surrogate marker for cellular glucose uptake. Tissue hypoxia is a potent stimulus for increased glucose utilization by the cardiomyocytes. High glycolytic activity from infiltrates of active inflammatory cells also increases glucose utilization in inflammation and infection. GLUT1 synthesis and cell membrane expression of GLUT1 receptors are upregulated in activated macrophages facilitate increased glucose utilization.[26] In addition, circulating cytokines and growth factors are thought to increase the affinity of glucose transporters for ^{18}F-FDG.[27] Once transported into the cells through GLUT1, GLUT3, and GLUT4 receptors,[28] ^{18}F-FDG is phosphorylated by hexokinase to ^{18}F-FDG-6-phosphate which is not metabolized any further. The trapped ^{18}F-FDG-6-phosphate within the cell[28] provides the imaging signal for metabolically active inflamed tissues. This chapter will focus on imaging of cardiac sarcoidosis and cardiovascular prosthetic infection using ^{18}F-FDG PET. (See Chapter 3 for further review of FDG.)

^{18}F-FDG PET/CT Imaging of Cardiac Sarcoidosis

Introduction

Sarcoidosis is an idiopathic, multisystem inflammatory disorder characterized by accumulation of non-caseating granulomas. These organized collections of macrophages, epithelioid cells, and lymphocytes are formed in response to inciting antigens and can eventually lead to organ damage. Both cardiac and neurologic sarcoidosis can occur in isolation without involvement of other organs.[29]

Cardiac sarcoidosis can involve virtually any part of the heart from endocardium to pericardium and both ventricles and atria.[30] The myocardium is most frequently affected, in particular, the left ventricular free wall at the base of the heart, followed by the basal interventricular septum.[31] Clinical manifestations range from arrhythmias to congestive heart failure to sudden death. Cardiac involvement represents the cause of death in up to 25% of fatal sarcoidosis in the United States. Early diagnosis is important as these complications are potentially preventable with early treatment. Until recently cardiac sarcoidosis was diagnosed using the criteria proposed by the Japanese Ministry of Health and Welfare, that included a histological diagnosis by endomyocardial biopsy or a clinical diagnosis by

Table 24-1
Japanese Ministry of Health and Welfare Guidelines for Diagnosis of Cardiac Sarcoidosis
Histologic diagnosis group
Cardiac sarcoidosis is confirmed when endomyocardial biopsy specimens demonstrate noncaseating epithelioid cell granulomas with histological or clinical diagnosis of extracardiac sarcoidosis.
Clinical diagnosis group
Although endomyocardial biopsy specimens do not demonstrate noncaseating epithelioid cell granulomas, extracardiac sarcoidosis is diagnosed histologically or clinically and satisfies the following conditions and more than 1 in 6 basic diagnostic criteria. 1. 2 or more of the 4 major criteria are satisfied. 2. 1 in 4 of the major criteria and 2 or more of the 5 minor criteria are satisfied.
Major criteria a. Advanced atrioventricular block. b. Basal thinning of the interventricular septum. c. Positive ^{67}gallium uptake in the heart. d. Depressed ejection fraction of the left ventricle (<50%).
Minor criteria a. Abnormal ECG findings: ventricular arrhythmias (ventricular tachycardia), multifocal or frequent PVCs, CRBBB, axis deviation, or abnormal Q-wave. b. Abnormal echocardiography: regional abnormal wall motion or morphological abnormality (ventricular aneurysm, wall thickening). c. Nuclear medicine: perfusion defect detected by ^{201}thallium or ^{99m}technetium myocardial scintigraphy. d. Gadolinium-enhanced CMR imaging: delayed enhancement of myocardium. e. Endomyocardial biopsy: interstitial fibrosis or monocyte infiltration over moderate grade.

Reproduced with permission from Tahara N, Tahara A, Nitta Y, et al. Heterogeneous myocardial FDG uptake and the disease activity in cardiac sarcoidosis. *JACC Cardiovasc Imaging.* 2010;3(12):1219–1228.

extracardiac biopsy-proven sarcoidosis in conjunction with major and minor criteria including findings on ECG, echocardiography, myocardial perfusion imaging with ^{201}thallium, ^{99m}technetium, ^{67}gallium, and CMR (Table 24-1). ^{18}F-FDG PET/CT, though not included in the Japanese criteria, plays a major role in the contemporary diagnosis and management of cardiac sarcoidosis.[32]

Indications for ^{18}F-FDG PET/CT

Diagnosis of Cardiac Sarcoidosis

The most definitive diagnosis of cardiac sarcoidosis, currently, is based on a positive endomyocardial biopsy. Endomyocardial biopsy is usually a blind procedure with several small samples taken from the right ventricular aspect of the interventricular septum (usual location). As sarcoidosis is a focal disease, endomyocardial biopsy is more prone to sampling error. In sarcoidosis, different parts of the myocardium may harbor granulomas in different stages of inflammation, fibrosis, or an admixture of inflammation and fibrosis. As only a minute portion of the myocardium from the interventricular septum is sampled randomly, assessment of disease activity in the whole heart is limited. ^{18}F-FDG-PET/CT overcomes these limitations. Inflammation is assessed in the entire heart. Furthermore, as shown in Table 24-2, an abnormal ^{18}F-FDG PET/CT clinches a diagnosis of cardiac sarcoidosis, without an endomyocardial biopsy, in individuals with a histological proof of extracardiac sarcoidosis and abnormal cardiac symptoms, examination findings, ECG findings, or LVEF <50%.[33]

Despite these advantages, when cardiac sarcoidosis is suspected, a CMR study is generally considered before ^{18}F-FDG PET/CT due to its high negative predictive value to exclude sarcoidosis[7] and the absence of ionizing radiation. ^{18}F-FDG PET/CT may be considered as the initial test, if CMR is contraindicated (ferromagnetic devices, glomerular filtration rate, GFR <30 mL/min), or if CMR is abnormal and a confirmation of active inflammation may change clinical management or if clinical suspicion of cardiac sarcoidosis remains high despite a normal CMR.[32] The sensitivity and specificity of ^{18}F-FDG PET for the diagnosis of cardiac sarcoidosis

Table 24-2

HRS Expert Consensus Recommendations on Criteria for the Diagnosis of Cardiac Sarcoidosis

There are 2 pathways to a diagnosis of cardiac sarcoidosis (CS):
1. Histological diagnosis from myocardial tissue
   CS is diagnosed in the presence of noncaseating granuloma on histological examination of myocardial tissue with no alternative cause identified (including negative organismal stains if applicable).
2. Clinical diagnosis from invasive and noninvasive studies:
   It is probable[a] that is CS if:
   (a) There is a histological diagnosis of extracardiac sarcoidosis
   and
   (b) One or more of following is present
   - Steroid +/− immunosuppressant responsive cardiomyopathy or heart block
   - Unexplained reduced LVEF (<40%)
   - Unexplained sustained (spontaneous or induced) VT
   - Mobitz type II 2nd-degree heart block or 3rd-degree heart block
   - Patchy uptake on dedicated cardiac PET (in a pattern consistent with CS)
   - Late gadolinium enhancement on CMR (in a pattern consistent with CS)
   - Positive gallium uptake (in a pattern consistent with CS)
   and
   (c) Other causes for the cardiac manifestation(s) have been reasonably excluded

[a]In general, "probable involvement" is considered adequate to establish a clinical diagnosis of CS.
Reproduced with permission from Birnie DH, Sauer WH, Bogun F, et al. HRS expert consensus statement on the diagnosis and management of arrhythmias associated with cardiac sarcoidosis. *Heart Rhythm.* 2014;11(7):1305–1323.

are summarized in Table 24-3.[34] Figure 24-3 outlines a proposed algorithm for CMR and ^{18}F-FDG PET/CT to diagnose cardiac sarcoidosis.

Assessment of Response to Treatment

The results of ^{18}F-FDG PET/CT can be useful to initiate, as well as to monitor response to anti-inflammatory therapy (Fig. 24-4). In individuals with ongoing or increasing inflammation an increase in dose or addition of new medications may be considered, while in those with decreased ^{18}F-FDG uptake on subsequent scans, medication dose may be tapered.[35] However, the utility of ^{18}F-FDG PET/CT to guide changes in anti-inflammatory therapy has not been validated in prospective clinical trials.

Table 24-3

Sensitivity and Specificity of ^{18}F-FDG PET for the Diagnosis of Cardiac Sarcoidosis

Study	Year	Number of Patients	Cohort	Diagnosis	Sensitivity (%)	Specificity (%)
Yamagishi	2003	17	Cardiac sarcoid	Histologic	100	n/a
Okumura	2004	22	Sarcoid	Histologic	100	91
Ishimaru	2005	32	Sarcoid	Clinical	100	82
Ohira	2008	21	Suspected cardiac sarcoid	ECG and Holter diagnosis	88	39
Langah	2009	65	Suspected cardiac sarcoid	Suspected sarcoid	85	90
Weighted mean		168			*89.9*	*81.4*
Mean		168			*91*	*75.5*

All studies with ^{18}F-FDG PET against gold standard of Japanese Ministry of Health and Welfare Guidelines.
Data from Ohira H, Tsujino I, Ishimaru S, et al. Myocardial imaging with 18F-fluoro-2-deoxyglucose positron emission tomography and magnetic resonance imaging in sarcoidosis. *Eur J Nucl Med Mol Imaging.* 2008;35(5):933–941.

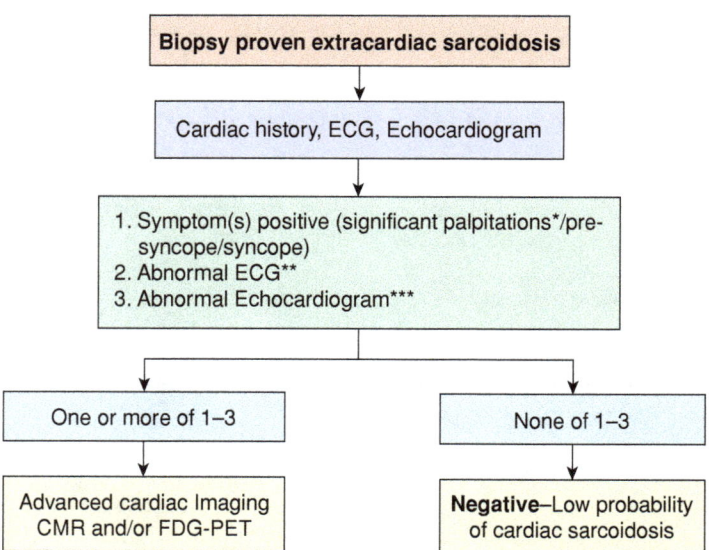

FIGURE 24-3 Proposed diagnostic algorithm for cardiac sarcoidosis.
*palpitations were defined as "prominent patient complaint lasting > 2 weeks"
**abnormal ECG defined as complete left or right bundle branch block and/or presence of unexplained pathological Q waves in 2 or more leads and/or sustained 2nd or 3rd degree AV block and/or sustained or non-sustained VT
***abnormal echocardiogram defined RWMA and/or wall aneurysm and/or basal septum thinning and/or LVEF <40% (Reproduced with permission from Birnie DH, Sauer WH, Bogun F, et al. HRS expert consensus statement on the diagnosis and management of arrhythmias associated with cardiac sarcoidosis. *Heart Rhythm.* 2014;11(7):1305–1323.)

Prognosis

Cardiac involvement in sarcoidosis carries a poor prognosis. In a study of 118 patients with suspected or known cardiac sarcoidosis, the presence of both a perfusion defect and myocardial ^{18}F-FDG uptake had the strongest association with death or sustained ventricular tachycardia when compared to those with normal studies or perfusion defects alone or myocardial ^{18}F-FDG uptake alone.[36] In addition, of the patients with PET/CT abnormalities, those with focal uptake in the right ventricle had an even higher adverse event rate. Cardiac PET/CT imaging of perfusion and metabolism, therefore, has the potential to risk stratify patients with cardiac sarcoidosis.[36]

Imaging Technique

Protocol

Radionuclide imaging protocols for cardiac sarcoidosis comprise of a rest myocardial perfusion imaging study along with cardiac and a limited whole-body ^{18}F-FDG imaging. Myocardial perfusion imaging can be performed with SPECT using ^{99m}Tc-sestamibi or ^{99m}Tc-tetrofosmin or with a PET using ^{13}N-ammonia or ^{82}rubidium. Table 24-4 outlines a summary protocol for the ^{18}F-FDG PET/CT study for cardiac sarcoidosis. Historically, ^{67}gallium SPECT was the mainstay for inflammation imaging and is included in the Japanese diagnostic criteria for cardiac sarcoidosis. But, due to the poor image resolution, long scan duration and limited sensitivity, in practice, this has largely been supplanted by ^{18}F-FDG PET/CT. PET-only imaging can also be performed on dedicated PET cameras with smaller field of views, but can be challenging to localize focal hotspots of ^{18}F-FDG. Fusion imaging with myocardial perfusion may help localize ^{18}F-FDG uptake. As with PET/CT, images should be reconstructed and displayed as short axis, horizontal long axis, and vertical long axis to correlate with myocardial perfusion imaging.

Dietary Preparation

The myocardium is a metabolic omnivore that consumes glucose or fatty acids for its metabolic needs, depending on the substrate abundance. The goal of dietary preparation is to suppress normal myocardial glucose utilization to be able to detect abnormal signal within the myocardium. This is accomplished by shifting myocardial metabolism to fatty acid use. Several approaches exist including prolonged fasting, specific diet (a high fat, low to zero carbohydrate, protein permitted diet), and intravenous unfractionated heparin (Table 24-5).

A retrospective study[37] from the Netherlands compared three methods: (1) fasting alone (>6 hours),

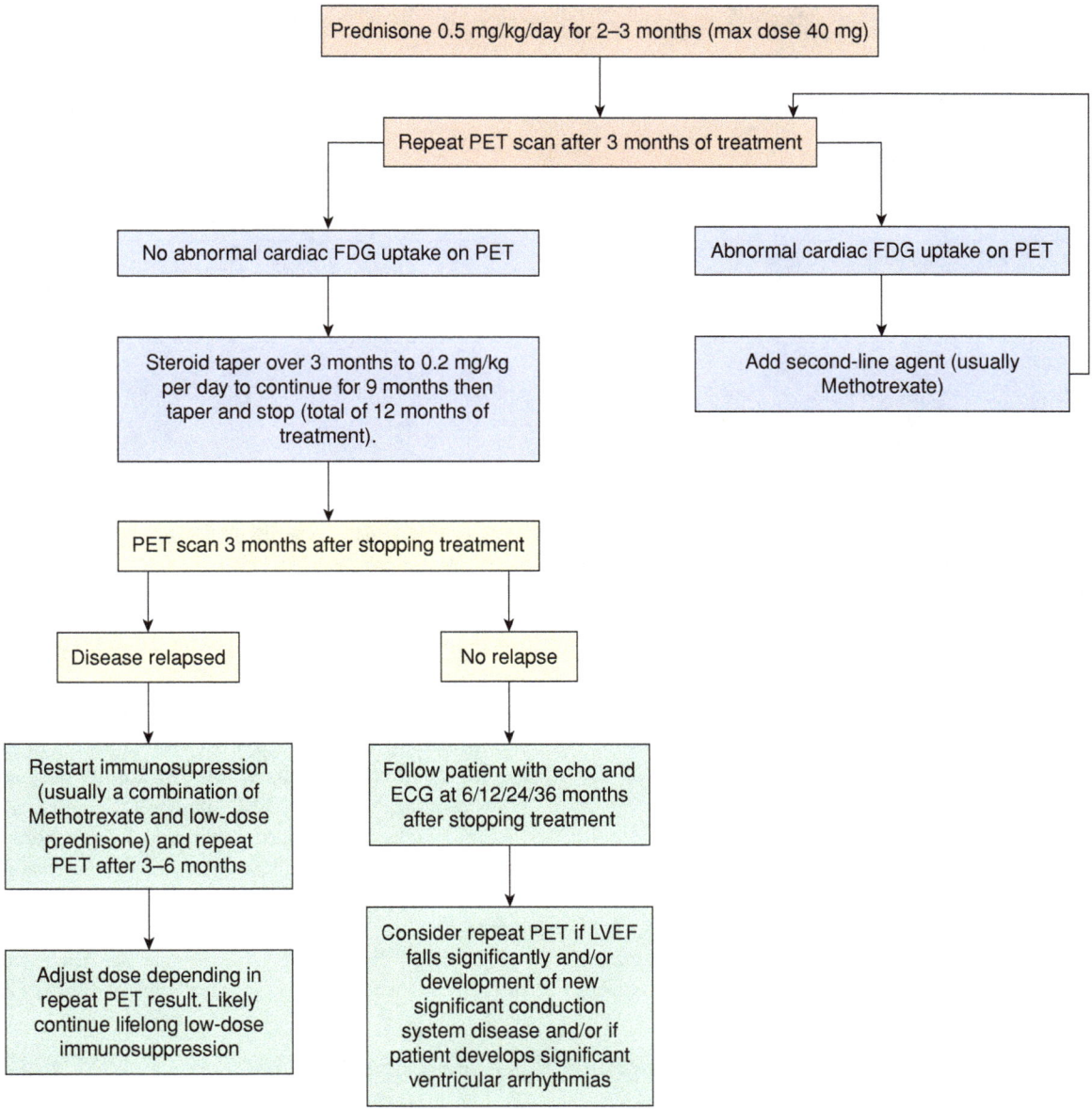

FIGURE 24-4 Proposed therapeutic algorithm for cardiac sarcoidosis based on ¹⁸F-FDG imaging. (Reproduced with permission from Birnie DH, Nery PB, Ha AC, et al. Cardiac sarcoidosis. *J Am Coll Cardiol.* 2016;68(4):411–421.)

(2) low carbohydrate, protein and fat permitted diet for 12 hours followed by 12-hour fasting, and (3) low carbohydrate diet, protein and fat permitted diet for 12 hours followed by 12-hour fasting and IV unfractionated heparin 50 IU/kg, 15 minutes prior to injection of ¹⁸F-FDG. This study showed that dietary preparation (method 1) outperformed fasting alone while the addition of IV unfractionated heparin to diet and fasting (method 3) outperformed diet and fasting (method 2) in terms of suppression of myocardial glucose utilization. However, this study did not include a high fat diet. A high fat, low to zero carbohydrate, protein permitted diet for two meals on the day prior followed by an overnight fast prior to the ¹⁸F-FDG PET examination currently remains the standard protocol for ¹⁸F-FDG PET for suppressing physiological

Table 24-4

Radionuclide Imaging Protocol for Cardiac Sarcoidosis

Patient preparation
High fat, low to zero carbohydrate diet (see Table 24-5) for at least 2 meals 24 hours prior to the test, followed by overnight fast
Avoid strenuous activity for at least 24 hours

Myocardial perfusion imaging
Rest myocardial perfusion imaging using standard protocols of ^{99m}Tc SPECT or ^{82}rubidium PET or ^{13}N-ammonia PET

^{18}F-FDG PET/CT Imaging

Radiopharmaceutical
10 mCi (3D PET) or 15 mCi (2D PET) ^{18}F-FDG administered intravenously

Uptake period
90-minute uptake phase following ^{18}F-FDG administration (keep same uptake period for follow-up scan as at baseline)
Patient should be kept in a quiet room that is shielded for radiation protection
No food intake during the uptake period
No exercise to avoid muscle uptake

Imaging protocol
Dedicated cardiac ^{18}F-FDG scan: 20-minute (2D) or 10-minute (3D) image acquisition in the cardiac bed position followed by limited whole-body ^{18}F-FDG scan: Base of skull through abdomen, 3 minutes per bed position for 3D PET.

---

myocardial glucose utilization for sarcoid, infection/inflammation protocol ^{18}F-FDG PET.[15] Table 24-6 lists some sample foods for the sarcoid ^{18}F-FDG PET diet.

Image Interpretation

Assessment/Diagnosis

Interpretation of the perfusion and ^{18}F-FDG integrated study involves four steps: (1) interpretation of perfusion images, (2) interpretation of cardiac ^{18}F-FDG PET/CT, (3) integration of perfusion and ^{18}F-FDG PET/CT data, and (4) interpretation of limited whole-body ^{18}F-FDG PET/CT. Images should be interpreted in conjunction with clinical data, ECG findings, and other results of imaging studies such as echocardiography and CMR. Interpretation of perfusion images is discussed separately in this book. For the purposes of cardiac sarcoidosis, perfusion imaging is approached the same way as for coronary artery disease.

Cardiac ^{18}F-FDG PET/CT images are reviewed in the standard cardiac imaging planes of short axis

Table 24-5

Summary of Different Approaches to Patient Preparation

Patient Preparation	Rationale	Advantages	Disadvantages
Prolonged fasting (5–18 hours)	In the fasting state, free fatty acids account for up to 90% of oxygen consumption in normal myocytes[35]	Easy to instruct patient	Variable myocardial suppression
High fat, zero- to low-carbohydrate diet (24 hours prior to the study) followed by fasting after midnight	Fatty acid loading suppresses glucose metabolism[36]	More reproducible myocardial suppression	Compliance can be difficult
Intravenous unfractionated heparin (15–50 IU/kg administered 15 minutes prior to ^{18}F-FDG injection)	Activates lipoprotein and hepatic lipases ultimately increasing plasma free fatty acid levels[37]	No special preparation necessary	May be contraindicated in some patients

Table 24-6

Sample Foods for High Fat, High Protein, Low Carbohydrate Diet

Foods Allowed	Food to Avoid
Coffee or tea WITHOUT milk/sugar/Splenda	
Sweet'n low (saccharin), Nutra-sweet (aspartame) or Equal (aspartame) is ok	Sugar (glucose, fructose, sucrose, etc.), Splenda (sucralose)
Fatty, unsweetened foods without breading (chicken, turkey, fish, red meat, bacon, fried eggs, meat only sausage)	Milk, cheese
Butter and oils	Carbohydrates (bread, rice, pasta, bagels, cereal, cookies, crackers)
Diet Pepsi or Diet Coke	Nuts, peanut butter Candy, gum, mint, cough drops Vegetables, beans Any kind of sauce other than pure oil Sausage with additives other than meat (e.g., casings containing carbohydrates)

(SA), vertical long axis (VLA), and horizontal long axis (HLA) as well in the standard radiological imaging planes of axial, sagittal, and coronal planes. ^{18}F-FDG uptake in the right ventricle (RV) and atria are evaluated on the fused ^{18}F-FDG emission and the CT transmission images. In individuals with adequate suppression of physiological myocardial glucose uptake, focally increased ^{18}F-FDG uptake with or without corresponding perfusion defects may represent myocardial inflammation. Lack of focal myocardial ^{18}F-FDG uptake may represent noninflamed tissue, including normal myocardium and scar. Patterns of myocardial perfusion and ^{18}F-FDG uptake and their interpretations are summarized in Figure 24-5. In a multivariate analysis, Blankstein et al.[36] found that a pattern of both abnormal perfusion and abnormal FDG had the strongest association with death or VT (Fig. 24-6).

Notably, hibernating myocardium could cause a similar pattern of perfusion–metabolism mismatch. Hence, significant epicardial coronary artery disease needs to be excluded, preferably, by coronary angiography (CT or invasive) or by rest and stress imaging. Indeed, local tissue hypoxia from microvascular perfusion abnormalities related to endothelial dysfunction or microvascular compression from sarcoid granulomas may account for some of the increased myocardial ^{18}F-FDG signal in active sarcoidosis. The limited whole-body ^{18}F-FDG PET/CT can be a valuable adjunct by providing evidence of active extracardiac sarcoidosis (or lack thereof) and potentially identifying a biopsy site. Individuals with sarcoidosis have a twofold higher risk of malignancy[38]; hence, the whole-body images are evaluated also for coexisting undiagnosed malignancy (Fig. 24-7). Knowledge of the normal biodistribution of ^{18}F-FDG is essential to understand normal variants and identify pathological uptake on the whole-body images. The spectrum of extracardiac ^{18}F-FDG PET/CT findings in sarcoidosis is beyond the scope of this text and readers are referred to an excellent review on this topic.[39]

Assessing Response to Treatment

Due to the serious side-effect profile with long-term use of anti-inflammatory medications (steroids, methotrexate, or the novel TNF alfa inhibitors), ^{18}F-FDG is frequently repeated several months after initiation of anti-inflammatory therapy to tailor medication dose. Interval decrease or complete resolution of ^{18}F-FDG uptake in the myocardium, compared to baseline study, could either mean resolution of inflammation or progression to fibrosis. Comparison with myocardial perfusion imaging is very important as a concomitant improvement in perfusion would support resolution of inflammation while worsening perfusion indicates a scar.[40] It is important to recognize that the images are normalized to the

Rest Perfusion	FDG	Frequency	Example Perfusion	Example FDG	Interpretation / Comment
Normal perfusion and metabolism					
Normal	Normal (negative)	32 (27%)	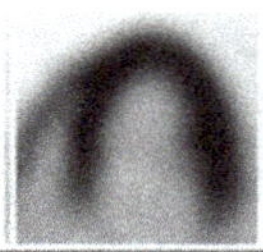	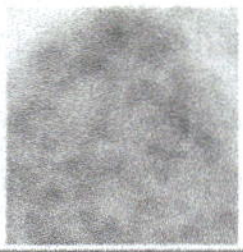	Normal
Normal	Diffuse (non-specific)	15 (12%)	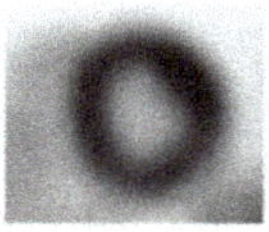	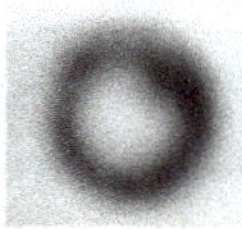	Diffuse FDG most likely due to failure to suppress FDG from normal myocardium
Abnormal perfusion or metabolism					
Normal	Focal	20 (17%)	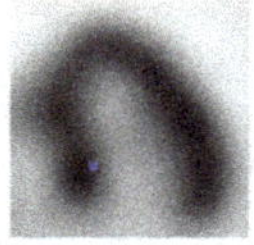	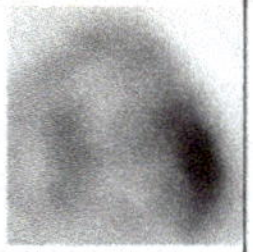	Nonspecific pattern; focal increase in FDG may represent early disease vs. normal variant
Positive	Negative	17 (14%)	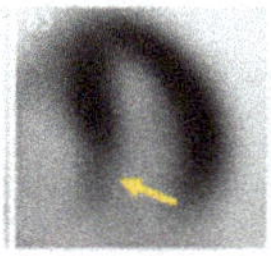	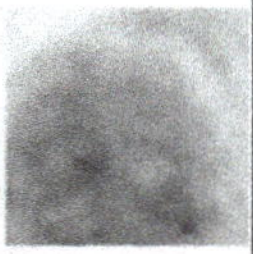	Rest perfusion defect may represent scar from cardiac sarcoidosis or other etiologies
Abnormal perfusion and metabolism					
Positive	Focal increase ("mismatch pattern")	23 (19%)	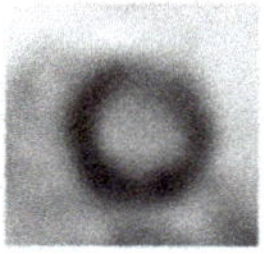	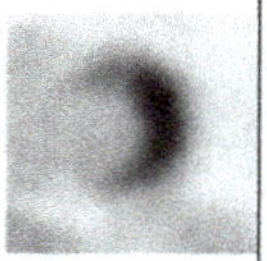	Presence of active inflammation ± scar in the same location
Positive	Focal on diffuse	6 (5%)	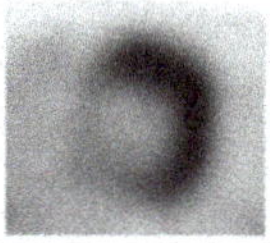	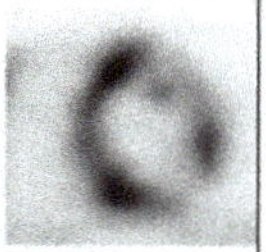	Similar to above but also areas of inability to suppress FDG from normal myocardium vs. diffuse inflammation
Positive	Focal increase (different area)	5 (4%)	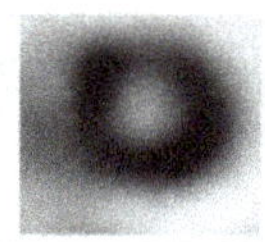	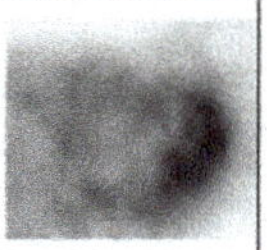	Presence of both scar and inflammation but in different segments

FIGURE 24-5 Normal perfusion and metabolism (Category 1), abnormal perfusion or metabolism (Category 2), abnormal perfusion and metabolism (Category 3). FDG, ^{18}F-fluorodeoxyglucose. (Reproduced with permission from Blankstein R, Osborne M, Naya M, et al. Cardiac positron emission tomography enhances prognostic assessments of patients with suspected cardiac sarcoidosis. *J Am Coll Cardiol.* 2014;63(4):329–336.)

hottest pixel and hence a purely visual assessment could be potentially misleading. Semi-quantitative metrics of standardized uptake value (SUV) (defined as the radioactivity activity concentration [kBq/mL] measured by the PET scanner within an ROI divided by decay-corrected amount of injected radiolabeled ^{18}F-FDG [kBq] per unit patient weight [g]), offer the advantage of absolute quantitation of tissue uptake. That being said, semi-quantitative analyses using SUVmax or SUV mean, though widely used clinically, are influenced by a number of factors,[41] and need further evaluation. With studies performed at

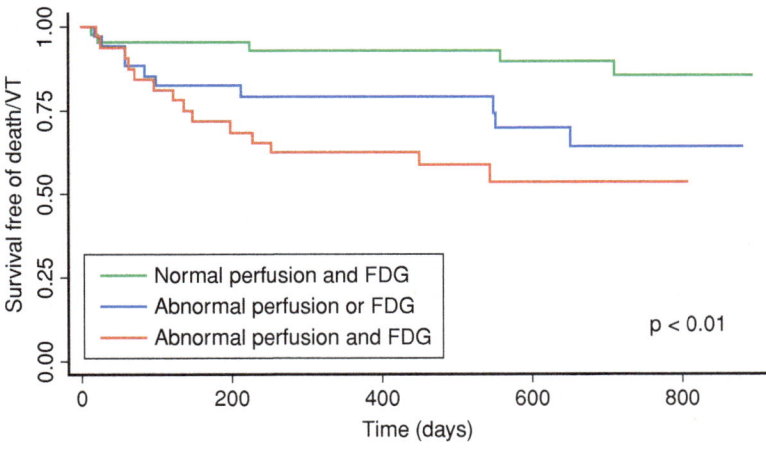

FIGURE 24-6 Survival free of death or ventricular tachycardia (VT) in individuals with suspected sarcoidosis stratified by cardiac ^{18}F-FDG PET and myocardial perfusion imaging results. (Reproduced with permission from Blankstein R, Osborne M, Naya M, et al. Cardiac positron emission tomography enhances prognostic assessments of patients with suspected cardiac sarcoidosis. *J Am Coll Cardiol.* 2014;63(4):329–336.)

the same institution with the same protocol, suggested methods include comparing mean (SUV mean) and maximum SUVs (SUVmax), measuring volume of inflamed tissue using an SUV threshold, and measuring target-to-background ratio comparing myocardial SUV to blood pool or cerebellum as outlined in Table 24-7.

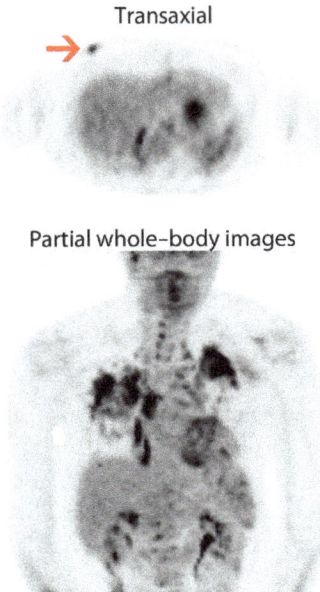

FIGURE 24-7 A 55-year-old man with known pulmonary sarcoidosis was referred for ^{18}F-FDG PET/CT imaging to evaluate for cardiac sarcoidosis activity. The ^{18}F-FDG PET/CT images demonstrated intense uptake in the lungs, myocardium and a focus of intense FDG uptake in the left subareolar region (*black arrow*). Biopsy of the subareolar lesion confirmed active sarcoid granulomas along with breast cancer.

Artifacts and Pitfalls

Several artifacts need to considered in interpreting ^{18}F-FDG PET/CT scans for cardiac sarcoidosis. A major potential pitfall in interpretation is insufficient suppression of physiological glucose utilization by normal myocardium. Diffuse myocardial ^{18}F-FDG uptake is more likely due to insufficient suppression of physiological uptake rather than cardiac sarcoidosis. Likewise, focal increase in ^{18}F-FDG uptake in the lateral wall, especially with normal perfusion in the lateral wall, may represent a normal variant.[36] In these scenarios, one should investigate possible dietary noncompliance, remedy accordingly and repeat the study if needed. Otherwise, only data from perfusion images and any extracardiac evidence of sarcoidosis on the ^{18}F-FDG PET/CT portion of the study can be used for interpretation. As mentioned above, there is evidence that the addition of IV unfractionated heparin to dietary preparation could result in improved suppression and the study can be redone using this protocol, if there are no contraindications to heparin.

Patient motion during image acquisition is another potential cause of artifact and care must be taken to ensure proper motion correction and registration to ensure accurate attenuation correction. Focal hotspots may pose a problem particularly in individuals with intracardiac devices, especially ICD. In those cases both the attenuation-corrected and non–attenuation-corrected images need to be reviewed or metal artifact reduction applied.

Some of these patients may be on corticosteroid therapy which could alter the biodistribution of

Table 24-7
Semi-Quantitative Methods for Assessment of ^{18}F-FDG Uptake

Reference	Method	Advantage
SUVmax[38]	Measure SUVmax in the myocardium using ROI tool	Maximal intensity of inflammation independent of extent
Volume of metabolically active myocardium	VOI tool tissue with uptake above a predefined threshold of SUV[39]	Extent of inflammation can be estimated
Target-to-background ratio	Myocardium to blood pool[40] (left atrium, aorta) Myocardium to liver Myocardium to cerebellum	No need for SUV measurements

^{18}F-FDG. In this case, using target-to-background ratio or ratio of SUV uptake in different organs can be helpful.

Other factors that alter biodistribution such as hyperglycemia and hyperinsulinemia should also be taken into consideration during interpretation. In general, patients with blood glucose >120–200 mg/dL based on various guidelines[42,43] should be rescheduled if possible as altered biodistribution from hyperglycemia could decrease the diagnostic specificity of ^{18}F-FDG PET/CT.

Reporting

The report should include all relevant clinical information (including prior echocardiography, CMR, ^{18}F-FDG PET/CT results, dose and type of anti-inflammatory medications), technique (including imaging protocol, dose of ^{18}F-FDG and uptake period, interval between injection and scan), the quality of the study (including adequacy of suppression of physiological glucose utilization), results of perfusion (including LV size, RV size, tracer uptake, perfusion defects), gated SPECT findings (including rest LVEF, LV volumes, wall motion, RV function), ^{18}F-FDG PET/CT cardiac and extracardiac findings as well as a final impression (presence of myocardial inflammation and concordance with perfusion defects, change from prior, LV function, evidence of extracardiac sarcoidosis).[44]

Conclusions

^{18}F-FDG PET/CT plays a critical role in the diagnosis and treatment of individuals with suspected or known cardiac sarcoidosis. Diagnosis of active inflammation and assessment of response to treatment are the two primary indications for ^{18}F-FDG PET/CT in cardiac sarcoidosis. While ^{18}F-FDG PET/CT is sensitive to detect myocardial inflammation, it is not specific; other noninflammatory or neoplastic processes that increase myocardial glucose utilization or even normal myocardium may exhibit increased ^{18}F-FDG uptake. Further studies are warranted to optimize patient preparation methods to suppress physiological myocardial ^{18}F-FDG uptake and improve the specificity of ^{18}F-FDG PET/CT in cardiac sarcoidosis. Finally, several studies are underway to evaluate more specific radiotracers including somatostatin receptor–binding agents, as well as novel more specific radiotracers for inflammation (^{11}C-PBR28).

^{18}F-FDG PET/CT IMAGING OF CARDIOVASCULAR INFECTIONS

Introduction

Cardiovascular prosthetic material/device infection significantly increases the risk of mortality. In the setting of suspected infection in cardiovascular devices such as prosthetic valves, vascular grafts, and implantable pacemakers/defibrillators, accurate diagnosis can be difficult due to atypical clinical presentations, frequently negative blood cultures, and limitations of anatomical imaging with echocardiography or cardiac CT. Several recent studies have shown the usefulness of ^{18}F-FDG PET/CT in detecting infections associated with devices and grafts as discussed in the recent European guidelines for the management of infective endocarditis.[45–49]

Indications

Pacer/ICDs

^{18}F-FDG PET/CT can be helpful in evaluating patients with suspected infection from an implantable pacer/defibrillator when anatomic imaging studies are uncertain or negative. In a prospective study of 66 patients, ^{18}F-FDG SUV values were found to be helpful in differentiating between active cardiac device infection and normal postoperative inflammatory changes 1 to 2 months' post implantation (SUV-max 4.4 ± 1.6 vs. 1.2 ± 1.4, $p < 0.001$) with a sensitivity of 89% and a specificity of 86%.[48] In the same study, they found that inflammatory changes and residual uptake typically resolve after 6 months. Figure 24-8 shows a proposed diagnostic and treatment algorithm for suspected cardiac device infection.

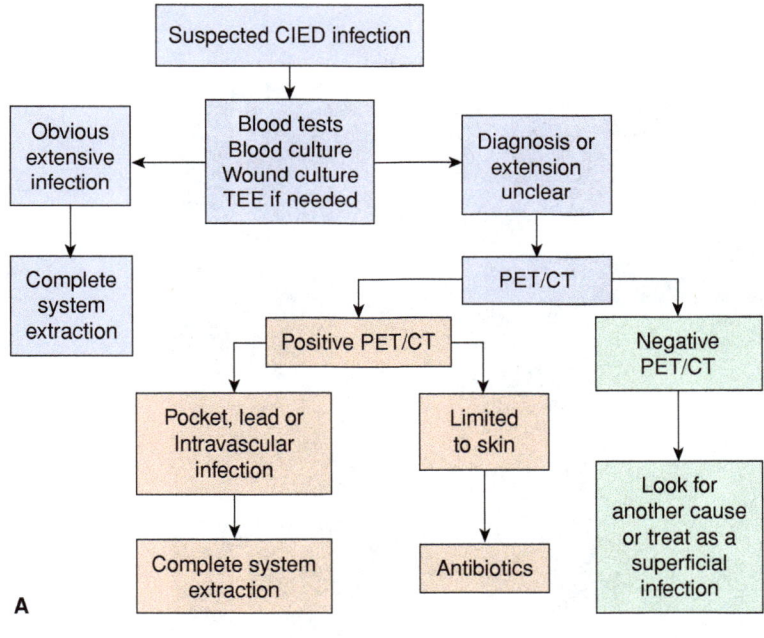

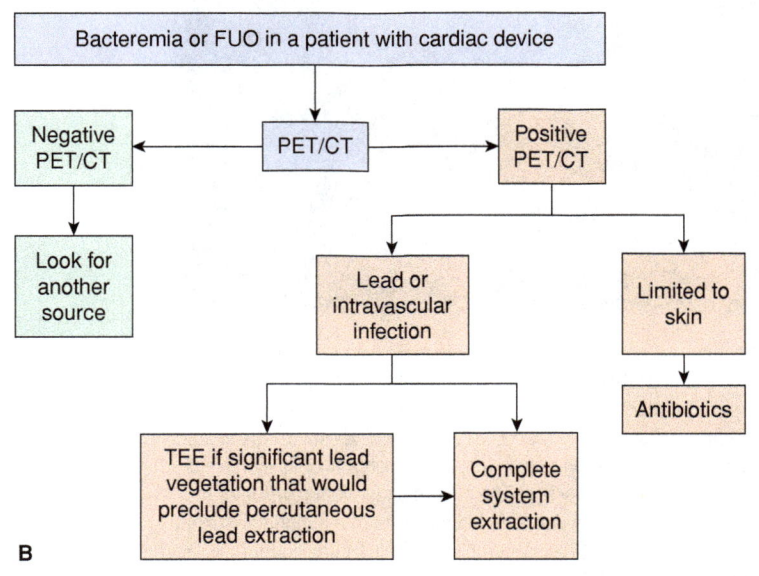

FIGURE 24-8 Proposed algorithms incorporating ^{18}F-FDG PET/CT in the evaluation and management of patients with either initial suspected CIED infection **(A)** or patients with a cardiac device and bacteremia or fever of unknown origin (FUO) **(B)**. CIED, cardiovascular implantable electronic device infection; FUO, fever of unknown origin. (Reproduced with permission from Sarrazin JF, Philippon F, Tessier M, et al. Usefulness of fluorine-18 positron emission tomography/computed tomography for identification of cardiovascular implantable electronic device infections. *J Am Coll Cardiol*. 2012;59(18):1616–1625.)

Left Ventricular Assist Devices

Use of left ventricular assist devices (LVAD) has been increasing due to shortage of donor hearts. They are used both as a bridge to transplant and as destination therapy. Infectious complications in these patients are common with sepsis developing in 42% of patients after 1 year and 52% of patients after 2 years.[19] All areas of the LVAD can be involved (Fig. 24-9). A recent retrospective study of 31 patients (total of 40 studies) with and without external signs of driveline infection showed 100% sensitivity and 80% specificity in detection of LVAD infection. Management was altered by ^{18}F-FDG PET/CT findings in 85% of patients.[44,50] This study also showed decreased FDG uptake related to response to therapy.

Prosthetic Valves

Prosthetic valve endocarditis (PVE) is associated with high morbidity and mortality. The current diagnostic gold standard for infective endocarditis, the modified

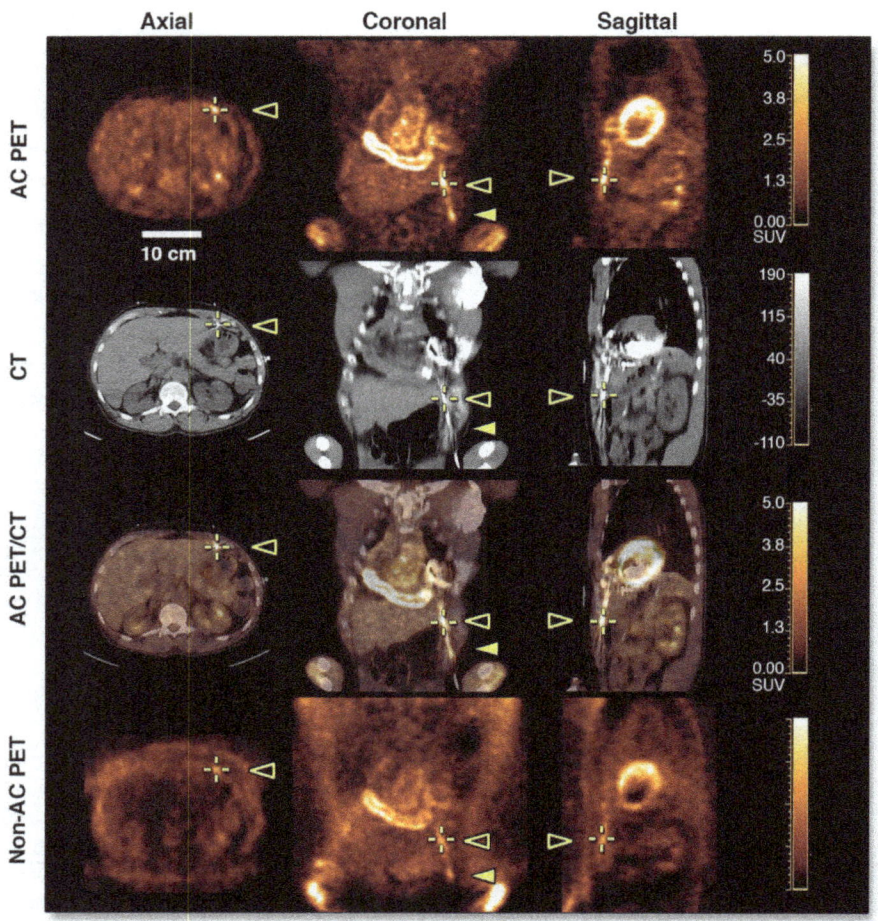

FIGURE 24-9 Driveline LVAD infection. An example of a 45-year-old male patient with familial nonischemic dilated cardiomyopathy status post-HeartWare LVAD implantation. At 6 months after implantation, the patient reported pain, purulent discharge, and nonhealing at the driveline exit site. The driveline culture revealed coagulase-negative *Staphylococcus aureus* and yeast. PET/CT images show intense linear FDG uptake along the driveline (*open arrowhead*) and percutaneous exit (*solid arrowhead*) that is compatible with driveline LVAD infection. The patient underwent revision of the driveline and subsequent urgent heart transplantation due to failed response to antibiotic treatment. (Reproduced with permission from Kim J, Feller ED, Chen W, et al. FDG PET/CT imaging for LVAD associated infections. *JACC Cardiovasc Imaging*. 2014;7(8):839–842.)

Duke criteria,[51] has limited sensitivity in the presence of prosthetic valves.[52] This is in part due to difficulty of echocardiographic assessment in these patients due to acoustic shadowing from the valve and difficulty in detecting small vegetations and abscesses. ^{18}F-FDG PET/CT is particularly helpful for reclassifying patients that fall under the *possible PVE* category under the modified Duke criteria[47] and identifying peripheral embolic and metastatic infectious foci (except in the brain, where high physiological uptake of ^{18}F-FDG may limit visualization of metastatic infectious foci).[45] Pizzi et al.[53] showed that the combination of modified Duke criteria and ^{18}F-FDG PET with cardiac CT angiography compared to cardiac CT without contrast reclassified an additional 20% of cases of possible endocarditis.

Vascular Grafts

Infection of vascular grafts is a serious complication that occurs in 0.5% to 5% of prostheses.[54] No consensus currently exists regarding diagnosis and management but a few studies have found ^{18}F-FDG PET/CT to be useful in diagnosing vascular prosthetic infection, particularly low-grade infections. In a prospective study of 76 patients, focal ^{18}F-FDG uptake and irregular graft boundary were found to be significant predictors of infection.[49]

Imaging Technique

Protocol and patient preparation including diet is identical to ^{18}F-FDG PET/CT for cardiac sarcoidosis.[44] For the whole-body images, scan from head to toes is recommended to evaluate for potential secondary embolic sources of infection. Myocardial perfusion images are not necessary for imaging cardiovascular infection. Imaging with hybrid PET/CT is preferred to localize region of focal ^{18}F-FDG uptake, and imaging with dedicated PET cameras can be challenging to localize the region of abnormal radiotracer uptake. Ideally, whole-body images should be done to also evaluate for potential secondary embolic sources of infection.

Image Interpretation

Assessment/Diagnosis

^{18}F-FDG accumulates in inflamed and infected tissue due to increased intracellular glucose metabolism in inflammatory cells that are responding to the infection (such as leukocytes and macrophages). Infection in general manifests higher SUV values than postprocedural inflammation. However, given the variability of SUV based on different factors there is currently no established cutoff for distinguishing postprocedural inflammation from infection. In general, the further out the PET/CT is from surgery/implantation (particularly >8 weeks), the more likely that the radiotracer uptake represents true infection in the proper clinical setting.

It is very important to evaluate the non–attenuation-corrected images. Devices have relatively higher attenuation than normal soft tissue or myocardium on CT. Attenuation correction with CT tends to overestimate focal radiotracer uptake in areas of high attenuation and artifactually increase tracer uptake in these regions. Non–attenuation-corrected images or metal artifact reduction methods may be used to distinguish inflammation from artifact. In instances where high specificity is desired, radiolabeled white blood cell scanning is recommended.[45]

Extracardiac Findings

As with sarcoidosis, the remainder of the scan should be evaluated for other possible embolic areas of infection or other abnormalities such as undiagnosed malignancy.

Response to Treatment

In general, treatment includes removal of infected devices followed by antibiotic therapy. In rare instances wherein the devices are not removed (e.g., aortic stent, prosthetic material in complex congenital heart disease patients), response to treatment can be evaluated by decreased ^{18}F-FDG uptake in the area of concern (Fig. 24-10). It is recommended to evaluate both the uptake (SUVmax) as well as the target-to-background ratio to account for possible differences in biodistribution between scans.

Artifacts and Pitfalls

Apart from attenuation artifact from the device itself, false-positive findings have been reported in Dacron grafts[48,50] and bland thrombi.[47] Patients who are immunosuppressed or on long-term antibiotics can

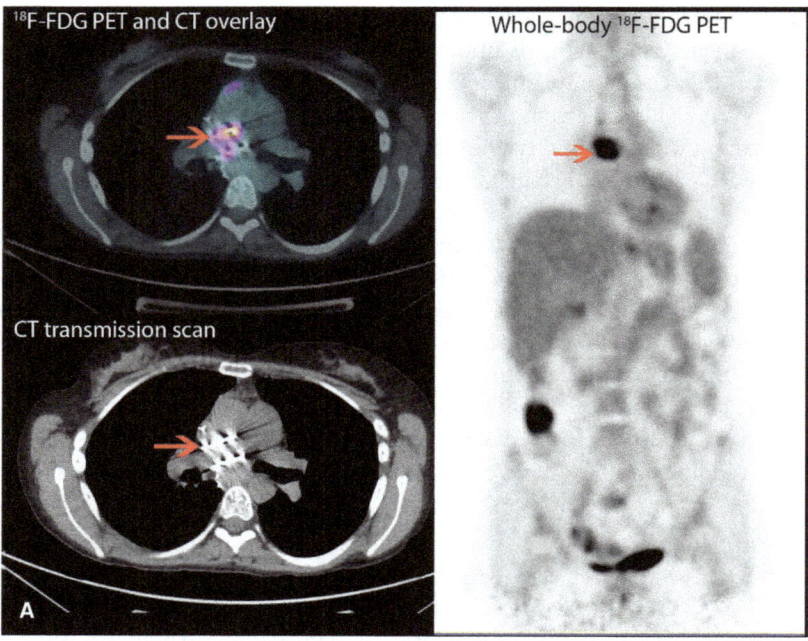

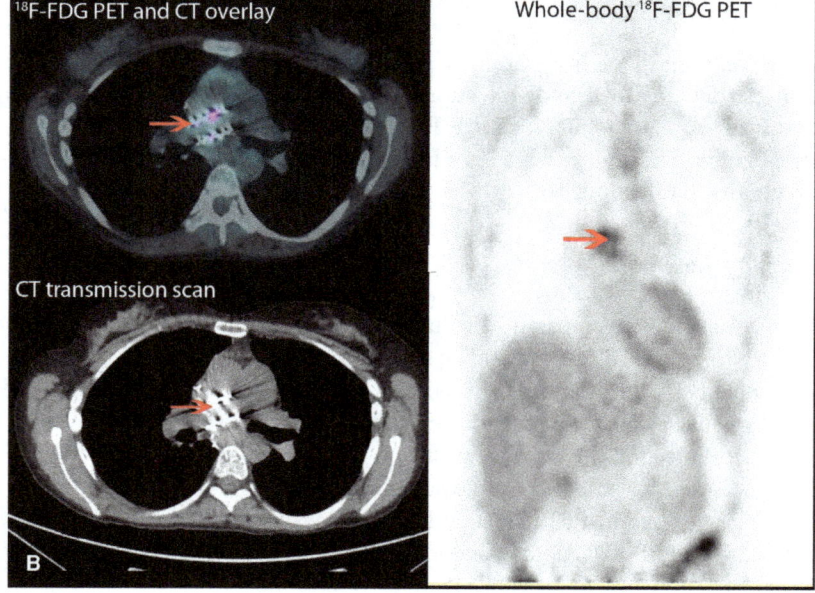

FIGURE 24-10 Pulmonary artery stent infection. An example of a 23-year-old female patient with a history of cystic fibrosis and status post bilateral lung transplant, 5 years prior, was referred to an ^{18}F-FDG PET scan to evaluate for positive blood cultures, a negative transesophageal echocardiogram, and persistent fevers with a clinical suspicion of infection of pulmonary artery stent. Images in panel **A** (before therapy) show focal intense ^{18}F-FDG uptake (SUVmax 10.4) in the region of the pulmonary artery stent (*red arrows*), while images in panel **B** (4 months after successful antibiotic therapy) show a persistent small focus of ^{18}F-FDG uptake (SUVmax 5.9) in the region of the pulmonary artery stent, but is significantly improved compared to baseline.

present as false negative due to relatively decreased immune cells in the region of infection.

Small and mobile infected lesions (endocarditis) may not be detected on ^{18}F-FDG PET/CT due to limited temporal resolution; in those instances a TEE may be superior to identify infection on the leads. Factors that alter biodistribution such as hyperglycemia and hyperinsulinemia should also be taken into consideration during interpretation. In general, patients with blood glucose >120–200 mg/dL based on various guidelines[42,43] should be rescheduled if possible as altered biodistribution from hyperglycemia could decrease the specificity of ^{18}F-FDG PET/CT. Although less of a concern, as with the sarcoid protocol, inadequate myocardial suppression can render a study uninterpretable if the area of concern is close to the myocardium.

Reporting

The report should include the indication, relevant clinical information (including date of surgery/device implantation and medications such as antibiotics or corticosteroids), technique (including type and dose of radiopharmaceuticals), the quality of the study, ^{18}F-FDG PET/CT cardiac and extracardiac findings as well as a final impression (presence of suspicious ^{18}F-FDG uptake, any unexpected findings).[44]

Conclusions

The main strength of ^{18}F-FDG PET/CT is its high sensitivity to detect infection, while its main limitation is its limited specificity. It is not useful in the early postoperative period (4–8 weeks) due to expected postoperative inflammation that could lead to false-positive findings on ^{18}F-FDG PET/CT. Certain types of devices and grafts can also cause false-positive results and low-grade infections can be missed. Development of more specific radiotracers for imaging infection[55] will be useful to improve the specific diagnosis of device infection.

REFERENCES

1. Chiu CZ, Nakatani S, Zhang G, et al. Prevention of left ventricular remodeling by long-term corticosteroid therapy in patients with cardiac sarcoidosis. *Am J Cardiol.* 2005;95:143–146.
2. Houston BA, Park C, Mukherjee M. A diagnostic and therapeutic approach to arrhythmias in cardiac sarcoidosis. *Curr Treat Options Cardiovasc Med.* 2016;18:16.
3. Falk RH, Alexander KM, Liao R, Dorbala S. AL (Light-Chain) cardiac amyloidosis: A review of diagnosis and therapy. *J Am Coll Cardiol.* 2016;68:1323–1341.
4. Rapezzi C, Merlini G, Quarta CC, et al. Systemic cardiac amyloidoses: Disease profiles and clinical courses of the 3 main types. *Circulation.* 2009;120:1203–1212.
5. Mohammed SF, Mirzoyev SA, Edwards WD, et al. Left ventricular amyloid deposition in patients with heart failure and preserved ejection fraction. *JACC Heart Failure.* 2014;2:113–122.
6. Ruberg FL, Berk JL. Transthyretin (TTR) cardiac amyloidosis. *Circulation.* 2012;126:1286–1300.
7. Falk RH, Quarta CC, Dorbala S. How to image cardiac amyloidosis. *Circ Cardiovasc Imaging.* 2014;7:552–562.
8. Bokhari S, Castano A, Pozniakoff T, Deslisle S, Latif F, Maurer MS. (99m)Tc-pyrophosphate scintigraphy for differentiating light-chain cardiac amyloidosis from the transthyretin-related familial and senile cardiac amyloidoses. *Circ Cardiovasc Imaging.* 2013;6:195–201.
9. Castano A, Haq M, Narotsky DL, et al. Multicenter study of planar technetium 99m pyrophosphate cardiac imaging: Predicting survival for patients with ATTR cardiac amyloidosis. *JAMA Cardiol.* 2016;1(8):880–889.
10. Gillmore JD, Maurer MS, Falk RH, et al. Nonbiopsy diagnosis of cardiac transthyretin amyloidosis. *Circulation.* 2016;133:2404–2412.
11. Hutt DF, Quigley AM, Page J, et al. Utility and limitations of 3,3-diphosphono-1,2-propanodicarboxylic acid scintigraphy in systemic amyloidosis. *European Heart Journal Cardiovascular Imaging.* 2014;15:1289–1298.
12. Rapezzi C, Quarta CC, Guidalotti PL, et al. Role of (99m)Tc-DPD scintigraphy in diagnosis and prognosis of hereditary transthyretin-related cardiac amyloidosis. *JACC Cardiovasc Imaging.* 2011;4:659–670.
13. Antoni G, Lubberink M, Estrada S, et al. In vivo visualization of amyloid deposits in the heart with 11C-PIB and PET. *J Nucl Med.* 2013;54:213–220.
14. Lee SP, Lee ES, Choi H, et al. (11)C-Pittsburgh B PET imaging in cardiac amyloidosis. *JACC Cardiovasc Imaging.* 2015;8:50–59.
15. Dorbala S, Vangala D, Semer J, et al. Imaging cardiac amyloidosis: A pilot study using (18)F-florbetapir positron emission tomography. *Eur J Nucl Med Mol Imaging.* 2014;41:1652–1662.
16. Osborne DR, Acuff SN, Stuckey A, Wall J. A routine PET/CT protocol with simple calculations for assessing cardiac amyloid using 18F-Florbetapir. *Frontiers in Cardiovascular Medicine.* 2015;2.
17. Law WP, Wang WY, Moore PT, Mollee PN, Ng AC. Cardiac amyloid imaging with 18F-florbetaben positron emission tomography: a pilot study. *J Nucl Med.* 2016.
18. Coutinho MC, Cortez-Dias N, Cantinho G, et al. Reduced myocardial 123-iodine metaiodobenzylguanidine uptake: a prognostic marker in familial amyloid polyneuropathy. *Circ Cardiovasc Imaging.* 2013;6:627–636.
19. Delahaye N, Dinanian S, Slama MS, et al. Cardiac sympathetic denervation in familial amyloid polyneuropathy assessed by iodine-123 metaiodobenzylguanidine scintigraphy and heart rate variability. *Eur J Nucl Med.* 1999;26:416–424.
20. Noordzij W, Glaudemans AW, van Rheenen RW, et al. (123)I-Labelled metaiodobenzylguanidine for the evaluation of cardiac sympathetic denervation in early stage amyloidosis. *Eur J Nucl Med Mol Imaging.* 2012;39:1609–1617.
21. Tanaka M, Hongo M, Kinoshita O, et al. Iodine-123 metaiodobenzylguanidine scintigraphic assessment of myocardial sympathetic innervation in patients with familial amyloid polyneuropathy. *J Am Coll Cardiol.* 1997;29:168–174.
22. Castano A, DeLuca A, Weinberg R, et al. Serial scanning with technetium pyrophosphate (99mTc-PYP) in advanced ATTR cardiac amyloidosis. *J Nucl Cardiol.* 2015.
23. Dorbala S, Kijewski MF, Park MA. Quantitative molecular imaging of cardiac amyloidosis: The journey has begun. *J Nucl Cardiol.* 2016;23(4):751–753.
24. Perugini E, Guidalotti PL, Salvi F, et al. Noninvasive etiologic diagnosis of cardiac amyloidosis using 99mTc-3,3-diphosphono-1,2-propanodicarboxylic acid scintigraphy. *J Am Coll Cardiol.* 2005;46:1076–1084.
25. http://www.asnc.org/files/Practice%20Resources/Practice%20Points/ASNC%20Practice%20Point-99mTechnetium PyrophosphateImaging2016.pdf. 2016. Accessed November 1, 2016.

26. Tzen KY, Oster ZH, Wagner HN, Jr, Tsan MF. Role of iron-binding proteins and enhanced capillary permeability on the accumulation of gallium-67. *J Nucl Med*. 1980;21:31–35.
27. Love C, Tomas MB, Tronco GG, Palestro CJ. FDG PET of infection and inflammation. *Radiographics*. 2005;25:1357–1368.
28. Depre C, Vanoverschelde JL, Taegtmeyer H. Glucose for the heart. *Circulation*. 1999;99:578–588.
29. Iannuzzi MC, Rybicki BA, Teirstein AS. Sarcoidosis. *N Engl J Med*. 2007;357:2153–2165.
30. Doughan AR, Williams BR. Cardiac sarcoidosis. *Heart*. 2006; 92:282–288.
31. Roberts WC, McAllister HA, Jr, Ferrans VJ. Sarcoidosis of the heart. A clinicopathologic study of 35 necropsy patients (group 1) and review of 78 previously described necropsy patients (group 11). *Am J Med*. 1977;63:86–108.
32. Hulten E, Aslam S, Osborne M, Abbasi S, Bittencourt MS, Blankstein R. Cardiac sarcoidosis-state of the art review. *Cardiovasc Diagn Ther*. 2016;6:50–63.
33. Birnie DH, Sauer WH, Bogun F, et al. HRS expert consensus statement on the diagnosis and management of arrhythmias associated with cardiac sarcoidosis. *Heart Rhythm*. 2014;11: 1305–1323.
34. Ohira H, Tsujino I, Ishimaru S, et al. Myocardial imaging with 18F-fluoro-2-deoxyglucose positron emission tomography and magnetic resonance imaging in sarcoidosis. *Eur J Nucl Med Mol Imaging*. 2008;35:933–941.
35. Tahara N, Tahara A, Nitta Y, et al. Heterogeneous myocardial FDG uptake and the disease activity in cardiac sarcoidosis. *JACC Cardiovasc Imaging*. 2010;3:1219–1228.
36. Blankstein R, Osborne M, Naya M, et al. Cardiac positron emission tomography enhances prognostic assessments of patients with suspected cardiac sarcoidosis. *J Am Coll Cardiol*. 2014;63:329–336.
37. Scholtens AM, Verberne HJ, Budde RP, Lam MG. Additional heparin preadministration improves cardiac glucose metabolism suppression over low-carbohydrate diet alone in 18 F-FDG PET Imaging. *J Nucl Med*. 2016;57:568–573.
38. Bonifazi M, Bravi F, Gasparini S, et al. Sarcoidosis and cancer risk: Systematic review and meta-analysis of observational studies. *Chest*. 2015;147:778–791.
39. Prabhakar HB, Rabinowitz CB, Gibbons FK, O'Donnell WJ, Shepard JA, Aquino SL. Imaging features of sarcoidosis on MDCT, FDG PET, and PET/CT. *AJR Am J Roentgenol*. 2008;190:S1–S6.
40. Skali H, Schulman AR, Dorbala S. (18)F-FDG PET/CT for the assessment of myocardial sarcoidosis. *Curr Cardiol Rep*. 2013; 15:352.
41. Thie JA. Understanding the standardized uptake value, its methods, and implications for usage. *J Nucl Med*. 2004;45: 1431–1434.
42. Jamar F, Buscombe J, Chiti A, et al. EANM/SNMMI guideline for 18F-FDG use in inflammation and infection. *J Nucl Med*. 2013;54:647–658.
43. Surasi DS, Bhambhvani P, Baldwin JA, Almodovar SE, O'Malley JP. (1)(8)F-FDG PET and PET/CT patient preparation: A review of the literature. *J Nucl Med Technol*. 2014;42:5–13.
44. Dilsizian V, Bacharach SL, Beanlands RS, et al. ASNC imaging guidelines/SNMMI procedure standard for positron emission tomography (PET) nuclear cardiology procedures. *J Nucl Cardiol*. 2016;23(5):1187–1226.
45. Habib G, Lancellotti P, Antunes MJ, et al. 2015 ESC Guidelines for the management of infective endocarditis: The Task Force for the Management of Infective Endocarditis of the European Society of Cardiology (ESC). Endorsed by: European Association for Cardio-Thoracic Surgery (EACTS), the European Association of Nuclear Medicine (EANM). *Eur Heart J*. 2015;36:3075–3128.
46. Ricciardi A, Sordillo P, Ceccarelli L, et al. 18-Fluoro-2-deoxyglucose positron emission tomography-computed tomography: An additional tool in the diagnosis of prosthetic valve endocarditis. *Int J Infect Dis*. 2014;28:219–224.
47. Saby L, Laas O, Habib G, et al. Positron emission tomography/computed tomography for diagnosis of prosthetic valve endocarditis: Increased valvular 18F-fluorodeoxyglucose uptake as a novel major criterion. *J Am Coll Cardiol*. 2013;61:2374–2382.
48. Sarrazin JF, Philippon F, Tessier M, et al. Usefulness of fluorine-18 positron emission tomography/computed tomography for identification of cardiovascular implantable electronic device infections. *J Am Coll Cardiol*. 2012;59:1616–1625.
49. Spacek M, Belohlavek O, Votrubova J, Sebesta P, Stadler P. Diagnostics of "non-acute" vascular prosthesis infection using 18F-FDG PET/CT: Our experience with 96 prostheses. *Eur J Nucl Med Mol Imaging*. 2009;36:850–858.
50. Dell'Aquila AM, Mastrobuoni S, Alles S, et al. Contributory role of fluorine 18-fluorodeoxyglucose positron emission tomography/computed tomography in the diagnosis and clinical management of infections in patients supported with a continuous-flow left ventricular assist device. *Ann Thorac Surg*. 2016;101:87–94; discussion 94.
51. Li JS, Sexton DJ, Mick N, et al. Proposed modifications to the Duke criteria for the diagnosis of infective endocarditis. *Clin Infect Dis*. 2000;30:633–638.
52. Habib G, Thuny F, Avierinos JF. Prosthetic valve endocarditis: Current approach and therapeutic options. *Prog Cardiovasc Dis*. 2008;50:274–281.
53. Pizzi MN, Roque A, Fernandez-Hidalgo N, et al. Improving the diagnosis of infective endocarditis in prosthetic valves and intracardiac devices with 18F-fluorodeoxyglucose positron emission tomography/computed tomography angiography: Initial results at an infective endocarditis referral center. *Circulation*. 2015;132:1113–1126.
54. Valentine RJ. Diagnosis and management of aortic graft infection. *Semin Vasc Surg*. 2001;14:292–301.
55. Tsopelas C. Radiotracers used for the scintigraphic detection of infection and inflammation. *Scientific World Journal*. 2015;2015:676719.

SECTION 5

ALTERNATIVE NONINVASIVE TESTING

Hybrid Imaging: SPECT–CT and PET–CT

CHAPTER 25

Patrycja Galazka, Sanjeev A. Francis, and Sharmila Dorbala

INTRODUCTION

There has been a significant growth in hybrid single-photon emission computed tomography and computed tomography (SPECT–CT) and positron emission tomography computed tomography (PET–CT) systems over the past decade, driven in large part by oncologic imaging. A fortuitous byproduct of this has been the development, application, and validation of myocardial perfusion imaging (MPI) using these hybrid systems. Cardiac hybrid SPECT–CT and PET–CT systems offer distinct advantages compared with traditional SPECT or PET MPI. The CT provides for excellent attenuation correction and improves the sensitivity and specificity of MPI, CT-derived coronary artery calcium (CAC) score adds substantial incremental diagnostic and prognostic information to MPI, and hybrid scanners offer the ability to combine a physiologic assessment of perfusion, function, or metabolism with an anatomic assessment of atherosclerosis and structural heart disease. By doing so, hybrid SPECT–CT and PET–CT imaging offers unprecedented opportunities for molecular cardiology research. The primary focus of this chapter is to discuss the clinical applications of hybrid radionuclide MPI with calcium scoring and coronary CTA.

SPECT–CT AND PET–CT

The hardware of SPECT–CT and PET–CT scanners comprises a conventional SPECT scanner or a PET scanner coupled with a CT scanner of various configurations. While all SPECT–CT and PET–CT scanners offer CT-based attenuation correction, calcium scoring (≥4 slice MDCT) and coronary CTA (≥64 slice MDCT) may be performed only on certain hybrid SPECT–CT and PET–CT scanners. Sample hybrid PET–CT and SPECT–CT protocols are shown in Figure 25-1A and B, respectively. The CAC score and/or coronary CTA study can be performed sequentially right before or after the SPECT or PET scan or at a separate setting.

ATTENUATION CORRECTION WITH CT FOR BOTH SPECT AND PET

Attenuation correction using transmission scanning employing external radioactive sources or cardiac CT improves the count uniformity of the image and helps distinguish attenuation artifacts from real defects. It also offers the possibility of stress-only imaging, with potential savings of time, cost, and radiation dose as discussed in more detail in Chapter 9. Also, accurate attenuation correction enables precise measurements of absolute radiotracer concentration in the myocardium making feasible noninvasive quantitative estimation of myocardial blood flow in mL/g/min.

External radionuclide source transmission scans pose some challenges including: (1) degradation of the radionuclide source over time which adversely impacts image quality, (2) longer acquisition time when compared with the CT transmission scans, and (3) a small additional radiation dose (in addition to the emission

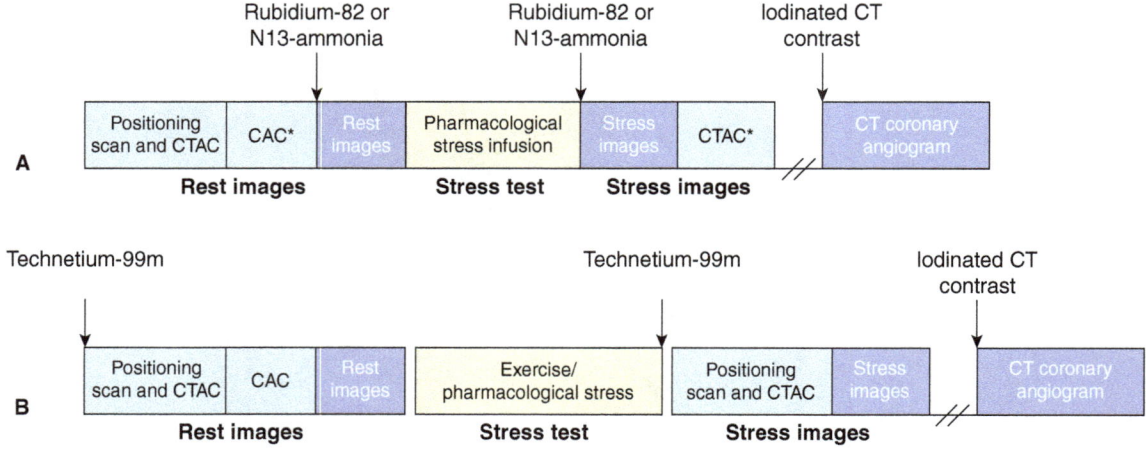

FIGURE 25-1 Sample protocols for PET/CT (Panel **A**) and SPECT/CT (Panel **B**) myocardial perfusion imaging. CTAC, CT for AC (10 mA, 120 keV, nongated free breathing); CAC, calcium score CT scan (300 mA, 140 keV, ECG-gated CT scan with breath hold). *, optional.

scan). CT attenuation correction, on the other hand, is rapid (takes a few seconds) and of excellent quality. SPECT–CT and PET–CT utilize a low-dose x-ray transmission computed tomogram for attenuation correction (CTAC). But, due to inherent differences in image resolution between CT and SPECT or PET MPI, the CTAC and SPECT or PET myocardial perfusion images may be misregistered (not appropriately aligned) resulting in artifacts. Accurate registration is critical for improving the diagnostic yield of CT attenuation-corrected MPI (Fig. 25-2A and B).

SPECT–CT MPI has been validated in patients with and without underlying CAD.[1,2] Multiple studies of SPECT MPI with radionuclide attenuation correction compared with non–attenuation-corrected images demonstrated that test specificity and normalcy are improved while maintaining sensitivity to detect obstructive CAD.[3-6] Importantly, attenuation correction of MPI increases the normalcy rate, a term used to define the percentage of normal studies in a low-risk cohort. Figure 25-3 demonstrates the effect of attenuation correction using a hybrid SPECT–CT system. Recent publications have demonstrated the improved prognostic capability of attenuation-corrected SPECT MPI.[7,8] However, radionuclide attenuation correction with SPECT MPI is not easy to use and widespread clinical adaptation of this technique has been slow.

In contrast, PET MPI with attenuation correction has been widely used clinically (Fig. 25-4) and for research applications, but PET MPI without attenuation correction is significantly degraded by attenuation and is not interpreted clinically or for research purposes.[9] Multiple studies demonstrated the excellent diagnostic[10] and prognostic value[11] of PET MPI. Furthermore, noninvasive quantitative assessment of myocardial blood flow with PET has emerged as a powerful tool to diagnose microvascular dysfunction, follow progression or regression or CAD, and identify localized ischemia, transplant vasculopathy, and balanced ischemia.[9] Absolute myocardial blood flow and coronary flow reserve assessed by PET accurately predicts future adverse cardiovascular outcomes; in particular, a normal coronary flow reserve offers excellent negative predictive value to exclude high risk CAD.[12-15]

CORONARY ARTERY CALCIFICATION AND CORONARY CT ANGIOGRAPHY

Advances in multidetector row CT scanners have tremendously improved the noninvasive diagnosis of CAD using CAC score, coronary CTA, combined imaging of myocardial perfusion and anatomy,[16] as well as CT-derived estimates of fractional flow reserve (CT-FFR).[17] For attenuation correction, low-resolution CT (nondiagnostic CT), 2-slice CT or ≥4-slice multidetector-row CT-based hybrid scanners can be used. For CAC scoring, at least 4-slice CT is required (≥6-slice recommended). For coronary CTA, at least a

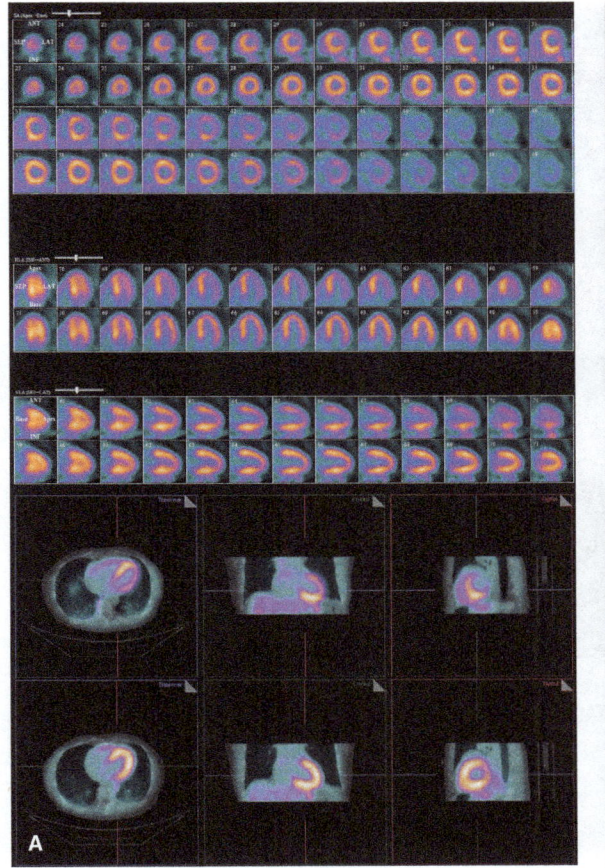
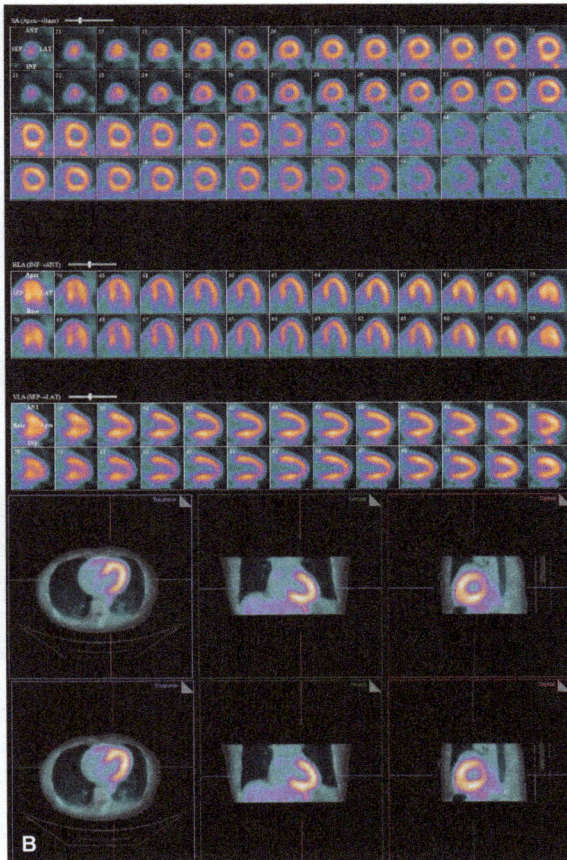

FIGURE 25-2 (**A** and **B**) The top panel demonstrates stress and rest rubidium-82 myocardial perfusion images. The bottom panel shows the overlay of the CT transmission and rubidium-82 emission images. In "**A**," the emission images demonstrate a reversible anterolateral myocardial perfusion defect, and the fusion images demonstrate that the stress transmission and emission images are misregistered. Using software, the transmission and emission images were realigned and the images reconstructed with a new appropriately registered attenuation map, resulting in normal myocardial perfusion images (**B**).

16-slice scanner is required (≥64-slice multidetector-row CT recommended), with imaging capability for slice width of 0.4 to 0.6 mm and temporal resolution of 500 ms or less (≤350 ms is preferred).[18]

Coronary artery calcification is a specific marker of coronary atherosclerosis and a powerful indicator of increased cardiovascular risk (see Chapter 28).[19,20] CAC score in addition to MPI can be of great value both to the clinician and the patient and stimulate further discussions regarding patient's risk factor management.[21] Likewise, extensive literature (as discussed in Chapter 28) supports the role of coronary CTA alone or in conjunction with MPI in the diagnosis and management of individuals with known or suspected CAD. Extensive coronary artery calcification, high or irregular heart rates, and high body mass index may limit the diagnostic accuracy of coronary CTA; ischemia evaluation may provide incremental diagnostic value in those instances. Furthermore, revascularization decisions guided by functional testing with SPECT MPI[22] or invasive fractional flow reserve[23] may improve clinical outcomes.

HYBRID CORONARY CT AND RADIONUCLIDE IMAGING

▶ Hybrid CAC Score and MPI

With hybrid SPECT/CT and PET/CT systems a prospectively gated calcium score scan can be acquired

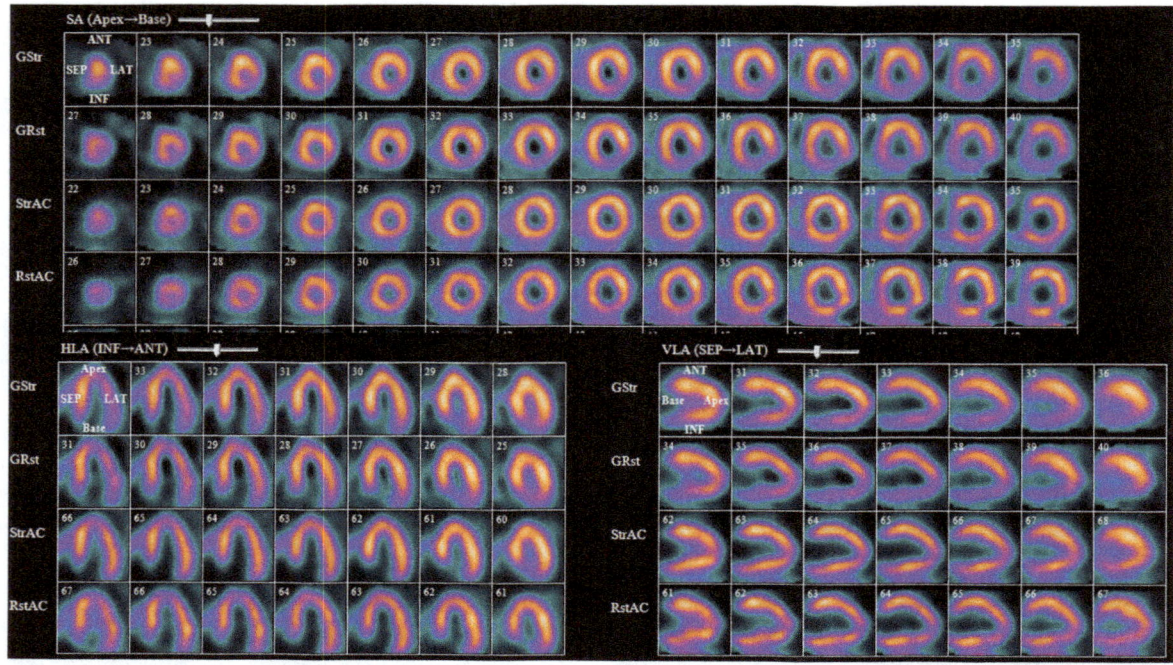

FIGURE 25-3 SPECT CT myocardial perfusion images demonstrating a fixed defect involving the entire inferior wall on the non–attenuation-corrected images (NAC) that resolved with AC (CTAC) suggesting diaphragmatic attenuation on the NAC images.

along with the MPI or the CTAC obtained during PET–CT or SPECT–CT MPI can be visually assessed for coronary artery calcification with good accuracy.[24,25] Several studies wherein subjects underwent both a CAC score study and MPI (at the same setting or at different settings) have demonstrated that subjects with normal MPI may have extensive underlying calcified atherosclerosis, and this finding may influence physicians to prescribe aspirin and lipid-lowering agents.[26] The frequency of ischemia in subjects with Agatston calcium score of >400 is high (>20%)[27–31]; a myocardial perfusion study is considered appropriate among individuals with CAC score >400 or among individuals with high CHD risk and CAC score 100 to 400 independent of symptoms.[32] As with CAC score, investigators[33] have evaluated the diagnostic and prognostic value of a zero CAC score in conjunction with stress SPECT MPI in patients presenting to the emergency room with chest pain. In that study, 0.8% of patients had an abnormal MPI (5/625 patients, four of whom had no CAD on subsequent invasive angiography), and 0.3 event rate (mildly elevated troponin, no cardiac death) over a mean follow-up of 7 months. These authors[33] concluded that most of the patients with chest pain in the ED have a calcium score of 0, which predicts both a normal stress SPECT result and an excellent short-term outcome. A recent meta-analysis by Bavishi et al.[34] confirmed that zero to low CAC scores were infrequently associated with ischemia, but there was a wide variance in the frequency of ischemia among patients with intermediate to high CAC scores (Tables 25-1 and 25-2).

Indeed, the broad range of CAC scores[27–31] among patients with both normal and abnormal perfusion scans in multiple studies, supports the concept that presence of calcified coronary atherosclerosis does not necessarily predict ischemia. Moreover, in subjects without overt CAD, the degree of CAC showed no relation[35] or a weak inverse relation to peak hyperemic myocardial blood flow and coronary flow reserve and direct relation to coronary vascular resistance.[36–38] The results of these studies suggest that CAC score and coronary microvascular function may provide biologically different information and could be complementary for risk assessment.

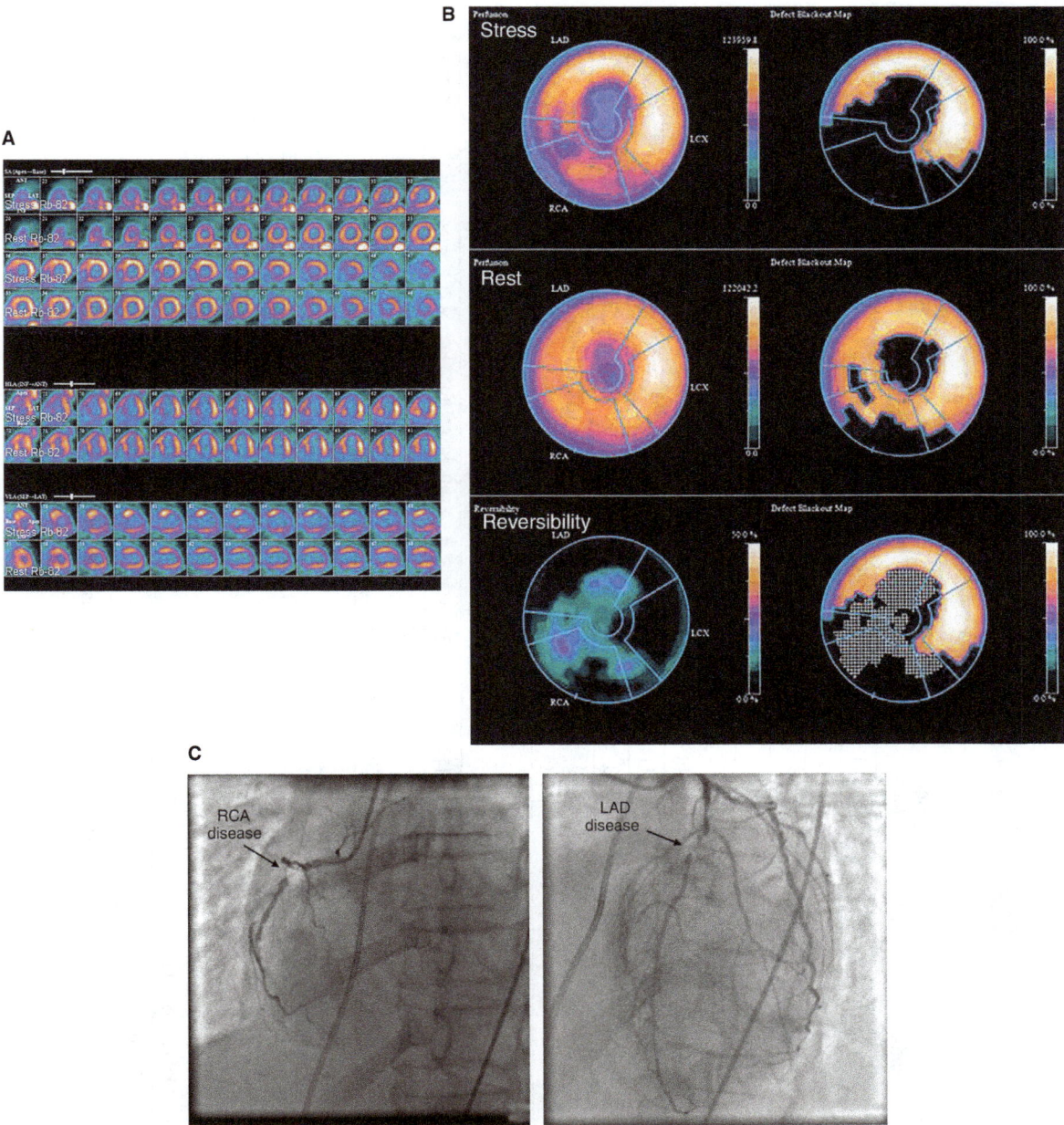

FIGURE 25-4 Dipyridamole stress and rest rubidium-82 PET–CT myocardial perfusion images demonstrate a large-sized and severe perfusion defect in the entire anteroseptal wall, the mid and apical anterior walls, and LV apex that was reversible, consistent with reversibility in the left anterior descending artery (Panel **A**). In addition, there was a medium-sized and severe perfusion defect in the entire inferior wall and the basal inferoseptal wall that was reversible consistent with reversibility in posterior descending artery. There was transient ischemic dilation of the left ventricle (TID ratio = 1.3) and a rest left ventricular ejection fraction of 26% that decreased to 21% during peak stress (high-risk features). Polar plots of perfusion are shown in panel **B**. Coronary angiography demonstrated severe disease in the right coronary artery, left anterior descending artery, and left circumflex artery (Panel **C**).

Table 25-1
A Listing of Studies That Reported on the Prevalence of CAC Score and Myocardial Ischemia

First Author	Year of Publication	Sample Size	Patient Characteristics	Age (years)	Male (%)	HTN (%)	DM (%)	HL (%)	CAC Categories	Ischemia Prevalence (%)
Anand	2004	220	Asymptomatic, suspected CAD	56 ± 11	72	35	30	30	100–399, ≥400	30
Anand	2006	180	Asymptomatic, Type II DM	53 ± 8	61	22	100	62	≤10, 11–100, 101–400, 401–1000, >1,000	31.7
Blumethal	2006	260	Siblings of premature CAD	51 ± 8	38	60	14	38	0, 1–10, 11–100, 101–399, ≥400	18.8
Chang	2015	946	Suspected CAD	58 ± 9	75	50	10	57	0–10, 11–100, 101–400, ≥400	10.9
Estevez	2008	80	Symptomatic, suspected CAD	62 ± 15	39	80	30	38	0, >0	15.5
Fathala	2011	157	Suspected CAD	64 ± 10	60	18	17	16	0, >10	31.8
Ghardi	2013	462	Known or suspected CAD	63 ± 11	68	53	17	40	0, >0	22.9
He	2000	411	Suspected CAD	53 ± 8	69	39	6	54	0, 1–10, 11–100, 101–399, ≥400	19.7
Ho	2007	703	Suspected CAD	59 ± 9	79	48	7	69	0–10, 11–100, 101–400, 401–1000, >1000	7.4
Moser	2003	102	Asymptomatic, suspected CAD	NR	NR	NR	NR	NR	0–100, 101–400, ≥400	18.6
Nishida	2005	83	Symptomatic, suspected CAD	68	66	63	27	48	0, >0	42.2
Piers	2008	531	Suspected CAD	55 ± 11	57	57	12	41	<10, 10–99, 100–399, ≥400	13.9
Ramakrishna	2007	835	Suspected CAD	55 ± 10	77	42	14	67	0, 1–10, 11–100, 101–400, >400	8.3
Rozanski	2007	1153	Suspected CAD	58 ± 10	74	38	8	65	0, 1–9, 10–99, 100–399, 400–999, ≥1,000	5.6
Rosman	2006	126	Asymptomatic, Suspected CAD	59 ± 11	67	39	10	72	0, 1–99, 100–399, 400–999, ≥1000	18.3
Schenker	2008	621	Suspected CAD patients	61 ± 11	40	74	28	54	0, 1–399, ≥400	28.8
Schepis	2007	77	Suspected CAD Patients	66 ± 9	62	73	18	NR	≤10, 11–100, 101–400, 401–1,000, ≥1000	
Scholte	2008	100	Asymptomatic, Type II DM	53 ± 10	65	51	100	53	0, 1–10, 11–100, 101–400, 401–1000, ≥1000	23
Seyahi	2011	35	Renal Transplant	37 ± 11	67	81	6	NR	101–400, ≥400	17.1
Yao	2004	73	Suspected CAD	53 ± 11	NR	NR	NR	NR	0, 1–10, 11–100, 101–399, ≥400	42.5

Reproduced with permission Bavishi C, Argulian E, Chatterjee S, et al. CACS and the frequency of stress-induced myocardial ischemia during MPI: A meta-analysis. *JACC Cardiovasc Imaging.* 2016;9(5):580–589.

Table 25-2
Pooled Prevalence and Odds Ratio for Ischemia by CAC Categories

CAC Categories	Patients (n)	Pooled Prevalence of Ischemia (%)	Range of Ischemia (%)	Pooled Odds Ratio (95% CI)
0	487	6.6	0.0–24.1	Reference
1–100	529	8.5	2.1–50.0	1.7 (1.04–8.2)
101–399	513	10.5	4.0–63.6	3.3 (1.4–8.2)
≥400	594	23.6	12.4–57.1	6.9 (3.5–13.4)

Reproduced with permission Bavishi C, Argulian E, Chatterjee S, et al. CACS and the frequency of stress-induced myocardial ischemia during MPI: A meta-analysis. *JACC Cardiovasc Imaging.* 2016;9(5):580–589.

When combined with SPECT or PET MPI, CAC score provides independent and complementary information about risk of death or myocardial infarction.[30,31] In a previous SPECT study, including a lower-risk cohort with some asymptomatic subjects, and normal MPI, calcium scores did not show an incremental prognostic value over MPI over a mean follow-up of 32 months.[39] In contrast, with a longer follow-up (mean follow-up of 6.9 years), Chang et al.[30] demonstrated that individuals with high calcium score had greater annualized cardiac event rates (3%), despite a normal MPI (Fig. 25-5). The addition of a CAC score to ^{82}Rb perfusion data provided incremental prognostic information in patients with both ischemic and nonischemic perfusion studies.[40] These combined data supports the concept that while a normal relative MPI may indicate excellent short-term prognosis a high CAC score may indicate a worse intermediate-term prognosis despite a normal MPI.

▶ Hybrid Coronary CTA and MPI

Imaging coronary atherosclerosis and its functional consequences with hybrid SPECT/CT and PET/CT

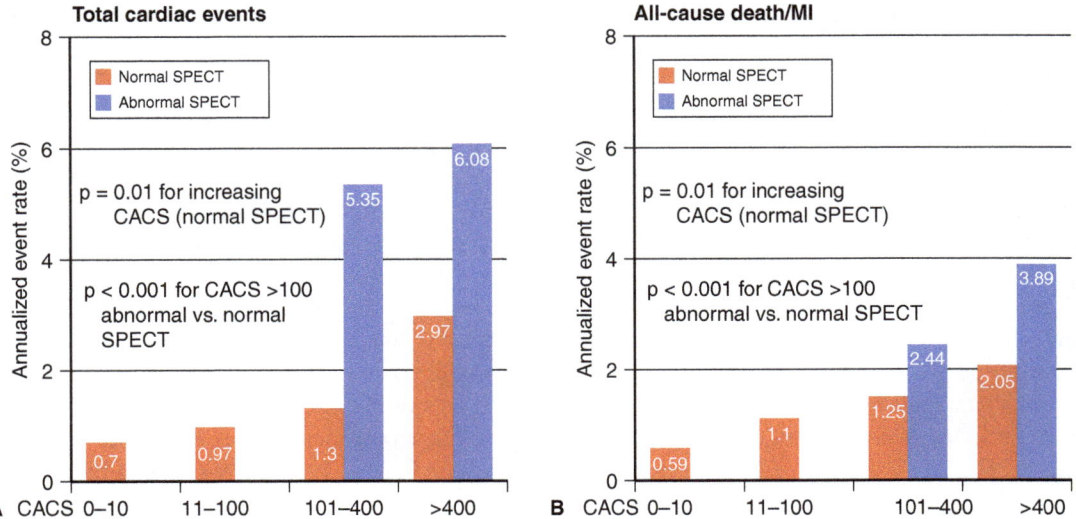

FIGURE 25-5 Adjusted annualized total cardiac death, MI, and coronary revascularization **(A)** and all-cause death/MI **(B)** event rates based on CACS and SPECT results. CACS, coronary artery calcium score; MI, myocardial infarction. (Reproduced with permission from Chang SM, Nabi F, Xu J, et al. The coronary artery calcium score and stress myocardial perfusion imaging provide independent and complementary prediction of cardiac risk. *J Am Coll Cardiol.* 2009;54(20):1872–1882.)

devices in a single or a sequential study is now a reality. When performed on the same day, coronary CTA is typically performed after completion of stress MPI, so that beta-blockers can be administered to slow the heart rate for the coronary CTA without affecting ischemia assessment on MPI. Radionuclide and coronary CTA images can be interpreted independently or together using one of several software options to fuse the images.

The relationship between anatomic assessment of CAD and functional assessment of perfusion is complex. Lesion severity as assessed by coronary angiography does not account for the degree of endothelial dysfunction or the effect of serial stenosis on vascular resistance. Multiple single-center studies with coronary CTA and MPI have demonstrated the relatively poor ability of coronary CTA to predict ischemia on perfusion imaging with a modest PPV ~30%.[41] Similarly, a normal myocardial perfusion scan is a relatively poor discriminator for the presence or absence of nonobstructive CAD.[42] In addition, the extent of CAD can often be underestimated due to reduced heterogeneity of flow in patients with underlying CAD and concomitant endothelial dysfunction. Given the imperfect relationship between anatomic lesion severity and the degree of ischemia, a hybrid approach of radionuclide MPI and coronary CTA may allow for a more comprehensive characterization of CAD burden. However, both coronary CTA and MPI may not be indicated in all patients. A strategy of sequential imaging with initial MPI followed by coronary CTA (if MPI is not normal or severely abnormal) may be considered in subjects with an intermediate to high pretest likelihood. In contrast, an initial coronary CTA followed by MPI (unless the coronary CTA demonstrates normal arteries or critical CAD) may be a better strategy in subjects with low or low intermediate pretest likelihood of CAD. Others have proposed a coronary CTA along with stress MPI. An example of how this hybrid approach can provide useful clinical information is demonstrated in Figure 25-6.

Several studies to date support the notion that both CAC score and coronary CTA offer incremental diagnostic and prognostic information to MPI. A few clinical scenarios wherein a hybrid approach of combined MPI along with coronary CTA may be helpful are: (1) to detect severe multivessel CAD in the setting of mild perfusion abnormalities when the clinical suspicion is high (balanced ischemia); (2) to diagnose microvascular dysfunction in subjects with abnormal MPI by excluding atherosclerosis; (3) to evaluate patients with structural abnormalities of the coronary arteries.[43] Discordant findings on MPI and coronary CTA can result from microvascular dysfunction (abnormal blood flow without obstructive epicardial CAD, calcified and nonobstructive CAD with normal perfusion or obstructive CAD that is not flow-limiting (due to hemodynamic or collateral changes), and imaging artifacts. Therefore, combined MPI and CTA can provide better characterization of the extent and severity of underlying CAD and potential benefit from revascularization than does either technique alone.[18] Indeed, one recent study showed that combining stress-only SPECT with coronary CTA in individuals presenting to the emergency room offers the added advantage of feasibility (no contraindications to SPECT), lower radiation dose when stress-only MPI was used, and higher prognostic value.[44] However, the coronary CTA approach was less costly, and none of the individuals with a 0 calcium score had significant CAD or cardiac event during follow-up.

There is also emerging evidence that diagnostic performance of SPECT or PET MPI and coronary CTA is superior than SPECT/PET MPI or coronary CTA alone (Table 25-3).[45-50] The EVINCI study, a multicenter study, included 292 symptomatic individuals with at least intermediate pretest likelihood of CAD, who underwent coronary CTA and at least one form of ischemia testing and were referred to invasive coronary angiography with an intention of evaluating FFR in intermediate lesions. These patients were followed up for 30 days and coronary revascularization was documented. Invasive coronary angiograms by QCA were considered obstructive with >50% stenosis in the left main or >70% stenosis in any of the other coronary arteries or 30% to 70% stenosis with an FFR ≤0.8. Majority of the individuals (70%) in the EVINCI study underwent SPECT MPI and the rest underwent PET MPI. Overall about 41% of the patients had normal hybrid imaging (MPI and coronary CTA normal) and 24% had a hybrid match (perfusion defect in the territory of a ste-

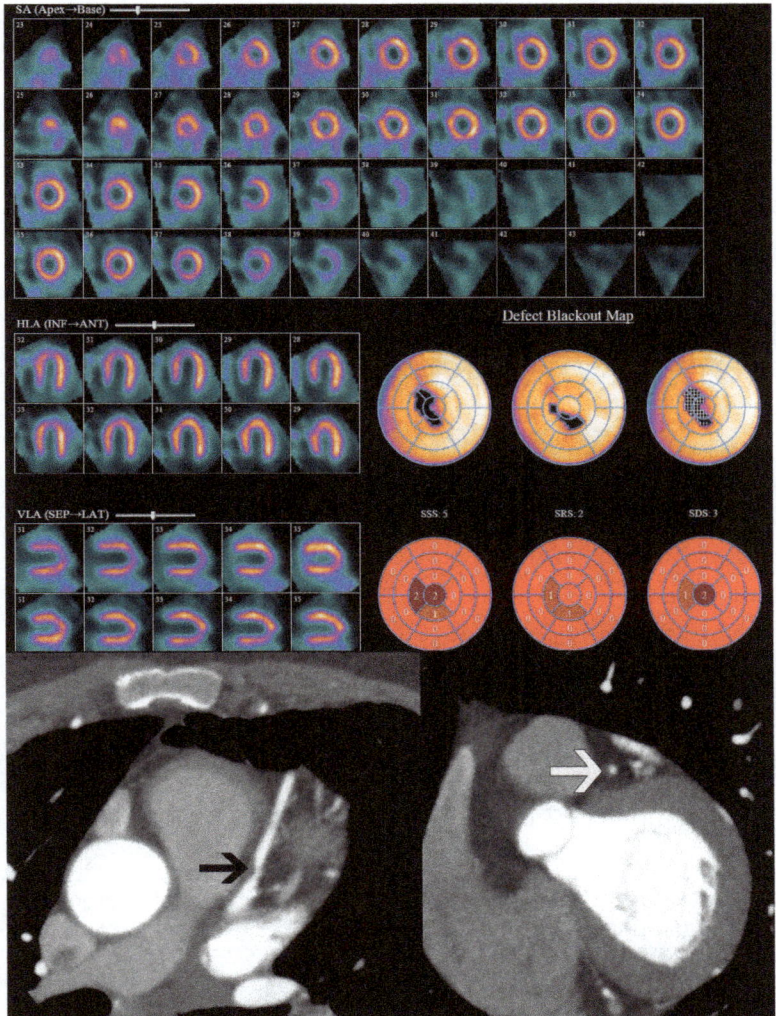

FIGURE 25-6 A 42-year-old female with hypertension and family history of premature coronary atherosclerosis presented with chest pain. Exercise myocardial perfusion SPECT images demonstrated a small defect of moderate intensity involving the apical septum and true apex that is completely reversible. Coronary CT angiogram reveals a noncalcified plaque involving the proximal left anterior descending artery (LAD; *black arrow* in axial plane, *white arrow* on short axis of LAD) with a severe stenosis of >70%. Invasive coronary angiography confirmed severe mid-LAD stenosis (bottom left panel shows long-axis views and the right panel shows short-axis views of the mid-LAD lesion) that was stented successfully.

notic artery). As in prior single-center studies,[51–54] rate of coronary revascularization was highest in the matched group (70%), intermediate in the mismatch group (36%), and least in the normal group (10%), $p < 0.001$. However, radiation dose with the hybrid imaging approach was high (PET/coronary CTA: 9.4 mSv and SPECT/coronary CTA: 18.5 mSv (range 6–31 mSv). Before advocating a combined imaging approach, larger studies with longer-term follow-up are necessary to determine the optimal strategy for hybrid imaging. Whether a combined imaging strategy improves patient outcomes by identification of patients who will benefit from revasculariza-

tion, avoidance of invasive angiography, or improved adherence to optimal medical therapy is still being determined.

▶ **Hybrid Cardiac CT and Radionuclide Imaging**

Cardiac Inflammation and Infection

Hybrid imaging is uniquely suited to localize radiotracer uptake in hotspot radionuclide imaging and for molecular imaging (Fig. 25-7). As discussed in Chapter 24,[18]F-FDG imaging is emerging as a valuable technique to diagnose and manage sarcoidosis and prosthetic valve or cardiac device infection, and provides incremental value to diagnose infective endocarditis in prosthetic valves and intracardiac devices wherein echocardiography, cardiac CT, and cardiac magnetic resonance imaging (CMR) may be inconclusive.

Complex Congenital Heart Disease

Hybrid imaging is well suited for imaging individuals with complex congenital heart disease.[55,56] In addition to improved image quality, and attenuation correct, the CT portion of the PET or SPECT MPI helps

Table 25-3

Diagnostic Accuracy of Integrated MPI and Coronary CTA: Vessel-Based Analysis in Identifying Obstructive CAD on Invasive Angiography

First Author/Year	N	Gold Standard (Definition of Significant CAD)	Sensitivity	Specificity	PPV	NPV	Hybrid Technique
Namdar (2005)[58]	25	Flow limiting coronary stenoses requiring revascularization (ICA + PET)	90	98	82	99	^{13}N-ammonia PET/4 slice CT
Rispler (2007)[46]	56	Flow limiting coronary stenoses (>50% stenosis on ICA and SPECT positive)	96	95	77	99	^{99m}Tc SPECT/16 slice CT
Groves (2009)[59]	33	>50% stenosis on ICA	88	100	97	99	^{82}Rb PET/64 slice CT
Sato (2010)[60]	130	>50% stenosis on ICA	94	92	85	97	^{99m}Tc SPECT/64 slice CT[c]
Kajander (2010)[61]	107	Flow limiting coronary stenoses (>50% stenosis on ICA + FFR)	93	99	96	99	^{15}O-water PET/64 slice CT
Danad (2013)[62]	120	Flow limiting coronary stenoses, CFR (>50% stenosis on ICA + FFR)	72	89	69	90	^{15}O-water PET/64 slice CT
Thomassen (2013)[63]	44	ICA, QCA, 50% stenoses	88	97	85	97	^{15}O-water PET/64 slice CT
Schaap (2013)[a54]	98	Flow limiting coronary stenoses (>50% stenosis on ICA + FFR)	96	95	96	95	^{99m}Tc SPECT/64 slice CT
Dong (2014)[64]	78	ICA/CTA ≥50% with ischemic SPECT defect	89	92	81	96	^{99m}Tc SPECT/16 slice CT
Winther[b] (2015)[65]	138	Flow limiting coronary stenoses (>50% stenosis on ICA)	67	86	57	90	^{99m}Tc SPECT/Dual source CT
Liga (2016)[57]	252	Flow limiting coronary stenoses ([>50% stenosis on ICA] or [30–50% stenosis on ICA and FFR +] and perfusion defect)	83	68	NA	NA	SPECT/PET/CTA

ICA, invasive coronary angiography; FFR, fractional flow reserve; QCA, quantitative coronary angiography; CFR, coronary flow reserve; CTA, CT angiography; PET, Positron Emission Tomography; SPECT, single photon emission computed tomography; Tc, Technetium; Rb, rubidium; CT, computed tomography.
[a]Patient-based analysis.
[b]Prerenal transplant patients, per patient analysis.
[c]Hybrid SPECT/coronary CTA only applied for nonevaluable arteries on coronary CTA.
Data from Gaemperli O, Bengel FM, Kaufmann PA. Cardiac hybrid imaging. *Eur Heart J.* 2011;32(17):2100–2108.

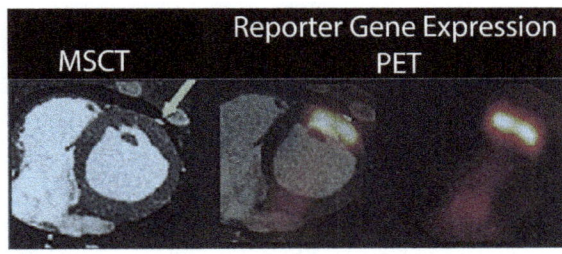

FIGURE 25-7 Positron emission tomography (PET)–computed tomographic (CT) imaging of morphology and biology. In a model of regional adenoviral transfer of the VEGF (121) gene to myocardium of healthy pigs, PET–CT using multiple molecular-directed radiotracers was employed. Representative short-axis tomographic images are shown. On the left is a short-axis image of contrast-enhanced multislice CT showing the location of titanium clip markings. On the right is PET image showing significant accumulation of the reporter probe [^{18}F]fluoro-hydroxymethylbutyl-guanine (FHBG). The middle image (overlay of PET and CT) shows that the FHBG accumulation colocalizes with clip markings in areas expressing the herpes simplex virus 1-sr39tk receptor gene. (Reproduced with permission from Wagner B, Anton M, Nekolla SG, et al. Noninvasive characterization of myocardial molecular interventions by integrated positron emission tomography and computed tomography. *J Am Coll Cardiol.* 2006;48(10):2107–2115.)

distinguish prosthetic material-related perfusion defects from fibrosis.

RADIATION EXPOSURE

Increased utilization of ionizing radiation in medical imaging, in large part attributable to CT scans and nuclear medicine studies, has led to increased scrutiny on the risk of radiation exposure from medical imaging.[57] Therefore, a chapter on hybrid SPECT–CT and PET–CT imaging must include a brief discussion on radiation risk and exposure, which is more completely addressed in Chapters 2 and 7. The estimated effective radiation doses for cardiac imaging studies are: coronary calcium CT 3 mSv, coronary CTA 2 to 18 mSv, ^{99m}Tc-sestamibi 9 mSv, ^{82}rubidium PET 5 mSv, and CT for attenuation correction 0.2 mSv.[31] The addition of a CAC score CT or a coronary CTA to an MPI study will further increase radiation dose.[57] The risk of this radiation exposure must be counterbalanced against the incremental diagnostic and prognostic information gained from the hybrid approach. Recently, measuring the cellular effects of radiation on DNA has emerged as an additional method of assessing radiation risk.[58,59] More research is needed to develop new agents to protect patients from the potential adverse effects of radiation and to decrease the radiation exposure.

SUMMARY

Hybrid SPECT–CT and PET–CT systems offer attenuation-corrected MPI that improves the image quality and diagnostic accuracy compared to non–attenuation-corrected MPI. In addition to attenuation correction, the CT component of hybrid scanners can provide an accurate measure of calcified atherosclerotic burden and additional diagnostic and prognostic information to guide risk factor management, particularly when MPI is normal. Incorporation of coronary CTA with relative stress MPI and quantitative myocardial blood flow imaging is providing an intricate anatomic and physiologic assessment of CAD in each individual patient and offers the potential to guide personalized management of CAD. Hybrid PET–CT imaging with ^{18}F-FDG PET–CT is breakthrough for imaging cardiac sarcoidosis, prosthetic valve and intracardiac device endocarditis, and molecular cardiology research. The ultimate transition to hybrid imaging with stress MPI and coronary CT angiography in clinical practice will be further defined and clarified with large, carefully designed and conducted clinical trials.

REFERENCES

1. Fricke E, Fricke H, Weise R, et al. Attenuation correction of myocardial SPECT perfusion images with low-dose CT: Evaluation of the method by comparison with perfusion PET. *J Nucl Med.* 2005;46:736–744.
2. Masood Y, Liu YH, Depuey G, et al. Clinical validation of SPECT attenuation correction using x-ray computed tomography-derived attenuation maps: Multicenter clinical trial with angiographic correlation. *J Nucl Cardiol.* 2005;12:676–686.
3. Ficaro EP, Fessler JA, Shreve PD, Kritzman JN, Rose PA, Corbett JR. Simultaneous transmission/emission myocardial perfusion tomography. Diagnostic accuracy of attenuation-corrected 99mTc-sestamibi single-photon emission computed tomography. *Circulation.* 1996;93:463–473.
4. Hendel RC, Berman DS, Cullom SJ, et al. Multicenter clinical trial to evaluate the efficacy of correction for photon attenuation and scatter in SPECT myocardial perfusion imaging. *Circulation.* 1999;99:2742–2749.
5. Kluge R, Sattler B, Seese A, Knapp WH. Attenuation correction by simultaneous emission-transmission myocardial

single-photon emission tomography using a technetium-99m-labelled radiotracer: Impact on diagnostic accuracy. *Eur J Nucl Med.* 1997;24:1107–1114.
6. Links JM, DePuey EG, Taillefer R, Becker LC. Attenuation correction and gating synergistically improve the diagnostic accuracy of myocardial perfusion SPECT. *J Nucl Cardiol.* 2002;9:183–187.
7. Baghdasarian SB, Noble GL, Ahlberg AW, Katten D, Heller GV. Risk stratification with attenuation corrected stress Tc-99m sestamibi SPECT myocardial perfusion imaging in the absence of ECG-gating due to arrhythmias. *J Nucl Cardiol.* 2009;16:533–539.
8. Garcia EV, Esteves FP. Attenuation corrected myocardial perfusion SPECT provides powerful risk stratification in patients with coronary artery disease. *J Nucl Cardiol.* 2009;16:490–492.
9. Dilsizian V, Bacharach SL, Beanlands RS, et al. ASNC imaging guidelines/SNMMI procedure standard for positron emission tomography (PET) nuclear cardiology procedures. *J Nucl Cardiol.* 2016.
10. Di Carli MF, Hachamovitch R. New technology for noninvasive evaluation of coronary artery disease. *Circulation.* 2007;115:1464–1480.
11. Dorbala S, Di Carli MF. Cardiac PET perfusion: Prognosis, risk stratification, and clinical management. *Semin Nucl Med.* 2014;44:344–357.
12. Herzog BA, Husmann L, Valenta I, et al. Long-term prognostic value of 26N-ammonia myocardial perfusion positron emission tomography added value of coronary flow reserve. *J Am Coll Cardiol.* 2009;54:150–156.
13. Murthy VL, Naya M, Foster CR, et al. Association between coronary vascular dysfunction and cardiac mortality in patients with and without diabetes mellitus. *Circulation.* 2012;126:1858–1868.
14. Fukushima K, Javadi MS, Higuchi T, et al. Impaired global myocardial flow dynamics despite normal left ventricular function and regional perfusion in chronic kidney disease: A quantitative analysis of clinical 82Rb PET/CT studies. *J Nucl Med.* 2012;53:887–893.
15. Ziadi MC, Dekemp RA, Williams KA, et al. Impaired myocardial flow reserve on rubidium-82 positron emission tomography imaging predicts adverse outcomes in patients assessed for myocardial ischemia. *J Am Coll Cardiol.* 2011;58:740–748.
16. Hulten E, Ahmadi A, Blankstein R. CT Assessment of Myocardial Perfusion and Fractional Flow Reserve. *Prog Cardiovasc Dis.* 2015;57:623–631.
17. Min JK, Leipsic J, Pencina MJ, et al. Diagnostic accuracy of fractional flow reserve from anatomic CT angiography. *JAMA.* 2012;308:1237–1245.
18. Dorbala S, Di Carli MF, Delbeke D, et al. SNMMI/ASNC/SCCT guideline for cardiac SPECT/CT and PET/CT 1.0. *J Nucl Med.* 2013;54:1485–1507.
19. Pletcher MJ, Tice JA, Pignone M, Browner WS. Using the coronary artery calcium score to predict coronary heart disease events: A systematic review and meta-analysis. *Arch Intern Med.* 2004;164:1285–1292.
20. Yeboah J, McClelland RL, Polonsky TS, et al. Comparison of novel risk markers for improvement in cardiovascular risk assessment in intermediate-risk individuals. *JAMA.* 2012;308:788–795.
21. Nasir K, Bittencourt MS, Blaha MJ, et al. Implications of Coronary Artery Calcium Testing Among Statin Candidates According to American College of Cardiology/American Heart Association Cholesterol Management Guidelines: MESA (Multi-Ethnic Study of Atherosclerosis). *J Am Coll Cardiol.* 2015;66:1657–1668.
22. Shaw LJ, Berman DS, Maron DJ, et al. Optimal medical therapy with or without percutaneous coronary intervention to reduce ischemic burden: Results from the Clinical Outcomes Utilizing Revascularization and Aggressive Drug Evaluation (COURAGE) trial nuclear substudy. *Circulation.* 2008;117:1283–1291.
23. De Bruyne B, Pijls NH, Kalesan B, et al; Investigators FT. Fractional flow reserve-guided PCI versus medical therapy in stable coronary disease. *N Engl J Med.* 2012;367:991–1001.
24. Einstein AJ, Johnson LL, Bokhari S, et al. Agreement of visual estimation of coronary artery calcium from low-dose CT attenuation correction scans in hybrid PET/CT and SPECT/CT with standard Agatston score. *J Am Coll Cardiol.* 2010;56:1914–1921.
25. Patchett ND, Pawar S, Miller EJ. Visual identification of coronary calcifications on attenuation correction CT improves diagnostic accuracy of SPECT/CT myocardial perfusion imaging. *J Nucl Cardiol.* 2016.
26. Thompson RC, McGhie AI, Moser KW, et al. Clinical utility of coronary calcium scoring after nonischemic myocardial perfusion imaging. *J Nucl Cardiol.* 2005;12:392–400.
27. Berman DS, Wong ND, Gransar H, et al. Relationship between stress-induced myocardial ischemia and atherosclerosis measured by coronary calcium tomography. *J Am Coll Cardiol.* 2004;44:923–930.
28. He ZX, Hedrick TD, Pratt CM, et al. Severity of coronary artery calcification by electron beam computed tomography predicts silent myocardial ischemia. *Circulation.* 2000;101:244–251.
29. Anand DV, Lim E, Raval U, Lipkin D, Lahiri A. Prevalence of silent myocardial ischemia in asymptomatic individuals with subclinical atherosclerosis detected by electron beam tomography. *J Nucl Cardiol.* 2004;11:450–457.
30. Chang SM, Nabi F, Xu J, et al. The coronary artery calcium score and stress myocardial perfusion imaging provide independent and complementary prediction of cardiac risk. *J Am Coll Cardiol.* 2009;54:1872–1882.
31. Ramakrishna G, Miller TD, Breen JF, Araoz PA, Hodge DO, Gibbons RJ. Relationship and prognostic value of coronary artery calcification by electron beam computed tomography to stress-induced ischemia by single photon emission computed tomography. *Am Heart J.* 2007;153:807–814.
32. Hendel RC, Berman DS, Di Carli MF, et al. ACCF/ASNC/ACR/AHA/ASE/SCCT/SCMR/SNM 2009 Appropriate Use Criteria for Cardiac Radionuclide Imaging: A Report of the American College of Cardiology Foundation Appropriate Use Criteria Task Force, the American Society of Nuclear Cardiology, the American College of Radiology, the American Heart Association, the American Society of Echocardiography, the Society of Cardiovascular Computed Tomography, the Society for Cardiovascular Magnetic Resonance, and the Society of Nuclear Medicine. Endorsed by the American College of Emergency Physicians. *J Am Coll Cardiol.* 2009;53:2201–2229.

33. Nabi F, Chang SM, Pratt CM, et al. Coronary artery calcium scoring in the emergency department: Identifying which patients with chest pain can be safely discharged home. *Ann Emerg Med.* 2010.
34. Bavishi C, Argulian E, Chatterjee S, Rozanski A. CACS and the Frequency of Stress-Induced Myocardial Ischemia During MPI: A Meta-Analysis. *JACC Cardiovasc Imaging.* 2016;9:580–589.
35. Pirich C, Leber A, Knez A, et al. Relation of coronary vasoreactivity and coronary calcification in asymptomatic subjects with a family history of premature coronary artery disease. *Eur J Nucl Med Mol Imaging.* 2004;31:663–670.
36. Curillova Z, Yaman BF, Dorbala S, et al. Quantitative relationship between coronary calcium content and coronary flow reserve as assessed by integrated PET/CT imaging. *Eur J Nucl Med Mol Imaging.* 2009.
37. Naya M, Murthy VL, Foster CR, et al. Prognostic interplay of coronary artery calcification and underlying vascular dysfunction in patients with suspected coronary artery disease. *J Am Coll Cardiol.* 2013;61:2098–2106.
38. Naya M, Murthy VL, Blankstein R, et al. Quantitative relationship between the extent and morphology of coronary atherosclerotic plaque and downstream myocardial perfusion. *J Am Coll Cardiol.* 2011;58:1807–1816.
39. Rozanski A, Gransar H, Wong ND, et al. Clinical outcomes after both coronary calcium scanning and exercise myocardial perfusion scintigraphy. *J Am Coll Cardiol.* 2007;49:1352–1361.
40. Schenker MP, Dorbala S, Hong EC, et al. Interrelation of coronary calcification, myocardial ischemia, and outcomes in patients with intermediate likelihood of coronary artery disease: A combined positron emission tomography/computed tomography study. *Circulation.* 2008;117:1693–1700.
41. Dorbala S, Hachamovitch R, Di Carli MF. Myocardial perfusion imaging and multidetector computed tomographic coronary angiography: Appropriate for all patients with suspected coronary artery disease? *J Am Coll Cardiol.* 2006;48:2515–2517.
42. Di Carli MF, Dorbala S, Curillova Z, et al. Relationship between CT coronary angiography and stress perfusion imaging in patients with suspected ischemic heart disease assessed by integrated PET-CT imaging. *J Nucl Cardiol.* 2007;14:799–809.
43. Di Carli MF. Hybrid imaging: Integration of nuclear imaging and cardiac CT. *Cardiol Clin.* 2009;27:257–263.
44. Nabi F, Kassi M, Muhyieddeen K, et al. Optimizing evaluation of patients with low-to-intermediate-risk acute chest pain: A randomized study comparing stress myocardial perfusion tomography incorporating stress-only imaging versus cardiac CT. *J Nucl Med.* 2016;57:378–384.
45. Gaemperli O, Schepis T, Valenta I, et al. Cardiac image fusion from stand-alone SPECT and CT: Clinical experience. *J Nucl Med.* 2007;48:696–703.
46. Rispler S, Keidar Z, Ghersin E, et al. Integrated single-photon emission computed tomography and computed tomography coronary angiography for the assessment of hemodynamically significant coronary artery lesions. *J Am Coll Cardiol.* 2007;49:1059–1067.
47. Santana CA, Garcia EV, Faber TL, et al. Diagnostic performance of fusion of myocardial perfusion imaging (MPI) and computed tomography coronary angiography. *J Nucl Cardiol.* 2009;16:201–211.
48. Sato A, Nozato T, Hikita H, et al. Incremental value of combining 64-slice computed tomography angiography with stress nuclear myocardial perfusion imaging to improve noninvasive detection of coronary artery disease. *J Nucl Cardiol.* 2010;17:19–26.
49. Slomka PJ, Cheng VY, Dey D, et al. Quantitative analysis of myocardial perfusion SPECT anatomically guided by coregistered 64-slice coronary CT angiography. *J Nucl Med.* 2009;50:1621–1630.
50. Schuijf JD, Wijns W, Jukema JW, et al. Relationship between noninvasive coronary angiography with multi-slice computed tomography and myocardial perfusion imaging. *J Am Coll Cardiol.* 2006;48:2508–2514.
51. Pazhenkottil AP, Nkoulou RN, Ghadri JR, et al. Prognostic value of cardiac hybrid imaging integrating single-photon emission computed tomography with coronary computed tomography angiography. *Eur Heart J.* 2011;32:1465–1471.
52. Pazhenkottil AP, Nkoulou RN, Ghadri JR, et al. Impact of cardiac hybrid single-photon emission computed tomography/computed tomography imaging on choice of treatment strategy in coronary artery disease. *Eur Heart J.* 2011;32:2824–2829.
53. Schaap J, de Groot JA, Nieman K, et al. Hybrid myocardial perfusion SPECT/CT coronary angiography and invasive coronary angiography in patients with stable angina pectoris lead to similar treatment decisions. *Heart.* 2013;99:188–194.
54. Schaap J, Kauling RM, Boekholdt SM, et al. Incremental diagnostic accuracy of hybrid SPECT/CT coronary angiography in a population with an intermediate to high pre-test likelihood of coronary artery disease. *Eur Heart J Cardiovasc Imaging.* 2013;14:642–649.
55. Partington SL, Valente AM, Landzberg M, Grant F, Di Carli MF, Dorbala S. Clinical applications of radionuclide imaging in the evaluation and management of patients with congenital heart disease. *J Nucl Cardiol.* 2016;23:45–63.
56. Grani C, Benz DC, Possner M, et al. Fused cardiac hybrid imaging with coronary computed tomography angiography and positron emission tomography in patients with complex coronary artery anomalies. *Congenit Heart Dis.* 2016.
57. Liga R, Vontobel J, Rovai D, et al; Investigators ES. Multicentre multi-device hybrid imaging study of coronary artery disease: Results from the EValuation of INtegrated Cardiac Imaging for the Detection and Characterization of Ischaemic Heart Disease (EVINCI) hybrid imaging population. *Eur Heart J Cardiovasc Imaging.* 2016;17:951–960.
58. Namdar M, Hany TF, Koepfli P, et al. Integrated PET/CT for the assessment of coronary artery disease: A feasibility study. *J Nucl Med.* 2005;46:930–935.
59. Groves AM, Goh V, Rajasekharan S, et al. CT coronary angiography: Quantitative assessment of myocardial perfusion using test bolus data-initial experience. *Eur Radiol.* 2008;18:2155–2163.
60. Sato A, Hiroe M, Tamura M, et al. Quantitative measures of coronary stenosis severity by 64-Slice CT angiography and relation to physiologic significance of perfusion in nonobese

patients: Comparison with stress myocardial perfusion imaging. *J Nucl Med*. 2008;49:564–572.
61. Kajander S, Joutsiniemi E, Saraste M, et al. Cardiac positron emission tomography/computed tomography imaging accurately detects anatomically and functionally significant coronary artery disease. *Circulation*. 2010.
62. Danad I, Raijmakers PG, Appelman YE, et al. Hybrid imaging using quantitative H215O PET and CT-based coronary angiography for the detection of coronary artery disease. *J Nucl Med*. 2013;54:55–63.
63. Thomassen A, Petersen H, Diederichsen AC, et al. Hybrid CT angiography and quantitative 15O-water PET for assessment of coronary artery disease: Comparison with quantitative coronary angiography. *Eur J Nucl Med Mol Imaging*. 2013; 40:1894–1904.
64. Dong W, Wang Q, Gu S, Su H, Jiao J, Fu Y. Cardiac hybrid SPECT/CTA imaging to detect "functionally relevant coronary artery lesion": A potential gatekeeper for coronary revascularization? *Ann Nucl Med*. 2014;28:88–93.
65. Winther S, Svensson M, Jorgensen HS, et al. Diagnostic performance of coronary CT angiography and myocardial perfusion imaging in kidney transplantation candidates. *JACC Cardiovasc Imaging*. 2015;8:553–562.

ECG Exercise Testing

CHAPTER 26

J. Wells Askew and Todd D. Miller

INTRODUCTION

Exercise electrocardiography testing has been a valuable noninvasive tool for many decades in the evaluation of patients with suspected or known coronary artery disease (CAD) and remains widely utilized. The primary goals of noninvasive stress testing are to aid in the diagnosis of obstructive CAD and to provide risk stratification in an attempt to estimate the probability of myocardial infarction (MI) or death. Although cardiac stress imaging can improve the diagnostic yield and enhance risk stratification beyond exercise electrocardiogram (ECG) variables alone, the standard exercise ECG stress test should play a key role in the evaluation of patients with suspected CAD. The exercise ECG continues to be of great value, especially as the CAD paradigm has shifted from an emphasis on diagnosis to the importance of risk stratification.

It is beyond the scope of this chapter to review the instrumentation, patient preparation, technical considerations, detailed instructions, and interpretation of exercise ECG testing; much of this material is discussed in Chapter 8. Additional information is available for review in prior publications from the American Heart Association.[1-4] As a general rule, exercise testing is most commonly performed on a treadmill using a standardized protocol that incrementally increases both the speed and grade of the treadmill in an attempt to achieve maximal cardiac stress. A variety of exercise protocols have been developed, with the Bruce protocol being the most commonly used. Despite the strong clinical validation of the Bruce protocol, the use of a singular protocol for all patients is not appropriate.

Exercise testing is generally a safe and well-tolerated procedure, yet clinical judgment and appropriate supervision should be employed. Death or MI may occur in up to 1 per 2500 tests.[2,5] Absolute and relative contraindications to exercise testing and indications for the termination of exercise testing are summarized in Chapter 8.[2]

DIAGNOSTIC TESTING

The standard criterion of an abnormal exercise ECG response is ST-segment depression (horizontal or down-sloping) ≥1 mm 80 ms after the J-junction. Using the standard 12-lead ECG, ST-segment depression in lead V_5 has the greatest diagnostic value for CAD, whereas ST-segment depression confined only to the inferior leads is of little value. ST-segment depression does not localize areas of ischemia. ST-segment elevation in leads without Q waves occurs infrequently. This finding represents transmural ischemia and, as a result, localizes ischemia and the culprit vessel. Exercise-induced ST-segment elevation in lead aVR has been utilized to improve detection of left main or ostial left anterior descending artery disease.[6]

It is well recognized that certain drugs (beta-blockers and nitrates) reduce test sensitivity, and resting baseline ECG abnormalities (left ventricular hypertrophy with strain, digoxin effect, and ST-segment depression) reduce test specificity and should be taken into consideration for test interpretation. Bayes' theorem states that the greatest yield of testing for diagnostic purposes occurs in patients who have intermediate (10–90%) pretest probability of CAD. Individuals at the extremes of pretest probability, either very low (younger women with atypical chest pain) or very high (older men with typical angina), derive little benefit from testing. The ACC/AHA Exercise Test guidelines[2] recommend against performing an exercise test for diagnostic purposes in these patient subsets. The ACC/AHA guidelines as well as other organizations generally discourage exercise testing with our without imaging in asymptomatic patients.[7,8]

There are multiple meta-analyses reviewing the diagnostic accuracy of exercise treadmill testing.[2,9–11] Sensitivity is generally in the range of 65% and specificity 80%. It is important to appreciate that these apparent values for sensitivity and specificity have not been corrected for referral bias (also called verification bias). Referral bias is a concept that addresses the preferential referral of patients with positive test results to coronary angiography, the subset of patients in whom sensitivity and specificity are determined. The net impact of referral bias is to artificially inflate test sensitivity and to artificially decrease test specificity. Approaches to overcome referral bias include catheterizing the entire population of patients who undergo evaluation for CAD[12] or adjusting the sensitivity and specificity values by applying mathematical corrections.[13] Posttest referral bias alters not only standard exercise treadmill test (ETT) results, but also stress imaging results.[14,15]

RISK STRATIFICATION

A multitude of valuable prognostic information can be obtained during an exercise ECG test. Variables obtained through the ETT may reflect overall cardiovascular and physical fitness as well as function of the autonomic nervous system. Exercise variables that have been shown to predict outcome include: exercise duration, chronotropic incompetence, heart rate recovery, exercise hypotension, exercise hypertension, and ventricular ectopy.[16,17] Exercise ST-segment depression contains prognostic information but generally is a weaker parameter than these other variables.

Exercise duration has been demonstrated in many studies to be the strongest prognostic variable (Fig. 26-1).[2,18–23] Several studies have demonstrated the relationship of exercise duration to myocardial ischemia and subsequent events. Patients achieving ≥10 metabolic equivalents (METS) have demonstrated a lower prevalence of myocardial ischemia by stress SPECT compared to patients achieving <7 METS and also low rates of nonfatal myocardial infarct (0.7%/year) or cardiac death (0.1%/year).[24,25] Available data on whether exercise hypertension (commonly defined as a systolic blood pressure during exercise >190–220 mm Hg) corresponds to an increased risk of cardiac events are unclear,[26,27] whereas exercise hypotension has been associated with an increased (threefold higher) risk of future cardiovascular events over a 2-year period.[28] Chronotropic incompetence is the failure of the heart rate to increase appropriately with exercise (defined as <80% of the predicted value) and the proportion of heart rate reserve used during exercise can be calculated by the formula: (heart rate^{peak} − heart rate^{rest})/(220 − age − heart rate^{rest}).[17] Chronotropic incompetence has been shown to predict all-cause mortality and cardiac death.[29,30] Impairment of heart rate recovery and heart rate variability have also been shown to predict all-cause mortality and cardiovascular events.[31,32] While sustained episodes of ventricular arrhythmias are uncommon and can be mediated by ischemia, shorter periods of ventricular ectopy (isolated ventricular premature complexes, couplets, or nonsustained ventricular tachycardia) during exercise or in the recovery period occur more often. The prognostic importance of these "short" episodes of ventricular ectopy is uncertain.[33] The relationship between exercise-induced ventricular ectopy, myocardial ischemia, and left ventricular systolic function remains ill defined.

Many prognostic scores have been developed and subsequently validated using combinations of the variables described above. The most commonly used score is the Duke treadmill score that is calculated using three exercise parameters (exercise duration, ST-segment depression, and angina). The Duke treadmill score = exercise time (minutes based on the Bruce protocol) − (5 × maximum ST-segment deviation [in millimeters]) − (4 × exercise angina [0 = none, 1 = non-limiting, and 2 = exercise limiting]). The Duke treadmill score stratifies patients into

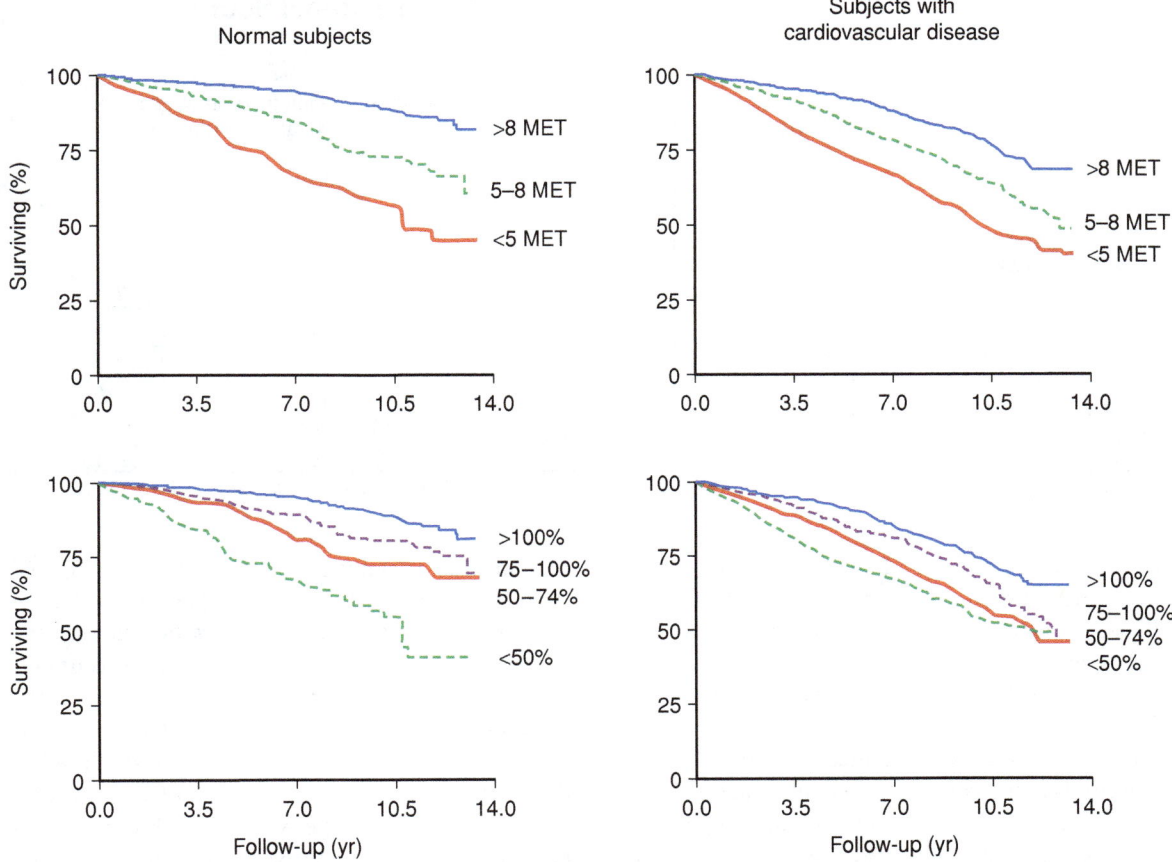

FIGURE 26-1 Survival curves for normal subjects stratified according to peak exercise capacity (*top left*) and according to the percentage of age-predicted exercise capacity achieved (*bottom left*) and survival curves for subjects with cardiovascular disease stratified according to peak exercise capacity (*top right*) and according to the percentage of age-predicted exercise capacity achieved (*bottom right*). The stratification according to exercise capacity discriminated among groups of subjects with significantly different mortality rates—that is, the survival rate was lower as exercise capacity decreased ($p < 0.001$). (Reproduced with permission from Myers J, Prakash M, Froelicher V, et al. Exercise capacity and mortality among men referred for exercise testing. *N Engl J Med*. 2002;346(11):793–801.)

low-risk (score ≥+5, annual cardiovascular mortality 0.25%), intermediate-risk (score +4 to −10, annual cardiovascular mortality 1.25%), or high-risk (score <−10, annual cardiovascular mortality 5%) categories (Fig. 26-2).[34,35] This score was initially developed using the Duke University treadmill database and has subsequently been validated by several other investigators.[36,37] Applying all available prognostic information and not just the three variables that comprise the Duke score enhances the accuracy of risk stratification.[38]

Comparison of ECG–ETT with Stress Imaging

The standard ETT and stress imaging study each has advantages compared to the other (Table 22-1). The major advantage of ETT is lower cost. The charge for an exercise stress SPECT study is approximately five to seven times higher than a standard ETT. Stress imaging does have several advantages over the standard ETT. In patients with significant abnormalities on the resting ECG (left bundle branch block, paced ventricular rhythm, ventricular pre-excitation, and

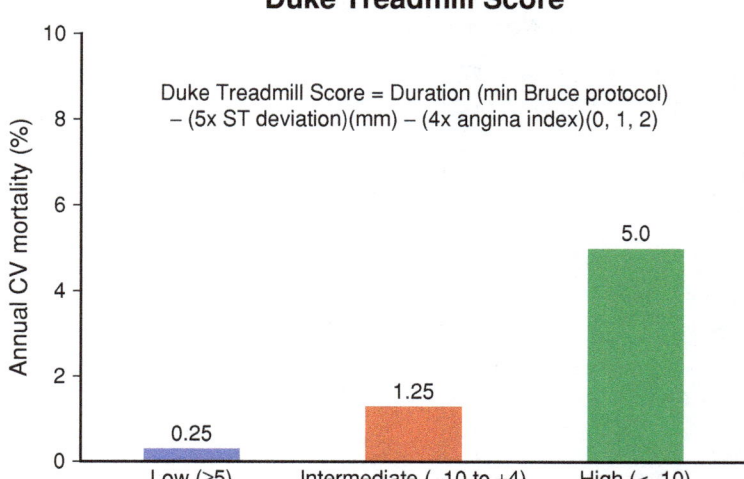

FIGURE 26-2 Duke treadmill score and stratification of outpatients into low-, intermediate-, and high-risk scores with observed annual cardiovascular mortality rates. (Data from Mark DB, Shaw L, Harrell FE, Jr, et al. Prognostic value of a treadmill exercise score in outpatients with suspected coronary artery disease. *N Engl J Med.* 1991;325(12):849–853.)

ST-segment depression ≥1 mm), the stress ECG will be either uninterpretable or inaccurate. Patients with percutaneous coronary intervention (PCI) and/or coronary artery bypass graft surgery (CABG) are more likely to have significant resting ECG abnormalities. In these patients another important clinical issue is localization of ischemia if further revascularization is being considered. Finally, the sensitivity of the stress ECG in patients who undergo pharmacologic stress, especially vasodilator stress, is very low. In these patients pharmacologic stress needs to be combined with imaging. The ACC/AHA guidelines[2,39] acknowledge these issues and recommend that stress imaging preferentially be performed instead of standard ETT as the initial stress modality in the following patients: (1) high pretest probability of CAD; (2) inability to exercise; or (3) significant resting ECG abnormalities.

Many studies have demonstrated that stress imaging also has higher sensitivity[40] and provides incremental prognostic accuracy[36,41–45] compared to the standard ETT. However, these studies did not indicate which subsets of patients benefit or what percentage of the population can be more accurately risk stratified. An important question is whether the standard ETT can identify a subset of patients whose event rate is so low that imaging fails to add additional prognostic information or is not cost effective.

To address this issue, several studies have compared the ability of an approach using just clinical and exercise ECG variables versus an approach using clinical, exercise ECG, and nuclear imaging variables to identify patients with severe (left main and/or three-vessel) CAD at angiography and to predict clinical outcome.[46–49] The study populations were restricted to patients with a normal resting ECG. The rationale for studying only patients with a normal resting ECG was twofold: (1) the majority of patients with a normal resting ECG have normal left ventricular ejection fraction (LVEF) and (2) the exercise ECG is more accurate

Table 26-1

Features of ECG ETT and Stress Imaging

ECG ETT	Imaging
• Lower cost • More widely available • Less influenced by technical processing	• Resting ECG abnormalities (LBBB, paced, ventricular pre-excitation, ≥1 mm ST) • Prior PCI or CABG • Unable to exercise • Higher sensitivity than ETT • Incremental prognostic value over ETT

if the resting ECG is normal. Approximately 95% of patients with a normal resting ECG undergoing evaluation for CAD have a normal LVEF when directly measured by a variety of imaging techniques.[50–53] In addition, in patients with a normal resting ECG, the specificity of the exercise ECG is much higher compared to those with resting ST-T abnormalities.[2]

In a study of 411 patients with a normal resting ECG who underwent exercise SPECT followed by coronary angiography within 6 months,[46] the clinical–exercise ECG–SPECT model correctly reclassified only an additional 14 patients (3% of the study population) for the presence or absence of severe angiographic CAD compared to the clinical–exercise ECG model alone (Fig. 26-3). Importantly, the addition of SPECT failed to identify more patients as high risk who had angiographic severe CAD. A cost-effectiveness analysis employing a conservative approach of Medicare RVUs revealed that the cost of each of these correctly reclassified patients exceeded $20,000. In addition, the follow-up component of this study revealed no difference in event rates between patients categorized as low or high risk by each model. These results are consistent with earlier studies comparing the clinical–exercise ECG-only approach to an approach using clinical–exercise ECG–exercise gated equilibrium radionuclide imaging.[47,49]

A very small number of patients with a normal resting ECG who have a low-risk treadmill score will have a subsequent event (a "false-negative" prognostic treadmill score). To determine if these patients can be identified by SPECT, 1461 patients with these characteristics (normal resting ECG and low-risk Duke treadmill score) who underwent exercise SPECT were followed up for 7 ± 1 years.[48] To further risk stratify this population, a clinical risk score previously demonstrated to predict a patient's risk of both severe angiographic CAD and clinical outcome[54–56] and different from the Diamond–Forrester method that assesses pretest probability of any CAD was applied. The majority (79%) of the population characterized as low risk by the clinical score had good clinical outcome (annual risk of cardiac death <0.5%), regardless of the SPECT image results (Fig. 26-4 [top panel]). In the minority (21%) of the population characterized as high risk by the clinical score, SPECT summed stress score (SSS) prognostic categories could risk stratify these patients.

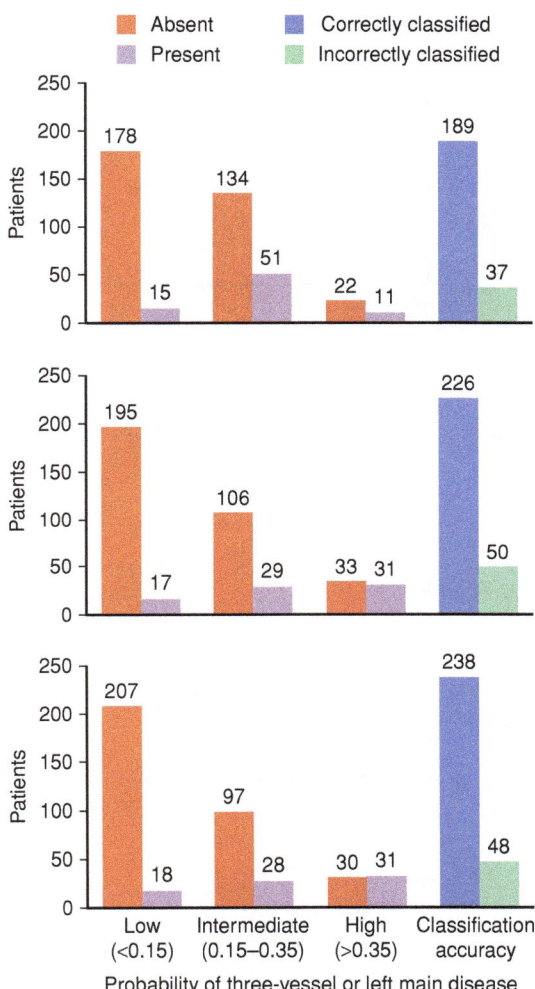

FIGURE 26-3 The anatomical results of patients classified as having a low, intermediate, or high probability of developing three-vessel or left main coronary artery disease by the use of multivariate models. (*Top*) Clinical variables only (diabetes, history of typical angina, sex, and age). (*Middle*) Clinical and exercise variables (heart rate–blood pressure product and the magnitude of exercise ST-segment depression were added independently). (*Bottom*) Clinical, exercise, and thallium-201 variables (the change in global score was added independently). (Reproduced with permission from Christian TF, Miller TD, Bailey KR, et al. Exercise tomographic thallium-201 imaging in patients with severe coronary artery disease and normal electrocardiograms. *Ann Intern Med.* 1994;121(11):825–832.)

Those with low- or intermediate-risk SSS had annual cardiac mortality <1%, whereas in those with high-risk SSS annual cardiac mortality approached 3% (Fig. 26-4 [bottom panel]).

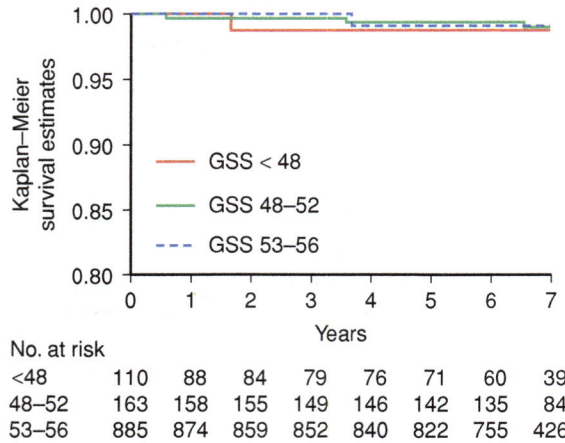

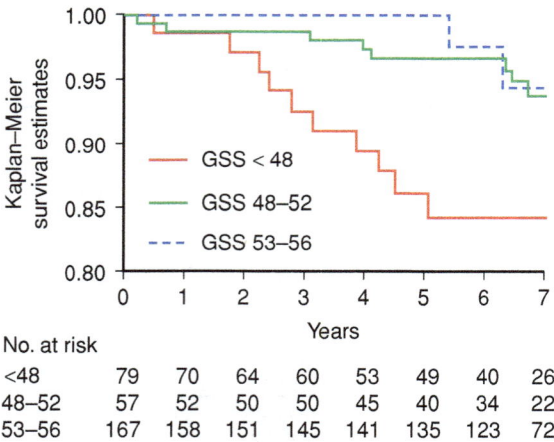

FIGURE 26-4 Survival to cardiac death in the group with a clinical score <5 (*top panel*). Survival to cardiac death in the group with a clinical score ≥5 (*bottom panel*). GSS, global stress score. (Reproduced with permission from Poornima IG, Miller TD, Christian TF, et al. Utility of myocardial perfusion imaging in patients with low risk treadmill scores. *J Am Coll Cardiol.* 2004;43:194–199.)

The results of these studies are generally in agreement with other studies examining this issue.[43,45,57] In a study using SPECT imaging, patients with normal gated SPECT LVEF were at low risk (annual cardiac death rate <1%), even if their SSS was severely abnormal.[57] In a more recent study, SPECT imaging could risk stratify 1136 patients with a normal resting ECG who had a low-risk Duke treadmill score.[43] The annual cardiac death/MI rate in patients with normal SPECT was 0.5% versus 2.9% for mildly abnormal SPECT and 3.5% for moderately severely abnormal SPECT. For patients with a low pretest probability of CAD, however, the cost-effectiveness analysis revealed that the cost per hard event detected by applying SPECT was $211,470.

Other studies suggest that certain patient subsets who are at higher risk on clinical grounds, which includes the "older" elderly (age ≥75 years), might be more effectively risk stratified by using stress SPECT instead of standard ETT.[58] Age is a major determinant of both pretest probability of CAD and risk of experiencing a clinical event. National guidelines recommend that high-risk patients preferentially undergo stress imaging as the initial stress modality.[39] However, specific recommendations addressing age have yet to be incorporated into national guidelines. More work in this field is necessary to clarify if such an approach is cost effective. Women represent an additional patient subset of interest as a result of lower test accuracy of the standard treadmill test, which in part is due to a lower prevalence of CAD in women compared to men. The WOMEN (What is the Optimal Method for Ischemia Evaluation in Women) trial randomized symptomatic women with an intermediate likelihood of CAD to standard ETT or exercise SPECT.[59] The cumulative costs were lower in women randomized to the standard ETT and importantly, the survival free of major adverse events was not significantly different between the groups (98% for ETT vs. 97.7% for exercise SPECT; $p = 0.59$) over 2 years of follow-up.

Additional cost savings may also be possible through using newer stress protocols with SPECT imaging performed as needed. As mentioned earlier, patients achieving ≥10 METS have demonstrated a lower prevalence of myocardial ischemia by stress SPECT compared to patients achieving <7 METS and also low rates of nonfatal myocardial infarct (0.7%/year) or cardiac death (0.1%/year).[24,25] Using the strategy of beginning with a standard ETT in select patients and avoiding SPECT imaging in those patients who achieve ≥10 METS, a satisfactory cardiac workload (usually defined as ≥85% maximal age-predicted heart rate, and without ischemic ST changes during exercise) may result in considerable cost savings when compared to exercise SPECT.[24] If patients were unable to achieve ≥10 METS, had worrisome

Table 26-2

Exercise Treadmill Testing—Appropriate Indications for Testing[a]

Symptomatic or Asymptomatic (without Symptoms or Ischemic Equivalent)
- Low pretest probability for CAD, interpretable ECG, and able to exercise (symptomatic)
- Intermediate pretest probability for CAD, interpretable ECG, and able to exercise (symptomatic)
- High global CAD risk, interpretable ECG, and able to exercise (asymptomatic)

Arrhythmia Evaluation
- Exercise-induced ventricular tachycardia or nonsustained ventricular tachycardia
- Frequent ventricular premature complexes
- Prior to initiation of antiarrhythmic therapy in high global CAD risk patients

Syncope without Ischemic Equivalent
- Intermediate or high global CAD risk

Sequential Testing (≤90 days): Abnormal Test/Study
- Abnormal prior CCTA calcium (Agatston score >100)

Follow-Up Testing (>90 Days): Asymptomatic or Stable Symptoms
- Abnormal prior CCTA calcium (Agatston score >400)

Follow-Up Testing: New or Worsening Symptoms
- Obstructive CAD on invasive coronary angiography
- Abnormal CCTA calcium (Agatston score >100)

Exercise Prescription
- No prior revascularization

Prior to Initiation of Cardiac Rehabilitation (Stand-Alone Indication): Able to Exercise
- Post revascularization (percutaneous coronary intervention or coronary artery bypass graft)
- Heart failure

[a]Appropriate indications for Exercise Treadmill testing based on the ACCF/AHA 2013 Multimodality Appropriate Use Criteria for the Detection and Risk Assessment of Stable Ischemic Heart Disease.

---

exercise-related symptoms, or ECG findings during exercise (i.e., ischemic ST changes or complex ventricular ectopy) then a strategy of SPECT imaging "on-demand" could be utilized with injection of the isotope during exercise followed by a decision regarding the need for subsequent resting SPECT images.

▶ Appropriate Use Criteria and ECG–ETT

The American College of Cardiology Foundation Appropriate Use Criteria (AUC) Task Force in conjunction with the American Heart Association and other societal organizations published appropriateness criteria for noninvasive testing modalities for the diagnosis of or evaluation for stable ischemic heart disease.[60] This multimodality AUC document assigns AUC ratings for exercise ECG as well as adjunct stress imaging modalities for the detection and risk assessment of stable ischemic heart disease patients. The ETT appropriate ratings for a variety of clinical scenarios evaluated in the AUC document are shown in Table 26-2. These AUC are partially consistent with the ACC/AHA Guideline Update for Exercise Testing[2] that address the use of standard ETT versus stress SPECT (Table 26-3). For patients at low pretest probability of CAD with a normal resting ECG who can adequately exercise, the appropriateness criteria document assigns an indication of rarely appropriate for SPECT imaging, based on the rationale that such patients should be evaluated with the standard ETT. For the patient at intermediate or high pretest probability of CAD and otherwise the same characteristics, the appropriateness criteria document assigns SPECT imaging a rating of appropriate.

Table 26-3
Exercise Treadmill Testing

Diagnosing CAD in Symptomatic Patients	2013 AUC for Multimodality of SIHD	2012 SIHD Guideline
Low pretest probability of CAD, interpretable ECG, able to exercise	Appropriate	Class IIa
Intermediate pretest probability of CAD, interpretable ECG, able to exercise	Appropriate	Class I
High pretest probability of CAD, interpretable ECG, able to exercise	May be appropriate	

AUC, appropriate use criteria; SIDH, stable ischemic heart disease.
Data from Fihn SD, Gardin JM, Abrams J, et al. 2012 ACCF/AHA/ACP/AATS/PCNA/SCAI/STS Guideline for the Diagnosis and Management of Patients With Stable Ischemic Heart Disease. *Circulation*. 2012;126(25):e354–471; Wolk MJ, Bailey SR, Doherty JU, et al. ACCF/AHA/ASE/ASNC/HFSA/HRS/SCAI/SCCT/SCMR/STS 2013 multimodality appropriate use criteria for the detection and risk assessment of stable ischemic heart disease. *J Am Coll Cardiol*. 2014;63(4):380–406.

CONCLUSION

The available literature suggests that the standard ETT can effectively detect or exclude the presence of CAD in a large number of patients, as well as successfully identify patients who are at low clinical risk. Numerous studies have demonstrated that annual event rates in these patients who have a low-risk ETT score are well below 1%. SPECT imaging in these patients either fails to identify additional patients who subsequently experience events or the cost of using SPECT to identify the small number of higher-risk patients missed by the standard ETT is prohibitive. Many patients being evaluated for CAD will have low-risk treadmill scores and can be appropriately reassured and will not require additional testing. The very small percentage of patients (most studies suggest <5%) with high-risk treadmill scores are candidates for proceeding directly to coronary angiography. The subset of patients classified as intermediate risk by the treadmill score will often require additional testing, which could include SPECT,[42] for refinement of risk stratification. In these patients this two-step approach of standard ETT followed by SPECT is less convenient than if only SPECT had been performed as the initial test. However, applying the standard ETT in the entire population initially may be a more cost-effective strategy overall, as most patients will be classified as low risk and will not require additional testing. The standard ETT should continue to play a major role in the initial stratification of CAD patients, especially in an area of increasingly constrained financial resources.

REFERENCES

1. Fletcher GF, Ades PA, Kligfield P, et al. Exercise standards for testing and training: A scientific statement from the American Heart Association. *Circulation*. 2013;128(8):873–934.
2. Gibbons RJ, Balady GJ, Bricker JT, et al. ACC/AHA 2002 guidelines update for exercise testing: A report of the American College of Cardiology/American Heart Association Task Force on Practice Guidelines (Committee on Exercise Testing). *Am Coll Cardiol*. http://wwwaccorg/clinical/guidelines/exercise/exercise_cleanpdf 2002. Accessed October 21, 2016.
3. Pina IL, Balady GJ, Hanson P, Labovitz AJ, Madonna DW, Myers J. Guidelines for clinical exercise testing laboratories: A statement for healthcare professionals from the Committee on exercise and cardiac rehabilitation, American Heart Association. *Circulation*. 1995;91(3):912–921.
4. Washington RL, Bricker JT, Alpert BS, et al. Guidelines for exercise testing in the pediatric age group. From the Committee on atherosclerosis and hypertension in children, Council on cardiovascular disease in the young, the American Heart Association. *Circulation*. 1994;90(4):2166–2179.
5. Stuart RJ, Jr, Ellestad MH. National survey of exercise stress testing facilities. *Chest*. 1980;77(1):94–97.
6. Uthamalingam S, Zheng H, Leavitt M, et al. Exercise-induced ST-segment elevation in ECG lead AVR is a useful indicator of significant left main or ostial lad coronary artery stenosis. *JACC: Cardiovascular Imaging*. 2011;4(2):176–186.
7. Greenland P, Alpert JS, Beller GA, et al. 2010 ACCF/AHA Guideline for assessment of cardiovascular risk in asymptomatic adults: A Report of the American College of Cardiology Foundation/American Heart Association Task Force on Practice Guidelines developed in collaboration with the American Society of Echocardiography, American Society of Nuclear Cardiology, Society of Atherosclerosis Imaging and Prevention, Society for Cardiovascular Angiography and Interventions, Society of Cardiovascular Computed Tomography, and Society for Cardiovascular Magnetic Resonance. *J Am Coll Cardiol*. 2010;56(25):e50–e103.
8. Moyer VA. Screening for Coronary Heart Disease With Electrocardiography: U.S. Preventive Services Task Force Recommendation Statement. *Ann Intern Med*. 2012;157(7):512–518.

9. Detrano R, Gianrossi R, Froelicher V. The diagnostic accuracy of the exercise electrocardiogram: A meta-analysis of 22 years of research. *Prog Cardiovasc Dis.* 1989;32(3):173–206.
10. Gianrossi R, Detrano R, Mulvihill D, et al. Exercise-induced ST depression in the diagnosis of coronary artery disease. A meta-analysis. *Circulation.* 1989;80(1):87–98.
11. Kwok Y, Kim C, Grady D, Segal M, Redberg R. Meta-analysis of exercise testing to detect coronary artery disease in women. *Am J Cardiol.* 1999;83:660–666.
12. Froelicher VF, Lehmann KG, Thomas R, et al. The electrocardiographic exercise test in a population with reduced workup bias: Diagnostic performance, computerized interpretation, and multivariable prediction. *Ann Intern Med.* 1998;128(1):965–974.
13. Morise AP, Diamond GA. Comparison of the sensitivity and specificity of exercise electrocardiography in biased and unbiased populations of men and women. *Am Heart J.* 1995;130(4):741–747.
14. Miller TD, Hodge DO, Christian TF, Milavetz JJ, Bailey KR, Gibbons RJ. Effects of adjustment for referral bias on the sensitivity and specificity of single photon emission computed tomography for the diagnosis of coronary artery disease. *Am J Med.* 2002;112:290–297.
15. Roger VL, Pellikka PA, Bell MR, Chow CW, Bailey KR, Seward JB. Sex and test verification bias: Impact on the diagnostic value of exercise echocardiography. *Circulation.* 1997;95(2):405–410.
16. Miller TD. The exercise treadmill test: Estimating cardiovascular prognosis. *Cleve Clin J Med.* 2008;75(6):424–430.
17. Kligfield P, Lauer MS. Exercise electrocardiogram testing: Beyond the ST segment. *Circulation.* 2006;114:2070–2082.
18. Blair SN, Kohl HW, 3rd, Paffenbarger RS, Jr, Clark DG, Cooper KH, Gibbons LW. Physical fitness and all-cause mortality. A prospective study of healthy men and women. *J Am Med Assoc.* 1989;262(17):2395–2401.
19. Roger VL, Jacobsen SJ, Pellikka PA, Miller TD, Bailey KR, Gersh BJ. Prognostic value of treadmill exercise testing: A population-based study in Olmsted County, Minnesota. *Circulation.* 1998;98(25):2836–2841.
20. Ekelund LG, Haskell WL, Johnson JL, Whaley FS, Criqui MH, Sheps DS. Physical fitness as a predictor of cardiovascular mortality in asymptomatic North American men. The Lipid Research Clinics Mortality Follow-up Study. *N Engl J Med.* 1988;319(21):1379–1384.
21. Mora S, Redberg RF, Cui Y, et al. Ability of exercise testing to predict cardiovascular and all-cause death in asymptomatic women: A 20-year follow-up of the lipid research clinics prevalence study. *J Am Med Assoc.* 2003;290(12):1600–1607.
22. Kodama S, Saito K, Tanaka S, et al. Cardiorespiratory fitness as a quantitative predictor of all-cause mortality and cardiovascular events in healthy men and women: A meta-analysis. *JAMA.* 2009;301(19):2024–2035.
23. Myers J, Prakash M, Froelicher VF, Do D, Partington S, Atwood JE. Exercise capacity and mortality among men referred for exercise testing. *N Engl J Med.* 2002;346(11):793–801.
24. Bourque JM, Holland BH, Watson DD, Beller GA. Achieving an exercise workload of > = 10 metabolic equivalents predicts a very low risk of inducible ischemia: Does myocardial perfusion imaging have a role? *J Am Coll Cardiol.* 2009;54(6):538–545.
25. Bourque JM, Charlton GT, Holland BH, Belyea CM, Watson DD, Beller GA. Prognosis in patients achieving ≥10 METS on exercise stress testing: Was SPECT imaging useful? *J Nucl Cardiol.* 2011;18(2):230–237.
26. Allison TG, Cordeiro MA, Miller TD, Daida H, Squires RW, Gau GT. Prognostic significance of exercise-induced systemic hypertension in healthy subjects. *Am J Cardiol.* 1999;83(3):371–375.
27. Lauer MS, Pashkow FJ, Harvey SA, Marwick TH, Thomas JD. Angiographic and prognostic implications of an exaggerated exercise systolic blood pressure response and rest systolic blood pressure in adults undergoing evaluation for suspected coronary artery disease. *J Am Coll Cardiol.* 1995;26(7):1630–1636.
28. Dubach P, Froelicher VF, Klein J, Oakes D, Grover-McKay M, Friis R. Exercise-induced hypotension in a male population. Criteria, causes, and prognosis. *Circulation.* 1988;78(6):1380–1387.
29. Lauer MS, Francis GS, Okin PM, Pashkow FJ, Snader CE, Marwick TH. Impaired chronotropic response to exercise stress testing as a predictor of mortality. *J Am Med Assoc.* 1999;281:524–529.
30. Lauer MS, Okin PM, Larson MG, Evans JC, Levy D. Impaired heart rate response to graded exercise: Prognostic implications of chronotropic incompetence in the Framingham Heart Study. *Circulation.* 1996;93:1520–1526.
31. Dewey FE, Freeman JV, Engel G, et al. Novel predictor of prognosis from exercise stress testing: Heart rate variability response to the exercise treadmill test. *Am Heart J.* 2007;153:281–288.
32. Myers J, Tan SY, Abella J, Aleti V, Froelicher VF. Comparison of the chronotropic response to exercise and heart rate recovery in predicting cardiovascular mortality. *Eur J Cardiovasc Prevent Rehabil.* 2007;14(2):215–221.
33. Beckerman J, Wu T, Jones S, Froelicher VF. Exercise test-induced arrhythmias. *Prog Cardiovasc Dis.* 2005;47(4):285–305.
34. Mark DB, Hlatky MA, Harrell FE, Jr, Lee KL, Califf RM, Pryor DB. Exercise treadmill score for predicting prognosis in coronary artery disease. *Ann Intern Med.* 1987;106(6):793–800.
35. Mark DB, Shaw L, Harrell FE, Jr, et al. Prognostic value of a treadmill exercise score in outpatients with suspected coronary artery disease. *N Engl J Med.* 1991;325(12):849–853.
36. Hachamovitch R, Berman DS, Kiat H, et al. Exercise myocardial perfusion SPECT in patients without known coronary artery disease: Incremental prognostic value and use in risk stratification. *Circulation.* 1996;93(5):905–914.
37. Kwok JM, Miller TD, Christian TF, Hodge DO, Gibbons RJ. Prognostic value of a treadmill exercise score in symptomatic patients with nonspecific ST-T abnormalities on resting ECG. *J Am Med Assoc.* 1999;282(11):1047–1053.
38. Lauer MS, Pothier CE, Magid DJ, Smith SS, Kattan MW. An externally validated model for predicting long-term survival after exercise treadmill testing in patients with suspected coronary artery disease and a normal electrocardiogram. *Ann Intern Med.* 2007;147(12):821–828.
39. Fihn SD, Gardin JM, Abrams J, et al. 2012 ACCF/AHA/ACP/AATS/PCNA/SCAI/STS Guideline for the diagnosis and management of patients with stable ischemic heart disease: A report of the American College of Cardiology Foundation/American Heart Association Task Force on Practice Guidelines, and the American College of Physicians, American

Association for Thoracic Surgery, Preventive Cardiovascular Nurses Association, Society for Cardiovascular Angiography and Interventions, and Society of Thoracic Surgeons. *J Am Coll Cardiol.* 2012;60(24):e44–e164.
40. Fleischmann KE, Hunink MG, Kuntz KM, Douglas PS. Exercise echocardiography or exercise SPECT imaging? A meta-analysis of diagnostic test performance. *JAMA.* 1998;280:913–920.
41. Kwok JM, Christian TF, Miller TD, Hodge DO, Gibbons RJ. Incremental prognostic value of exercise single-photon emission computed tomographic (SPECT) thallium 201 imaging in patients with ST-T abnormalities on their resting electrocardiograms. *Am Heart J.* 2005;149(1):145–151.
42. Gibbons RJ, Hodge DO, Berman DS, et al. Long-term outcome of patients with intermediate-risk exercise electrocardiograms who do not have myocardial perfusion defects on radionuclide imaging. *Circulation.* 1999;100:2140–2145.
43. Hachamovitch R, Berman DS, Kiat H, Cohen I, Friedman JD, Shaw LJ. Value of stress myocardial perfusion single photon emission computed tomography in patients with normal resting electrocardiograms: An evaluation of incremental prognostic value and cost-effectiveness. *Circulation.* 2002;105(7):823–829.
44. Sharir T, Germano G, Kang X, et al. Prediction of myocardial infarction versus cardiac death by gated myocardial perfusion SPECT: Risk stratification by the amount of stress-induced ischemia and the poststress ejection fraction. *J Nucl Med.* 2001;42(6):831–837.
45. Ladenheim ML, Kotler TS, Pollock BH, Berman DS, Diamond GA. Incremental prognostic power of clinical history, exercise electrocardiography and myocardial perfusion scintigraphy in suspected coronary artery disease. *Am J Cardiol.* 1987;59(4):270–277.
46. Christian TF, Miller TD, Bailey KR, Gibbons RJ. Exercise tomographic thallium-201 imaging in patients with severe coronary artery disease and normal electrocardiograms. *Ann Intern Med.* 1994;121(11):825–832.
47. Gibbons RJ, Zinsmeister AR, Miller TD, Clements IP. Supine exercise electrocardiography compared with exercise radionuclide angiography in noninvasive identification of severe coronary artery disease [see comments]. *Ann Intern Med.* 1990;112(10):743–749.
48. Poornima IG, Miller TD, Christian TF, Hodge DO, Bailey KR, Gibbons RJ. Utility of myocardial perfusion imaging in patients with low risk treadmill scores. *J Am Coll Cardiol.* 2004;43:194–199.
49. Simari RD, Miller TD, Zinsmeister AR, Gibbons RJ. Capabilities of supine exercise electrocardiography versus exercise radionuclide angiography in predicting coronary events. *Am J Cardiol.* 1991;67(7):573–537.
50. Christian TF, Miller TD, Chareonthaitawee P, Hodge DO, O'Connor MK, Gibbons RJ. Prevalence of normal resting left ventricular function with normal rest electrocardiograms. *Am J Cardiol.* 1997;79(9):1295–1298.
51. O'Keefe JH, Jr, Zinsmeister AR, Gibbons RJ. Value of normal electrocardiographic findings in predicting resting left ventricular function in patients with chest pain and suspected coronary artery disease. *Am J Med.* 1989;86(6 Pt 1):658–662.
52. Rihal CS, Davis KB, Ward Kennedy J, Gersh BJ. The utility of clinical, electrocardiographic, and roentgenographic variables in the prediction of left ventricular function. *Am J Cardiol.* 1995;75(4):220–223.
53. Talreja D, Gruver C, Sklenar J, Dent J, Kaul S. Efficient utilization of echocardiography for the assessment of left ventricular systolic function. *Am Heart J.* 2000;139(3):394–398.
54. Hubbard BL, Gibbons RJ, Lapeyre AC, III, Zinsmeister AR, Clements IP. Identification of severe coronary artery disease using simple clinical parameters. *Arch Intern Med.* 1992;152:309–312.
55. Ho KT, Miller TD, Hodge DO, Bailey KR, Gibbons RJ. Use of a simple clinical score to predict prognosis of patients with normal or mildly abnormal resting electrocardiographic findings undergoing evaluation for coronary artery disease. *Mayo Clin Proc.* 2002;77:515–521.
56. Miller TD, Roger VL, Hodge DO, Gibbons RJ. A simple clinical score accurately predicts outcome in a community-based population undergoing stress testing. *Am J Med.* 2005;118(8):866–872.
57. Sharir T, Germano G, Kavanagh PB, et al. Incremental prognostic value of post-stress left ventricular ejection fraction and volume by gated myocardial perfusion single photon emission computed tomography. *Circulation.* 1999;100(10):1035–1042.
58. Valeti US, Miller TD, Hodge DO, Gibbons RJ. Exercise single-photon emission computed tomography provides effective risk stratification of elderly men and elderly women. *Circulation.* 2005;111:1771–1776.
59. Shaw LJ, Mieres JH, Hendel RH, et al. Comparative effectiveness of exercise electrocardiography with or without myocardial perfusion single photon emission computed tomography in women with suspected coronary artery disease: Results from the what is the optimal method for ischemia evaluation in women (women) trial. *Circulation.* 2011;124(11):1239–1249.
60. Wolk MJ, Bailey SR, Doherty JU, et al. ACCF/AHA/ASE/ASNC/HFSA/HRS/SCAI/SCCT/SCMR/STS 2013 multimodality appropriate use criteria for the detection and risk assessment of stable ischemic heart disease: A report of the American College of Cardiology Foundation Appropriate Use Criteria Task Force, American Heart Association, American Society of Echocardiography, American Society of Nuclear Cardiology, Heart Failure Society of America, Heart Rhythm Society, Society for Cardiovascular Angiography and Interventions, Society of Cardiovascular Computed Tomography, Society for Cardiovascular Magnetic Resonance, and Society of Thoracic Surgeons. *J Am Coll Cardiol.* 2014;63(4):380–406.

Echocardiography

CHAPTER 27

Zeina Ibrahim, Elizabeth A. Grier, and Vera H. Rigolin

INTRODUCTION

Echocardiography is a widely used cardiac imaging modality that is often the first-choice test for assessing cardiac structure and function. It provides a detailed structural assessment of the myocardium, valves, pericardium, and portions of the surrounding vasculature, which includes the thoracic aorta, pulmonary artery, pulmonary veins, inferior vena cava, and superior vena cava. With real-time evaluation, echocardiography provides an assessment of the systolic and diastolic function of the myocardium, as well as a measurement of intracardiac hemodynamics and the severity of valvular disease. Compared to other cardiac imaging modalities, echocardiography is relatively less expensive, does not expose the patient to ionizing radiation, and is generally well tolerated by the patient.

The two primary echocardiographic techniques include transthoracic echocardiography (TTE) and transesophageal echocardiography (TEE). With TTE, the ultrasound probe is placed on the patient's chest and several views of the heart are obtained from various angles. In TEE, a flexible ultrasound transducer is introduced into the esophagus and can be rotated or flexed at varying levels in the esophagus to allow for imaging of the cardiac structures. Compared to TTE, TEE has better image quality for posterior cardiac structures due to the closer proximity of the transducer to the heart. TEE is especially useful in the evaluation of endocarditis, valvular dysfunction, and interatrial septal defects.[1] Since its introduction to clinical medicine, echocardiograpjy has undergone significant technological advances. As a result, echocardiography is an essential imaging tool in clinical medicine.

Echocardiographic images are obtained with an ultrasound transducer which emits sound waves that are transmitted through the internal structures and then reflected back to the transducer to create an image.[2] In standard TTE, the available modalities include M mode, two-dimensional (2D), and three-dimensional (3D). M mode is the most basic method which evaluates cardiac structures in a one-dimensional (1D) view along a single-scan line, which places depth on the y-axis and time on the x-axis. This is ideal for making fine linear measurements. M mode also has excellent temporal and spatial resolution and is thus useful to assess motion and timing.[2] 2D is the most utilized echocardiographic modality, and produces cross-sectional images of the heart by emitting numerous signals that are repeatedly generated to create moving images in real time. The most common standard 2D views are the parasternal long-axis, parasternal short-axis, and the apical and subcostal views (Fig. 27-1). Off-axis imaging may then be necessary to evaluate more complex structures. Newer machines are also able to generate 3D images of the cardiac structures through the use of matrix-array transducers to provide detailed structural assessments.[3] Compared to 2D echocardiography, 3D imaging provides more accurate quantification of ventricular volumes (Fig. 27-2), generates unique views of valve structures (Fig. 27-3), and demonstrates improved visualization of spatial relationships between cardiac structures.[3]

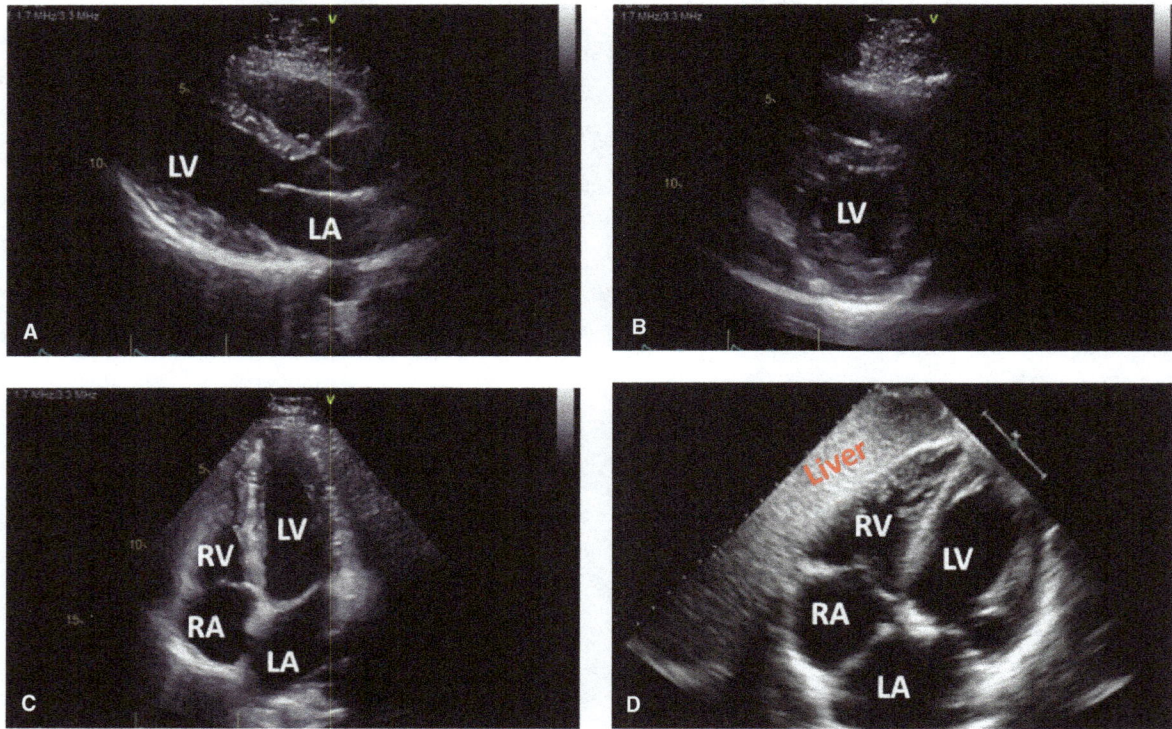

FIGURE 27-1 Transthoracic echocardiographic images from multiple views. Panels **A** and **B** are parasternal long- and short-axis views, respectively. They show the LV in long axis (**A**) and short axis (**B**). Panel **C** is a four-chamber view that is typically obtained from the apex. Panel **D** is a subcostal view, and similarly shows a four-chamber view of the cardiac chambers. LV, left ventricle; LA, left atrium; RV, right ventricle; RA, right atrium.

Another echocardiographic imaging technique that helps to improve image resolution is tissue harmonic imaging. When an ultrasound wave is transmitted through tissues, the signal becomes distorted and generates additional frequencies. These are harmonics of the fundamental frequency, and the energy of these frequencies increases with the distance of propagation.[2] In echocardiography, a great deal of the image artifacts is due to scattering at the chest wall, where there is little harmonic frequency

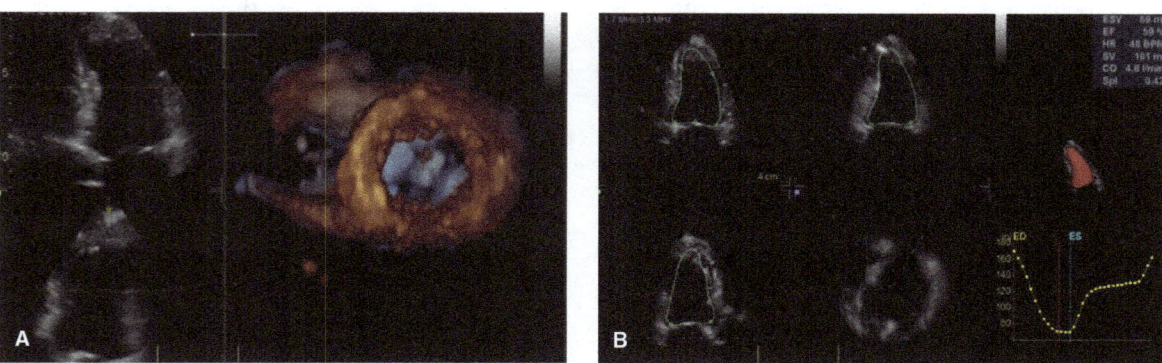

FIGURE 27-2 Three-dimensional evaluation of the left ventricle via transthoracic echocardiography. Cropping the 3D image set (panel **A**) avoids foreshortening of the LV and so allows more accurate assessment of LV volume and ejection fraction (panel **B**). LV, left ventricle.

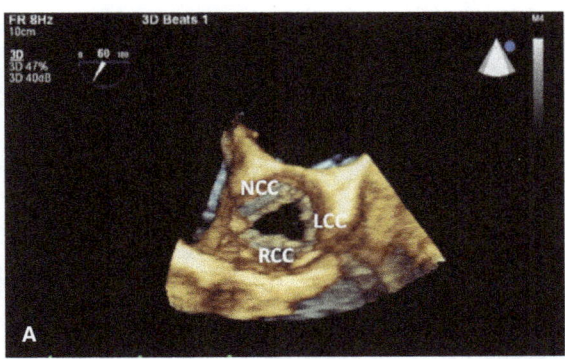 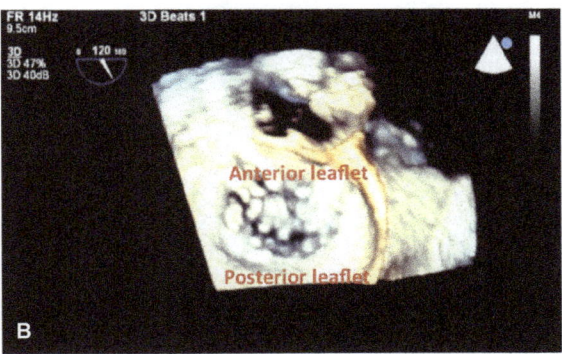

FIGURE 27-3 Three-dimensional transesophageal echocardiography. Panel **A** shows an enface view of the aortic valve; the three aortic leaflets are shown open in systole. Panel **B** shows a three-dimensional view of the mitral valve from the atrial side; the anterior and posterior mitral leaflets are visible. NCC, noncoronary cusp; LCC, left coronary cusp; RCC, right coronary cusp.

energy. Therefore, if the imaging is limited to only the harmonic range, a significant amount of the artifact is eliminated and a higher-quality image is obtained.[4] This technique has the greatest benefit in patients who have technically limited studies with poor image quality.[4]

One of the primary reasons for ordering an echocardiogram is to evaluate the left ventricular systolic function. In 2D echocardiography, the most common method for determining ejection fraction is the use of the biplane method of disks summation (modified Simpson's rule) (Fig. 27-4).[5] In this method, the

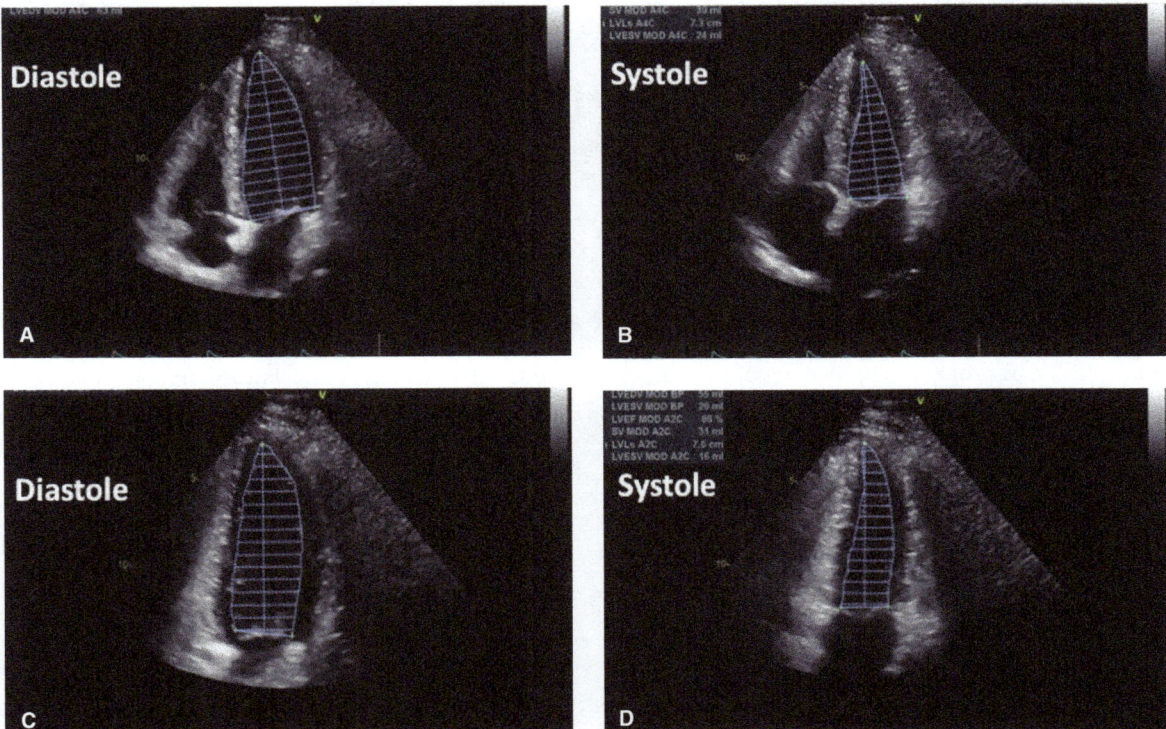

FIGURE 27-4 Two-dimensional volume measurement of the left ventricle using the biplane method of discs (modified Simpson's rule). The endocardial borders are traced in the apical four-chamber (panels **A** and **B**) and apical two-chamber (panels **C** and **D**) views at end diastole and end systole, in order to calculate the ejection fraction. The papillary muscles should be excluded from the cavity in the tracing.

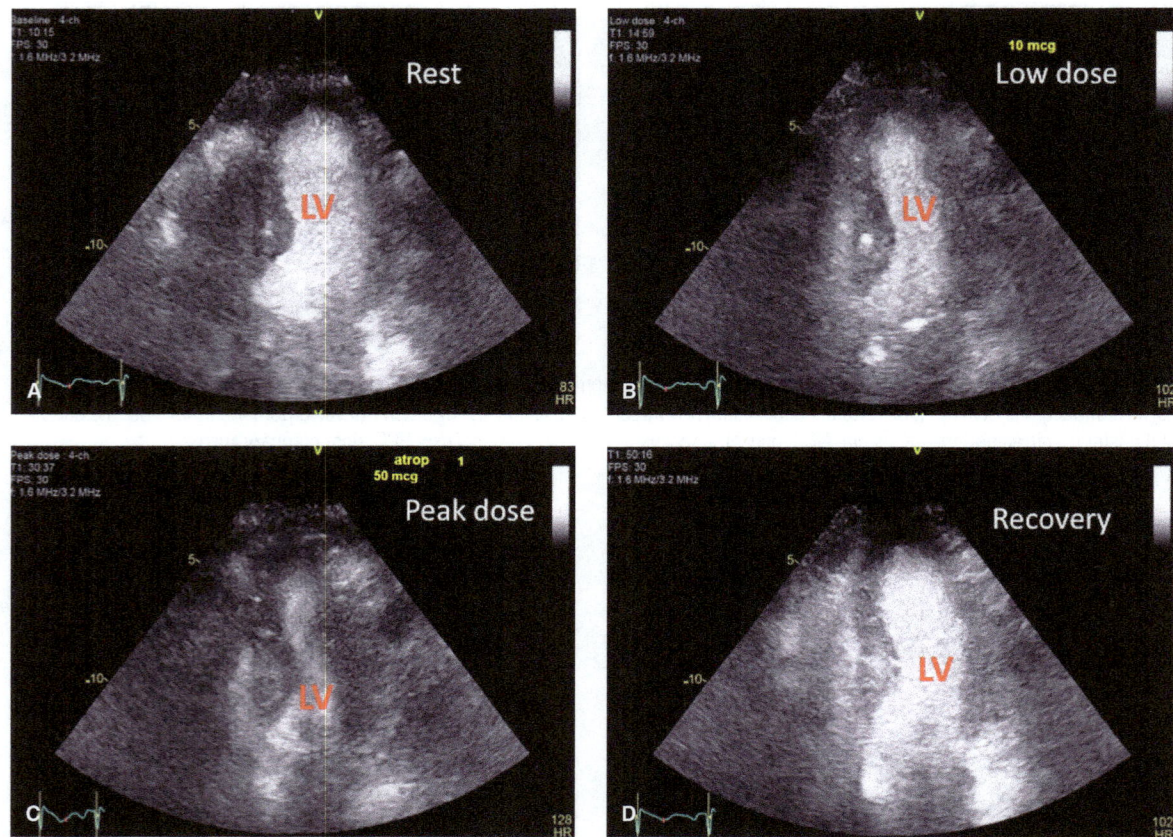

FIGURE 27-5 Normal dobutamine stress echocardiography showing the LV in the four-chamber view. Contrast was administered to improve endocardial border visualization. Normal response is seen with increasing doses of dobutamine; wall-motion contractility increases globally, and the LV decreases in size. Panel **A**, Rest stage; Panel **B**, Low dose dobutamine; Panel **C**, Peak dose dobutamine; Panel **D**, Recovery stage. LV, left ventricle.

reader manually traces the endocardial border, with the left ventricular volume calculated as the summation of a stack of elliptical disks filling the space. This approach can be prone to error in cases of poor image quality where the endocardial borders are difficult to delineate, and can become less accurate if foreshortening of the ventricle occurs in the apical views. By making the borders easier to identify, the use of an echo contrast agent improves the accuracy and reproducibility of 2D echocardiography.[6] Echocardiographic contrast reduces both inter- and intraobserver variability,[6] which has traditionally been one of the disadvantages of echocardiography when compared to other imaging modalities (Fig. 27-5).

Ultrasound images can also be used to assess cardiac blood flow and myocardial movement through the use of Doppler. This is based on the principle that the frequency of the reflected signal emitted from a moving object will be perceived differently depending on whether the object is moving toward or away from the observer.[2,7] In echocardiography, the moving objects being tracked are typically red blood cells. The two primary types of spectral Doppler imaging are pulsed-wave (PW) and continuous-wave (CW) Doppler (Fig. 27-6).[7] In PW Doppler, discrete intermittent bursts of ultrasound are reflected off the moving red blood cells at a specific depth within the heart. The common applications for this modality include the measurement of cardiac output, assessment of regurgitant volumes, and the evaluation of diastolic function.[8] This technique is limited by its inability to accurately detect signals at higher velocities. With CW Doppler on the other hand, continuous ultrasound is emitted from the transducer and continuously

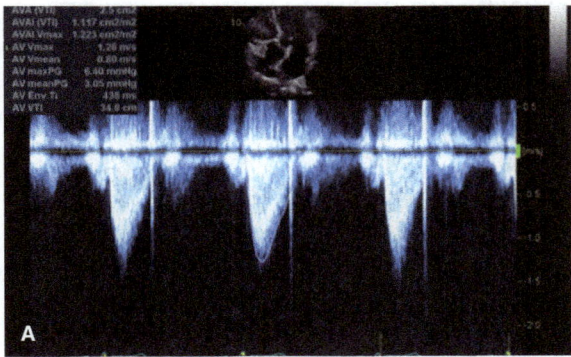 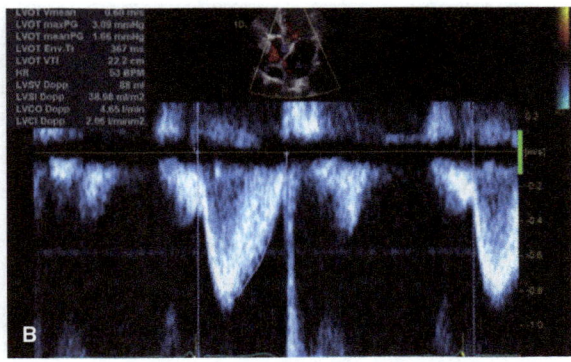

FIGURE 27-6 Doppler hemodynamic assessment of the aortic valve. Panels **A** and **B** show continuous and pulsed Doppler waves across a normally functioning aortic valve. Tracing these waves allows the assessment of peak velocity, mean pressure gradient, and calculated aortic valve area.

analyzed. This allows for the assessment of higher velocities, though at the expense of decreased precision in localization. CW Doppler is best suited for evaluation of high-velocity flow across stenotic or regurgitant valvular orifices.[8] The combination of PW and CW can be used to calculate intracardiac and valvular flows and gradients that allow for a comprehensive hemodynamic assessment of the heart. Color-flow Doppler is an additional technique that is based on PW Doppler, and involves color-coding of flow based on velocity and direction. Red represents blood flow toward the transducer, while blue represents blood flowing away. High velocity and turbulent blood flow show a mosaic color pattern, making color-flow Doppler ideal for evaluating flow in abnormal valves (Fig. 27-7).

Another application for Doppler echocardiography is tissue Doppler imaging (TDI). In contrast to the previously described traditional Doppler techniques that focus on the high-frequency motion of red blood cells, tissue Doppler assesses the higher-amplitude and lower-velocity signals generated from myocardial movement.[9] TDI is particularly useful in the assessment of diastolic function, which develops in the setting of impaired myocardial relaxation and increased LV chamber stiffness (Fig. 27-8).[10]

During the normal cardiac cycle the apex remains relatively fixed, with the mitral annulus moving toward the apex in systole and away in diastole. The shortening of the left ventricle during systole can be demonstrated by the descent of the annulus, and thus TDI of mitral annular motion provides a good representation of left ventricular systolic function.[11]

TDI waveforms reflect the systolic velocity (S'), early diastolic velocity (e'), and late diastolic velocity (a') of the mitral annulus. Combining these measurements with the mitral inflow velocities in early diastole (E) and late diastole (A) provides for an assessment of diastolic function. Specifically, peak E and A velocities, E/A ratio, e' velocity, and E/e' ratio are all important measurements in the determination of diastolic dysfunction. Other echocardiographic parameters, including left atrial size, pulmonary vein systolic to diastolic ratio, and peak velocity of tricuspid regurgitation (TR) signal, can also be integrated to help determine the degree of diastolic impairment (Fig. 27-9).[10] One of the main weaknesses of TDI is the inability of the technique to differentiate myocardium that is actively contracting from one that is dyskinetic or akinetic, but appears to be contracting because it is tethered to a moving segment. Myocardial deformation imaging, on the other hand, is a newer technique that does not have this limitation. Deformation indices such as strain and strain rate provide quantitative, and thus more objective, measures of regional myocardial performance.

Simply put, strain represents the percentage change in the length of a myocardial fiber during contraction relative to its original dimension, and strain rate is its temporal derivative (1/second). Thus, these strain-derived parameters allow assessment of the extent of myocardial thickening in addition to its timing. Because these methods evaluate each myocardial segment individually, they are relatively less susceptible to tethering and translational motion.

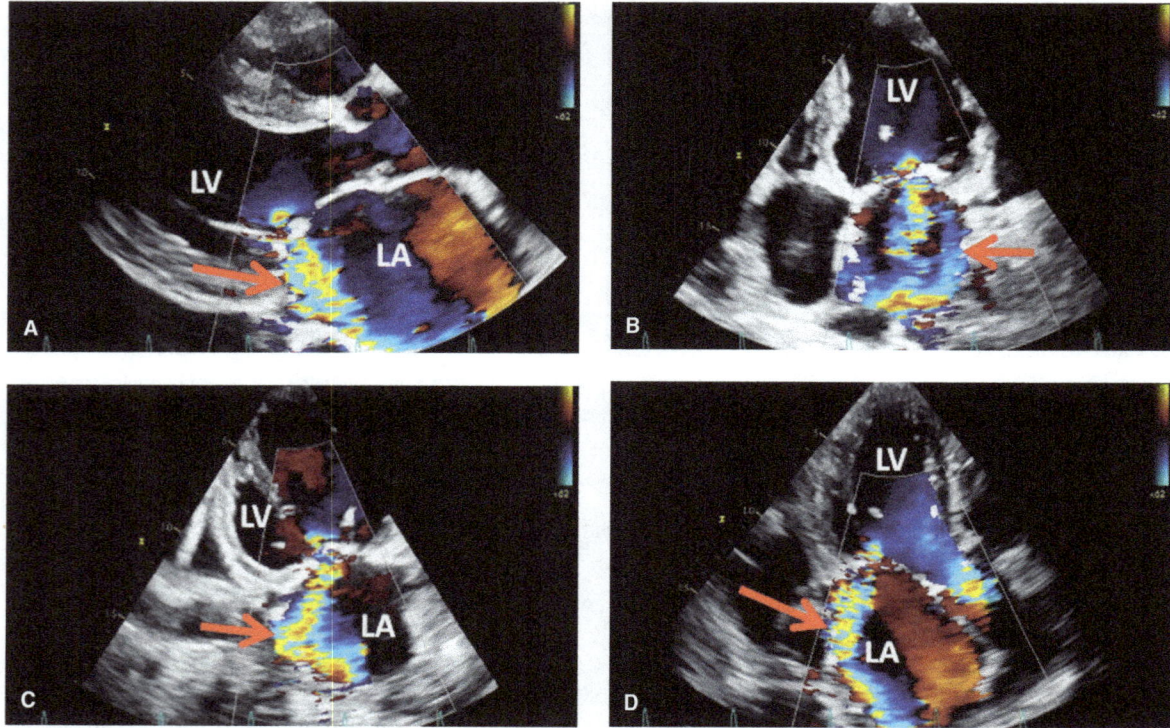

FIGURE 27-7 Transthoracic echocardiogram of a patient with ischemic cardiomyopathy and a restricted posterior mitral leaflet. Color Doppler assessment of the mitral valve in multiple views shows severe mitral regurgitation (*red arrows*). Panel **A**, parasternal long-axis view; panel **B**, four-chamber view; panel **C**, two-chamber view; panel **D**, three-chamber view. LV, left ventricle; LA, left atrium.

Strain and strain rate may be derived from TDI, which requires the direction of wall motion to be along the scan line of the ultrasound, and therefore is angle-dependent.[12] Alternatively, speckle-tracking echocardiography, which tracks the unique speckle patterns of the myocardium, is not dependent on the Doppler angle. This allows for strain analysis in multiple different planes, including longitudinal, circumferential, radial, and rotational strain.[12,13]

In addition to these advances in 2D echocardiography, 3D imaging also allows for a high-quality assessment of systolic function. 3D echocardiography

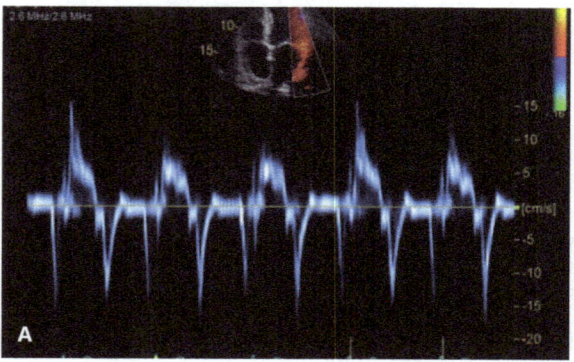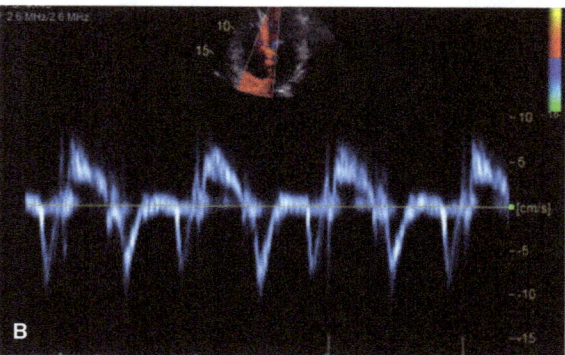

FIGURE 27-8 Tissue Doppler evaluation at the mitral annulus. Panel **A** shows the evaluation of the lateral mitral annulus, and panel **B** shows evaluation of the septal mitral annulus.

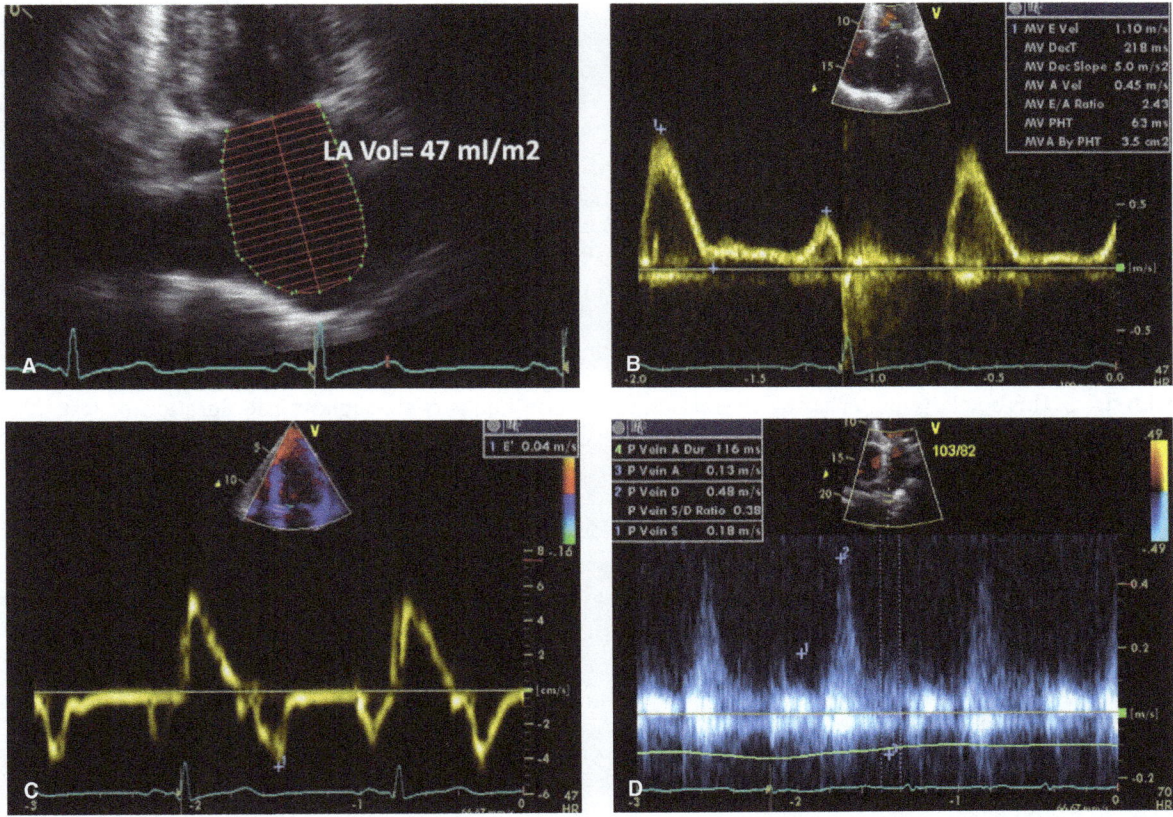

FIGURE 27-9 2D, Doppler, and tissue Doppler transthoracic echocardiographic views used in combination, for diastolic evaluation. Panel **A** shows a dilated left atrium. Mitral inflow evaluation by pulsed Doppler (panel **B**) shows an E/A >2. Panel **C** shows depressed septal tissue Doppler velocity, and Panel **D** shows a pulmonary vein inflow pattern suggestive of advanced diastolic disease (diastolic predominance and prominent atrial flow reversal). The E/'e = 27.5. In combination, this is diagnostic of restrictive diastolic dysfunction (grade 3) with elevated filling pressures. LA, left atrium; vol, volume.

does not require geometric assumptions about left ventricular shape, and therefore provides a more accurate measure of left ventricular volumes compared to standard 2D imaging, especially in patients with asymmetric ventricles or with wall-motion abnormalities after a myocardial infarction (MI).[14] 3D echocardiography has been shown to provide comparable volume measurements to radionuclide angiography,[15] which has long been one of the preferred noninvasive methods for estimating left ventricular ejection fraction. Similarly, when compared to standard 2D imaging, 3D echocardiography demonstrates a greater correlation to the volume measurements obtained with cardiac magnetic resonance imaging (CMR),[16] which is generally considered to be the gold standard for measuring ejection fraction. With 3D echocardiography becoming more widely available, it appears to be a reasonable alternative to CMR imaging for accurate and noninvasive assessment of left ventricular systolic function in patients with optimal image quality.

Stress Echocardiography

General Principles

Stress echocardiography (SE) is primarily used to evaluate for myocardial ischemia through the assessment of regional wall-motion abnormalities. It can also be used as a prognostic tool in patients with known CAD, to predict outcomes after coronary revascularization, and to assess the severity of valvular heart disease (VHD). While stress testing has traditionally involved patients undergoing aerobic exercise, pharmacologic stress agents can also elicit a similar cardiovascular response in patients unable to participate in a usual exercise protocol.

In the normal response to either a physical or inotropic stress, the left ventricle demonstrates increased endocardial excursion and myocardial thickening, which subsequently leads to an increase in ejection fraction and reduced cavity size at end systole. As a result, the myocardial oxygen demand and uptake increases with stress. This uptake is influenced by several factors, including heart rate, contractility, and left ventricular wall stress. Coronary blood flow increases in a linear fashion alongside myocardial oxygen uptake, up to a fivefold higher flow than at baseline.[17] In patients who have obstructive CAD, however, coronary blood flow is unable to satisfy the metabolic demands of the myocardium during stress. This results in myocardial ischemia from a regional mismatch between the myocardial oxygen demand and the reduced supply from arterial stenosis. In SE, this is generally represented by new or worsening wall-motion abnormalities, as well as increasing left ventricular cavity size with stress and decreased ejection fraction.

Techniques

Prior to initiating the stress portion of the examination, baseline echocardiographic images are obtained with the patient at rest. Standard M-mode and 2D imaging is performed to assess all segments of the left ventricle. An overall assessment of other cardiac structures is also performed. Evaluation of the left ventricle using harmonic imaging can improve endocardial border definition, which is critical for the assessment of wall motion.[18] Typically the parasternal long- and short-axis views are obtained, as well as at least two and preferably three apical views. The baseline images should be evaluated for any resting abnormalities that may be indicative of a prior infarct. Other cardiac structures, such as the valves, pericardium, and aortic root, can also be evaluated for any pathology or contraindications to stress testing.

To assess for myocardial ischemia with echocardiographic stress testing, several modalities are available, including exercise, pharmacologic, and pacing. When patients are physically able to exercise, this is the preferred method for stress testing as it provides additional information regarding exercise capacity, which has been shown to be a predictor of mortality.[19] With standard protocols, baseline echo images are obtained at rest prior to the patient exercising, and then again at peak exercise or immediately after peak exercise.

Exercise SE is most commonly performed using a treadmill and less often a supine bicycle. In both modalities, the patient gradually increases exercise intensity throughout the duration of test. The Bruce protocol, which is the most common treadmill protocol in use, involves incremental increases in treadmill speed and grade in 3-minute intervals. Both bicycle and treadmill exercises allow for the determination of exercise capacity and peak metabolic equivalents (METs) achieved. In treadmill SE, the patient is moved quickly from the treadmill to the imaging bed after the termination of exercise to obtain post-exercise images (Fig. 27-10). In order to obtain the most accurate evaluation for ischemia, post-exercise images need to be captured within the first minute of cessation of exercise. Even so, during this time period, the transient echocardiographic findings indicative of ischemia may already be resolving, which can reduce the sensitivity of the test. With supine bicycle testing, echo images are obtained during exercise, which allows capture of exercise images at a higher heart rate. When comparing supine bicycle echocardiography to traditional treadmill stress testing with the capture of immediate post-exercise images, supine bicycle stress testing has a higher sensitivity for detecting ischemia.[20]

For patients who are unable to exercise, pharmacologic stress testing is an available alternative. The most commonly used agent is dobutamine, with graded infusions uptitrated in 3-minute increments starting from 5 or 10 μg/kg/min up to a peak dose of 40 μg/kg/min, as discussed in greater detail in Chapter 8 (Fig. 27-11).[21] This increases the myocardial oxygen consumption by increasing inotropic state, heart rate, and blood pressure.[22] The goal is to increase the heart rate to at least 85% of the age-predicted maximum, which is the target of both the exercise and pharmacologic protocols.

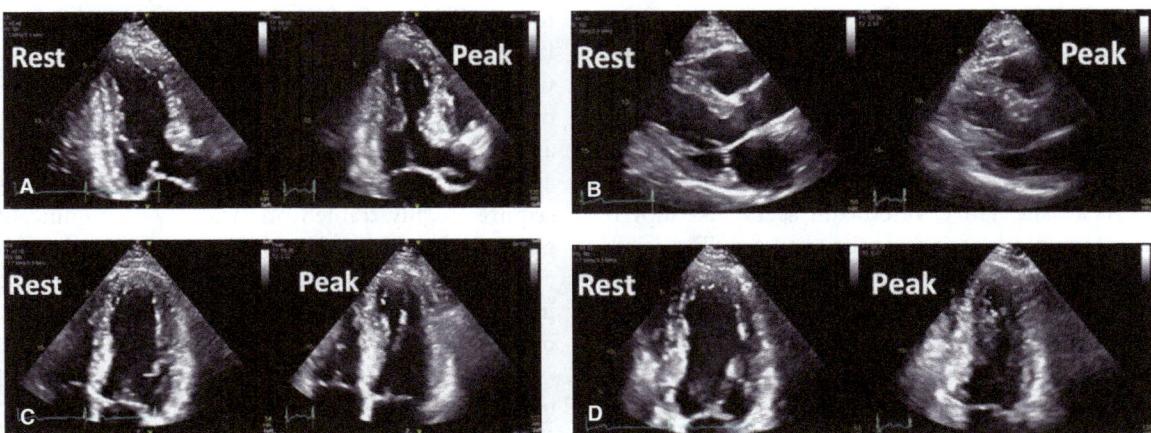

FIGURE 27-10 A normal exercise-stress echocardiographic test is shown. Baseline echocardiographic views are obtained at rest showing normal wall motion. This is followed by obtaining peak images after maximal exercise on a treadmill. Peak images show normal response with hypercontractile wall motion and decreased left ventricular cavity size. Panel **A**, three-chamber view; panel **B**, parasternal long-axis view; panel **C**, four-chamber view; panel **D**, two-chamber view.

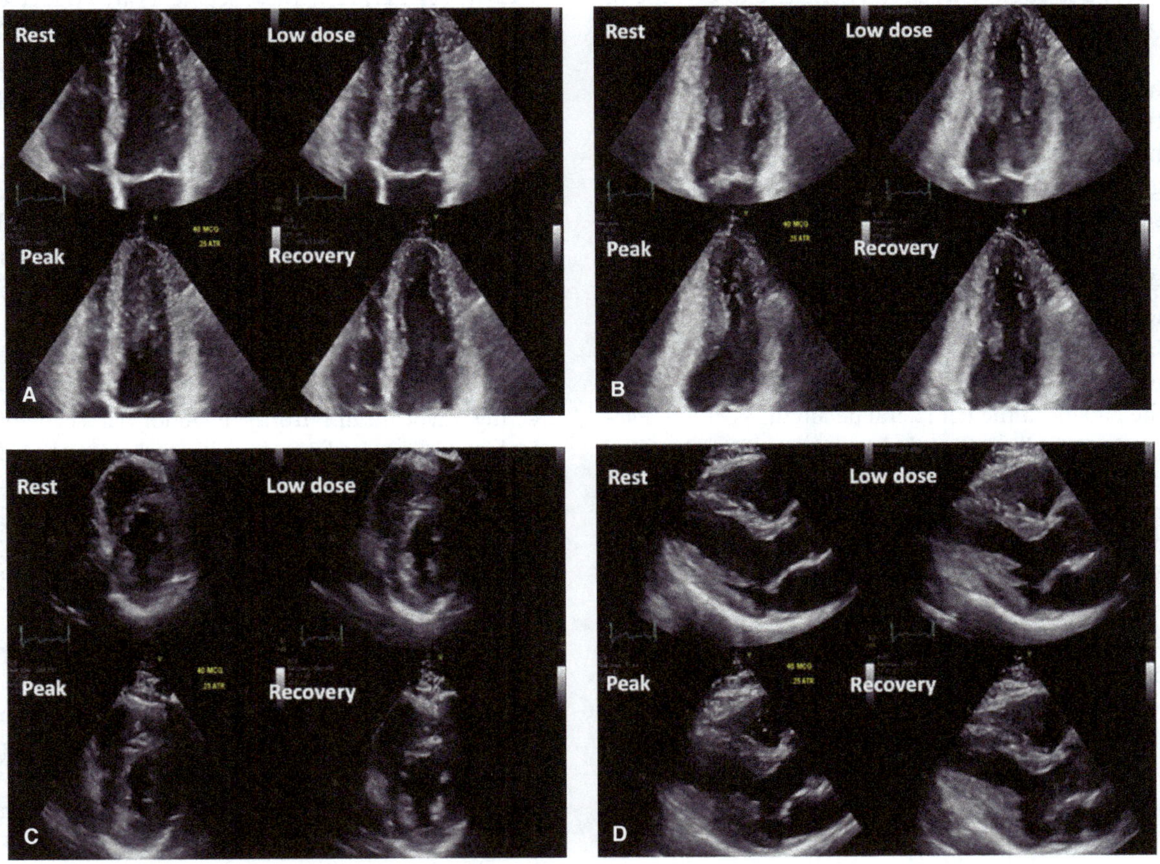

FIGURE 27-11 A normal dobutamine stress echocardiographic test is shown. All images are at end systole. As the dobutamine is infused, the myocardial contractility increases and the left ventricular cavity size decreases until the target heart rate is achieved. Recovery images are obtained after the infusion is stopped and the heart rate recovers back to baseline. Panel **A**, four-chamber view; panel **B**, two-chamber view; panel **C**, short-axis view; panels **D**, parasternal long-axis view.

Dobutamine SE (DSE) can also be used to assess for myocardial viability. In this technique, the starting dose of dobutamine is 2.5 µg/kg/min up to a peak dose of 20 µg/kg/min. Higher doses of dobutamine can be given if the detection of ischemia, in addition to viability, is needed.[21]

As an alternative, vasodilator agents like dipyridamole and adenosine can be used for SE as well. These function by inducing coronary steal, which occurs in the setting of significant coronary artery disease. The choice of pharmacologic agent is driven by several factors, including expertise at the facility and patient characteristics. Adenosine is usually avoided in asthmatics, and dobutamine needs to be used with caution in patients with arrhythmias or severe hypertension. Dobutamine remains the preferred agent for pharmacologic stress testing when assessing wall-motion abnormalities.

A less-commonly used alternative to exercise or pharmacologic stress testing is pacing SE. This can be accomplished in patients who already have an implanted pacemaker, or by atrial pacing through transesophageal echocardiography. In patients who have a permanent pacemaker, the pacing rate can be gradually increased until target heart rate is achieved, sometimes in conjunction with the use of dobutamine. This pacemaker stress technique has been shown to have similar diagnostic accuracy for CAD when compared to pharmacologic or exercise SE.[23] In transesophageal SE, the pacing catheter can be placed either orally or nasally and is advanced with the patient in the left lateral decubitus position. Pacing is typically initiated above the patient's baseline heart rate and increased every few minutes until the patient's target heart rate is reached.[24] This technique has been shown to have good agreement with DSE for the detection of myocardial ischemia.[24] When compared to exercise or pharmacologic stress testing, the primary advantage of pacing is the rapid return to baseline conditions at the cessation of the test, which helps to prevent a prolonged period of myocardial ischemia.

Image Analysis

For image analysis, the rest and stress images are displayed side by side to allow for direct comparison. When image quality is poor and two or more myocardial segments cannot be adequately visualized, intravenous echo contrast agents can be used. Contrast has been shown to increase the percentage of wall segments visualized, improve image quality, and increase the confidence of interpretation, both at rest and at peak stress (Fig. 27-5).[25] Image analysis requires highly trained physicians with significant experience in the field. For less-experienced readers, the use of contrast agents along with harmonic imaging improves both the accuracy and efficiency of the reader.[26]

For image analysis, the myocardium is divided into several different segments, which are all evaluated independently. Per the 2015 American Society of Echocardiography chamber quantification guidelines, the LV can be divided into 17 segments, as with SPECT and PET, which includes an "apical cap" that represents the myocardium beyond the end of the LV cavity (Fig. 27-12).[5] These segments are evaluated for endocardial excursion and wall thickening, with motion evaluated in several different views. A grade is assigned to each segment based on the following scoring system: (1) normal or hyperkinetic, (2) hypokinetic (reduced thickening), (3) akinetic (absent or negligible thickening), and (4) dyskinetic (systolic thinning or stretching) (Table 27-1). The rest and stress images can then be compared to evaluate for stress-induced changes suggestive of myocardial viability and/or ischemia (Fig. 27-13).

When assessing wall-motion abnormalities, the reader must be careful to differentiate normally contracting myocardium from an abnormal segment which may appear to be moving because it is tethered to a normal segment, but does not in fact demonstrate the typical thickening that would be expected of normally functioning myocardium. In addition, it is important to consider the clinical context and medical history of each individual patient, as several nonischemic etiologies of stress-induced wall-motion abnormalities are possible.

During evaluation of the SE images, attention should also be paid to the size of the left ventricular cavity. Not only should the LV become hypercontractile with stress, but the cavity should also shrink in size. An increase in LV volume with stress is generally indicative of extensive coronary artery disease.[2] One exception is with supine bicycle stress testing, where left ventricular cavity size may increase at peak

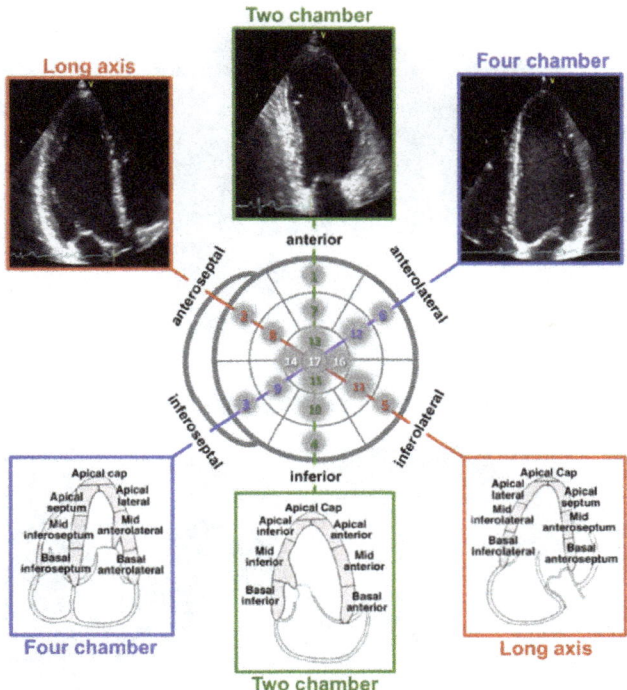

FIGURE 27-12 The 17-segment representation of the left ventricle. In the center is the bull's-eye depiction of the segments, with the corresponding apical long-axis, apical two-chamber, and apical four-chamber TTE views shown above. Below the bull's eye are schematic representations of the left ventricle showing how these segments are imaged in the three views. (Reproduced with permission from Lang RM, Badano LP, Mor-Avi V, et al. Recommendations for cardiac chamber quantification by echocardiography in adults: an update from the American Society of Echocardiography and the European Association of Cardiovascular Imaging. *J Am Soc Echocardiogr*. 2015;28(1):1–39.)

stress due to increased venous return from leg elevation. However, this quickly resolves with the cessation of exercise.

Diagnostic Accuracy

The accuracy of SE, expressed in sensitivity and specificity varies between different studies, depending on the study's angiographic cutoff for significant disease, the criteria used for a positive test, the pretest probability, and the prevalence of disease in the study population. For the detection of CAD, sensitivity in the general population is around 74% to 97% for exercise echocardiography, 61% to 95% for dobutamine, and 61% to 81% for dipyridamole/adenosine while specificity is 64% to 86%, 51% to 95%, and 90% to 94%, respectively.[22]

There are several factors that alter the sensitivity and specificity of stress echo. Interpretation of

Table 27-1
Echocardiographic Responses to the Administration of Dobutamine during Pharmacologic Stress Testing

Interpretation	Rest/Baseline	Low-Dose Stress	Peak Stress
Normal	Normal	Normal or hyperkinetic	Hyperkinetic
Ischemic	Normal	Normal or hypokinetic/akinetic	Hypokinetic/akinetic
Ischemic	Hypokinetic	Hypokinetic/akinetic	Hypokinetic/akinetic (when compared to baseline)
Ischemic with viability	Resting WMA	Improved WMA	Hypokinetic/akinetic (when compared to baseline)
Nonischemic with viability	Resting WMA	Improved WMA	Further improved WMA
Infarction	Resting WMA	No charge	No change

WMA, wall-motion abnormalities.

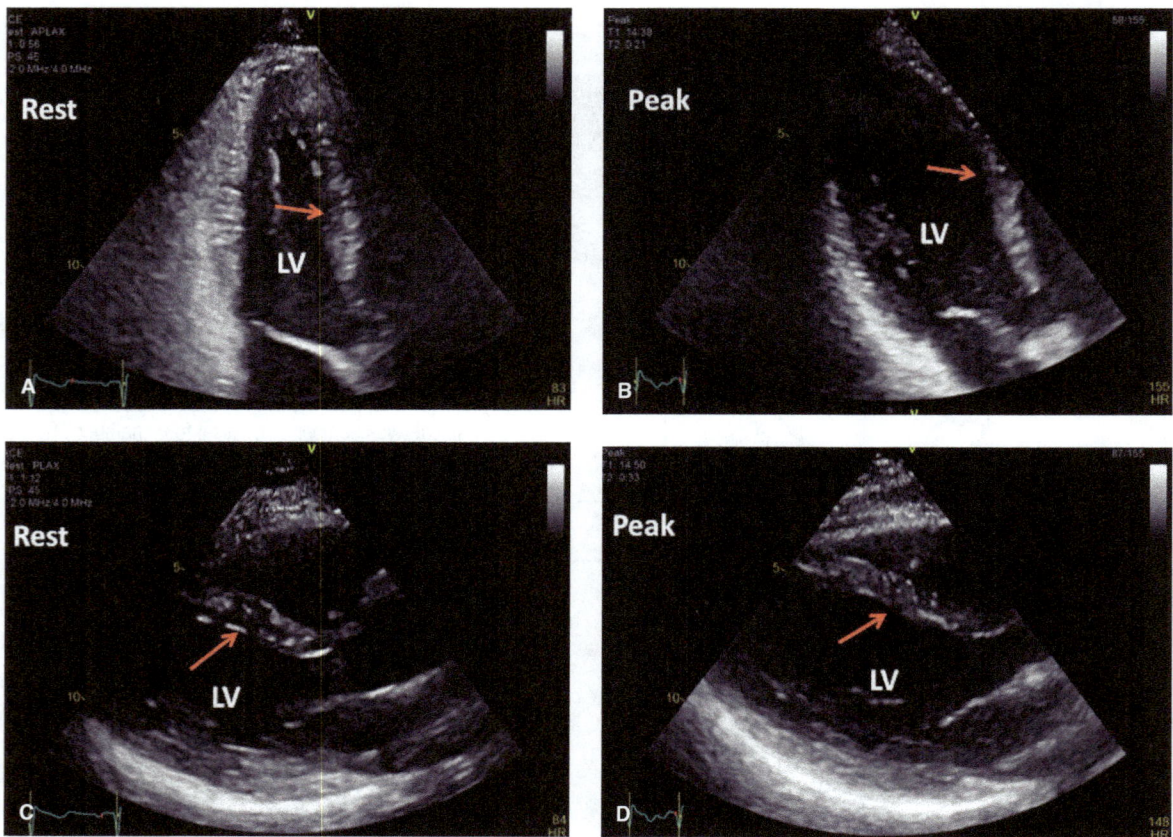

FIGURE 27-13 Abnormal exercise-stress echocardiography: Panels **A** and **C** show normal wall motion at rest, both in the three-chamber view **(A)** and parasternal long-axis view **(C)**. However, at peak exercise (panels **B** and **D**), the mid-anteroseptal wall becomes hypokinetic (*red arrow*), suggesting a stenosis in the left anterior descending coronary artery. In addition, the left ventricular cavity dilates during peak stress. LV, left ventricle.

stress-echo tests is dependent on the induction of ischemia, the adequacy of stress, image quality, and expertise of the interpreting physician. Thus, many factors are pivotal for accurate and sensitive results. The primary causes for a false-negative test are inability to reach target heart rate (e.g., due to poor exercise capacity, use of a beta blocker, or delay in capturing post-exercise images), poor image quality, a small area of ischemia, single-vessel disease, distal coronary disease, or other pre-existing conditions such as significant LV hypertrophy or a hyperdynamic state.[22] Poor-quality images or suboptimal acoustic windows can result from large body habitus or chronic obstructive lung disease. However, with the use of contrast echocardiography there is excellent feasibility of stress echo in obese patients.[27,28] In a recent study of 209 patients with morbid obesity, the use of contrast allowed the attainability of diagnostic images in almost 99% of patients.[29]

A marked hypertensive response, nonischemic cardiomyopathy, left bundle branch block (LBBB), pulmonary hypertension, and translational cardiac motion can all cause wall-motion abnormalities with stress and may lead to a false-positive test.[22] In patients with LBBB, there is abnormal septal motion which is aggravated further by tachycardia. This leads to reduction in the diagnostic accuracy of SE in this group of patients.[30] Similarly, right ventricular pacing may lead to false-positive apical wall-motion abnormalities. A hypertensive response during an SE can also falsely cause LV dilation and systolic dysfunction.

The overall accuracy of nuclear perfusion imaging and SE have been shown to be similar in meta-analyses; the superior sensitivity nuclear perfusion is balanced by the superior specificity of SE.[31-35] The higher sensitivity of myocardial perfusion imaging is explained by the fact that it works by detecting a relative reduction in myocardial blood volume that occurs earlier than wall-thickening abnormality in the ischemic cascade. In a pooled analysis of 18 studies in 1304 patients who underwent exercise or pharmacologic SE in conjunction with thallium- or technetium-labeled radioisotope imaging, sensitivity and specificity were 80% and 86% for echocardiography and 84% and 77% for myocardial perfusion imaging, respectively.[33,21] Local expertise, cost, exposure to radiation, and specific patient characteristics are all important factors in determining which imaging modality to use.

Prognostic Value

SE has valuable prognostic information in risk stratification in various patient populations including suspected or known CAD, post-myocardial infarction, and in patients undergoing noncardiac surgery. In general, a negative stress test portends a very low risk (<1% per year) of cardiovascular events for the subsequent 4 to 5 years.[36] However, the risk is slightly higher in patients with diseases associated with accelerated atherogenesis, such as patients with diabetes or chronic kidney disease. A positive test, on the other hand, indicates elevated risk for future cardiac events. An abnormal SE in a patient with intermediate risk factors, carries a 1-year cardiac event rate of 10% to 30%. Other stress data need to be integrated as well, including functional capacity, blood pressure response, ischemic threshold, location and extent of wall-motion abnormality, heart rate recovery, and ST segment response.[37,38]

One study showed the long-term (>10 years) prognostic value of DSE in a high-risk cohort of 3381 patients. Patients with abnormal DSE had a higher mortality rate compared to those with normal DSE (44% vs. 35% at 15 years' follow-up).[39] Yao et al.[40] studied 4566 patients with low-intermediate 10-year risk and low- or high-lifetime risk of cardiovascular disease who underwent dobutamine or exercise-stress echo. An SE showing three or more new ischemic segments compared to one showing less than three ischemic segments was associated with higher risk of nonfatal MI and death in the low-lifetime risk group (3.3% vs. 0.3% per year) and high-lifetime risk group (2% vs. 0% per year). Thus, SE can further refine risk stratification, even in patients with low-intermediate short-term risk. SE for both preoperative and post-myocardial infarction studies have been primarily carried out with pharmacologic stress, which appears to be as useful for prognostication as exercise testing. The positive predictive value of a positive stress test ranges from 7% to 35% for hard events, while the negative predictive value ranges 93% to 100%. Several studies have evaluated the role of DSE in patients with an increased perioperative cardiovascular risk, particularly those undergoing vascular surgery (abdominal aortic or peripheral vascular surgery). DSE appears safe and feasible as part of a preoperative assessment. Overall, the ability of a positive test result to predict an event (nonfatal MI or death) in this population ranged from 0% to 37%, and the negative predictive value ranged from 90% to 100%.[41-44]

▶ Myocardial Viability

Myocardial viability denotes dysfunctional myocardium at rest that has the potential to improve or recover. One of the most widely available techniques to detect viability is low-dose DSE.[45] As the dobutamine is administered, the initial low dose causes increased myocardial perfusion and thus, increased myocardial contractility. If sufficient myocardial contractile reserve is present, then the myocardial contractility will be augmented in segments with resting dysfunction. However, as the dose of dobutamine is increased, there is a demand–supply mismatch, and a subsequent deterioration in contractility is seen. This so-called "biphasic response" has the best value of all the possible responses to dobutamine in predicting improvement in LV function following revascularization (Fig. 27-14).

In comparison to nuclear techniques for viability detection, DSE is less sensitive but more specific in predicting functional recovery.[46,47] In a meta-analysis of 52 studies that included 1367 patients with ischemic LV dysfunction, the comparison of different imaging tests for predicting recovery of segmental function after revascularization showed the following:

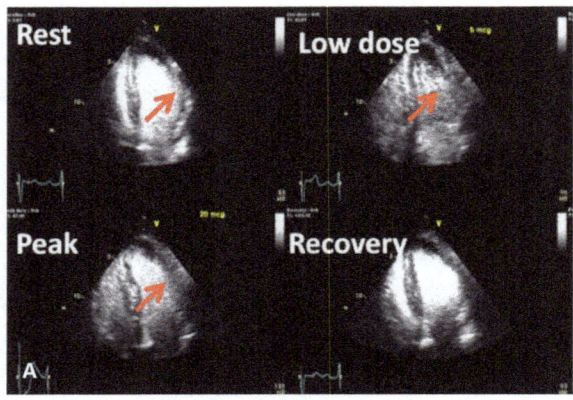 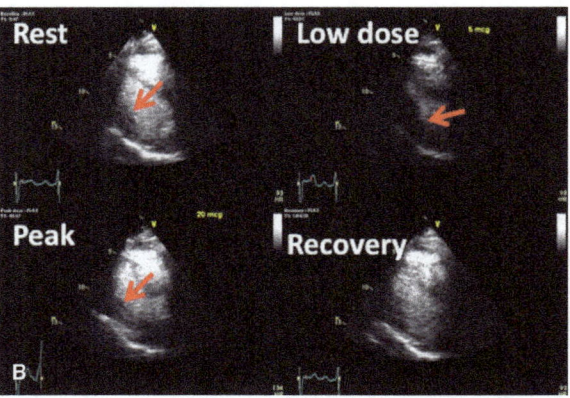

FIGURE 27-14 An example of the biphasic response on dobutamine stress echocardiography. With low dose of dobutamine, there is augmentation of the anterolateral and inferolateral walls (*red arrows*) seen on the four-chamber view **(A)** and the parasternal long-axis view **(B)**. This is followed by deterioration of contractility in these areas at peak dobutamine dose. This suggests viability and ischemia in the LCX territory.

DSE had the highest positive predictive value, and had a similar negative predictive value compared to FDG-PET and reinjection thallium SPECT.[48] This difference in sensitivity and specificity likely is secondary to the fact that at least 50% viable myocardium is required in a given segment for a contractile response to be seen following dobutamine administration.[49] While on the other hand thallium measures cell membrane activity, so even a minor amount of tissue viability can be identified.

A large body of evidence, including two meta-analysis studies, confirmed the association between myocardial viability and improved survival after revascularization while the absence of viability predicted similar outcomes, irrespective of treatment strategy.[50,51] This is in contrast to the findings in the STICH trial, which failed to identify patients with a differential survival benefit from coronary surgery versus optimal medical therapy regardless of the presence of myocardial viability.[52] Thus, more studies are needed to determine the role of myocardial viability identification through cardiac imaging in clinical decision making.[53]

▶ Role of Stress Echocardiography in Nonischemic Cardiac Conditions

SE has an important role in the evaluation of VHD, particularly in situations where there is a discrepancy between the severity of the valvular disease and patients' symptoms.[54,55] By using exercise echocardiography, a patient's true functional class can be teased out, therefore either verifying a patient's truly asymptomatic state from a severe valve lesion, or on the other hand, revealing the underlying symptoms secondary to the valve disease. With the aid of Doppler assessment, exercise-induced hemodynamic changes can be unmasked in borderline valvular lesions, and correlated with the patient's exertional symptoms. Both treadmill and bicycle protocols may be used as the exercise method, although Doppler signals are more easily and continuously acquired with the bicycle test.[21] Specific clinical scenarios where stress echo has been found to be useful include mitral stenosis and mitral regurgitation. Low-dose dobutamine is also useful for evaluating low-flow, low-gradient aortic stenosis (Fig. 27-15).

Information obtained from echocardiography and stress echo is invaluable in hypertrophic cardiomyopathy (HCM). Resting echo identifies maximal wall thickness and distribution, as well as left ventricular outflow (LVOT) gradient. Exercise echocardiography can identify patients with obstructive HCM if the LVOT gradient increases to above 30 mm Hg even if there is no resting gradient. In addition, exercise testing can provide information on functional class, exercise-induced arrhythmia, and blood pressure response.[56]

If the resting echo cannot explain the patient's exertional symptoms, then diastolic exercise-stress testing is indicated.[10] In individuals with normal

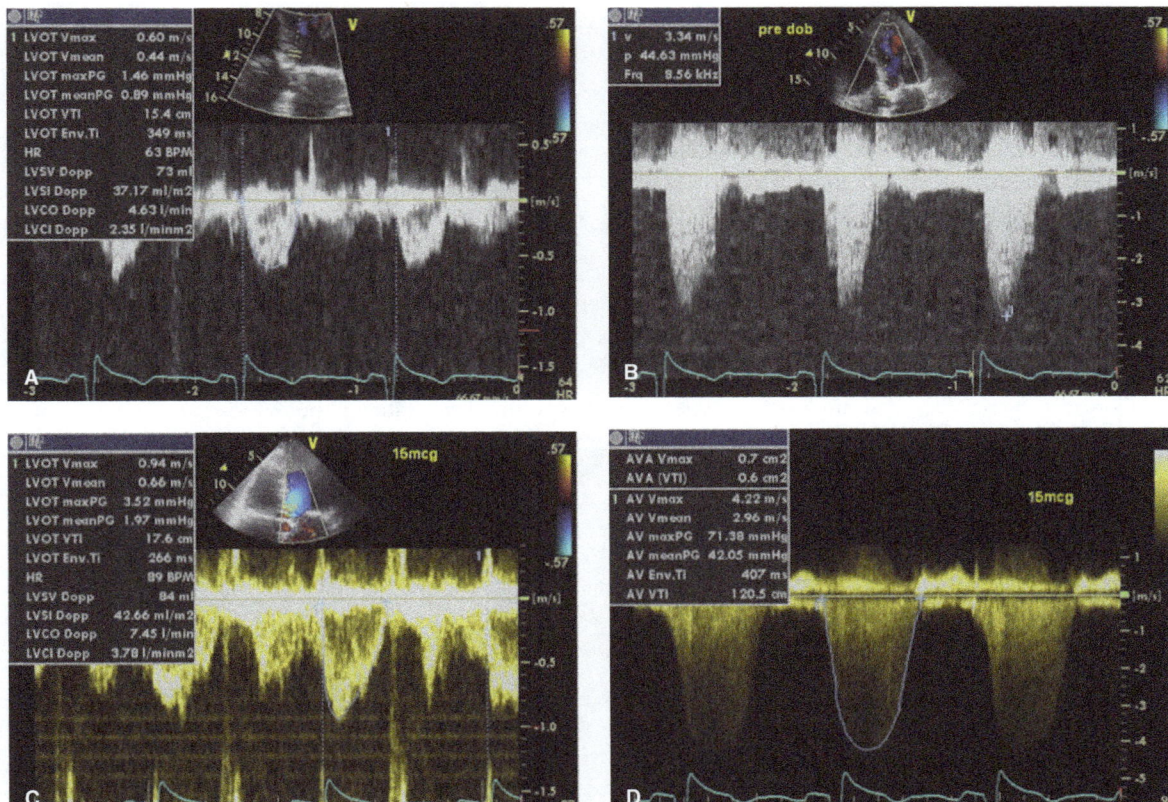

FIGURE 27-15 A low-dose dobutamine echo was performed in the assessment for low-flow, low-gradient aortic stenosis in the setting of low-ejection fraction. At rest, the stroke volume indexed is 35 mL/m², the mean gradient across the aortic valve is 20 mm Hg, and the calculated aortic area is 0.92 cm² (panel **A**, PW LVOT; panel **B**, CW across AV). With increasing doses of dobutamine (panels **C** and **D**), there is an increase in the cardiac output (stroke volume indexed 45 mL/m²) and flow across the aortic valve (mean gradient 42.05 mm Hg). The calculated AV is 0.75 cm², confirming severe aortic stenosis. PW LVOT, pulsed wave Doppler across left ventricular outflow tract; CW, continuous wave Doppler; AV, aortic valve.

myocardial relaxation, the E and e' velocities increase proportionally during exercise so that the E/e' ratio remains the same or is reduced. On the other hand, in those with impaired myocardial relaxation, the e' velocity increases less than E velocity so that the E/e' increases during exercise. However, there is still a paucity of data regarding the prognostic utility of diastolic stress testing.

Novel Developments in Echocardiography

Contrast

One of the main limitations affecting diagnostic accuracy in echo is image quality, or lack thereof, because of poor acoustic windows such as those seen in patients with increased body mass index or obstructive lung disease. Ultrasound contrast agents improve the ability to adequately visualize the endocardial borders, thus allowing the detection of LV wall motion and global systolic function, and aiding in decreasing interobserver variability in SE interpretation (Fig. 27-5).[57,58]

The currently utilized intravenous contrast agents are perfluorocarbon-containing microspheres that can cross the pulmonary vascular bed and thus provide LV opacification. The current American Society of Echocardiography guidelines for the use of contrast for LV opacification recommend its use when two or more contiguous myocardial segments are not adequately visualized.[57,58] The clinical benefit of enhanced endocardial border detection using contrast administration in DSE was seen in a randomized trial of 101 patients undergoing both noncontrast- and contrast-enhanced studies. The use of contrast showed significantly improved endocardial visualization at both rest and peak stress, leading to both a higher confidence of interpretation and greater diagnostic accuracy as compared with angiography (66% vs. 53%, $p = 0.02$). The highest impact on DSE accuracy with contrast enhancement was seen in the patients with the poorest image quality.[59]

Contrast agents can also aid in the assessment of myocardial perfusion. A continuous infusion of a contrast agent is administered and myocardial perfusion is observed with real-time imaging. This is followed by an ultrasound impulse of high intensity (high mechanical index, MI >1.5) which destroys the microbubbles within the myocardium. If the myocardium perfusion is normal, then the microbubbles will be replenished within 5 to 7 cardiac cycles. On the other hand, if there is no or decreased perfusion, the contrast will not be replenished normally and the myocardial area will appear dark or patchy.[60] Several studies have demonstrated the incremental predictive value of myocardial perfusion imaging over wall-motion analysis during pharmacological or exercise SE.[61–63] However, many technical and clinical issues still need to be resolved before myocardial contrast perfusion echocardiography becomes routine clinical practice. Use of contrast for myocardial perfusion is not yet approved by the U.S. Food and Drug Administration.

Myocardial Deformation Analysis

As mentioned previously, one of the major drawbacks of SE is its subjectivity and dependence on good image quality and reader expertise. In addition, translational motion of the myocardium, for example, in the case of adjacent tethering of an akinetic segment, can be erroneously interpreted as true motion. Myocardial deformation indices such as strain and strain rate provide quantitative and thus more objective measures of regional myocardial performance. (Fig. 27-16).

So how does this translate into early detection of ischemia? Ischemia decreases the extent or amplitude of contraction of the myocardial fibers and also slows the onset of contraction and delays the start of relaxation. Furthermore, the layer most susceptible to ischemia is the subendocardial layer, which mostly consists of longitudinal fibers, thus allowing longitudinal strain assessment to detect ischemia earlier. Another more recent parameter that has been used is post-systolic shortening (PSS), which reflects myocardial thickening after aortic valve closure (after the end of systole). PSS has been shown to be an extremely sensitive and early marker of ischemia.[13] Thus in acute ischemia, the systolic strain and peak systolic strain rate will be reduced and the PSS component will increase.

There is growing body of literature supporting the diagnostic value and accuracy of strain in the detection of ischemia. In a very recent study of 52 patients with chest pain and intermediate pretest probability of obstructive CAD, the value of strain in the evaluation of the presence and extent of ischemia was assessed. Strain, strain rate, and post-systolic strain index (PSI), which is post-systolic strain divided by peak strain, were measured by speckle tracking during DSE. All patients also underwent PET perfusion imaging and invasive angiography. The authors found that increased PSI and reduced strain during early recovery were the strongest predictors of obstructive CAD and can help in the detection of hemodynamically significant coronary stenosis compared with visual analysis alone.[64]

In another study of 197 patients undergoing DSE, strain analyses using speckle tracking, echocardiography was found to be feasible, accurate, and more sensitive in detecting CAD in the patients with confirmatory coronary angiography, compared to wall-motion scoring alone (84% vs. 75%, $p = 0.03$).[65] Similarly, a study by Hanekom et al.[66] showed that regional–longitudinal strain had high-diagnostic accuracy for angiographically significant CAD comparable to wall-motion analysis alone.

Resting global longitudinal strain (GLS) may also have a role in predicting coronary artery disease. In their study, Gaibazzi et al.[67] demonstrated that rest GLS has similar accuracy compared with stress-echo regional wall-motion analysis alone for the prediction of obstructive CAD. Further studies, however, are needed to validate these findings with prospective testing, and to determine its clinical role.

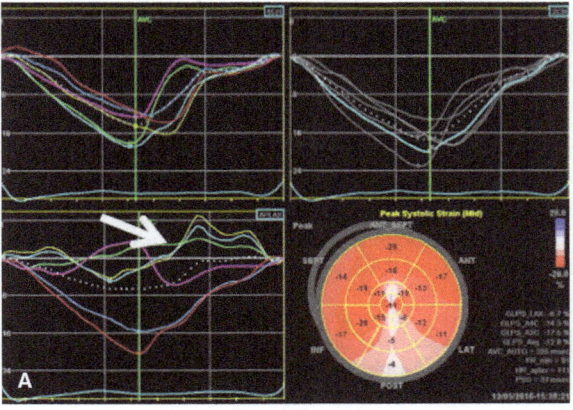
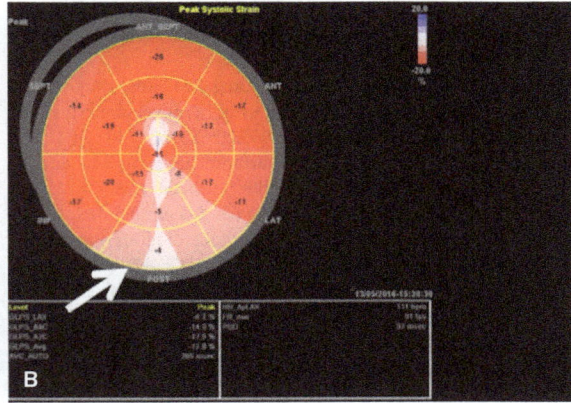
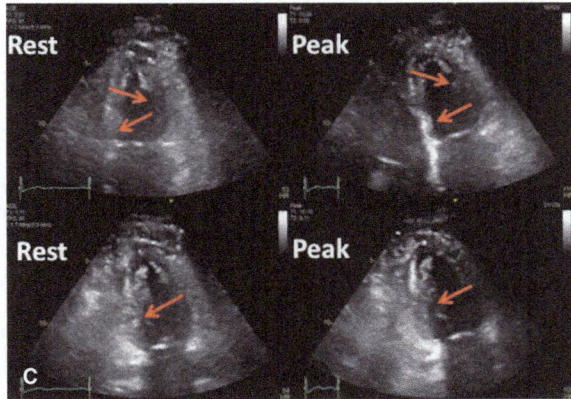

FIGURE 27-16 An example of abnormal strain on stress echocardiography. Immediately post exercise, both 2D and strain images were obtained. Strain images (panels **A** and **B**) show abnormal strain in the inferior, inferolateral, and anterolateral walls (*white arrows*). This correlates with wall-motion abnormalities at peak exercise in 2D imaging (*red arrows* in panel **C**). The ischemia is in the distribution of the LCX/RCA territories.

3D Stress Echocardiography

Three-dimensional SE can offer incremental value to 2D imaging. Advantages of 3D imaging include better visualization of the left ventricular apex, thereby avoiding foreshortening which is frequently a problem with 2D imaging. In addition, because 3D echo is able to evaluate multiple myocardial segments from different planes from a single data set, rapid acquisition of peak stress images before the heart rate declines is attainable.[68,69] More recently, integrated 2D/3D SE has been suggested to offer advantages over either modality alone. In a study of 25 patients who underwent combined 2D and 3D SE, 3D imaging was found to be superior in visualizing the anterior and anterolateral basal regions, while 2D remained superior in imaging the mid-inferior and inferoseptal segments.[70] Further refinement of 3D SE technology and methodology is needed prior to its integration into routine clinical practice.

CONCLUSIONS

Echocardiography is useful for the diagnosis and management of multiple cardiac disorders at rest and with stress. SE is invaluable for the assessment of patients with ischemic and nonischemic heart disease. Standard 2D echo and Doppler techniques remain the bedrock of echo imaging. More recently, novel modalities such as echo contrast, 3D echo, tissue Doppler, and deformation analysis have expanded the utility and improved the accuracy of echo imaging in a variety of cardiac disorders.

REFERENCES

1. Hahn RT, Abraham T, Adams MS, et al. Guidelines for performing a comprehensive transesophageal echocardiographic examination: Recommendations from the American Society of Echocardiography and the Society of Cardiovascular Anesthesiologists. *J Am Soc Echocardiogr.* 2013;26:921–964.

2. Armstrong WF, Ryan T, Feigenbaum H. *Feigenbaum's Echocardiography*. 7th ed. Philadelphia, PA: Wolters Kluwer Health/Lippincott Williams & Wilkins; 2010.
3. Sugeng L, Weinert L, Thiele K, Lang RM. Real-time three-dimensional echocardiography using a novel matrix array transducer. *Echocardiography*. 2003;20:623–635.
4. Thomas JD, Rubin DN. Tissue harmonic imaging: why does it work? *J Am Soc Echocardiogr*. 1998;11(8):803–808.
5. Lang RM, Badano LP, Mor-Avi V, et al. Recommendations for cardiac chamber quantification by echocardiography in adults: An update from the American Society of Echocardiography and the European Association of Cardiovascular Imaging. *J Am Soc Echocardiogr*. 2015;28:1–39.
6. Malm S, Frigstad S, Sagberg E, et al. Accurate and reproducible measurement of left ventricular volume and ejection fraction by contrast echocardiography: A comparison with magnetic resonance imaging. *J Am Coll Cardiol*. 2004;44:1030–1035.
7. Solomon S, Wu J, Gillam L. Echocardiography. In: Mann DL, Zipes DP, Libby P, Bonow RO, eds. *Braunwald's Heart Disease: A Textbook of Cardiovascular Medicine*. 10th ed. Philadelphia, PA: Saunders/Elsevier; 2015:179–251.
8. Quinones MA, Otto CM, Stoddard M, et al. Recommendations for quantification of Doppler echocardiography: A report from the Doppler quantification task force of the Nomenclature and Standards Committee of the American Society of Echocardiography. *J Am Soc Echocardiogr*. 2002;15:167–184.
9. Ho CY, Solomon SD. A clinician's guide to tissue Doppler imaging. *Circulation*. 2006;113:e396–e398.
10. Nagueh SF, Smiseth OA, Appleton CP, et al. Recommendations for the evaluation of left ventricular diastolic function by echocardiography: An update from the American Society of Echocardiography and the European Association of Cardiovascular Imaging. *J Am Soc Echocardiogr*. 2016;29(4):277–314.
11. Gulati VK, Katz WE, Follansbee WP, Gorcsan JI. Mitral annular descent velocity by tissue Doppler echocardiography as an index of global left ventricular function. *Am J Cardiol*. 1996;77:979–984.
12. Gorcsan JI, Tanaka H. Echocardiographic assessment of myocardial strain. *J Am Coll Cardiol*. 2011;58:1401–1413.
13. Blessberger H, Binder T. Two dimensional speckle tracking echocardiography: Clinical applications. *Heart*. 2010;96:2032–2040.
14. Arai K, Hozumi T, Matsumura Y, et al. Accuracy of measurement of left ventricular volume and ejection fraction by new real-time three-dimensional echocardiography in patients with wall motion abnormalities secondary to myocardial infarction. *Am J Cardiol*. 2004;94:552–558.
15. Gopal AS, Shen Z, Sapin PM, et al. Assessment of cardiac function by three-dimensional echocardiography compared with conventional noninvasive methods. *Circulation*. 1995;92:842–853.
16. Jenkins C, Bricknell K, Chan J, Hanekom L, Marwick TH. Comparison of two- and three-dimensional echocardiography with sequential magnetic resonance imaging for evaluating left ventricular volume and ejection fraction over time in patients with healed myocardial infarction. *Am J Cardiol*. 2007;99:300–306.
17. Fletcher GF, Ades PA, Kligfield P, et al. Exercise standards for testing and training: A scientific statement from the American Heart Association. *Circulation*. 2013;128:873–934.
18. Main ML, Asher CR, Rubin DN, et al. Comparison of tissue harmonic imaging with contrast (sonicated albumin) echocardiography and Doppler myocardial imaging for enhancing endocardial border resolution. *Am J Cardiol*. 1999;83:218–222.
19. Blair SN, Kohl HW III, Paffenbarger RS Jr, et al. Physical fitness and all-cause mortality: A prospective study of healthy men and women. *JAMA*. 1989;262:2395–2401.
20. Badruddin SM, Ahmad A, Mickelson J, et al. Supine bicycle versus post-treadmill exercise echocardiography in the detection of myocardial ischemia: A randomized single-blind crossover trial. *J Am Coll Cardiol*. 1999;33:1485–1490.
21. Pellikka PA, Nagueh SF, Elhendy AA, et al. American Society of Echocardiography recommendations for performance, interpretation, and application of stress echocardiography. *J Am Soc Echocardiogr*. 2007;20(9):1021–1041.
22. Marwick TH. Stress echocardiography. *Heart*. 2003;89:113–118.
23. Picano E, Alaimo A, Chubuchny V, et al. Noninvasive pacemaker stress echocardiography for diagnosis of coronary artery disease: a multicenter study. *J Am Coll Cardiol*. 2002;40:1305–1310.
24. Lee C, Pellikka PA, McCully RB, Mahoney DW, Seward JB. Non exercise stress transthoracic echocardiography: Transesophageal atrial pacing versus dobutamine stress. *J Am Coll Cardiol*. 1999;33:506–511.
25. Rainbird AJ, Mulvagh SL, Oh JK, et al. Contrast dobutamine stress echocardiography: Clinical practice assessment in 300 consecutive patients. *J Am Soc Echocardiogr*. 2001;14:378–385.
26. Vlassak I, Rubin DN, Odabashian JA. Contrast and harmonic imaging improves the accuracy and efficiency of novice readers for dobutamine stress echocardiography. *Echocardiography*. 2002;19:483–488.
27. Supariwala A, Makani H, Kahan J, et al. Feasibility and prognostic value of stress echocardiography in obese, morbidly obese, and super obese patients referred for bariatric surgery. *Echocardiography*. 2014;31(7):879–885.
28. Lerakis S, Kalogeropoulos AP, El-Chami MF, et al. Transthoracic dobutamine stress echocardiography in patients undergoing bariatric surgery. *Obes Surg*. 2007;17(11):1475–1481.
29. Shah BN, Zacharias K, Pabla JS, et al. The clinical impact of contemporary stress echocardiography in morbid obesity for the assessment of coronary artery disease. *Heart*. 2016;102(5):370–375.
30. Mordi I, Tzemos N. Non-invasive assessment of coronary artery disease in patients with left bundle branch block. *Int J Cardiol*. 2015;184:47–55.
31. Quiñones MA, Verani M, Haichin R, Mahmarian JJ, Suarez J, Zoghbi WA. Exercise echocardiography versus 201Tl single-photon emission computed tomography in evaluation of coronary artery disease: Analysis of 292 patients. *Circulation*. 1992;85:1217–1218.
32. Fleischmann K, Hunink M, Kuntz K, et al. Exercise echocardiography or exercise SPECT imaging? A meta-analysis of diagnostic test performance. *JAMA*. 1998;280:913–920.
33. Schinkel R, Bax J, Geleijnse M, et al. Noninvasive evaluation of ischemic heart disease: Myocardial perfusion imaging or stress echocardiography? *Eur Heart J*. 2003;24:789–800.
34. Smart S, Bhatia A, Hellman R, et al. Dobutamine-atropine stress echocardiography and dipyridamole sestamibi scintigraphy for the detection of coronary artery disease: Limitations and concordance. *J Am Coll Cardiol*. 2000;36:1265–1273.

35. Marwick T, D'Hondt A, Baudhuin T, et al. Optimal use of dobutamine stress for the detection and evaluation of coronary artery disease: Combination with echocardiography or scintigraphy, or both? *J Am Coll Cardiol*. 1993;22:159–167.
36. McCully RB, Roger VL, Mahoney DW, et al. Outcome after normal exercise echocardiography and predictors of subsequent cardiac events: Follow-up of 1,325 patients. *J Am Coll Cardiol*. 1998;31(1):144–149.
37. Marwick TH, Case C, Vasey C, et al. Prediction of mortality by exercise echocardiography: A strategy for combination with the Duke treadmill score. *Circulation*. 2001;103:2566–2571.
38. Poldermans D, Arnese M, Fioretti PM, et al. Improved cardiac risk stratification in major vascular surgery with dobutamine-atropine stress echocardiography. *J Am Coll Cardiol*. 1995;26:648–653.
39. Van der Sijde JN, Boiten H, van Domburg RT, Schinkel AF. Long-term (>10 years) prognostic value of dobutamine stress echocardiography in a high-risk cohort. *Am J Cardiol*. 2016;117(1):1078–1083.
40. Yao SS, Supariwala A, Yao A, Dukkipati S. Prognostic value of stress echocardiography in patients with low-intermediate or high short-term (10 years) versus low (<39%) or high (≥39%) lifetime predicted risk of cardiovascular disease according to the American College of Cardiology/American Heart Association 2013 Cardiovascular Risk Calculator. *Am J Cardiol*. 2015;116(5):725–729.
41. Ballal RS, Kapadia S, Secknus MA, et al. Prognosis of patients with vascular disease after clinical evaluation and dobutamine stress echocardiography. *Am Heart J*. 1999;137:469–475.
42. Dávila-Román VG, Waggoner AD, Sicard GA, et al. Dobutamine stress echocardiography predicts surgical outcome in patients with an aortic aneurysm and peripheral vascular disease. *J Am Coll Cardiol*. 1993;21:957–963.
43. Eichelberger JP, Schwarz KQ, Black ER, et al. Predictive value of dobutamine echocardiography just before noncardiac vascular surgery. *Am J Cardiol*. 1993;72:602–607.
44. Fleisher LA, Fleischmann KE, Auerbach AD, et al. 2014 ACC/AHA guideline on perioperative cardiovascular evaluation and management of patients undergoing noncardiac surgery: A report of the American College of Cardiology/American Heart Association Task Force on practice guidelines. *J Am Coll Cardiol*. 2014;64:e77–e137.
45. Bax JJ, Cornel JH, Vissner FC, et al. Prediction of recovery or regional left ventricular dysfunction following revascularization: Comparison of F18-fluorodeoxyglucose SPECT, thallium stress-reinjection SPECT and dobutamine echocardiography. *J Am Coll Cardiol*. 1996;28:558–564.
46. Bonow RO. Identification of viable myocardium. *Circulation*. 1996;94(11):2674–2680.
47. Bax JJ, Wijns W, Cornel JH, et al. Accuracy of currently available techniques for prediction of functional recovery after revascularization in patients with left ventricular dysfunction due to chronic coronary artery disease: Comparison of pooled data. *J Am Coll Cardiol*. 1997;30(6):1451–1460.
48. Bax JJ, Poldermans D, Elhendy A, Boersma E, Rahimtoola SH. Sensitivity, specificity, and predictive accuracies of various noninvasive techniques for detecting hibernating myocardium. *Curr Probl Cardiol*. 2001;26:141–188.
49. deFillipe CR, Willet DR, Irani WN, et al. Comparison of myocardial contrast echocardiography and low dose dobutamine stress echocardiography in predicting recovery of left ventricular function after revascularization after coronary revascularization in chronic ischemic heart disease. *Circulation*. 1995;91:990–998.
50. Allman KC, Shaw LJ, Hachamovitch R, Udelson JE. Myocardial viability testing and impact of revascularization on prognosis in patients with coronary artery disease and left ventricular dysfunction: A meta-analysis. *J Am Coll Cardiol*. 2002;39:115–118.
51. Camici PG, Prasad SK, Rimoldi OE. Stunning, hibernation, and assessment of myocardial viability. *Circulation*. 2008;117:103–114.
52. Bonow RO, Maurer G, Lee KL, et al. Myocardial viability and survival in ischemic left ventricular dysfunction. *N Eng J Med*. 2011;364:1617–1625.
53. Cortigiani L, Bigi R, Sicari R. Is viability still viable after the STICH trial? *Eur Heart J Cardiovasc Imaging*. 2012;13(3):219–224.
54. Nishimura RA, Otto CM, Bonow RO, et al. AHA/ACC guideline for the management of patients with valvular heart disease: A report of the American College of Cardiology/American Heart Association Task Force on Practice Guidelines. *J Thorac Cardiovasc Surg*. 2014;148:e1–e132.
55. Vahanian A, Alfieri O, Andreotti F, et al. Guidelines on the management of valvular heart disease. *Eur Heart J*. 2012;33:2451–2496.
56. Gersh BJ, Maron BJ, Bonow RO, et al. 2011 ACCF/AHA guideline for the diagnosis and treatment of hypertrophic cardiomyopathy: A report of the American College of Cardiology Foundation/American Heart Association Task Force on Practice Guidelines. *Circulation*. 2011;124.
57. Mulvagh SL, Rakowski H, Vannan MA, et al. American Society of Echocardiography Consensus Statement on the Clinical Applications of Ultrasonic Contrast Agents in Echocardiography. *J Am Soc Echocardiogr*. 2008;21(11):1179–1201.
58. Porter TR, Abdelmoneim S, Belcik JT, et al. Guidelines for the cardiac sonographer in the performance of contrast echocardiography: a focused update from the American Society of Echocardiography. *J Am Soc Echocardiogr*. 2014;27(8):797–810.
59. Plana JC, Mikati IA, Dokainish H, et al. A randomized crossover study for evaluation of the effect of image optimization with contrast on the diagnostic accuracy of dobutamine echocardiography in coronary artery disease. The OPTIMIZE trial. *JACC Cardiovasc Imaging*. 2008;1:145–150.
60. Porter TR, Xie F, Myocardial perfusion imaging with contrast ultrasound. *J Am Coll Cardiol Img*. 2010;3(2):176–187.
61. Gaibazzi N, Reverberi C, Lorenzoni V, et al. Prognostic value of high-dose dipyridamole stress myocardial contrast perfusion echocardiography. *Circulation*. 2012;126:1217–1224.
62. Dawson D, Kaul S, Peters D, et al. Prognostic value of dipyridamole stress myocardial contrast echocardiography: Comparison with single photon emission computed tomography. *J Am Soc Echocardiogr*. 2009;22:954–960.
63. Miszalski-Jamka T, Kuntz-Hehner S, Schmidt H, et al. Myocardial contrast echocardiography enhances long-term prognostic value of supine bicycle stress two-dimensional echocardiography. *J Am Soc Echocardiogr*. 2009;22:1220–1227.
64. Uusitalo V, Luotoahti M, Pietila M, et al. Two-dimensional speckle-tracking during dobutamine stress echocardiography

in the detection of myocardial ischemia in patients with suspected coronary artery disease. *J Am Soc Echocardiogr.* 2016;29(5):470-447.
65. Ingul CB, Stoylen A, Slordahl SA, et al. Automated analysis of myocardial deformation at dobutamine stress echocardiography: An angiographic validation. *J Am Coll Cardiol.* 2007;49:1651-1659.
66. Hanekom L, Cho GY, Leano R, Jeffriess L, Marwick TH. Comparison of two-dimensional speckle and tissue Doppler strain measurement during dobutamine stress echocardiography: An angiographic correlation. *Eur Heart J.* 2007;28:1765-1772.
67. Gaibazzi N, Pigazzani F, Reverberi C, Porter TR. Rest global longitudinal 2D strain to detect coronary artery disease in patients undergoing stress echocardiography: A comparison with wall-motion and coronary flow reserve responses. *Echo Res Pract.* 2014;1(2):61-70.
68. Lang RM, Badano LP, Tsang W. EAE/ASE recommendations for image acquisition and display using three-dimensional echocardiography. *J Am Soc Echocardiogr.* 2012;25:3-46.
69. Abusaid GH, Ahmad M. Real time three-dimensional stress echocardiography advantages and limitations. *Echocardiography.* 2012;29(2):200-206.
70. Johri AM, Chitty DW, Hua L, Marincheva G, Picard MH. Assessment of image quality in real time three-dimensional dobutamine stress echocardiography: An integrated 2D/3D approach. *Echocardiography.* 2015;32(3):496-507.

Coronary Calcium Scoring and Coronary CT Angiography

CHAPTER 28

Subhi J. Al'Aref, Khalil Anchouche,
Sarah J. Rinehart, Fay Y. Lin, and James K. Min

INTRODUCTION

Coronary artery calcium (CAC) scoring and cardiac computed tomographic angiography (CCTA) are comparatively new noninvasive imaging modalities that have experienced a rapid accumulation of scientific evidence for their clinical utility in the diagnosis, prognosis, and therapeutic planning for coronary heart disease. This technology offers a wide range of clinical applications and has value for a diverse range of patients.

CORONARY CALCIUM SCORING

Quantitation of coronary artery calcification by noncontrast cardiac computed tomography (CCT) for CAC scoring predicts future cardiovascular events in asymptomatic patients beyond what is conferred by assessment using traditional clinical risk-score calculators. The evaluation of coronary artery calcification has been widely accepted by the medical community as a powerful noninvasive screening tool due to the fact that atherosclerosis remains the only pathology known to be associated with coronary calcification (Fig. 28-1).[1] Furthermore, the correlation between the degree of vessel calcification and the overall atherosclerotic burden is well established, both through histopathologic determination and invasive imaging modalities such as intravascular ultrasound imaging.[2-5]

Scanning Protocols

CAC quantification may be performed by noncontrast electron beam computed tomography (EBCT) or multidetector row computed tomography (MDCT) scanners using electrocardiographic (ECG) gating. The standardized CAC protocol calls for axial imaging with prospective ECG triggering, with tube voltage of 120 kVp and tube current set at 120 to 150 milliampere-seconds (mAs), with the field of view limited to the heart and lungs using a scan length defined by the carina and the base of the heart. CAC scoring requires only a few seconds of scanning time and the overall study may be performed in 10 to 15 minutes. CAC scoring generally remains a screening tool; as such, patients selected for CAC evaluation with MDCT scanners should have minimal radiation exposure. The use of prospective ECG triggering enables performance of CAC scoring with very low-radiation doses that are less than the environmental exposure to radiation due to background radon exposure for an individual living at sea level for a year. The dose–length product (DLP) and effective radiation dose (E) should be maintained at less than 200 mGy × cm and 3.0 mSv, respectively.[6] Performed within guideline-suggested parameters, imaging results in a total radiation exposure that should average 1 to 1.5 mSv.[2]

Calculation of Coronary Artery Calcium Score

The Agatston score is the most commonly used tool for CAC scoring and best supported by the literature. The Agatston score is a semi-automated tool to calculate a weighted sum of the area of coronary calcification, wherein each calcified area is multiplied by a local density factor determined by the Hounsfield

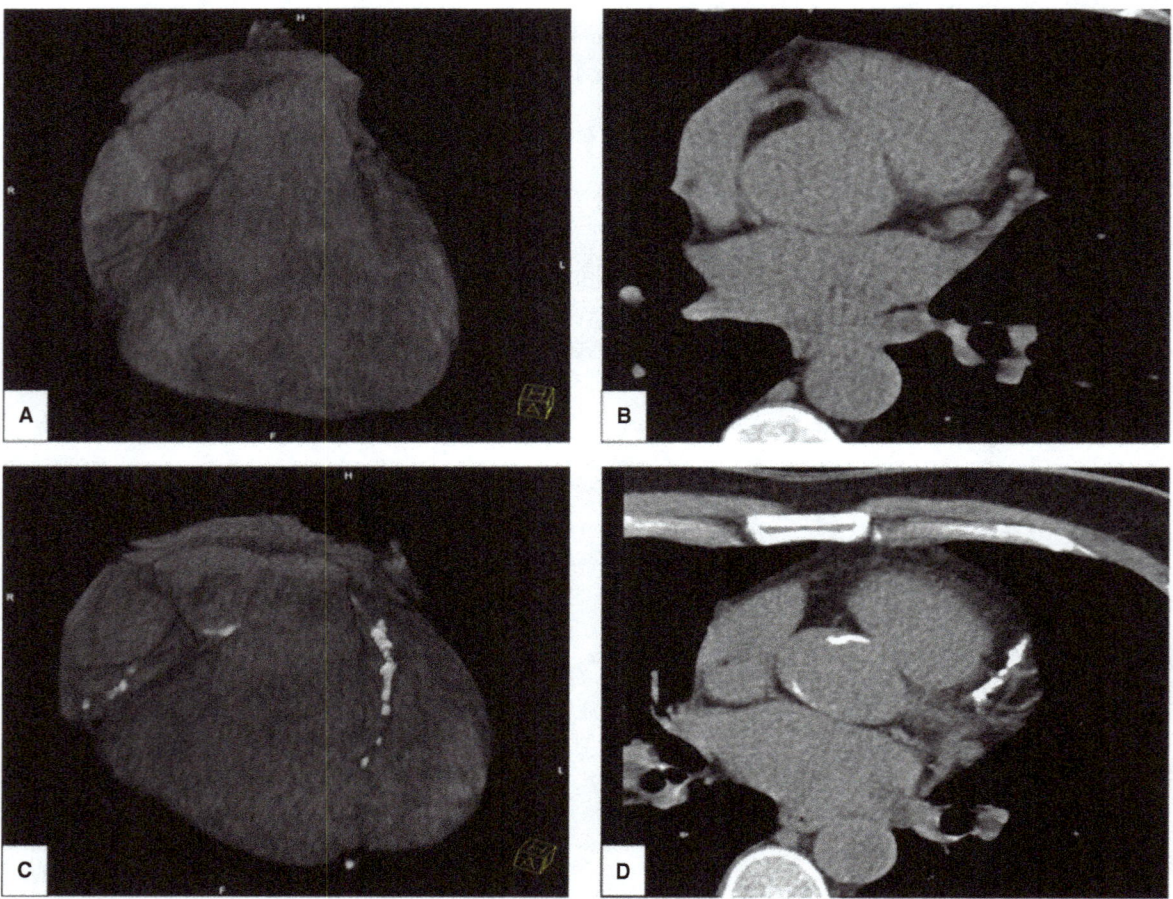

FIGURE 28-1 Computed tomography showing absence **(A,B)** and presence **(C,D)** of coronary artery calcium, used to compute a coronary calcium score. Figures A and C are volume rendered, while figures B and D are axial cross-sectional images.

unit (HU) of the calcium (0:0–129 HU; 1:130–199 HU; 2:200–299 HU, 3:300–399 HU; 4:>400 HU). There may be significant interscan variability in the Agatston score due to partial-volume effects and differences in attenuation coefficients between scanners. Other CAC scoring methods, such as the volume and mass scores, exhibit less-interscan variability, but have yet to be prognostically validated in large-scale clinical studies.[2] One potential mitigating factor to the routine use of Agatston CAC scoring is the integration of coronary calcium relative to HU density into the overall score. Prior studies have observed that lower-density calcifications confer greater risk for future major adverse cardiovascular events (MACE), while higher-density calcifications may somehow be protective. In this regard, the inability to extricate the HU density from the CAC score may lessen the CAC score as calculated by the method of Agatston.[7,8] Nevertheless, the Agatston CAC score has been validated for its predictive ability in an array of studies, and presently serves as the prognostic "gold standard" for CAC scoring. Importantly, technological improvements in newer-generation scanners have resulted in adequate CAC score reproducibility despite the technical limitations of the Agatston method.[9] CAC scoring has also been evaluated as an "add-on" for other imaging methods. In particular, single-photon emission computed tomography (SPECT) and positron emission tomography (PET) often use very low-dose CT scanning for attenuation correction. Despite these images not being acquired specifically for CAC scores, they nevertheless enable the quantification of CAC scores with generally high fidelity.[10] CAC scores are often similarly classified across clinical studies, with the following categorizations generally accepted for absent (CAC = 0 Agatston units), mild (CAC = 1–100 Agatston units), moderate (CAC = 101–400 Agatston units), and severe (CAC >400 Agatston units) coronary calcification. Based on the population-based multi-ethnic study of atherosclerosis (MESA), a CAC score of >300 Agatston units can also be considered to be severe.[11–13]

Diagnostic Performance

As a noncontrast study, CAC is unable to visualize noncalcified plaque or luminal stenosis encroachment by atherosclerotic plaque, and is thus unsuited for diagnosis of obstructive coronary artery disease (CAD). As a marker of overall atherosclerosis, severely elevated CAC score is associated with a higher likelihood of obstructive CAD among patients undergoing evaluation for stable chest pain. As an example, in a recent study evaluating the MESA population cohort of 6814 individuals, the mean CAC mass score for patients with nonobstructive (<50% stenosis), moderately obstructive (50–70% stenosis), and obstructive (>70% stenosis) CAD in the left anterior descending (LAD) artery were 105, 175, and 302 mg. A proportional association of total Agatston CAC score was observed for the number of obstructive stenosis in coronary arteries.[14] The negative predictive value (NPV) of the CAC score for the exclusion of obstructive CAD is excellent, as a CAC score of 0 carries an NPV of 99% for greater than 70% stenosis.[15] In distinction, for symptomatic patients, a negligible CAC score does not exclude the presence of obstructive stenosis. It has been shown that up to a fifth of patients referred for angiography had obstructive CAD despite having no coronary calcium detected by noninvasive imaging.[16,17]

Prognostic Value of Coronary Artery Calcium Score

CAC scores are population dependent and thus vary with age, gender, race, ethnicity, and socioeconomic status.[7,18,19] Yet in the MESA study, a similar overall relationship was observed for CAC in all populations, with CAC consistently associated with adverse clinical outcomes. This study, designed to investigate the prevalence, correlates and progression of subclinical cardiovascular disease in white, black, Hispanic, and Asian Americans of Chinese descent, demonstrated the consistent prognostic value of CAC score across each subgroup examined.[20] Agatston CAC scores of 0 predicted very low rates of downstream major coronary events, with a 4.6-year follow-up of 0.2%. In contrast, those individuals exhibiting a CAC 1 to 100, 101 to 300, and >300 experienced major coronary event rates of 1.4%, 3.2%, and 3.8%; these correlated to increased hazard ratios of 3.89, 7.08, and 6.84. Importantly, the prognostic utility of CAC scores is an independent factor incremental to traditional cardiovascular risk factors, and can correctly risk-stratify, discriminate, and reclassify patients with CAD. Indeed, the net reclassification improvement (NRI) based on CAC can be used to reclassify individuals to low-risk categories as well as high-risk categories. Individuals with CAC <100 can be reclassified as low risk 21.7% of the time, while individuals with CAC ≥400 can be reclassified as high risk 30.6% of the time.[21]

Clinical Utility of Coronary Artery Calcium Score

On the basis of the large body of evidence supporting its clinical utility, CAC scoring has been adopted as a useful risk-stratification tool in preventive cardiology guidelines. Notably, CAC scoring is considered useful in the following patient populations: (1) asymptomatic adults with intermediate-cardiovascular risk (class IIa); (2) asymptomatic adults with low–intermediate risk (class IIb); (3) asymptomatic diabetics age >40 (class IIa). In the recent risk-stratification guidelines proposed by the ACCF/American Heart Association (AHA), it is recommended that CAC scoring may be considered in the decision to prescribe statins for patients with an estimated cardiovascular event rate between 5% and 7.5%, calculated using the pooled-cohort equations, while patient groups with either higher- or lower-estimated event rates are recommended for treatment strategies regardless of CAC scores.[22–24] Such recommendations have also been echoed by the 2013 appropriate use criteria (AUC), which state that it may be appropriate to perform a CAC score in the evaluation of asymptomatic patients determined to be at intermediate-to-high risk for CAD.[25]

CAC scoring has also proven to be useful in select populations at a particularly high risk of adverse cardiovascular events. As an example, in asymptomatic diabetics, it has recently been shown that a CAC = 0 carries a very favorable 5-year prognosis, similar to that of nondiabetics. However, the mortality risk at 15 years of follow-up increases dramatically regardless of the initial prognosis, suggesting a limited "warranty period" for this high-risk patient population.[26]

Finally, while CAC progression has correlated with traditional cardiovascular risk factors, serial measurements of CAC are currently not recommended because the clinical understanding of progression of coronary calcification is not clearly understood, nor is it apparent what the effect of pharmacologic or behavioral modification of cardiovascular risk is on CAC progression.[12] In addition, such measurements involve increased costs and exposure (albeit small) to radiation, with unclear management implications. Among asymptomatic patients, the "warranty period" of a CAC = 0 transitioning to a CAC >0 appears to be approximately 4 years, with the clinical "warranty period" of event-free survival extending to nearly 15 years.[27]

CORONARY CT ANGIOGRAPHY

Computed tomography (CT) has been in clinical use since the 1970s, when Sir Godfrey Hounsfield utilized x-ray CT to construct axial images of the human body.[28] During the ensuing decade, CT was employed in evaluating noncardiac organs, given the need for greater temporal, spatial, and contrast resolution in imaging a moving organ. In 1981, ECG-gated cardiac CT was first utilized to directly image the myocardium and the chambers of the heart and in 1997, coronary luminal visualization was achieved using ECG-gated contrast-enhanced electron beam CT (EBCT).[29,30] Since the introduction of 64-detector row CT scanners in 2005, coronary CT angiography (CCTA) has been established as the definitive noninvasive imaging modality for visualization of native coronary arteries and coronary artery bypass grafts.

Cardiac CT images have traditionally been acquired through either EBCT or multidetector (MDCT) scanners. The clinical application of EBCT is limited to the noninvasive detection and evaluation of CAC. EBCT scanners have low spatial resolution, are expensive, and consequently are no longer used.[31] MDCT scanners, on the other hand, allow for superior imaging of the cardiovascular system through improved spatial resolution, as well as the ability to acquire volumetric data that now allow for image acquisition of the entire heart within 1 second. While inferior to the temporal resolution of EBCT scanners, MDCT methods have improved the temporal resolution, with the most contemporary scanners achieving resolutions as low as 70 milliseconds. Technological advances for improving temporal resolution are achieved with faster gantry rotation as well as different methods of image acquisition that do not require full helical imaging. The pitch, defined as the table movement in one 360-degree gantry rotation divided by the slice (or beam) width, can also be increased to this effect (e.g., fast-pitch helical modes). Furthermore, spatial resolution has been improved using different detector elements to achieve sub-millimeter isotropic voxels. In addition, whole-volume coverage of MDCT using 320-detector row scanners for 1-second cardiac imaging minimizes misregistration artifacts that are common in 64-detector row MDCT scanners.

CCTA is well tolerated by most patients, and generally requires minimal preparation. It is recommended that patients abstain from caffeinated beverages for at least 12 hours prior to imaging in order to prevent a rise in heart rate and avoid diuresis. Some institutions also recommend that patients undergoing CCTA abstain from food for 2 or more hours prior to imaging due to the risk of contrast-induced nausea, vomiting, and subsequent aspiration. While patients should continue to use their routinely prescribed medications on the day of examination, those on metformin and phosphodiesterase type 5 (PDE_5) inhibitors are instructed to abstain from them due to their unique side-effect profile. Though rare, there is concern for the development of lactic acidosis as a result of contrast-induced nephropathy with metformin use. Likewise, PDE_5 inhibitors are contraindicated due to the risk of hypotension when combined with nitroglycerin. Indeed, in the hours prior to imaging, patients typically receive an oral beta-blocker, such as metoprolol, to reduce the heart rate. Administration of this agent is then followed by use of sublingual nitroglycerin in the minutes immediately preceding initiation of the scan. While in the scanner, patients are instructed to hold their breath to prevent the development of image artifact. Nevertheless, despite such measures, imaging quality can be limited as a result of significant heart rate variability or ectopy (such as atrial fibrillation or the presence of premature contractions). In addition, the presence of advanced renal insufficiency or contrast intolerance/allergy limits the ability to administer contrast and reduces the quality of the acquired images.

▶ Noninvasive Coronary Imaging with Cardiac Computed Tomography Angiography

The primary application of MDCT cardiac imaging involves characterization of coronary anatomy for assessment of stenosis severity as well as atherosclerosis extent, severity, and location (Fig. 28-2). These findings are useful for aiding the prediction of future adverse cardiovascular events.[32,33]

Based on the recommendations of the 2008 AHA scientific statement on noninvasive coronary artery imaging, the 2010 Expert Consensus Document on CCTA and the 2012 American College of Cardiology (ACC)/AHA stable ischemic heart disease (SIHD) guidelines[34–36]:

1. CCTA should not be used to screen for CAD in the absence of signs or symptoms suggestive of CAD.
2. CCTA is not recommended in patients with either low pretest likelihood of CAD (due to concerns of radiation exposure) or a high pretest likelihood of CAD (such patients are likely to require invasive coronary angiography anyway).
3. CCTA is a reasonable option for patients with intermediate pretest probability of CAD who are unable to perform other noninvasive modalities (exercise-stress test, nuclear perfusion scar, or echocardiography).
4. CCTA might be reasonable for symptomatic patients who are at intermediate risk for CAD after initial risk stratification.
5. CCTA or cardiac MRI is suggested to evaluate patients with congenital or acquired coronary anomalies.

Importantly, in a departure from prior recommendations, the 2013 appropriate use criteria (AUC) guidelines deemed CCTA appropriate for follow-up testing within 90 days in the setting of uncertain prior ECG or

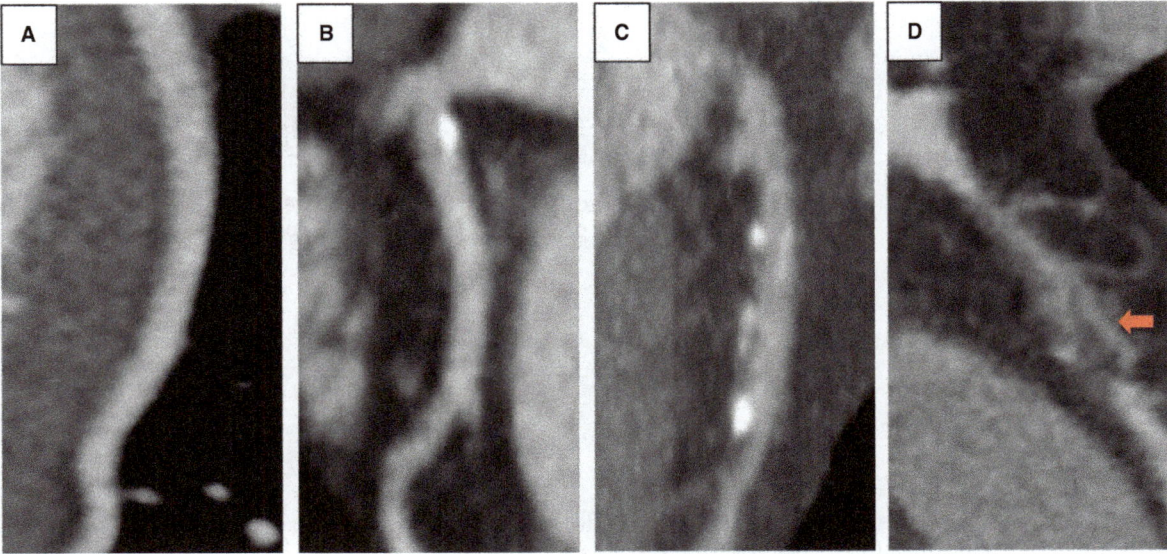

FIGURE 28-2 Coronary computed tomography angiography use in delineation of atherosclerotic disease burden. Curved multiplanar reformatted images demonstrating: normal coronary artery **(A)**, mildly stenotic calcified plaque **(B)**, moderately stenotic partially calcified plaque **(C)**, and **(D)**, a noncalcified occlusive plaque with bridging collaterals (*red arrow*).

stress imaging study results. In addition, the recommendation for the use of CCTA in symptomatic and preoperative patients has been weakened, in accordance with the most recent perioperative and SIHD guidelines.[25]

▶ Technical Aspects of Coronary CT Angiography

Image Acquisition Modes

ECG gating is applied in cardiac CT to synchronize image acquisition to the cardiac cycle, in order to minimize motion artifact in the beating heart. ECG gating can be performed prospectively or retrospectively (Fig. 28-3).[33] Prospective ECG gating involves initiation of image acquisition at a prespecified interval during the cardiac cycle (typically diastole). As a result, the projection data are acquired for only a short part of the complete gantry rotation. Once the desired data are acquired, the table is shifted to the next bed position and the scanner acquires more projections. This cycle repeats until the entire scan length is covered. In contrast, retrospective ECG gating involves continuous image acquisition throughout the cardiac cycle with significant overlap. Retrospective gating typically involves low scan pitch, defined as the relationship of the scan coverage to the table speed, which ensures contiguous sampling with the absence of gaps. In addition, retrospective gating permits image reconstruction at multiple points in the cardiac cycle, as opposed to the fixed point of acquisition used with prospective gating protocols.

The number of detector rows is an important aspect of image acquisition, since an increase in the number of detectors allows for a large portion of the heart to be covered per gantry rotation. For example, each detector row acquires data simultaneously in the z direction with each gantry rotation in multi-detector CT scanners. In a 64-slice detector CT with each detector measuring 0.625 mm in width, a typical cardiac region ranging between 120 and 150 mm in length can be covered in three to four gantry rotations (with each gantry rotation scanning approximately 40 mm). As a result, less acquisition time is required, decreasing the time required for breath holding and minimizing motion artifacts (which are major limitations in hospitalized patients).

Radiation Reduction Strategies

The rise of cardiac CT during a period of dramatic increase in radiation exposure from medical

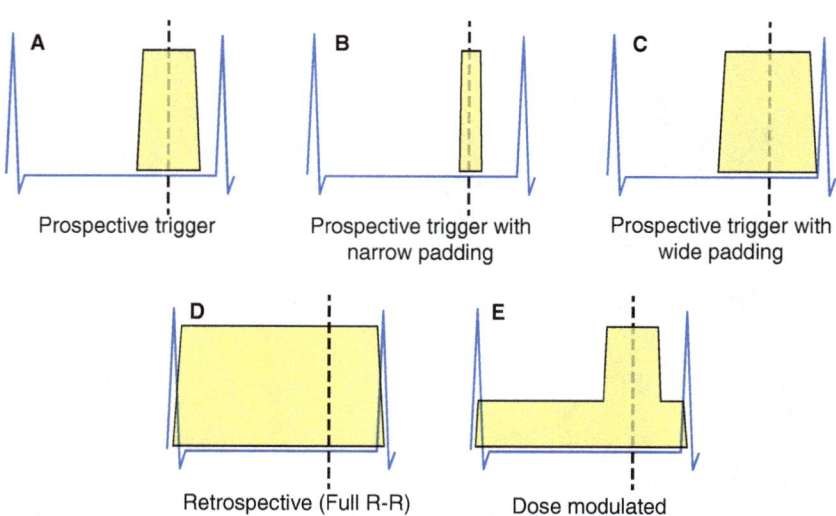

FIGURE 28-3 ECG-gating techniques. ECG-gated image acquisition can be performed prospectively (**A,C**) or retrospectively (**D,E**). Prospective gating involves data acquisition during a specified portion of the cardiac cycle (**A**), with the ability to narrow (**B**) or widen (**C**) the acquisition interval. Retrospective gating involves data acquisition throughout the cardiac cycle (**D**), with the existence of techniques to reduce radiation exposure (**E**).

procedures, coupled with an increased recognition of the associated stochastic and deterministic effects of radiation, has led to intense scrutiny of the radiation burden associated with this new technology (see Chapter 7). For example, a chest x-ray results in an effective dose exposure of 0.1 mSv, while CCTA results in an effective exposure of 3 to 4 mSv (and can be as high as 8–22 mSv in retrospectively gated scans) and 8 to 12 mSv for technetium myocardial perfusion scans. The 2011 Society of Cardiovascular Computed Tomography (SCCT) guidelines provide recommendations regarding interpretation of radiation dose indices and predictors of risk, appropriate use of scanner acquisition modes and settings (Fig. 28-3), development of algorithms for dose optimization, and establishment of procedures for dose monitoring.[37] Some of the commonly adopted techniques for radiation dose reduction include[38]:

1. Prospectively gated imaging (estimated dose reduction up to 83%) as a result of image acquisition during a short period in diastole.
2. ECG-gated (estimated dose reduction 30–50%) image acquisition is coupled with the cardiac cycle with high tube current applied only during diastole.
3. High-pitch scanning mode (estimated dose reduction up to 80%) requires dual-source scanners in order to obtain the projection data by the second detector to avoid gaps due to rapid table movement.
4. Low tube voltage (kVp) (estimated dose reduction up to 30%) results in decreased photon emission. Image quality is maintained due to differences in contrast level. Structures with high atomic number maintain contrast difference over those with low atomic number.
5. Anatomy-based tube-current modulation (estimated dose reduction 20–60%) involves adjustment of the tube current for each projection angle according to patients' anatomic structures.
6. Iterative reconstruction algorithms (estimated dose reduction up to 40%) employ computational techniques that enable improved image quality at lower-radiation doses while reducing image noise.

Contrast-Enhanced Techniques

The use of contrast media in CCTA aims for maximal opacification of the coronary arteries and the left ventricle. The determination of the volume of contrast to be administered is an important aspect of the examination. Initially, a test bolus of contrast is followed by an intravenous saline injection at a prespecified rate. Sequential axial scans at the proximal aorta are obtained to determine timing of peak opacification. The total contrast volume during actual image acquisition is calculated by adding the time required for peak aortic opacification to the time required to cover the scan length, multiplied by the infusion rate. As a result, the need for contrast media use for coronary artery opacification limits the usage of CCTA in patients with advanced renal impairment.

▶ Anatomic Evaluation

Stable Ischemic Heart Disease

Since the inception of 64-detector row MDCT scanners, debate has centered on CCTA's ability to determine coronary stenosis severity as compared to an invasive angiographic "gold standard." Three prospective multicenter studies have addressed this question (Table 28-1). In the first published ACCURACY study, 230 individuals with suspected but without known CAD underwent both CCTA and invasive angiography. Per-patient sensitivity and specificity to detect and exclude obstructive CAD were 95% and 83%.[39] This compared similarly to the study by Meijboom et al.[40] who evaluated 360 symptomatic patients with both acute and stable chest pain who underwent CCTA and invasive angiography. With more than two-thirds of patients exhibiting a coronary stenosis ≥50%, the sensitivity and specificity of CCTA versus invasive angiography was 99% and 64% respectively. In contrast, Miller et al.[41] evaluated a mixed population of patients with and without known CAD and observed a lower sensitivity of 85% with a higher specificity of 90%.

Acute Chest Pain/Emergency Department Evaluation

The diagnostic performance of CCTA in the evaluation of patients presenting with chest pain has been an area of active research and investigation. The use of CCTA in the emergency department (ED) features prominently in the 2015 ACR/ACC/AHA AUC, as

Table 28-1

Diagnostic Performance of CCTA in Patients with Stable Ischemic Heart Disease

Trial	Year	Sample Size	Patient Population	Variable Evaluated	Accuracy
Leschka et al.[42] *Eur Heart J*	2005	67	Patients with suspected coronary artery disease or prior to coronary artery bypass	≥50% stenosis	Per Segment Analysis Se 94%, Sp 97%, PPV 87%, NPV 99%
Raff et al.[43] *J Am Coll Cardiol*	2005	70	Patients scheduled to undergo coronary angiography	≥50% stenosis	Per Patient Analysis Se 95%, Sp 90%, PPV 93%, NPV 93% Per Vessel Analysis Se 91%, Sp 92%, PPV 80%, NPV 97%
Ehara et al.[44] *Circ J*	2006	69	Patients with suspected or proven coronary artery disease, or prior stenting	≥50% stenosis	Per Patient Analysis Se 98%, Sp 86%, PPV 98%, NPV 86% Per Vessel Analysis Se 90%, Sp 94%, PPV 89%, NPV 95%
Schujif et al.[45] *Am J Cardiol*	2006	60	Patients scheduled to undergo invasive angiography	≥50% stenosis	Per Patient Analysis Se 94%, Sp 97%, PPV 97%, NPV 93% Per Vessel Analysis Se 87%, Sp 96%, PPV 87%, NPV 96%
ACCURACY trial[39] *J Am Coll Cardiol*	2008	230	No history of coronary artery disease	≥50% or ≥70% stenosis	≥50% Stenosis Se 95%, Sp 83%, PPV 64%, NPV 99% ≥70% Stenosis Se 94%, Sp 83%, PPV 48%, NPV 99%
Meijboom et al.[40] *J Am Coll Cardiol*	2008	360	Stable or unstable anginal syndrome	≥50% stenosis	Per Patient Analysis Se 99%, Sp 64%, PPV 86%, NPV 97% Per Vessel Analysis Se 95%, Sp 77%, PPV 59%, NPV 98%
Miller et al.[41] *N Engl J Med*	2008	291	Suspected symptomatic coronary artery disease	≥50% stenosis	Per Patient Analysis Se 85%, Sp 90%, PPV 91%, NPV 83% Per Vessel Analysis Se 75%, Sp 93%, PPV 82%, NPV 89%
Brodoefel et al.[46] *Eur J Radiol*	2008	102	Known or suspected coronary artery disease	≥50% stenosis	Per Segment Analysis Se 91%, Sp 99%, PPV 95%, NPV 98%

Se, sensitivity; Sp, specificity; PPV, positive predictive value; NPV, negative predictive value.

a result of its favorable accuracy in detecting ≥50% coronary artery stenosis.[47] In the early assessment pathway, the use of CCTA is considered appropriate in patients presenting with chest pain when there is low–intermediate pretest likelihood of non–ST-segment elevation MI (NSTEMI) (through normal value of initial cardiac biomarkers, absence of ischemic changes on ECG, or low TIMI risk score) or when there is equivocal initial diagnosis of NSTEMI. The utility of CCTA in such a clinical setting stems from its high sensitivity (86–100%) and NPV (93–100%). The use of CCTA, on the other hand, is considered rarely appropriate in patients with positive initial evaluation of NSTEMI, since such patients will ultimately need to undergo invasive coronary angiography for diagnostic and therapeutic purposes. Furthermore, the positive predictive value (PPV) of CCTA is limited (50–90%), since CCTA has low accuracy in patients with extensive coronary calcification, which is a marker of advanced atherosclerosis

Table 28-2
Comparison of Outcomes in Patients Undergoing CCTA for Evaluation of Acute Chest Pain in the Emergency Department Setting

Randomized Trial	Year	Sample Size	Comparison Modality	Follow-up Period	Comparison of Clinical Outcomes
Goldstein et al.[48] J Am Coll Cardiol	2007	197 (99 CCTA)	Standard care	6 months	Death (0% CCTA vs. 0% standard care) AMI (0% CCTA vs. 0% standard care) PCI (4% CCTA vs. 1% Standard care, $p = 0.37$)
Beigel et al.[49] Am J Cardiol	2009	699 (340 CCTA)	MPI	3 months	Death (0.4% CCTA vs. 0% MPI, $p = 0.46$) ACS (0% CCTA vs. 1.3% MPI, $p = 0.13$) PCI (0% CCTA vs. 3% MPI, $p = 0.005$)
CT-STAT trial[45] J Am Coll Cardiol	2011	699 (361 CCTA)	MPI	6 months	Death (0% CCTA vs. 0% MPI) AMI (0% CCTA vs. 0% MPI) Revascularization (0.3% CCTA vs. 0% MPI, $p = 1.0$)
Litt et al.[50] N Engl J Med	2012	1370 (908 CCTA)	Standard care	30 days	Death (0% CCTA vs. 0% standard care) AMI (1% CCTA vs. 1% standard care) Revascularization (3% CCTA vs. 1% standard care)
ROMICAT II trial[51] N Engl J Med	2012	1000 (501 CCTA)	Standard care	28 days	MACE (0.4% CCTA vs. 1.2% standard care, $p = 0.18$)

AMI, acute myocardial infarction; PCI, percutaneous coronary intervention; MPI, myocardial perfusion imaging; ACS, acute coronary syndrome.

and results in increased risk of adverse cardiovascular events.

Three major randomized trials evaluated the utility of incorporating CCTA in the initial evaluation of patients with low-to-intermediate likelihood of acute coronary syndrome (ACS) in the ED setting (Table 28-2).[48,50,51] The ROMICAT II trial was a multicenter trial that randomized 1000 patients with chest pain (or anginal equivalent), but without ischemic electrocardiographic changes or an initial positive troponin level to early CCTA or to standard evaluation in the ED.[51] Incorporation of CCTA into a triage strategy was found to improve the efficiency of clinical decision making, as compared with a standard evaluation, through achievement of shorter length of stay without missing ACS events and a similar 28-day MACE rate between both arms. A disadvantage of using CCTA was that it resulted in an increase in downstream testing and radiation exposure with no decrease in the overall costs of care. Litt et al.[50] reinforced the notion that utilization of CCTA is safe in the evaluation of low-to-intermediate risk patients presenting to the ED with chest pain (30-day MI event rate of 1.1% in both the CCTA arm and the traditional care arm). Furthermore, patients undergoing CCTA evaluation were discharged earlier than patients undergoing traditional care (overall length of stay of 18.0 hours vs. 24.8 hours, respectively). Similar findings were reported in the CT-STAT trial where CCTA was compared to myocardial perfusion imaging (MPI).[48] As such, the use of CCTA for the evaluation of acute low-risk chest pain has been widely adopted as a safe alternative, compared to standard evaluation, and associated with reduced length of stay.

Atherosclerosis Evaluation

CCTA has the unique capability of noninvasively evaluating coronary atherosclerosis features such as plaque composition (Fig. 28-4). Prospective validation studies comparing CCTA plaque characteristics to IVUS-derived virtual histology (IVUS-VH) have observed that low-density noncalcified plaque (LD-NCP) identified by CCTA corresponds to necrotic core and fibrofatty tissue on IVUS-VH, while high-density noncalcified plaque (HD-NCP) corresponds to fibrous tissue on IVUS-VH.[52]

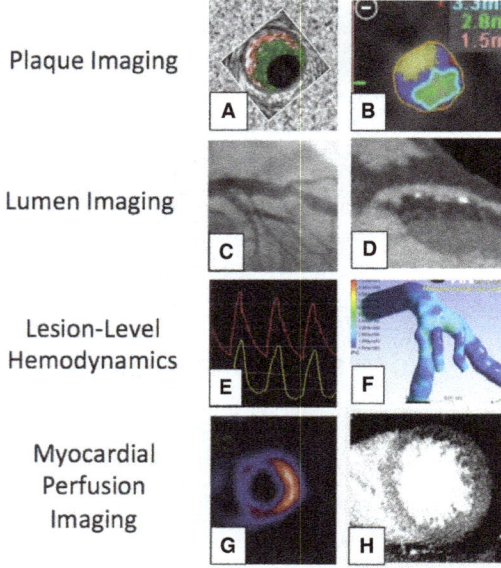

FIGURE 28-4 Correlation between anatomic and physiologic measurements in CCTA and other imaging modalities. Plaque imaging is demonstrated by intravascular ultrasound with radiofrequency backscatter **(A)** and coronary computed tomography angiography (CCTA) **(B)**. Luminal imaging is demonstrated by invasive coronary angiogram **(C)** and CCTA **(D)**. Lesion-level hemodynamics is demonstrated by invasive fractional flow reserve (FFR) **(E)** and CCTA-derived FFR measurement **(F)**. Myocardial perfusion imaging is demonstrated by nuclear SPECT **(G)** and CT perfusion **(H)**.

CCTA studies have established two major plaque characteristics found in culprit lesions within the ACS population: positive-arterial remodeling and low attenuation plaque as a surrogate measure of necrotic core.[53] Patients with more than one feature had a much higher incidence of future ACS. Subsequent studies have additionally established the significance of a "napkin-ring" sign, defined as a ring of high attenuation around coronary arterial plaque, and which has also been associated with higher risk of cardiac events (Fig. 28-5).[54]

Changes in atherosclerosis occur as a result of medical therapy for CAD, and early pilot studies have examined these changes for both atherosclerotic progression and lesion composition. In a small cohort of 32 patients, the effect of statin therapy was assessed by serial CCTA.[55] On follow-up CCTA, patients on statin therapy were noted to have a decrease in total plaque volume and low attenuation plaque volume, suggesting that the addition of statin therapy results in improvement in features associated with plaque instability.

Patency of Stents and Bypass Grafts

Patients frequently develop recurrent cardiovascular symptoms after revascularization procedures, necessitating the evaluation of patency of venous or arterial

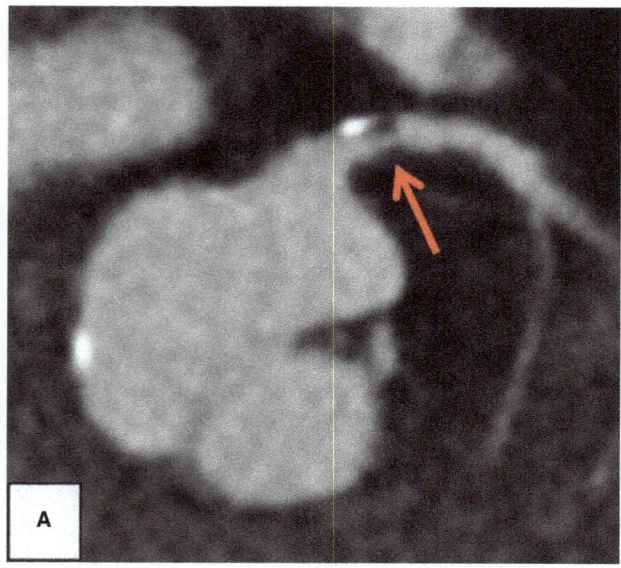
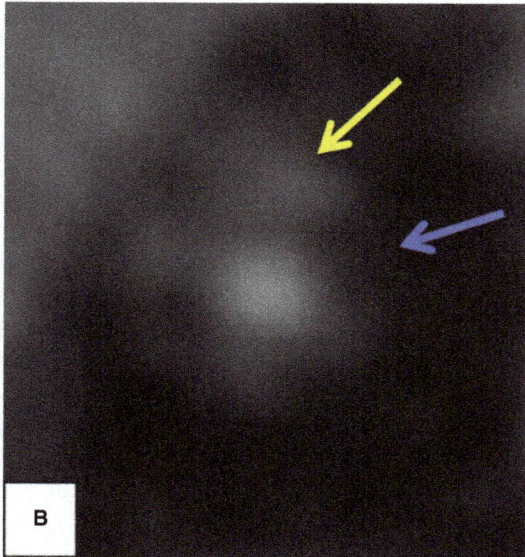

FIGURE 28-5 Napkin-ring sign. CCTA demonstrating severe stenosis in the left main artery (*red arrow*) with high-risk plaque features of napkin-ring sign (*yellow arrow*) and low attenuation plaque (*blue arrow*).

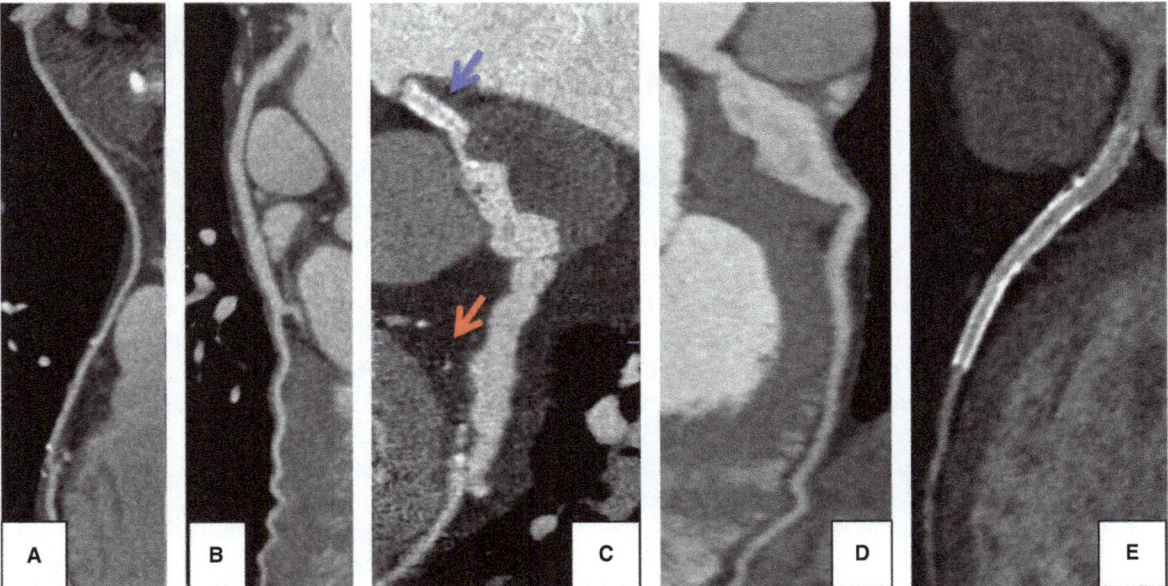

FIGURE 28-6 Utility of CCTA in evaluating bypass grafts and intracoronary stents. **(A)** Curved multiplanar reformatted images depicting patent LIMA to left anterior descending artery, **(B)** patent SVG to the obtuse marginal artery, **(C)** aneurysmal SVG to the obtuse marginal artery (*blue arrow* shows a patent stent in the proximal portion of the graft and *red arrow* shows the occluded native coronary artery), **(D)** aneurysmal native coronary artery with thrombus, and **(E)** patent stents in the left anterior descending artery.

bypass grafts or newly implanted coronary artery stents (Fig. 28-6). Invasive coronary angiography is often cumbersome and associated with significant contrast dye administration, while nuclear perfusion scans appear to have limited accuracy in detecting graft disease.[56] CCTA has been established as a reliable noninvasive tool for evaluating graft patency in symptomatic patients. Early studies utilizing 64-slice CCTA were useful for accurate exclusion of greater than 50% graft stenosis, but detection of distal anastomotic stenosis was limited.[57] This is a very important point, as the utility of CCTA in this population appears to be constrained to whether or not graft disease exists, and less so for comprehensive evaluation of bypass grafts and native CAD. Subsequent use of dual-source CCTA for the detection or exclusion of significant stenosis in arterial and venous grafts revealed an accuracy of 100%, with limited ability to image obstructive disease in distal runoffs and native coronary arteries.[58]

Improvements in the spatial resolution of current generation CT scanners have expanded the ability to visualize and evaluate the intracoronary space, particularly for in-stent restenosis in patients with previous percutaneous revascularization.

Evaluation of in-stent restenosis by CCTA is limited due to "blooming" or partial-volume artifacts conferred by metallic stent struts. To a degree, 64-slice CCTA enables detection of in-stent restenosis, quantification of neointimal hyperplasia, and correlates moderately with quantitative coronary angiography and IVUS ($r = 0.794$, $p < 0.001$, and $r = 0.943$, $p < 0.0001$, respectively).[59] Clinically, the accuracy of multidetector CT is favorable in large stents (diameter ≥3.0 mm) and has limited accuracy in smaller stents for the evaluation of in-stent restenosis.[60,61] Indeed, the 2013 AUC highlights that CCTA is rarely useful in the assessment of asymptomatic patients postrevascularization with CABG or PCI; it may be useful, however, in follow-up evaluation of patients with left-main disease, as well as in those who remain symptomatic despite intervention.[25]

▶ CT Myocardial Perfusion

One of the limitations of CCTA is the frequent lack of correlation between anatomic findings and functional significance, as the presence of an anatomic lesion does not necessarily correlate to a functional abnormality.

The combination of an anatomic assessment with CCTA and a functional assessment with SPECT perfusion imaging could provide essential direction for guiding clinical management and assessment of long-term prognosis. The advent of myocardial computed tomography perfusion (CTP) does, in theory, enable acquisition of both anatomic and physiologic information through assessment of myocardial perfusion and the presence of ischemia or infarction. Prior studies have observed that a combined CCTA/CTP study is superior for detection of hemodynamically significant atherosclerotic lesions compared with CCTA alone.[62] In addition, a combined CTP/CCTA study could provide a plethora of information regarding coronary anatomy, perfusion, ventricular function, and the presence of scar (with delayed-enhancement imaging) that is equivalent to radiation exposure in a SPECT study (average radiation dose of 12.7 mSv).[63] In a study involving patients at high risk for CAD, combining CTP/CCTA (compared to CCTA) for the detection of >50% stenosis increased sensitivity from 83% to 91%, specificity from 71% to 91%, PPV from 66% to 86%, and NPV from 87% to 93%.[64] However, such a strategy carries the inconvenience of performing two separate tests along with significant radiation exposure and thus is rarely used clinically and is still considered largely investigational.

Fractional Flow Reserve Derived from CT

While noninvasive cardiac imaging modalities are used to identify symptomatic patients who subsequently require invasive coronary angiography, nearly two-thirds of such patients are ultimately found to have nonobstructive CAD. A significant limitation of anatomic imaging methods, such as CCTA and invasive coronary angiography, is the inability to determine the physiologic significance of a given coronary stenosis. At present, fractional flow reserve (FFR) is widely considered the "gold" standard for evaluation of the physiologic significance of a coronary artery stenosis. Importantly, FFR requires a coupling of both anatomic as well as physiologic assessment, wherein an anatomic stenosis detected by invasive angiography is subsequently evaluated by FFR. FFR, defined as the ratio of hyperemic pressure distal to a stenosis to the hyperemic pressure proximal to a stenosis, has been established a prognostic "gold" standard as FFR-guided PCI results in improved event-free survival over anatomic stenosis-guided PCI alone.[65]

FFR_{CT} is an emerging novel method for evaluation of ischemia. In contrast to stress-testing methods that evaluate myocardial perfusion or stress-induced regional wall-motion abnormalities, FFR_{CT} proffers the ability to improve specificity of ischemia identification by interrogation of specific coronary stenosis for their ischemia-causing nature. Importantly, FFR_{CT} does not require any additional image acquisition, radiation exposure, or medications. Calculation of FFR_{CT} is done through three-dimensional modeling of the coronary tree, determination of rest and stress flow, and application of computational fluid dynamics to solve for coronary pressure, velocity, and flow (Fig. 28-7). An array of prospective multicenter international studies evaluating FFR_{CT} have been reported, including the DISCOVER-FLOW, DeFACTO, and NXT trials. In the most recent NXT trial, whose primary endpoint was discrimination of ischemia compared to invasive FFR by the area under the receiver-operating characteristics (ROC) curve, FFR_{CT} significantly improved discrimination for the diagnosis of hemodynamically significant CAD when compared to anatomic methods alone (ROC of 0.68; 95% CI, 0.62–0.74 for CCTA vs. ROC of 0.81; 95% CI, 0.75–0.86; $p < 0.01$ for FFR_{CT}).[66] Importantly, similar to the use of invasive FFR, adoption of FFR_{CT} encourages changes in clinical practice that improve clinical outcome and reduce resource utilization and costs. In the recently reported PLATFORM trial, FFR_{CT} was evaluated in comparison to standard of care in order to determine its effects on the rate of "normalcy" at the time of invasive angiography. In this study, the use of FFR_{CT} in symptomatic patients at intermediate risk reduced the rate of nonobstructive CAD during invasive coronary angiography from 73% to 12% with no differences in MACE, radiation exposure, or revascularization. Importantly, the rates of coronary revascularization were unchanged in the FFR_{CT} groups as compared to the standard-of-care groups, which suggest that FFR_{CT} may appropriately identify the "right" individuals who require coronary revascularization.[67]

Prognostic Utility of CCTA

CCTA has been established as a noninvasive imaging modality that enables visualization of atherosclerotic

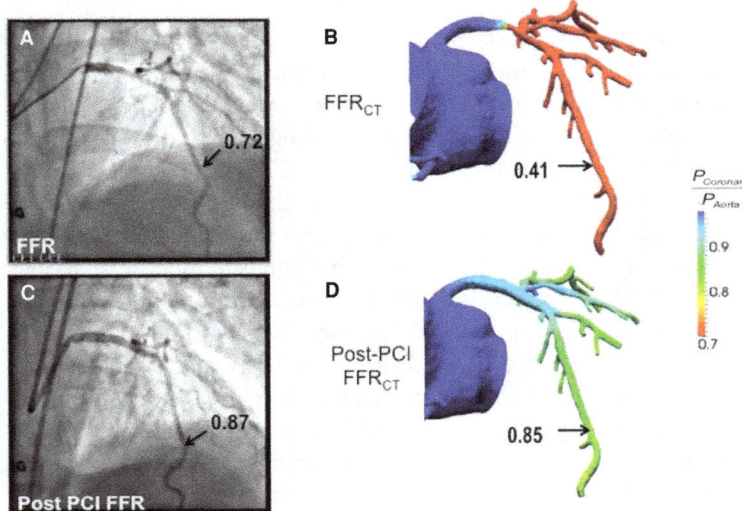

FIGURE 28-7 Case example of a patient who underwent CCTA, FFR$_{CT}$, invasive angiography, and invasive FFR. **(A)** Invasive angiogram demonstrating a stenosis in the proximal portion of the left anterior descending (LAD) artery that causes ischemia, with an invasive FFR value of <0.80. **(B)** CCTA demonstrating a similar high-grade stenosis in the proximal LAD, with FFR$_{CT}$ demonstrating similar ischemia. **(C)** FFR value after percutaneous coronary intervention has improved and the ischemia is resolved, with a value of >0.80. **(D)** Post-PCI FFR$_{CT}$ also demonstrates resolution of ischemia with a value of 0.85. (Based on concepts from Kim KH, Doh JH, Koo BK, et al. A novel noninvasive technology for treatment planning using virtual coronary stenting and computed tomography-derived computed fractional flow reserve. *JACC Cardiovasc Interv.* 2014;7(1):72–78.)

plaques with high diagnostic performance for identification and exclusion of CAD. These anatomic findings provide robust prognostic value for the prediction of all-cause mortality, nonfatal myocardial infarction, and MACE in an array of subgroups that include both men and women; younger and older patients; diabetic patients; patients with low cardiovascular risk, as measured by Framingham risk scores or presence of treatable CAD risk factors; patients with a family history of premature CAD; active or prior smokers; and hypertensive patients (Fig. 28-8).[68] While generally used for symptomatic patients with

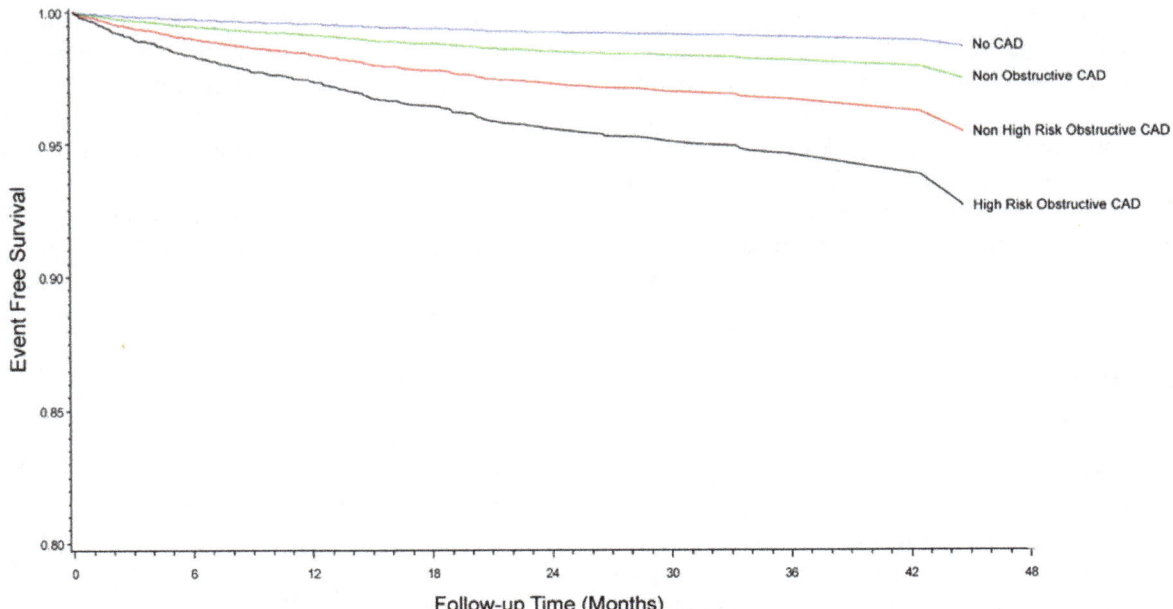

FIGURE 28-8 Prognostic utility of CCTA in coronary artery disease. Data from the CONFIRM registry demonstrating increasing incidence of major adverse cardiovascular events stratified by CAD severity (normal, nonobstructive, non–high-risk obstructive or high-risk obstructive CAD). (Reproduced with permission from Chow BJ, Small G, Yam Y, et al. Incremental prognostic value of cardiac computed tomography in coronary artery disease using CONFIRM. *Circ Cardiovasc Imaging.* 2011;4(5):463–472.)

suspected CAD, CCTA is sometimes performed for asymptomatic individuals for CAD risk assessment. In this population, CCTA findings are incrementally prognostic for individuals with moderately elevated CAC score (CAC between 101 and 400), but not for low (CAC <100) or high CAC score (CAC >400).[69]

CCTA may play an essential role in the evaluation of high-risk patient subsets. In a meta-analysis of 6225 diabetic patients undergoing CCTA with a follow-up period ranging from 20 to 66 months, the annualized cardiovascular event rate was 0.1% for no CAD, 4.5% for nonobstructive CAD, and 17.1% for obstructive CAD. The ability of CCTA to detect nonobstructive CAD, which might otherwise go unnoticed by other noninvasive imaging modalities, can help further risk-stratify diabetic patients. This is particularly important in light of the elevated annualized event rate of 4.5% in this patient population.[70] Another high-risk group of patients are those with left-main or triple-vessel CAD, where CCTA has been shown to have a sensitivity, specificity, PPV, and NPV of 95%, 83%, 53%, and 99%, respectively. Such diagnostic performance in excluding left-main or triple-vessel CAD is notable, given the fact that only 56% of patients with angiographically proven left-main disease exhibit moderate or severe ischemia by nuclear perfusion imaging, while nearly one in seven individuals exhibit no perfusion abnormalities.[71]

Finally, it is noteworthy to mention that the short-term, postimaging clinical management of patients without a history of CAD with an intermediate-to-high likelihood of CAD undergoing noninvasive imaging was evaluated in the SPARC trial, which revealed that up to 44% of patients with high-risk findings were undertreated with aspirin, statin, or a beta-blocker.[72]

▶ Coronary CT Angiography versus Radionuclide Perfusion Imaging

The performance of CCTA compared to that of other noninvasive imaging modalities has been assessed in several prospective studies. In a European multicenter study enrolling patients with stable chest pain and intermediate likelihood of CAD, CCTA exhibited the highest discriminatory performance compared to invasive angiography, with the ROC curve being 0.91 as compared to an ROC of 0.74 for MPI for the detection of obstructive CAD.[73] In the most contemporary study to date, Danad et al.[74] evaluated the diagnostic performance of an array of CAD imaging tests to diagnose coronary ischemia. Evaluating myocardial perfusion by SPECT or cardiac magnetic resonance imaging, stress echocardiography and invasive coronary angiography, and CCTA, the highest sensitivities noted were for CCTA and FFR_{CT}, while specificity for ischemia-causing CAD was highest for CMR and FFR_{CT}. However, such diagnostic superiority has yet to translate into improved clinical outcomes. The Prospective Multicenter Imaging Study for Evaluation of Chest Pain (PROMISE) trial compared anatomic with functional testing in 10,003 symptomatic patients. It showed that an initial anatomic assessment with CCTA, as compared with a functional assessment with SPECT, stress echocardiography, or exercise electrocardiography, did not improve cardiovascular outcomes (composite of death, MI, hospitalization for unstable angina, or major procedural complications) over a median follow-up period of 2 years, but was associated with lower-radiation exposure (10.0 mSv vs. 11.3 mSv) and less-invasive angiography demonstrating nonobstructive CAD (3.4% vs. 4.3%).[75] Overall, these results show that efficacy and safety endpoints were similar between a CCTA-based assessment and a SPECT-based assessment.

Finally, patients enrolled in the SPARC trial and undergoing an anatomic assessment with CCTA, compared with those undergoing a functional assessment using PET or SPECT, were more likely to be referred to invasive coronary angiography after normal or mildly abnormal study findings.[72] These findings highlight the clinical utility of CCTA performance in intermediate-risk patients, where a positive or a negative finding may lead to change in the clinical management strategy.

CONCLUSION

In the past several years, improvements in CT technology have enabled reliable and accurate evaluation of CAD. The introduction of novel technologies, such as FFR_{CT}, offers a new paradigm of combined anatomic and physiologic imaging, which is associated with salutary outcomes and improved performance measures at the time of invasive angiography.

Conflicts of interest: Dr. Min is a consultant to Heartflow Inc., and receives institutional research support from GE Healthcare.

REFERENCES

1. Simpson CL, Lindley S, Eisenberg C, et al. Toward cell therapy for vascular calcification: Osteoclast-mediated demineralization of calcified elastin. *Cardiovasc Pathol.* 2007;16(1):29–37.
2. Budoff MJ, Achenbach S, Blumenthal RS, et al. Assessment of coronary artery disease by cardiac computed tomography: A scientific statement from the American Heart Association Committee on Cardiovascular Imaging and Intervention, Council on Cardiovascular Radiology and Intervention, and Committee on Cardiac Imaging, Council on Clinical Cardiology. *Circulation.* 2006;114(16):1761–1791.
3. Blankenhorn D. Coronary arterial calcification, a review. *Am J Med Sci.* 1961;242:1–9.
4. Simons DB, Schwartz RS, Edwards WD, Sheedy PF, Breen JF, Rumberger JA. Noninvasive definition of anatomic coronary artery disease by ultrafast computed tomographic scanning: A quantitative pathologic comparison study. *J Am Coll Cardiol.* 1992;20(5):1118–1126.
5. Mintz GS. Pichard AD, Popma JJ, et al. Determinants and correlates of target lesion calcium in coronary artery disease: A clinical, angiographic and intravascular ultrasound study. *J Am Coll Cardiol.* 1997;29(2):268–274.
6. Voros S, Rivera JJ, Berman DS, et al. Guideline for minimizing radiation exposure during acquisition of coronary artery calcium scans with the use of multidetector computed tomography: A report by the Society for Atherosclerosis Imaging and Prevention Tomographic Imaging and Prevention Councils in collaboration with the Society of Cardiovascular Computed Tomography. *J Cardiovasc Comput Tomogr.* 2011;5(2):75–83.
7. Bild DE, Detrano R, Peterson DO, et al. Ethnic differences in coronary calcification: The Multi-Ethnic Study of Atherosclerosis (MESA). *Circulation.* 2005;111(10):1313–1320.
8. Criqui MH, Denenberg JO, Ix JH, et al. Calcium density of coronary artery plaque and risk of incident cardiovascular events. *JAMA.* 2014;311(3):271–278.
9. Budoff MJ, McClelland RL, Chung H, et al. Reproducibility of coronary artery calcified plaque with cardiac 64-MDCT: The Multi-Ethnic Study of Atherosclerosis. *AJR Am J Roentgenol.* 2009;192(3):613–617.
10. Einstein AJ, Johnson LL, Bokhari S, et al. Agreement of visual estimation of coronary artery calcium from low-dose CT attenuation correction scans in hybrid PET/CT and SPECT/CT with standard Agatston score. *J Am Coll Cardiol.* 2010;56(23):1914–1921.
11. Detrano R, Guerci AD, Carr JJ, et al. Coronary calcium as a predictor of coronary events in four racial or ethnic groups. *N Engl J Med.* 2008;358(13):1336–1345.
12. Greenland P, Bonow RO, Brundage BH, et al. ACCF/AHA 2007 clinical expert consensus document on coronary artery calcium scoring by computed tomography in global cardiovascular risk assessment and in evaluation of patients with chest pain: A report of the American College of Cardiology Foundation Clinical Expert Consensus Task Force (ACCF/AHA Writing Committee to Update the 2000 Expert Consensus Document on Electron Beam Computed Tomography) developed in collaboration with the Society of Atherosclerosis Imaging and Prevention and the Society of Cardiovascular Computed Tomography. *J Am Coll Cardiol.* 2007;49(3):378–402.
13. Yeboah J, Young R, McClelland RL, et al. Utility of nontraditional risk markers in atherosclerotic cardiovascular disease risk assessment. *J Am Coll Cardiol.* 2016;67(2):139–147.
14. Rosen BD, Fernandes V, McClelland RL, et al. Relationship between baseline coronary calcium score and demonstration of coronary artery stenoses during follow-up MESA (Multi-Ethnic Study of Atherosclerosis). *JACC Cardiovasc Imaging.* 2009;2(10):1175–1183.
15. Sarwar A, Shaw LJ, Shapiro MD, et al. Diagnostic and prognostic value of absence of coronary artery calcification. *JACC Cardiovasc Imaging.* 2009;2(6):675–688.
16. Villines TC, Hulten EA, Shaw LJ, et al. Prevalence and severity of coronary artery disease and adverse events among symptomatic patients with coronary artery calcification scores of zero undergoing coronary computed tomography angiography: Results from the CONFIRM (Coronary CT Angiography Evaluation for Clinical Outcomes: An International Multicenter) registry. *J Am Coll Cardiol.* 2011;58(24):2533–2540.
17. Gottlieb I, Miller JM, Arbab-Zadeh A, et al. The absence of coronary calcification does not exclude obstructive coronary artery disease or the need for revascularization in patients referred for conventional coronary angiography. *J Am Coll Cardiol.* 2010;55(7):627–634.
18. McClelland RL, Chung H, Detrano R, Post W, Kronmal RA, et al. Distribution of coronary artery calcium by race, gender, and age: Results from the Multi-Ethnic Study of Atherosclerosis (MESA). *Circulation.* 2006;113(1):30–37.
19. Roux AV, Detrano R, Jackson S, et al. Acculturation and socioeconomic position as predictors of coronary calcification in a multiethnic sample. *Circulation.* 2005;112(11):1557–1565.
20. Bild DE, Bluemke DA, Burke GL, et al. Multi-ethnic study of atherosclerosis: Objectives and design. *Am J Epidemiol.* 2002;156(9):871–881.
21. Erbel R, Möhlenkamp S, Moebus S, et al. Coronary risk stratification, discrimination, and reclassification improvement based on quantification of subclinical coronary atherosclerosis: The Heinz Nixdorf Recall study. *J Am Coll Cardiol.* 2010;56(17):1397–1406.
22. Taylor AJ, Cerqueira M, Hodgson JM, et al. ACCF/SCCT/ACR/AHA/ASE/ASNC/NASCI/SCAI/SCMR 2010 appropriate use criteria for cardiac computed tomography. A report of the American College of Cardiology Foundation Appropriate Use Criteria Task Force, the Society of Cardiovascular Computed Tomography, the American College of Radiology, the American Heart Association, the American Society of Echocardiography, the American Society of Nuclear Cardiology, the North American Society for Cardiovascular Imaging, the Society for Cardiovascular Angiography and Interventions, and the Society for Cardiovascular Magnetic Resonance. *J Cardiovasc Comput Tomogr.* 2010;4(6):407.
23. Goff DC, Lloyd-Jones DM, Bennett G, et al. 2013 ACC/AHA guideline on the assessment of cardiovascular risk: A report of the American College of Cardiology/American Heart Association Task Force on Practice Guidelines. *J Am Coll Cardiol.* 2014;63(25 Pt B):2935–2959.
24. Greenland P, Alpert JS, Beller GA, et al. 2010 ACCF/AHA guideline for assessment of cardiovascular risk in asymptomatic adults: A Report of the American College of Cardiology Foundation/American Heart Association Task Force on Practice Guidelines developed in collaboration with the American

Society of Echocardiography, American Society of Nuclear Cardiology, Society of Atherosclerosis Imaging and Prevention, Society for Cardiovascular Angiography and Interventions, Society of Cardiovascular Computed Tomography, and Society for Cardiovascular Magnetic Resonance. *J Am Coll Cardiol.* 2010;56(25):2182–2199.
25. Wolk MJ, Bailey SR, Doherty JU, et al. ACCF/AHA/ASE/ASNC/HFSA/HRS/SCAI/SCCT/SCMR/STS 2013 multimodality appropriate use criteria for the detection and risk assessment of stable ischemic heart disease: A report of the American College of Cardiology Foundation Appropriate Use Criteria Task Force, American Heart Association, American Society of Echocardiography, American Society of Nuclear Cardiology, Heart Failure Society of America, Heart Rhythm Society, Society for Cardiovascular Angiography and Interventions, Society of Cardiovascular Computed Tomography, Society for Cardiovascular Magnetic Resonance, and Society of Thoracic Surgeons. *J Am Coll Cardiol.* 2014;63(4):380–406.
26. Valenti V, Hartaigh B, Heo R, et al. A 15-year warranty period for asymptomatic individuals without coronary artery calcium: A prospective follow-up of 9,715 individuals. *JACC Cardiovasc Imaging.* 2015;8(8):900–909.
27. Min JK, Lin FY, Gidseg DS, et al. Determinants of coronary calcium conversion among patients with a normal coronary calcium scan: What is the "warranty period" for remaining normal? *J Am Coll Cardiol.* 2010;55(11):1110–1117.
28. Hounsfield GN. Historical notes on computerized axial tomography. *J Can Assoc Radiol.* 1976;27(3):135–142.
29. Lackner K, Thurn P. Computed tomography of the heart: ECG-gated and continuous scans. *Radiology.* 1981;140(2):413–420.
30. Chernoff DM, Ritchie CJ, Higgins CB. Evaluation of electron beam CT coronary angiography in healthy subjects. *AJR Am J Roentgenol.* 1997;169(1):93–99.
31. Baumgart D, Schmermund A, Goerge G, et al. Comparison of electron beam computed tomography with intracoronary ultrasound and coronary angiography for detection of coronary atherosclerosis. *J Am Coll Cardiol.* 1997;30(1):57–64.
32. Burrill J, Dabbagh Z, Gollub F, Hamady M. Multidetector computed tomographic angiography of the cardiovascular system. *Postgrad Med J.* 2007;83(985):698–704.
33. Cody DD, Mahesh M. AAPM/RSNA physics tutorial for residents: Technologic advances in multidetector CT with a focus on cardiac imaging. *Radiographics.* 2007;27(6):1829–1837.
34. Bluemke DA, Achenbach S, Budoff M, et al. Noninvasive coronary artery imaging: Magnetic resonance angiography and multidetector computed tomography angiography: A scientific statement from the American heart association committee on cardiovascular imaging and intervention of the council on cardiovascular radiology and intervention, and the councils on clinical cardiology and cardiovascular disease in the young. *Circulation.* 2008;118(5):586–606.
35. Mark DB, Berman DS, Budoff MJ, et al. ACCF/ACR/AHA/NASCI/SAIP/SCAI/SCCT 2010 expert consensus document on coronary computed tomographic angiography: A report of the American College of Cardiology Foundation Task Force on Expert Consensus Documents. *J Am Coll Cardiol.* 2010;55(23):2663–2699.
36. Fihn SD, Blankenship JC, Alexander KP, et al. 2012 ACCF/AHA/ACP/AATS/PCNA/SCAI/STS guideline for the diagnosis and management of patients with stable ischemic heart disease: A report of the American College of Cardiology Foundation/American Heart Association Task Force on Practice Guidelines, and the American College of Physicians, American Association for Thoracic Surgery, Preventive Cardiovascular Nurses Association, Society for Cardiovascular Angiography and Interventions, and Society of Thoracic Surgeons. *J Am Coll Cardiol.* 2012;60(24):e44–e164.
37. Halliburton SS, Abbara S, Chen MY, et al. SCCT guidelines on radiation dose and dose-optimization strategies in cardiovascular CT. *J Cardiovasc Comput Tomogr.* 2011;5(4):198–224.
38. Sabarudin A, Sun Z. Coronary CT angiography: Dose reduction strategies. *World J Cardiol.* 2013;5(12):465–472.
39. Budoff MJ, Dowe D, Jollis JG, et al. Diagnostic performance of 64-multidetector row coronary computed tomographic angiography for evaluation of coronary artery stenosis in individuals without known coronary artery disease: Results from the prospective multicenter ACCURACY (Assessment by Coronary Computed Tomographic Angiography of Individuals Undergoing Invasive Coronary Angiography) trial. *J Am Coll Cardiol.* 2008;52(21):1724–1732.
40. Meijboom WB, Meijs MF, Schuijf JD, et al. Diagnostic accuracy of 64-slice computed tomography coronary angiography: A prospective, multicenter, multivendor study. *J Am Coll Cardiol.* 2008;52(25):2135–2144.
41. Miller JM, Rochitte CE, Dewey M, et al. Diagnostic performance of coronary angiography by 64-row CT. *N Engl J Medicine.* 2008;359(22):2324–2336.
42. Leschka S, Alkadhi H, Plass A, et al. Accuracy of MSCT coronary angiography with 64-slice technology: first experience. *Eur Heart J.* 2005;26(15):1482–1487.
43. Raff GL, Gallagher MJ, O'Neill WW, et al. Diagnostic accuracy of noninvasive coronary angiography using 64-slice spiral computed tomography. *J Am Coll Cardiol.* 2005;46(3):552–557.
44. Ehara M, Surmely JF, Kawai M, et al. Diagnostic accuracy of 64-slice computed tomography for detecting angiographically significant coronary artery stenosis in an unselected consecutive patient population: comparison with conventional invasive angiography. *Circ J.* 2006;70(5):564–571.
45. Schuijf JD, Pundziute G, Jukema JW, et al. Diagnostic accuracy of 64-slice multislice computed tomography in the noninvasive evaluation of significant coronary artery disease. *Am J Cardiol.* 2006;98(2):145–148.
46. Brodoefel H, Reimann A, Burgstahler C, et al. Noninvasive coronary angiography using 64-slice spiral computed tomography in an unselected patient collective: effect of heart rate, heart rate variability and coronary calcifications on image quality and diagnostic accuracy. *Eur J Radiol.* 2008;66(1):134–141.
47. Rybicki FJ, Udelson JE, Peacock WF, et al. 2015 ACR/ACC/AHA/AATS/ACEP/ASNC/NASCI/SAEM/SCCT/SCMR/SCPC/SNMMI/STR/STS appropriate utilization of cardiovascular imaging in emergency department patients with chest pain: A joint document of the American College of Radiology Appropriateness Criteria Committee and the American College of Cardiology Appropriate Use Criteria Task Force. *J Am Coll Cardiol.* 2016;67(7):853–879.
48. Goldstein JA, Chinnaiyan KM, Abidov A, et al. The CT-STAT (Coronary Computed Tomographic Angiography for Systematic Triage of Acute Chest Pain Patients to Treatment) trial. *J Am Coll Cardiol.* 2011;58(14):1414–1422.

49. Beigel R, Oieru D, Goitein O, et al. Usefulness of routine use of multidetector coronary computed tomography in the "fast track" evaluation of patients with acute chest pain. *Am J Cardiol.* 2009;103(11):1481–1486.
50. Litt HI, Gatsonis C, Snyder B, et al. CT angiography for safe discharge of patients with possible acute coronary syndromes. *New England Journal of Medicine.* 2012;366(15):1393–1403.
51. Hoffmann U, Truong QA, Schoenfeld DA, et al. Coronary CT angiography versus standard evaluation in acute chest pain. *New England Journal of Medicine.* 2012;367(4):299–308.
52. Voros S, Rinehart S, Qian Z, et al. Prospective validation of standardized, 3-dimensional, quantitative coronary computed tomographic plaque measurements using radiofrequency backscatter intravascular ultrasound as reference standard in intermediate coronary arterial lesions: Results from the ATLANTA (assessment of tissue characteristics, lesion morphology, and hemodynamics by angiography with fractional flow reserve, intravascular ultrasound and virtual histology, and noninvasive computed tomography in atherosclerotic plaques) I study. *JACC Cardiovasc Interv.* 2011;4(2):198–208.
53. Motoyama S, Sarai M, Narula J, et al. Coronary CT angiography and high-risk plaque morphology. *Cardiovasc Interv Ther.* 2013;28(1):1–8.
54. Otsuka K, Fukuda S, Tanaka A, et al. Napkin-ring sign on coronary CT angiography for the prediction of acute coronary syndrome. *JACC Cardiovasc Imaging.* 2013;6(4):448–457.
55. Inoue K, Motoyama S, Sarai M, et al. Serial coronary CT angiography-verified changes in plaque characteristics as an end point: Evaluation of effect of statin intervention. *JACC Cardiovasc Imaging.* 2010;3(7):691–698.
56. Al Aloul B, Mbai M, Adabag S, et al., Utility of nuclear stress imaging for detecting coronary artery bypass graft disease. *BMC Cardiovasc Disord.* 2012;12:62.
57. Feuchtner, GM, Schachner T, Bonatti J, et al. Diagnostic performance of 64-slice computed tomography in evaluation of coronary artery bypass grafts. *AJR Am J Roentgenol.* 2007;189(3):574–580.
58. Weustink AC, Nieman K, Pugliese F, et al., Diagnostic accuracy of computed tomography angiography in patients after bypass grafting: Comparison with invasive coronary angiography. *JACC Cardiovasc Imaging.* 2009;2(7):816–824.
59. Andreini D, Pontone G, Bartorelli AL, et al. Comparison of feasibility and diagnostic accuracy of 64-slice multidetector computed tomographic coronary angiography versus invasive coronary angiography versus intravascular ultrasound for evaluation of in-stent restenosis. *Am J Cardiol.* 2009;103(10):1349–1358.
60. Andreini D, Pontone G, Mushtaq S, et al. Multidetector computed tomography coronary angiography for the assessment of coronary in-stent restenosis. *Am J Cardiol.* 2010;105(5):645–655.
61. Wykrzykowska JJ, Arbab-Zadeh A, Godoy G, et al. Assessment of in-stent restenosis using 64-MDCT: Analysis of the CORE-64 Multicenter International Trial. *AJR Am J Roentgenol.* 2010;194(1):85–92.
62. Techasith T, Cury RC. Stress myocardial CT perfusion: An update and future perspective. *JACC Cardiovasc Imaging.* 2011;4(8):905–916.
63. Blankstein, R, Shturman LD, Rogers IS, et al. Adenosine-induced stress myocardial perfusion imaging using dual-source cardiac computed tomography. *J Am Coll Cardiol.* 2009;54(12):1072–1084.
64. Rocha-Filho JA, Blankstein R, Shturman LD, et al. Incremental value of adenosine-induced stress myocardial perfusion imaging with dual-source CT at cardiac CT angiography. *Radiology.* 2010;254(2):410–419.
65. Min JK. Taylor CA, Achenbach S, et al. Noninvasive fractional flow reserve derived from coronary CT angiography: Clinical data and scientific principles. *JACC Cardiovasc Imaging.* 2015;8(10):1209–1222.
66. Min JK, Leipsic J, Pencina MJ, et al. Diagnostic accuracy of fractional flow reserve from anatomic CT angiography. *JAMA.* 2012;308(12):1237–1245.
67. Douglas PS, Pontone G, Hlatky MA, et al. Clinical outcomes of fractional flow reserve by computed tomographic angiography-guided diagnostic strategies vs. usual care in patients with suspected coronary artery disease: The prospective longitudinal trial of FFR(CT): Outcome and resource impacts study. *Eur Heart J.* 2015;36(47):3359–3367.
68. Otaki Y, Arsanjani R, Gransar H, et al. What have we learned from CONFIRM? Prognostic implications from a prospective multicenter international observational cohort study of consecutive patients undergoing coronary computed tomographic angiography. *J Nucl Cardiol.* 2012;19(4):787–795.
69. Cho I. Chang HJ, Hartaigh BÓ, et al. Incremental prognostic utility of coronary CT angiography for asymptomatic patients based upon extent and severity of coronary artery calcium: Results from the COronary CT Angiography EvaluatioN For Clinical Outcomes InteRnational Multicenter (CONFIRM) study. *Eur Heart J.* 2015;36(8):501–8.
70. Celeng C, Maurovich-Horvat P, Ghoshhajra BB, et al. Prognostic value of coronary computed tomography angiography in patients with diabetes: A meta-analysis. *Diabetes Care.* 2016;39(7):1274–1280.
71. Berman DS, Kang X, Slomka PJ, et al. Underestimation of extent of ischemia by gated SPECT myocardial perfusion imaging in patients with left main coronary artery disease. *J Nucl Cardiol.* 2007;14(4):521–528.
72. Hachamovitch R, Nutter B, Hlatky MA, et al.; SPARC Investigators. Patient management after noninvasive cardiac imaging results from SPARC (Study of myocardial perfusion and coronary anatomy imaging roles in coronary artery disease). *J Am Coll Cardiol.* 2012;59(5):462–474.
73. Neglia D, Rovai D, Caselli C, et al. Detection of significant coronary artery disease by noninvasive anatomical and functional imaging. *Circ Cardiovasc Imaging.* 2015;8(3). doi: 10.1161/CIRCIMAGING.114.002179.
74. Danad I, Szymonifka J, Twisk JWR, et al. Diagnostic performance of cardiac imaging methods to diagnose ischaemia-causing coronary artery disease when directly compared with fractional flow reserve as a reference standard: A meta-analysis. *Eur Heart J.* 2017;38(13):991–998.
75. Douglas PS, Hoffmann U, Patel MR, et al. Outcomes of anatomical versus functional testing for coronary artery disease. *N Engl J Med.* 2015;372(14):1291–1300.

Cardiovascular Magnetic Resonance

CHAPTER 29

Jamieson M. Bourque and Christopher M. Kramer

INTRODUCTION

Cardiovascular magnetic resonance is an advanced noninvasive cardiovascular imaging technique that has become well established but continues to evolve. It has some advantages over SPECT myocardial perfusion imaging (MPI) in the evaluation of ischemic heart disease but also has limitations that restrict the potential patient population. Technical advances in hardware and software protocols are unlocking new diagnostic and prognostic possibilities. In many areas of cardiovascular disease, it is the reference standard. The versatility of CMR allows one scan to provide information on cardiovascular structure, function, fibrosis, perfusion, and tissue characterization. CMR is a robust technique for evaluating ischemic heart disease and cardiomyopathies and has a role to play in evaluating other conditions, such as valvular and pericardial disease. We will provide a brief overview of the methods of CMR imaging, discuss its advantages and limitations, and outline its use in specific disease states.

CMR METHODS AND ADVANTAGES

Magnetic resonance imaging is performed by having a patient lie in the bore of a large hollow magnet in which a magnetic field is generated, typically at 1.5 Tesla. The hydrogen atoms in the body, predominately in water and fat, behave like magnets and possess "spin." When the hydrogen protons are exposed to the magnetic field they align their spins.[1,2] Radiofrequency pulses are generated by the magnet and excite the protons in specific planes of predetermined size and location so that their spins are aligned in a higher-energy state. Relaxation of the hydrogen nuclei to the lower-energy state gives off an electromagnetic signal that is detected by the scanner and processed into an image through a technique known as Fourier transformation.

There are many substantive advantages of CMR compared with other imaging modalities, including its high spatial resolution and high signal-to-noise ratio. CMR can also provide a 3D assessment of the heart, allowing the selection of any imaging plane, and is not susceptible to attenuation artifacts. Using different CMR sequences can also aid in tissue characterization, allowing multiple aspects of the myocardium to be assessed in one study (Table 29-1).

LIMITATIONS/CONTRAINDICATIONS

There are several limitations to the routine use of CMR. Despite recent improvements, there continues to be limited hardware availability, and cardiac-specific software is necessary. CMR remains an expensive imaging modality; this is challenging in the era of cost containment, although stress CMR and stress radionuclide imaging (RNI) are fairly similar in cost. Functional images are acquired over multiple beats gated to the electrocardiogram, which prolongs study times. Study times can be lengthy and are typically on the order of 40 to 60 minutes. Electrocardiographic gating can also result in artifacts in the setting of

Table 29-1
Advantages and Limitations of Cardiovascular Magnetic Resonance Imaging

Advantages	Limitations
• High spatial resolution	• Contraindicated with many implanted devices
• High signal-to-noise ratio	• Restricted in severe chronic kidney disease
• Infinite imaging planes possible	• Compliance issues due to lengthy studies, small tube bore, and breath-holds required
• No ionizing radiation	• Limited hardware availability
• Not susceptible to attenuation artifacts	• Operator dependent
• Tissue characterization possible through unique imaging sequences	• Expensive
• Multiple attributes evaluable with one study (function, perfusion, fibrosis)	

arrhythmias, particularly irregular rhythms such as atrial fibrillation and frequent premature ventricular contractions. Gating can be more difficult at higher field strengths. Patients must lie still, as all images are dependent on a fixed position relative to the magnetic field and RF coils. This can create compliance issues. Patients must hold their breath for most sequences, which can be challenging for symptomatic patients with limited respiratory reserve and also results in reduced compliance.[1] The confined nature of the magnet bore may be an issue for morbidly obese patients and can trigger claustrophobia, which can accentuate all of these issues. The magnetic field can interact with implanted devices. Some newer devices are potentially MRI compatible, but careful patient selection, well-defined safety protocols, and additional large-scale testing are needed prior to the widespread use of CMR in this population and in those without MRI-compatible devices. Performing protocols on the MRI machine and software requires highly trained staff. Adequate training is also required to perform the image processing that is required to quantify volumes and function. However, newer software is allowing these processes to be increasingly automated.[3] The use of gadolinium-based contrast agents (GBCAs) are contraindicated in patients with stage 4 and 5 kidney disease due to the association with nephrogenic systemic fibrosis.[4] Finally, in all but a few specialized laboratories, stress imaging can only be performed with pharmacologic stress, eliminating the most powerful prognostic marker in stress imaging, exercise capacity.[5] Rapid advances in CMR hardware, software, and MR sequences have the potential to improve many of these limitations in the near future.

CMR SEQUENCES

A CMR study is made up of a series of specific sequences that reveal different aspects of the heart and vascular system. The ordering physician supplies a clinical question and the performing laboratory determines the optimal CMR protocol to answer that question. Unique sequences can assess heart structure, myocardial function, tissue characterization, perfusion, valvular function, and angiography.

▶ Structure and Function

Steady-State Free Precession Cine Imaging

CMR is the gold standard for measuring left ventricular (LV) mass and LV and right ventricular (RV) chamber volumes and ejection fraction. Steady-state free precession (SSFP) imaging sequences are most commonly used to assess volumes and function, as they have excellent spatial and temporal resolution, a high signal-to-noise ratio, and short breath hold times.[6] Stacking multiple short-axis slices together allows precise volume and function assessment without geometric assumptions.[1] The endocardial and epicardial borders are traced in end-diastole and end-systole, and the myocardial mass, stroke volume and ejection fraction can be calculated (Fig. 29-1).[6,7] Regional function can be quantified using a 17-segment model based on coronary distribution.[8]

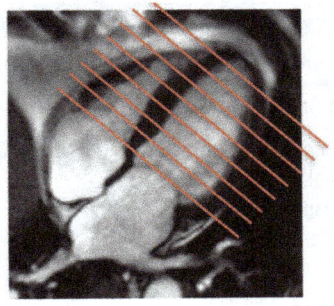
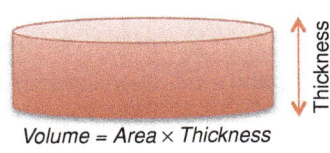
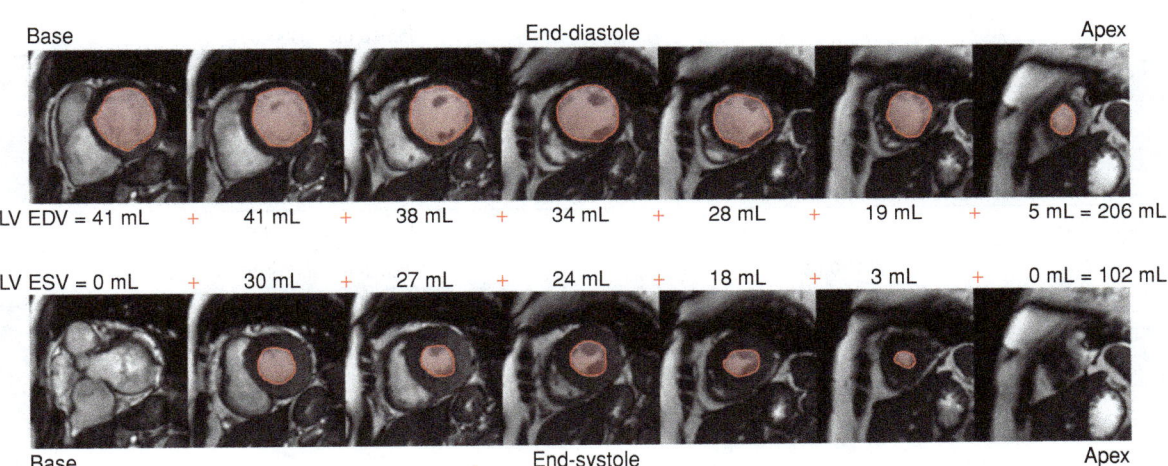

FIGURE 29-1 Quantification of left ventricular volumes and function from stacked short-axis steady-state free precession (SSFP) cine images. Endocardial contours are drawn at end-diastole and end-systole and summed across slices to give the left ventricular end-diastolic volume (LV EDV) and LV end-systolic volume (ESV). The stroke volume is calculated as the difference (LV EDV − LV ESV), and the ejection fraction by dividing the stroke volume by the LV EDV and multiplying by 100. These same calculations can be performed for the right ventricle. (Reproduced with permission from Lopez-Mattei JC, Shah DJ. The role of cardiac magnetic resonance in valvular heart disease. *Methodist Debakey Cardiovasc J.* 2013;9(3):142–148.)

In a comparison of LVEF between CMR, radionuclide ventriculography, and 2D echocardiography, the closest limits of agreement were with radionuclide ventriculography, which has also been considered a gold standard.[9] There are wide variances with 2D and 3D echo, with systematic underestimation by 3D echo due to insufficient definition of endocardial trabeculae.[10] CMR can orient the heart in any direction to assess function and precisely quantify RV and atrial function. CMR is particularly well suited for repeated studies for disease progression monitoring compared with echocardiography due to its accuracy and reproducibility, and RNI for the lack of radiation exposure.[3]

Several techniques are available to assess regional myocardial function and strain include myocardial tagging, harmonic phase imaging (HARP), and cine displacement encoded with stimulated echoes (DENSE).[3,6] Dobutamine CMR with tagging improves the identification of significant coronary lesions.[11] HARP is a low spatial resolution approach to tag analysis that has been used widely in population studies.[12] Cine DENSE has higher temporal and spatial resolution and will likely become dominant as the technology matures (Table 29-2).[13]

▶ **Tissue Characterization**

T1-, T2-, and T2*-Weighted (W) Imaging

Adjustment of the electrical gradients, RF pulses, and timing of signal acquisition can emphasize different properties of the myocardium and aid in tissue

Table 29-2
Cardiovascular Attributes, Disease Conditions, and the Sequences Used to Evaluate Them

Attributes	Sequences Used	Disease Conditions Evaluated
Structure and function	Steady-state free precession (SSFP) cine imaging Strain imaging (tagging, HARP, DENSE)	Ischemic heart disease Myocardial viability Cardiomyopathies Valvular heart disease Pericardial disease Ischemic heart disease Cardiomyopathies Pericardial disease
Tissue characterization	T1-weighted imaging T2-weighted imaging T2* imaging Late gadolinium enhancement (LGE)	Ischemic heart disease Myocardial viability Cardiomyopathies Pericardial disease Cardiac masses
Blood flow	Velocity-encoded imaging (VENC)	Valvular heart disease
Perfusion	First-pass perfusion imaging	Ischemic heart disease Cardiac masses
Angiography	SSFP imaging	Ischemic heart disease Congenital heart disease

characterization. The time it takes tissue to recover from excitation, the T1 relaxation time, is prolonged in fibrotic tissue and reduced in lipid-rich myocardium.[14] T2 describes the time for the proton spins to lose their alignment in adjacent tissue (spin–spin relaxation time). T2-W accentuates tissue with a high water content, such as edema in early states of myocardial injury.[15] T2* sequences can identify iron overload, such as in hemochromatosis or in conditions such as thalassemia after multiple transfusions.[16] T1, T2, and T2* mapping are rapidly replacing static images due to their quantitative nature and robustness to artifacts.[17,18]

Late Gadolinium Enhancement

Late gadolinium enhancement (LGE) is a method of scar assessment useful in assessing ischemic heart disease and cardiomyopathies. Patterns of gadolinium uptake during specific time periods following injection can help identify pathology. An absence of gadolinium uptake on delayed imaging indicates severe perfusion defects such as from microvascular obstruction after acute myocardial infarction (MI).[19] Increased gadolinium uptake and delayed washout occur in infarcted myocardium due to intracellular accumulation in injured myocytes due to ruptured cell walls and in fibrotic scar due to its small intracellular fraction.[19]

Blood Flow

Blood flow quantification is performed in CMR through velocity-encoded imaging. Protons at motion develop a specific phase shift directly proportional to their velocity. Velocity-encoded imaging (also called phase-contrast) produces images with signal proportional to the velocity and direction of each individual pixel.[7] Cumulative antero- or retrograde flows through specific vessels can be calculated by assessing blood flow through the region of interest over the entire cardiac cycle. Forward and regurgitant flow can be quantified and the regurgitant fraction calculated (Fig. 29-2).

Myocardial Perfusion

CMR perfusion imaging involves administering GBCAs and performing first-pass imaging, typically in several short-axis slices. Imaging is performed

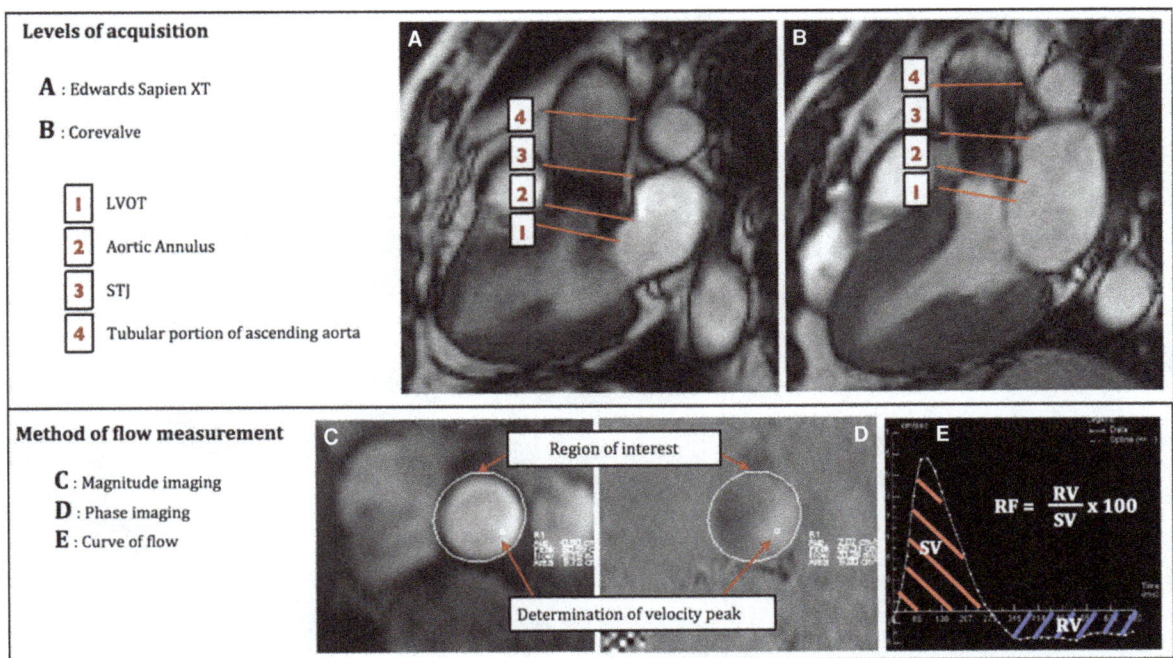

FIGURE 29-2 Velocity-encoded imaging (phase contrast mapping) to assess trans- and paravalvular regurgitation after transcatheter aortic valve replacement (TAVR). Multiple levels of acquisition are taken perpendicular to aortic flow for the Edwards Sapien XT (**A**) and Corevalve (**B**) prostheses. The aortic outflow tract cross section is planimetered on both magnitude (**C**), for localization and phase (**D**), for velocity information) images, throughout the cardiac cycle and a curve of forward and regurgitant flow is graphed (**E**). The regurgitant fraction (RF) is calculated as the regurgitant volume (RV) divided by the stroke volume (SV) × 100. (Reproduced with permission from Salaun E, Jacquier A, Theron A, et al. Value of CMR in quantification of paravalvular aortic regurgitation after TAVI. *Eur Heart J Cardiovasc Imaging.* 2016;17(1):41–50.)

at rest and after stress (typically using a vasodilator agent) to assess for ischemia. Images are typically assessed qualitatively for visible defects. However, quantitative perfusion analysis can be performed and improves differentiation of moderate and severe stenoses and improves the identification of three-vessel CAD.[20] In combination with LGE imaging, ischemia and infarct can be differentiated with high accuracy (Fig. 29-3).[21] The direct imaging of scar with LGE is an advantage over nuclear imaging.

CMR Coronary Angiography

SSFP imaging is used for coronary evaluation without contrast given the high blood T2/T1 ratio.[22] SSFP is not susceptible to calcium, allowing imaging with heavy calcification. Images are limited by reduced spatial resolution (1–1.5 mm) and long imaging times requiring free-breathing imaging with respiratory gating.

DISEASE STATES

Ischemic Heart Disease

Although relatively new in the evaluation of ischemic heart disease, stress CMR has many unique advantages and a rapidly expanding literature base supporting its use. Its high spatial resolution allows CMR to detect small subendocardial perfusion defects often missed by other techniques.[6] The standard CMR-guided evaluation of ischemic heart disease includes assessments of function, perfusion, extent and location of scar, and myocardial viability. Advanced techniques such as absolute flow assessment and angiography are also available in centers with expertise in these areas.

Function

Resting global systolic left ventricular function and segmental wall-motion can be assessed readily by

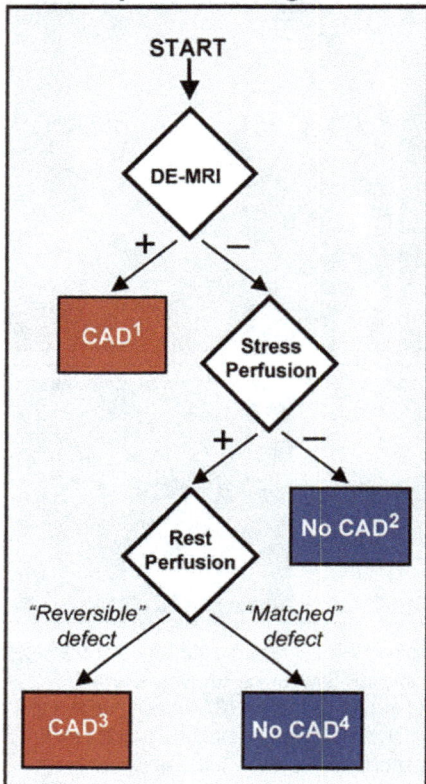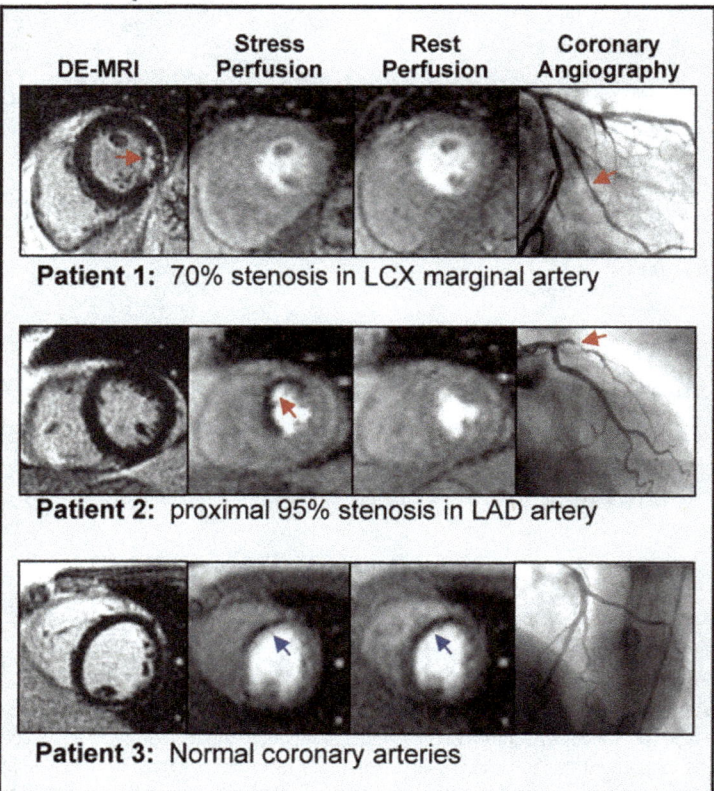

FIGURE 29-3 Interpretation algorithm combining late gadolinium enhancement (LGE, here marked DE-MRI) with rest and stress perfusion to improve the detection of coronary artery disease (CAD). The algorithm **(A)** involves assessing for LGE. If it is present, the patient has a prior myocardial infarction (CAD[1]). If it is negative and stress imaging is negative, they have no CAD[2]. If they have abnormal stress and rest imaging but no LGE, then this is considered artifactual. If they have abnormal stress but normal rest imaging, then this is consistent with ischemia (CAD[3]). (Reproduced with permission from Kim HW, Klem I, Kim RJ. Detection of myocardial ischemia by stress perfusion cardiovascular magnetic resonance. *Magn Reson Imaging Clin N Am.* 2007;15(4):527–540). The algorithm is illustrated in the patient examples **(B)**. The patient in the top row had a small inferolateral region of LGE and normal perfusion, consistent with myocardial infarction. The middle row patient had a classic ischemic perfusion defect and had obstructive CAD. The bottom row shows a "dark rim" artifact with normal LGE, consistent with artifact. Invasive coronary angiography was negative in this case. (Reproduced with permission from Klem I, Heitner JF, Shah DJ, et al. Improved detection of coronary artery disease by stress perfusion cardiovascular magnetic resonance with the use of delayed enhancement infarction imaging. *J Am Coll Cardiol.* 2006;47(8):1630–1638.)

CMR and can assist in differentiating acute coronary syndromes from noncardiac conditions. The improved spatial resolution and lack of attenuation from ribs and other structures can be particularly useful in assessing certain regions like the posterior wall.[23]

Quantitative strain analysis can also be useful to assess function in ischemic heart disease.[24]

Stress-induced wall-motion abnormalities have high diagnostic accuracy for CAD. Exercise stress CMR is challenging logistically and is only performed in a handful of centers. Dobutamine is a sympathomimetic drug that increases myocardial blood flow and contractility through chronotropic and inotropic effects and can be used in stress CMR.[25] A meta-analysis of 1183 patients showed a sensitivity of 83% and a specificity of 86% of dobutamine stress CMR for CAD at the patient level, which is higher than studies with stress echocardiography.[26,27] The prognostic impact of inducible wall-motion abnormalities on stress CMR was studied in patients in a bicenter study by Kelle et al.[28] Patients without abnormalities had a 0.9% rate of cardiac death/nonfatal MI. Inducible WMAs were an independent predictor with hazard ratio of 6.5, $p < 0.001$. Dobutamine functional stress CMR has largely been replaced at most centers by vasodilator stress perfusion CMR due to the short half-life of the vasodilators, patient comfort, as well as the use of GBCAs to assess LGE.

Perfusion

Stress CMR perfusion imaging has replaced dobutamine stress at most centers due to its high diagnostic accuracy, short vasodilator half-life, patient comfort, and excellent scar analysis. A meta-analysis of 166 articles (including 37 analyzing CMR) found an excellent patient-level sensitivity of 89% and specificity of 76% for the identification of 50% stenosis of an epicardial coronary artery.[29] The sensitivity of CMR was comparable to SPECT (88%) and PET (84%). However, the specificity was substantially improved over SPECT (61%). The CE-MARC trial compared stress SPECT MPI and CMR in 752 patients with suspected angina and at least one risk factor. In this study, while specificity was similar, sensitivity was increased with CMR (86.5% vs. 66.5%, $p < 0.001$).[30]

The degree of inducible ischemia is prognostically significant. Shah et al.[31] examined 815 consecutive patients undergoing stress CMR and showed that inducible ischemia was strongly associated with MACE (HR 14.66, $p < 0.0001$) and reclassified 91.5% of patients at moderate pretest risk to low risk (65.7%, MACE 0.3%/year) or high risk (25.8%, MACE 4.9%/year). A negative stress CMR is associated with a very low risk of cardiovascular death and MI (0.8%/year).[32] A recent analysis of follow-up data in the CE-MARC trial population showed no difference in major adverse cardiovascular event rates between the CMR and SPECT groups and similar rates of unnecessary coronary angiography.[33]

A substantial potential benefit of stress CMR over SPECT MPI and stress echocardiography is the ability to quantify absolute blood flow and calculate myocardial flow reserve with values similar to PET MPI.[34] Reduced absolute stress flow and flow reserve are associated with multivessel disease and increased cardiac events.[35,36] The high resolution of CMR imaging allows quantification of absolute flow across the layers of the myocardium.[6] The limitations of operator expertise and long postprocessing times will be reduced through automated software, allowing more mainstream adoption.

Assessment of Scar

The presence, location, and extent of scar are critical for diagnosing prior infarction and for risk stratification. LGE has been shown to correlate closely with the distribution of myocardial necrosis by TTC staining and microsphere analysis in animal models.[37] In contrast, ischemic myocardium that is not irreversibly damaged does not exhibit LGE.[38] Wagner et al.[39] performed both LGE CMR and SPECT in 91 patients. Although SPECT identified all patients with nearly transmural infarction, it did not identify subendocardial infarction in 47% of segments and 13% of patients. Although PET and CMR infarct size correlated well ($r = 0.81$, $p < 0.0001$), a small number of segments read as normal on PET MPI had evidence of LGE on CMR.[40] Scar location can also be used to identify optimal lead location in cardiac resynchronization therapy and likelihood of functional recovery.[14] Kwong et al.[41] showed that the presence of LGE in patients without known prior MI has incremental prognostic value beyond clinical factors, coronary stenosis, and left ventricular function. This same group found that diabetic patients with silent MI have increased mortality.[42]

Myocardial Viability

Noninvasive imaging can help identify which areas of myocardium are viable postinfarction. Kim et al.[43] performed CMR with LGE in 50 patients with left ventricular dysfunction. In an analysis of all 804 dysfunctional segments, there was a stepwise decrease in likelihood of functional improvement with increasing transmurality of LGE (Fig. 29-4). There have not been studies of long-term outcomes stratified by extent of viability identified on CMR imaging, though similar studies in patients undergoing SPECT and PET have been favorable.[44,45] The complementary information provided in the identification of metabolically active myocardium by FDG-PET and scar by CMR suggests there may be benefit to a comprehensive hybrid PET-MR viability assessment.[19]

Another index of viability available by CMR is the end-diastolic wall thickness. The high resolution

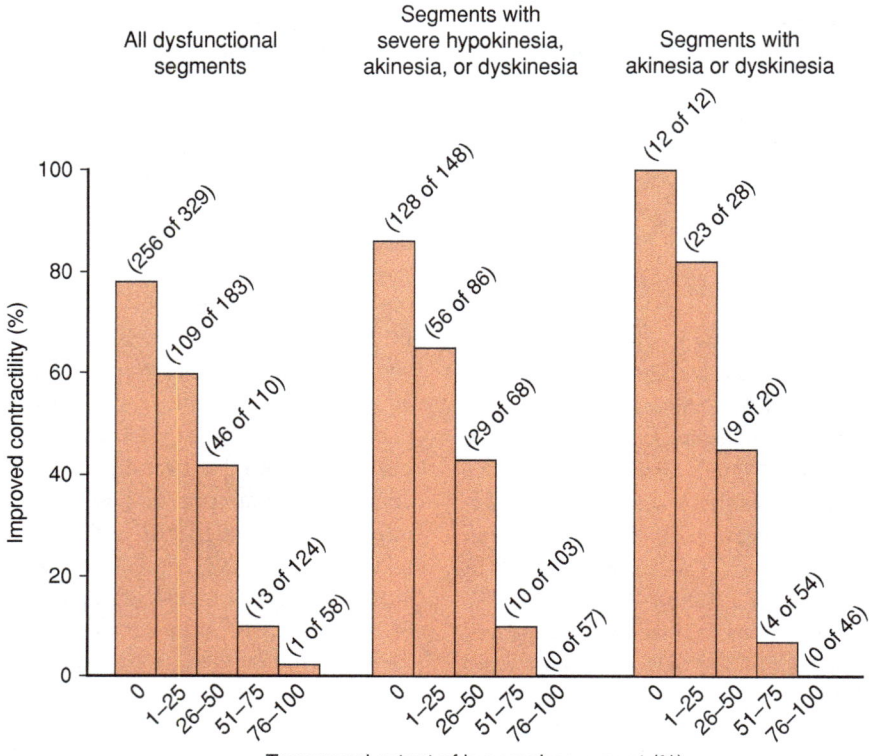

FIGURE 29-4 Likelihood of improved function after revascularization based on transmural extent of late gadolinium enhancement (LGE). Data are given in all dysfunctional segments (n = 804), segments with at least severe hypokinesis (n = 462), and segments that are akinetic or dyskinetic (n = 160). There is a stepwise decrease in likelihood of functional recovery as the transmural extent of LGE increases, with little recovery above 50% LGE. (Reproduced with permission from Kim RJ, Wu E, Rafael A, et al. The use of contrast-enhanced magnetic resonance imaging to identify reversible myocardial dysfunction. *N Engl J Med*. 2000;343(20):1445–1453.)

of CMR allows assessment of end-diastolic wall thickness, with values ≤5.5 mm associated with a low likelihood of myocardial viability.[46] Low-dose dobutamine induces inotropy that recruits stunned and hibernating myocardium but not necrotic tissue.[25] Multiple studies comparing LGE and contractile reserve assessment by CMR disagree on the best method to predict wall-motion improvement after revascularization. A meta-analysis by Romero et al.[47] found LGE to have the highest sensitivity and negative predictive value and dobutamine contractile reserve to have the highest specificity and positive predictive value. In particular, dobutamine contractile reserve appears to be beneficial in those with intermediate LGE thickness 1% to 75%, in which LGE is less definitive.[48]

Tissue Characterization

Tissue characterization by CMR can be particularly helpful in the setting of acute or subacute MI.[19] T2-W imaging can identify myocardial edema in areas with acute injury. The combination of this tool with LGE can help differentiate acute from chronic MI.[49] The extent of T2 enhancement identifies the area at risk in acute injury, and the area without subsequent LGE represents salvaged myocardium.[50,51] These findings are comparable to SPECT estimates of area at risk.[52] T2-W imaging acutely postinfarction can also identify dark zones of intramyocardial hemorrhage from particularly severe ischemic damage.[53] Intramyocardial hemorrhage is associated with adverse long-term left ventricular remodeling.[25,54]

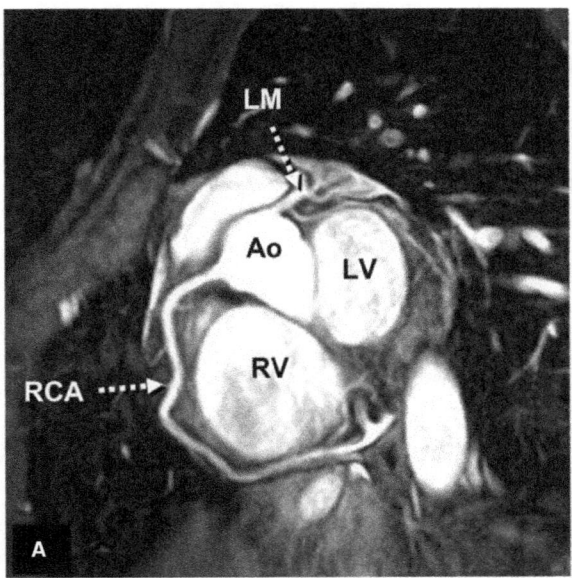 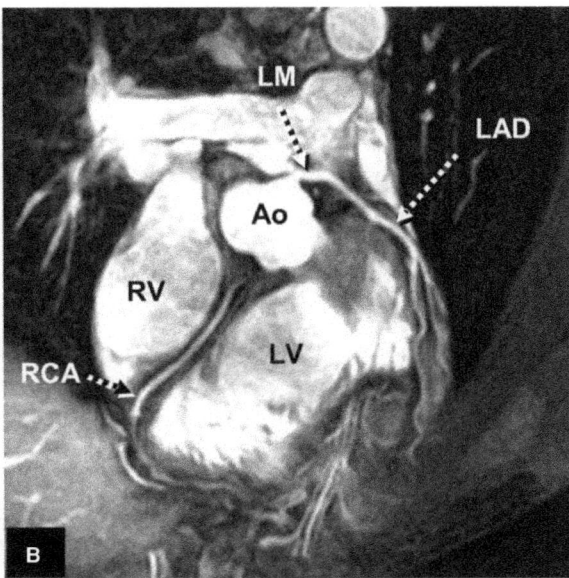

FIGURE 29-5 CMR angiography of the right **(A)** and left **(B)** coronary systems in two healthy adult patients. Images were steady-state free precession (SSFP) obtained during free-breathing with respiratory navigator. Ao, aorta; LM, left main; LV, left ventricle; RCA, right coronary artery; RV, right ventricle. (Reproduced with permission from Stuber M, Weiss RG. Coronary magnetic resonance angiography. *J Magn Reson Imaging*. 2007;26(2):219–234.)

▶ MR Coronary Angiography

MR coronary angiography can be combined with stress perfusion imaging to provide a comprehensive anatomic and functional assessment of ischemic heart disease. The absence of susceptibility to calcium artifacts is a substantial advantage, and CMR coronary angiography may have improved diagnostic accuracy in patients with high calcium scores.[55] Poor spatial resolution and long imaging times limit full coronary evaluation currently. These limitations have resulted in a rating of "inappropriate" for the exclusion of significant CAD in patients at intermediate risk with chest pain.[56] However, the sites of origin and proximal courses of the coronaries can be evaluated quickly and with sufficient accuracy.[22] Therefore, clinical use currently centers on the identification of anomalous coronary arteries and evaluation of coronary artery aneurysms in Kawasaki disease.[22] However, future advantages such as use of high field-strength 3T MRI, 32-channel coils, and high parallel imaging factors may allow full coronary evaluation with diagnostic accuracy similar to that obtained with a 64-slice CT scan (Fig. 29-5).[57]

▶ Heart Failure/Cardiomyopathies

CMR is considered "appropriate" in the 2013 ACC/AHA Appropriate Utilization of Cardiovascular Imaging in Heart Failure guidelines for evaluation in newly suspected or diagnosed heart failure, as well as in those meeting criteria for ICD or CRT implantation.[58] It plays an important role in multiple etiologies of heart failure, including dilated (DCM), hypertrophic (HCM), and restrictive cardiomyopathies (RCM), arrhythmogenic right ventricular cardiomyopathy (ARVC), iron overload, and left ventricular noncompaction.

LV and RV volumes and function may be ascertained with a lack of radiation, which facilitates repeat testing to monitor disease course and effects of therapy. The high spatial resolution facilitates the detection of LV thrombus and identification of LV noncompaction.[14,59] Excellent RV wall visualization aids in identifying global dysfunction and focal segmental abnormalities in ARVC.[23]

In DCM, tissue characterization and patterns of LGE can aid in differentiation of ischemic from nonischemic cardiomyopathy, suggest etiology, and inform prognosis (Fig. 29-6). In 90 patients with DCM, all with CAD had subendocardial LGE, while those

Hyperenhancement Patterns

Ischemic

A. Subendocardial infarct

B. Transmural infarct

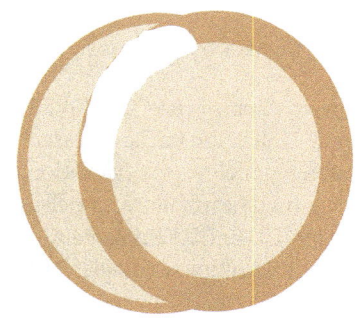

Nonischemic

A. Mid-wall HE

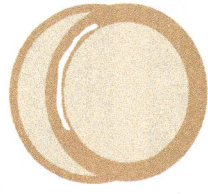

- Idiopathic dilated cardiomyopathy
- Myocarditis

- Hypertrophic cardiomyopathy
- Right ventricular pressure overload (e.g., congenital heart disease, pulmonary HTN)

- Sarcoidosis
- Myocarditis
- Anderson-Fabry
- Chagas disease

B. Epicardial HE

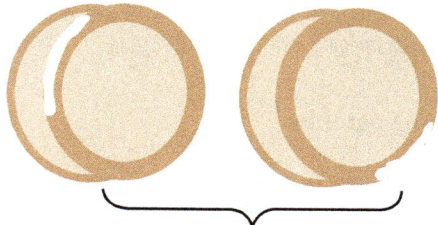

- Sarcoidosis, myocarditis, Anderson-Fabry, Chagas disease

C. Global Endocardial HE

- Amyloidosis, systemic sclerosis, post cardiac transplantation

FIGURE 29-6 Patterns of late gadolinium enhancement (LGE) in ischemic and nonischemic cardiomyopathies. The portion of the wall involved and global versus segmental distribution can help differentiate ischemic versus nonischemic and among the nonischemic etiologies. (Reproduced with permission from Edelman RR, Hesselink JR, Zlatkin MB, et al. *Clinical Magnetic Resonance Imaging,* 3rd ed. New York: Elsevier Press; 2005.)

with a nonischemic etiology had no enhancement (59%) or midwall or epicardial LGE.[60] LGE in DCM is associated with increased mortality and risk of sudden cardiac death.[61] CMR can identify myocarditis with moderate sensitivity (67%) and excellent specificity (91%) using edema presence and LGE patterns.[62] Nuclear MPI can assess LV, and to a lesser extent RV function and assess the microvasculature, but there is currently minimal role for the assessment of nonischemic DCM using this modality.[63]

CMR structural imaging can identify the multiple patterns of HCM, including classic asymmetric septal involvement, but also atypical midwall and apical variants that can be missed by echocardiography. T1 mapping can identify the extent of fibrosis.[64,65] LGE is often present with patchy midwall involvement.[66] In a recent meta-analysis of 1063 patients, LGE was present in 60% with HCM and was closely associated with increased cardiovascular mortality.[67] LGE involvement may predict sudden cardiac death and its prognostic role is being further evaluated in a large, multicontinent NIH-funded study.[68]

CMR structural assessment readily demonstrates the diffuse hypertrophy and biatrial enlargement in RCM. Amyloid can present with multiple LGE patterns, but the characteristic diffuse subendocardial involvement has 80% sensitivity and 94% specificity for amyloid and indicates a worse prognosis with increased 1-year mortality.[69,70] In similar fashion to Tc-pyrophosphate imaging, T1 mapping by CMR can differentiate between ATTR and AL amyloid subtypes.[71] LGE uptake in a noncoronary distribution is also present in some patients with cardiac sarcoidosis (13% and 26% in studies by Nagai et al. and Greulich et al., respectively).[72,73] LGE has been shown to be one of the best predictors of prognosis in this population, including death, defibrillator shocks, and need for a pacemaker.[73,74] In contrast to the scar identified by CMR LGE evaluation, ^{18}F-FDG PET imaging assesses active inflammation, which is more useful for assessment of a patient's current clinical status or response to therapy. There is some evidence that T2-W CMR imaging could play a similar role.[75]

Valvular Heart Disease

Echocardiography remains the primary means of evaluating valvular heart disease, but CMR has a role in certain circumstances. CMR can provide a highly detailed anatomic assessment in any plane, assisting in mechanism evaluation.[7] It is particularly helpful in evaluating right-sided valves, which are not evaluated well by echocardiography. CMR is beneficial in assessing valvular disease severity, particularly regurgitant volume and fraction by velocity-encoded imaging, in which it is superior to echocardiography.[76] The precise quantification of chamber volumes by SSFP imaging provides ideal assessment of the valvular disease consequences.

Cardiac Masses and Pericardial Disease

The combination of high spatial resolution for SSFP images and tissue characterization make CMR the ideal study to assess cardiac masses and pericardial disease. Combinations of T1- and T2-W imaging, perfusion, and LGE help identify the type of tumor and correctly classify 95% as benign or malignant.[77] Invasion of tumors from surrounding tissue is readily apparent. Spin echo sequences with T1-weighting visualize the extent and thickness of the pericardium, while T2-W images assess pericardial effusions and edema of the pericardium in cases such as inflammatory pericarditis.[78] Real-time SSFP images assess ventricular interdependence and myocardial tagging evaluates reduced myocardial–pericardial slippage in constriction.[78,79] LGE can be used both to assess inflammation in the pericardium, but also to assess myocardial involvement in myopericarditis.[80]

SUMMARY

The multiple sequences available in CMR imaging harness advantages including high spatial resolution and signal-to-noise ratio and limitless imaging planes to provide a comprehensive assessment of anatomy, function, perfusion, and tissue characterization of the myocardium and associated structures. CMR assesses ischemic heart disease with similar accuracy to nuclear MPI and has a robust and growing prognostic literature. In other conditions such as noninvasive evaluation of heart failure and cardiac masses, CMR is the gold standard. While some limitations with CMR imaging remain, including claustrophobia and restrictions in renal dysfunction, many are decreasing with hardware and software advances. Given these advances, CMR is playing an increasing role in the routine evaluation of cardiovascular disease.

REFERENCES

1. Pfeiffer MP, Biederman RW. Cardiac MRI: A general overview with emphasis on current use and indications. *Med Clin North Am.* 2015;99:849–861.

2. Rodgers CT, Robson MD. Cardiovascular magnetic resonance: Physics and terminology. *Progress in Cardiovascular Diseases*. 2011;54:181–190.
3. Grover S, Leong DP, Selvanayagam JB. Evaluation of left ventricular function using cardiac magnetic resonance imaging. *J Nucl Cardiol*. 2011;18:351–365.
4. Perazella MA. Nephrogenic systemic fibrosis, kidney disease, and gadolinium: Is there a link? *Clin J Am Soc Nephrol*. 2007;2:200–202.
5. Myers J, Prakash M, Froelicher V, Do D, Partington S, Atwood JE. Exercise capacity and mortality among men referred for exercise testing. *N Eng J Med*. 2002;346:793–801.
6. Isbell DC, Kramer CM. Cardiovascular magnetic resonance: Structure, function, perfusion, and viability. *J Nucl Cardiol*. 2005;12:324–336.
7. Lopez-Mattei JC, Shah DJ. The role of cardiac magnetic resonance in valvular heart disease. *Methodist Debakey Cardiovasc J*. 2013;9:142–148.
8. Cerqueira MD, Weissman NJ, Dilsizian V, et al.; American Heart Association Writing Group on Myocardial S, Registration for Cardiac I. Standardized myocardial segmentation and nomenclature for tomographic imaging of the heart. A statement for healthcare professionals from the cardiac imaging committee of the Council on Clinical Cardiology of the American Heart Association. *Circulation*. 2002;105:539–542.
9. Bellenger NG, Burgess MI, Ray SG, et al. Comparison of left ventricular ejection fraction and volumes in heart failure by echocardiography, radionuclide ventriculography and cardiovascular magnetic resonance; are they interchangeable? *Eur Heart J*. 2000;21:1387–1396.
10. Mor-Avi V, Jenkins C, Kuhl HP, et al. Real-time 3-dimensional echocardiographic quantification of left ventricular volumes: Multicenter study for validation with magnetic resonance imaging and investigation of sources of error. *JACC Cardiovasc Imaging*. 2008;1:413–423.
11. Kuijpers D, Ho KY, van Dijkman PR, Vliegenthart R, Oudkerk M. Dobutamine cardiovascular magnetic resonance for the detection of myocardial ischemia with the use of myocardial tagging. *Circulation*. 2003;107:1592–1597.
12. Osman NF, Kerwin WS, McVeigh ER, Prince JL. Cardiac motion tracking using cine harmonic phase (HARP) magnetic resonance imaging. *Magn Reson Med*. 1999;42:1048–1060.
13. Spottiswoode BS, Zhong X, Lorenz CH, Mayosi BM, Meintjes EM, Epstein FH. Motion-guided segmentation for cine dense MRI. *Med Image Anal*. 2009;13:105–115.
14. Gonzalez JA, Kramer CM. Role of imaging techniques for diagnosis, prognosis and management of heart failure patients: Cardiac magnetic resonance. *Curr Heart Fail Rep*. 2015;12:276–283.
15. Abdel-Aty H, Simonetti O, Friedrich MG. T2-weighted cardiovascular magnetic resonance imaging. *J Magn Reson Imaging*. 2007;26:452–459.
16. He T. Cardiovascular magnetic resonance T2* for tissue iron assessment in the heart. *Quant Imaging Med Surg*. 2014;4:407–412.
17. Moon JC, Messroghli DR, Kellman P, et al.; Society for Cardiovascular Magnetic Resonance I, Cardiovascular Magnetic Resonance Working Group of the European Society of Cardiology. Myocardial T1 mapping and extracellular volume quantification: A Society for Cardiovascular Magnetic Resonance (SCMR) and CMR working group of the European Society of Cardiology consensus statement. *J Cardiovasc Magn Reson*. 2013;15:92.
18. Verhaert D, Thavendiranathan P, Giri S, et al. Direct T2 quantification of myocardial edema in acute ischemic injury. *JACC Cardiovasc Imaging*. 2011;4:269–278.
19. Arai AE. The cardiac magnetic resonance (CMR) approach to assessing myocardial viability. *J Nucl Cardiol*. 2011;18:1095–1102.
20. Patel AR, Antkowiak PF, Nandalur KR, et al. Assessment of advanced coronary artery disease: Advantages of quantitative cardiac magnetic resonance perfusion analysis. *J Amer Coll Cardiol*. 2010;56:561–569.
21. Kim HW, Klem I, Kim RJ. Detection of myocardial ischemia by stress perfusion cardiovascular magnetic resonance. *Magn Reson Imaging Clin N Am*. 2007;15:527–540, vi.
22. Sakuma H. Coronary CT versus MR angiography: The role of MR angiography. *Radiology*. 2011;258:340–349.
23. West AM, Kramer CM. Cardiovascular magnetic resonance imaging of myocardial infarction, viability, and cardiomyopathies. *Curr Probl Cardiol*. 2010;35:176–220.
24. Gotte MJ, van Rossum AC, Twisk JW, Kuijer JP, Marcus JT, Visser CA. Quantification of regional contractile function after infarction: Strain analysis superior to wall thickening analysis in discriminating infarct from remote myocardium. *J Am Coll Cardiol*. 2001;37:808–817.
25. Guaricci AI, Brunetti ND, Marra MP, Tarantini G, di Biase M, Pontone G. Diagnosis and prognosis of ischemic heart disease: The framework of cardiac magnetic resonance. *J Cardiovasc Med*. 2015;16:653–662.
26. Nandalur KR, Dwamena BA, Choudhri AF, Nandalur MR, Carlos RC. Diagnostic performance of stress cardiac magnetic resonance imaging in the detection of coronary artery disease: A meta-analysis. *J Am Coll Cardiol*. 2007;50:1343–1353.
27. Nagel E, Lehmkuhl HB, Bocksch W, et al. Noninvasive diagnosis of ischemia-induced wall motion abnormalities with the use of high-dose dobutamine stress MRI: Comparison with dobutamine stress echocardiography. *Circulation*. 1999;99:763–770.
28. Kelle S, Nagel E, Voss A, et al. A bi-center cardiovascular magnetic resonance prognosis study focusing on dobutamine wall motion and late gadolinium enhancement in 3,138 consecutive patients. *J Am Coll Cardiol*. 2013;61:2310–2312.
29. Jaarsma C, Leiner T, Bekkers SC, et al. Diagnostic performance of noninvasive myocardial perfusion imaging using single-photon emission computed tomography, cardiac magnetic resonance, and positron emission tomography imaging for the detection of obstructive coronary artery disease: A meta-analysis. *J Am Coll Cardiol*. 2012;59:1719–1728.
30. Greenwood JP, Maredia N, Younger JF, et al. Cardiovascular magnetic resonance and single-photon emission computed tomography for diagnosis of coronary heart disease (CE-MARC): A prospective trial. *Lancet*. 2012;379:453–460.
31. Shah R, Heydari B, Coelho-Filho O, et al. Stress cardiac magnetic resonance imaging provides effective cardiac risk reclassification in patients with known or suspected stable coronary artery disease. *Circulation*. 2013;128:605–614.
32. Lipinski MJ, McVey CM, Berger JS, Kramer CM, Salerno M. Prognostic value of stress cardiac magnetic resonance imaging in patients with known or suspected coronary artery

disease: A systematic review and meta-analysis. *J Am Coll Cardiol.* 2013;62:826-838.
33. Greenwood JP, Ripley DP, Berry C, et al. Effect of care guided by cardiovascular magnetic resonance, myocardial perfusion scintigraphy, or nice guidelines on subsequent unnecessary angiography rates: The CE-MARC 2 randomized clinical trial. *JAMA.* 2016;316:1051-1060.
34. Qayyum AA, Hasbak P, Larsson HB, et al. Quantification of myocardial perfusion using cardiac magnetic resonance imaging correlates significantly to rubidium-82 positron emission tomography in patients with severe coronary artery disease: A preliminary study. *Eur J Radiol.* 2014;83:1120-1128.
35. Ziadi MC, Dekemp RA, Williams K, et al. Does quantification of myocardial flow reserve using rubidium-82 positron emission tomography facilitate detection of multivessel coronary artery disease? *J Nucl Cardiol.* 2012;19:670-680.
36. Murthy VL, Naya M, Foster CR, et al. Association between coronary vascular dysfunction and cardiac mortality in patients with and without diabetes mellitus. *Circulation.* 2012;126:1858-1868.
37. Kim RJ, Fieno DS, Parrish TB, et al. Relationship of MRI delayed contrast enhancement to irreversible injury, infarct age, and contractile function. *Circulation.* 1999;100:1992-2002.
38. Fieno DS, Kim RJ, Chen EL, Lomasney JW, Klocke FJ, Judd RM. Contrast-enhanced magnetic resonance imaging of myocardium at risk: Distinction between reversible and irreversible injury throughout infarct healing. *J Am Coll Cardiol.* 2000;36:1985-1991.
39. Wagner A, Mahrholdt H, Holly TA, et al. Contrast-enhanced MRI and routine single photon emission computed tomography (SPECT) perfusion imaging for detection of subendocardial myocardial infarcts: An imaging study. *Lancet.* 2003;361:374-379.
40. Klein C, Nekolla SG, Bengel FM, et al. Assessment of myocardial viability with contrast-enhanced magnetic resonance imaging: Comparison with positron emission tomography. *Circulation.* 2002;105:162-167.
41. Kwong RY, Chan AK, Brown KA, et al. Impact of unrecognized myocardial scar detected by cardiac magnetic resonance imaging on event-free survival in patients presenting with signs or symptoms of coronary artery disease. *Circulation.* 2006;113:2733-2743.
42. Kwong RY, Sattar H, Wu H, et al. Incidence and prognostic implication of unrecognized myocardial scar characterized by cardiac magnetic resonance in diabetic patients without clinical evidence of myocardial infarction. *Circulation.* 2008;118:1011-1020.
43. Kim RJ, Wu E, Rafael A, et al. The use of contrast-enhanced magnetic resonance imaging to identify reversible myocardial dysfunction. *N Engl J Med.* 2000;343:1445-1453.
44. Allman KC, Shaw LJ, Hachamovitch R, Udelson JE. Myocardial viability testing and impact of revascularization on prognosis in patients with coronary artery disease and left ventricular dysfunction: A meta-analysis. *J Am Coll Cardiol.* 2002;39:1151-1158.
45. Beanlands RS, Nichol G, Huszti E, et al; Investigators P-. F-18-fluorodeoxyglucose positron emission tomography imaging-assisted management of patients with severe left ventricular dysfunction and suspected coronary disease: A randomized, controlled trial (PARR-2). *J Am Coll Cardiol.* 2007;50:2002-2012.
46. Klem I, Heitner JF, Shah DJ, et al. Improved detection of coronary artery disease by stress perfusion cardiovascular magnetic resonance with the use of delayed enhancement infarction imaging. *J Am Coll Cardiol.* 2006;47:1630-1638.
47. Romero J, Xue X, Gonzalez W, Garcia MJ. CMR imaging assessing viability in patients with chronic ventricular dysfunction due to coronary artery disease: A meta-analysis of prospective trials. *JACC Cardiovasc Imaging.* 2012;5:494-508.
48. Wellnhofer E, Olariu A, Klein C, et al. Magnetic resonance low-dose dobutamine test is superior to scar quantification for the prediction of functional recovery. *Circulation.* 2004;109:2172-2174.
49. Abdel-Aty H, Zagrosek A, Schulz-Menger J, et al. Delayed enhancement and T2-weighted cardiovascular magnetic resonance imaging differentiate acute from chronic myocardial infarction. *Circulation.* 2004;109:2411-2416.
50. Aletras AH, Tilak GS, Natanzon A, et al. Retrospective determination of the area at risk for reperfused acute myocardial infarction with T2-weighted cardiac magnetic resonance imaging: Histopathological and displacement encoding with stimulated echoes (DENSE) functional validations. *Circulation.* 2006;113:1865-1870.
51. Friedrich MG, Abdel-Aty H, Taylor A, Schulz-Menger J, Messroghli D, Dietz R. The salvaged area at risk in reperfused acute myocardial infarction as visualized by cardiovascular magnetic resonance. *J Am Coll Cardiol.* 2008;51:1581-1587.
52. Carlsson M, Ubachs JF, Hedstrom E, Heiberg E, Jovinge S, Arheden H. Myocardium at risk after acute infarction in humans on cardiac magnetic resonance: Quantitative assessment during follow-up and validation with single-photon emission computed tomography. *JACC Cardiovasc Imaging.* 2009;2:569-576.
53. Ganame J, Messalli G, Dymarkowski S, et al. Impact of myocardial haemorrhage on left ventricular function and remodelling in patients with reperfused acute myocardial infarction. *Eur Heart J.* 2009;30:1440-1449.
54. Masci PG, Ganame J, Strata E, et al. Myocardial salvage by CMR correlates with LV remodeling and early ST-segment resolution in acute myocardial infarction. *JACC Cardiovasc Imaging.* 2010;3:45-51.
55. Liu X, Zhao X, Huang J, et al. Comparison of 3D free-breathing coronary MR angiography and 64-MDCT angiography for detection of coronary stenosis in patients with high calcium scores. *AJR Am J Roentgenol.* 2007;189:1326-1332.
56. Hendel RC, Patel MR, Kramer CM, et al.; American College of Cardiology Foundation Quality Strategic Directions Committee Appropriateness Criteria Working G, American College of R, Society of Cardiovascular Computed T, Society for Cardiovascular Magnetic R, American Society of Nuclear C, North American Society for Cardiac I, Society for Cardiovascular A, Interventions, Society of Interventional R. ACCF/ACR/SCCT/SCMR/ASNC/NASCI/SCAI/SIR 2006 appropriateness criteria for cardiac computed tomography and cardiac magnetic resonance imaging: A report of the American College of Cardiology Foundation quality strategic directions committee appropriateness criteria working group, American College of Radiology, Society of Cardiovascular Computed Tomography, Society for Cardiovascular Magnetic Resonance, American Society of Nuclear Cardiology, North American Society for Cardiac Imaging, Society for Cardiovascular Angiography

and Interventions, and Society of Interventional Radiology. *J Am Coll Cardiol.* 2006;48:1475–1497.
57. Yang Q, Li K, Liu X, et al. Contrast-enhanced whole-heart coronary magnetic resonance angiography at 3.0-T: A comparative study with X-ray angiography in a single center. *J Am Coll Cardiol.* 2009;54:69–76.
58. Patel MR, White RD, Abbara S, et al.; American College of Radiology Appropriateness Criteria C, American College of Cardiology Foundation Appropriate Use Criteria Task F. 2013 ACCF/ACR/ASE/ASNC/SCCT/SCMR appropriate utilization of cardiovascular imaging in heart failure: A joint report of the American College of Radiology appropriateness criteria committee and the American College of Cardiology Foundation appropriate use criteria task force. *J Am Coll Cardiol.* 2013;61:2207–2231.
59. Kassi M, Nabi F. Role of cardiac MRI in the assessment of non-ischemic cardiomyopathies. *Methodist Debakey Cardiovasc J.* 2013;9:149–155.
60. McCrohon JA, Moon JC, Prasad SK, et al. Differentiation of heart failure related to dilated cardiomyopathy and coronary artery disease using gadolinium-enhanced cardiovascular magnetic resonance. *Circulation.* 2003;108:54–59.
61. Gulati A, Jabbour A, Ismail TF, et al. Association of fibrosis with mortality and sudden cardiac death in patients with non-ischemic dilated cardiomyopathy. *JAMA.* 2013;309:896–908.
62. Friedrich MG, Sechtem U, Schulz-Menger J, et al.; International Consensus Group on Cardiovascular Magnetic Resonance in M. Cardiovascular magnetic resonance in myocarditis: A JACC white paper. *J Am Coll Cardiol.* 2009;53:1475–1487.
63. Neglia D. Positron emission tomography: An additional prognostic tool in dilated cardiomyopathy? *J Nucl Cardiol.* 2016;23:768–772.
64. Salerno M, Kramer CM. Prognosis in hypertrophic cardiomyopathy with contrast-enhanced cardiac magnetic resonance: The future looks bright. *J Am Coll Cardiol.* 2010;56:888–889.
65. Dass S, Suttie JJ, Piechnik SK, et al. Myocardial tissue characterization using magnetic resonance noncontrast T1 mapping in hypertrophic and dilated cardiomyopathy. *Circ Cardiovasc Imaging.* 2012;5:726–733.
66. Rudolph A, Abdel-Aty H, Bohl S, et al. Noninvasive detection of fibrosis applying contrast-enhanced cardiac magnetic resonance in different forms of left ventricular hypertrophy relation to remodeling. *J Am Coll Cardiol.* 2009;53:284–291.
67. Chan RH, Maron BJ, Olivotto I, et al. Prognostic value of quantitative contrast-enhanced cardiovascular magnetic resonance for the evaluation of sudden death risk in patients with hypertrophic cardiomyopathy. *Circulation.* 2014;130:484–495.
68. Kramer CM, Appelbaum E, Desai MY, et al. Hypertrophic cardiomyopathy registry: The rationale and design of an international, observational study of hypertrophic cardiomyopathy. *Am Heart J.* 2015;170:223–230.
69. Vogelsberg H, Mahrholdt H, Deluigi CC, et al. Cardiovascular magnetic resonance in clinically suspected cardiac amyloidosis: Noninvasive imaging compared to endomyocardial biopsy. *J Am Coll Cardiol.* 2008;51:1022–1030.
70. Austin BA, Tang WH, Rodriguez ER, et al. Delayed hyperenhancement magnetic resonance imaging provides incremental diagnostic and prognostic utility in suspected cardiac amyloidosis. *JACC Cardiovasc Imaging.* 2009;2:1369–1377.
71. Fontana M, Banypersad SM, Treibel TA, et al. Native T1 mapping in transthyretin amyloidosis. *JACC Cardiovasc Imaging.* 2014;7:157–165.
72. Nagai T, Kohsaka S, Okuda S, Anzai T, Asano K, Fukuda K. Incidence and prognostic significance of myocardial late gadolinium enhancement in patients with sarcoidosis without cardiac manifestation. *Chest.* 2014;146:1064–1072.
73. Greulich S, Deluigi CC, Gloekler S, et al. CMR imaging predicts death and other adverse events in suspected cardiac sarcoidosis. *JACC Cardiovasc Imaging.* 2013;6:501–511.
74. Patel MR, Cawley PJ, Heitner JF, et al. Detection of myocardial damage in patients with sarcoidosis. *Circulation.* 2009;120:1969–1977.
75. Vignaux O, Dhote R, Duboc D, et al. Detection of myocardial involvement in patients with sarcoidosis applying T2-weighted, contrast-enhanced, and cine magnetic resonance imaging: Initial results of a prospective study. *J Comput Assist Tomogr.* 2002;26:762–767.
76. Chai P, Mohiaddin R. How we perform cardiovascular magnetic resonance flow assessment using phase-contrast velocity mapping. *J Cardiovasc Magn Reson.* 2005;7:705–716.
77. Fussen S, De Boeck BW, Zellweger MJ, Bremerich J, Goetschalckx K, Zuber M, Buser PT. Cardiovascular magnetic resonance imaging for diagnosis and clinical management of suspected cardiac masses and tumours. *Eur Heart J.* 2011;32:1551–1560.
78. Bogaert J, Francone M. Cardiovascular magnetic resonance in pericardial diseases. *J Cardiovasc Magn Reson.* 2009;11:14.
79. Francone M, Dymarkowski S, Kalantzi M, Bogaert J. Real-time cine MRI of ventricular septal motion: A novel approach to assess ventricular coupling. *J Magn Reson Imaging.* 2005;21:305–309.
80. Taylor AM, Dymarkowski S, Verbeken EK, Bogaert J. Detection of pericardial inflammation with late-enhancement cardiac magnetic resonance imaging: Initial results. *Eur Radiol.* 2006;16:569–574.

Review Questions

SECTION 6

1. The radiations typically used to image ^{201}Tl are polyenergetic because:
   a. electron capture creates multiple γ-ray emissions.
   b. ^{201}Hg K- and L-shell electrons have different binding energies.
   c. there are multiple γ-ray emissions from ^{201}Hg.
   d. ^{201}Tl γ-ray emissions are more abundant than x rays.

2. In the decay of ^{99m}Tc, internal conversion is responsible for:
   a. characteristic x rays.
   b. Auger electrons.
   c. β$^+$ emissions.
   d. particulate emissions.

3. Photons undergoing Compton scatter in tissue:
   a. can be identified by their energy.
   b. are less abundant than the photoelectrons.
   c. are not considered in radiation safety.
   d. are more abundant than Compton electrons.

4. As the thickness of tissue overlying the heart increases:
   a. the percentage of transmitted photons increases.
   b. the number of photoelectrons decreases.
   c. the amount of characteristic x rays decreases.
   d. the number of energy-degraded photons increases.

5. The international unit for describing dose equivalent is:
   a. Coulomb/kg
   b. Air Kerma
   c. Gray
   d. Sievert

6. The US population receives approximately how much annual radiation from natural background?
   a. 3.1 mSv
   b. 6.2 mSv
   c. 9.3 mSv
   d. 12.4 mSv

7. The occupational worker annual whole-body radiation dose limit is the following:
   a. 0.05 Sv
   b. 0.15 Sv
   c. 0.5 Sv
   d. 5 Sv

8. The Nuclear Regulatory Commission recommended whole-body ALARA II investigational level is the following:
   a. 1.25 mSv per calendar quarter
   b. 3.75 mSv per calendar quarter
   c. 12.5 mSv per calendar quarter
   d. 37.5 mSv per calendar quarter

9. Effects from radiation that increase in severity after a threshold is exceeded are termed:
   a. Stochastic
   b. Deterministic
   c. Linear nonthreshold
   d. Carcinogenic

10. A radiation source is measured at 20 mR/hr at a distance of 2 m. What is the calculated measure of the source at 3 m?
    a. 2.2 mR/hr
    b. 6.7 mR/hr
    c. 8.9 mR/hr
    d. 10.0 mR/hr

11. Occupational workers are required to be issued a radiation-monitoring device under the following condition:
    a. The employee is a full-time occupational radiation worker.
    b. The employee is an undeclared pregnant worker.
    c. The employee is likely to receive 5% of the annual radiation dose limit.
    d. The employee is likely to receive 10% of the annual radiation dose limit.

12. Disposal of waste using the decay-in-storage method requires the following condition prior to disposal:
    a. Waste is held for a minimum of 5 half-lives.
    b. Waste is held for a minimum of 10 half-lives.
    c. Waste is held for a minimum of 10 half-lives and is indistinguishable from background radiation.
    d. Waste must be held for 10 half-lives and is less than two times background radiation.

13. A radioactive package containing 10 mCi of ^{99m}Tc with a surface exposure reading of 0.4 mR/hr and a wipe test of 6600 dpm/300 cm^2 should be returned with the following package label:
    a. Excepted Package Limited Quantity
    b. Radioactive I White
    c. Radioactive II Yellow
    d. Radioactive III Yellow

14. A radioactive package containing 10 mCi of ^{99m}Tc with a surface exposure reading of 1.0 mR/hr and a wipe test of 6600 dpm/300 cm^2 should be returned with the following package label:
    a. Excepted Package Limited Quantity
    b. Radioactive I White
    c. Radioactive II Yellow
    d. Radioactive III Yellow

15. Following an intravenous injection of ^{99m}Tc-sestamibi at stress, which of the following organs receive the highest radiation dose (target organ)?
    a. Kidneys
    b. Heart
    c. Upper large intestine
    d. Gallbladder

16. What are the respective corresponding physical half-lives of rubidium-82, N-13 ammonia, and O-15 water?
    a. 76 seconds, 9.8 minutes, and 2 minutes, respectively
    b. 25.5 days, 2 minutes, and 110 minutes, respectively
    c. 76 seconds, 2 minutes, and 110 minutes, respectively
    d. 2 minutes, 9.8 minutes, and 6 hours, respectively

17. Which of the following statements on PET imaging agent is FALSE?
    a. Rubidium-82 is the only clinical PET radiotracer produced by a generator.
    b. N-13 ammonia has a lower first-pass extraction fraction than rubidium-82.
    c. O-15 water is considered the gold standard for clinical noninvasive myocardial blood-flow measurements.
    d. Rubidium-82 has the lowest-image spatial resolution among the other available PET myocardial perfusion imaging agents.

18. Which of the following myocardial perfusion imaging radiotracers is NOT a cation or cationic complex?
    a. O-15 water
    b. Thallium-201
    c. ^{99m}Tc tetrofosmin
    d. ^{99m}Tc sestamibi

19. The OSEM iterative reconstruction is a:
    a. stepwise algorithm for estimating the source activity from a set of projection data based on a model.
    b. process for correcting for attenuation correction.
    c. reconstruction approach that uses Fourier transforms to produce a 3D reconstruction from a set of projection data.
    d. process for correcting for resolution recovery.

20. Which of these attenuation artifacts is specific to line-source attenuation correction?
    a. Misregistration artifact
    b. Downscatter into the photopeak window
    c. Implanted metal artifact
    d. Breathing artifact

21. 3D imaging in PET is used to:
    a. improve the resolution of a PET scan.
    b. allow for tomographic imaging in PET.
    c. enable flow imaging with PET.
    d. improve the sensitivity of the PET system.

22. At what frequency should a SPECT uniformity flood be routinely performed?
    a. Daily
    b. Weekly
    c. Monthly
    d. Quarterly

23. At what frequency should a SPECT system resolution and linearity be performed?
    a. Daily
    b. Weekly
    c. Monthly
    d. Quarterly

24. At what frequency should a PET system blank scan be performed?
    a. Daily
    b. Weekly
    c. Monthly or quarterly
    d. Annually

25. At what frequency should a PET system normalization be performed?
    a. Daily
    b. Weekly
    c. Monthly or quarterly
    d. Annually

26. When performing attenuation correction using gadolinium-153 or germanium-68 sealed sources, at what frequency should a reference scan be performed?
    a. Daily
    b. Weekly
    c. Monthly
    d. Quarterly

27. Which of the following answers best describes the goal(s) of quality assurance and improvement programs in nuclear cardiology?
    a. Radioisotope administration evaluation
    b. Camera image quality, image processing, image interpretation examination
    c. All aspects of nuclear cardiology from patient selection to downstream testing and patient outcomes
    d. Examination of compliance of the final report with current guidelines and standards

28. Accreditation of nuclear cardiology laboratories in the United States:
    a. is available only through the American College of Radiology.
    b. is required for Medicare reimbursement for myocardial perfusion imaging studies.
    c. is good for 10 years once accredited.
    d. requires that all physician interpreters be board-certified in nuclear cardiology.

29. Use of benchmarks is an important part of a quality assurance program. Which of the following is true regarding benchmarks?
    a. Benchmarks provide a mechanism to compare your laboratory to other similar laboratories regarding performance measures.
    b. Benchmarks lead to only high-risk patient selection.
    c. Benchmarks are widely available for nuclear cardiology testing.
    d. Benchmarks are only used by payers to determine reimbursement for testing.

30. Which of the following are commonly used tracers in Nuclear Cardiology:
    a. F-18 FDG
    b. Thallium-201
    c. Technetium-99m sestamibi
    d. Rubidium-82

    Please list in order of radiation exposure to patients (mSv), highest to lowest:
    A. a, c, d, b
    B. c, d, a, b
    C. b, c, a, d
    D. a, b, d, c

31. Utilizing which of the following techniques would **NOT** incur lower-radiation exposure compared to standard rest–stress technetium-sestamibi?
    a. Ordered subset expectation minimization (OSEM) algorithms
    b. Anger camera
    c. Stress-first protocols
    d. Careful screening of patients prior to testing

32. The American Society of Nuclear Cardiology has recommended a maximum radiation exposure to patients during a nuclear cardiology study be <9 mSv per patient. Latest data demonstrate what percentage of US laboratories is following this recommendation?
    a. 23%
    b. 75%
    c. 10%
    d. 1%

33. Stress-only (or stress-first) imaging protocols are advantageous to reduce radiation exposure because data indicate the percentage of all nuclear cardiology studies which demonstrate either infarction or ischemia is estimated to be:
    a. 36% to 55%
    b. 20% to 35%
    c. 8% to 15%
    d. 1% to 7%

34. When performing dipyridamole-stress testing to establish the presence or absence of ischemic heart disease, which of the following medications may be given within 12 hours before the test?
    a. Theophylline
    b. Dipyridamole
    c. Beta blockers
    d. Caffeine

35. Exercise SPECT myocardial perfusion imaging is recommended for which of the following patients?
    a. A 65-year-old man within 48 hours of a confirmed diagnosis of an acute coronary syndrome.
    b. A 71-year-old asymptomatic man who had a stent to LAD performed 18 months ago.
    c. A 62-year-old diabetic woman with new jaw pain.
    d. A 78-year-old man with dyspnea and LBBB on ECG.

36. Which of the following pharmacologic protocols is *not* endorsed by guidelines?
    a. 3-minute adenosine infusion
    b. A graded dobutamine infusion up to 50 mcg/min
    c. 0.56 mg/kg of diyridamole given over 4 minutes
    d. Adjunctive exercise with adenosine

37. Regadenoson:
    a. may be used safely in patients with asthma and/or COPD.
    b. rarely causes headaches.
    c. is frequently associated with complete heart block.
    d. requires the use of an infusion pump.

38. The Duke treadmill score does *not* depend on which of the following?
    a. Exercise time
    b. Severity of angina
    c. Blood pressure changes
    d. Magnitude of ST depression

39. What is the recommended ratio of low dose to high dose of Tc^{99m} tracers?
    a. 1:4
    b. 1:2
    c. 1:3
    d. 1:5

40. Which protocol has the highest radiation dose to the patient?
    a. Tl-201 stress–rest
    b. Tc^{99m} sestamibi rest–stress
    c. Tl-201 rest–Tc^{99m} stress (dual-isotope)
    d. Tc^{99m} stress-only

41. The half-life of Tl-201 is:
    a. 18.7 hours
    b. 6 hours
    c. 73.2 hours
    d. 76.3 hours

42. Which tracer has the fastest liver clearance?
    a. Tc^{99m} sestamibi
    b. Tc^{99m} tetrofosmin
    c. Tl-201
    d. All have a similar clearance rate

43. A 69-year-old male with atypical chest pain, diabetes, and hypertension who recently developed back pain undergoes pharmacologic stress Rb-82 imaging. The below images represent:
    a. three-vessel ischemia with TID.
    b. false positive due to misregistration.
    c. good prognosis.
    d. single-vessel disease, medical therapy.

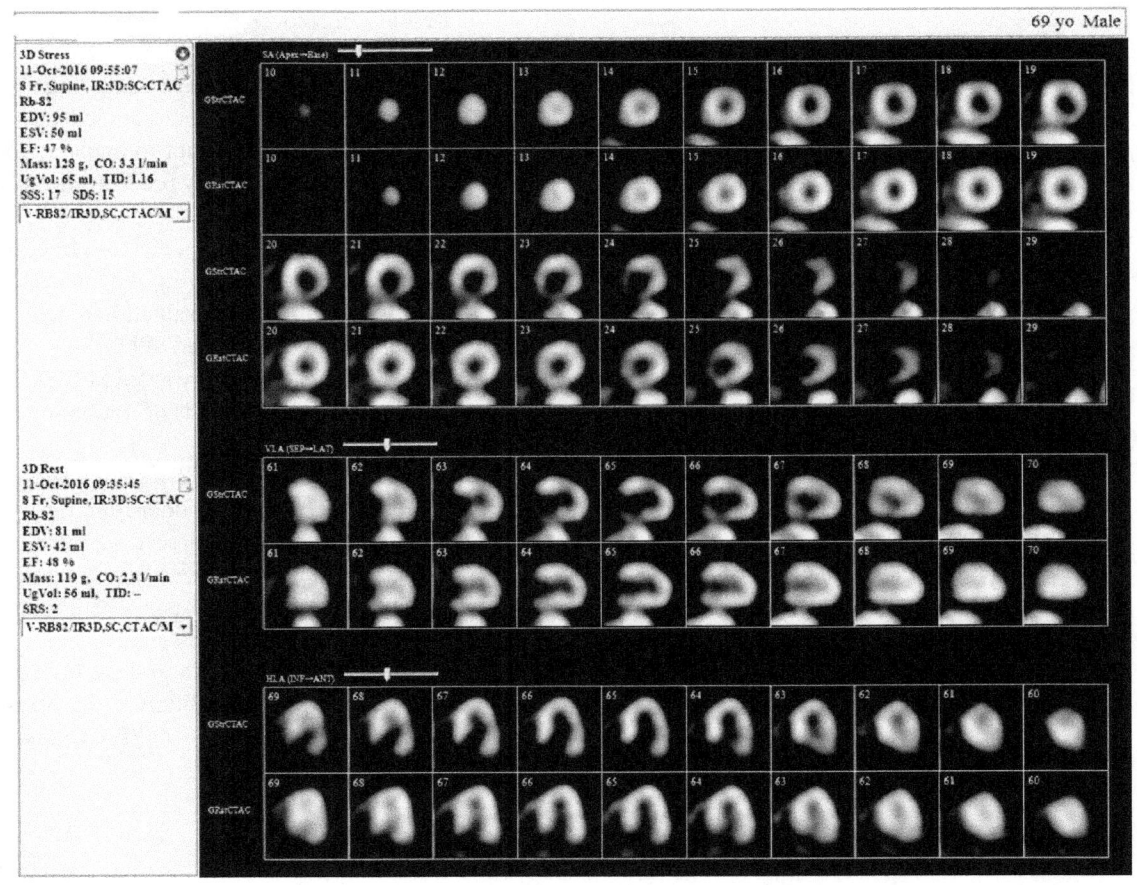

44. PET imaging is emerging as a very useful diagnostic tool, and offers benefit in comparison to standard SPECT. Which of the following is *not* an example of an advantage PET imaging?
    a. PET imaging is able to detect reversible wall-motion abnormalities at peak hyperemia.
    b. Exercise PET is currently available and routinely performed.
    c. PET perfusion imaging protocols are short (30–45 minutes).
    d. PET imaging demonstrates higher spatial resolution when compared to SPECT imaging.

45. Due to the advantages of PET, many patients may be more recommended to undergo a PET study instead of a SPECT study. All of the following indications are appropriate for PET except:
    a. a 54-year-old female with hypertension/chest pain and previous equivocal SPECT study.
    b. a 68-year-old female with a history of CABG, new chest pain and unable to exercise.
    c. a 75-year-old male with a history of smoking presents for preoperative evaluation prior to a fem-pop bypass surgery.
    d. a 35-year-old female with HTN, a 12 pack/yr history of tobacco use, and normal-resting ECG with atypical chest pain.

46. There are two PET perfusion tracers available commercially. Of these, the most often used is Rb-82. Of the following, which is not a characteristic of Rb-82?
    a. Provides rapid sequence between stress and rest imaging
    b. On-site cyclotron is necessary
    c. Image quality is high
    d. Radiation exposure is 3 to 5 mSv/patient

47. Myocardial blood flow (MBF) offers additional information beyond perfusion imaging by estimating flow reserve. CFR can provide additional information for all of the following conditions except:
    a. reduce likelihood of obstructive CAD with normal MPI and MBF reserve.
    b. endothelial dysfunction by the presence of regional reduction of MBF reserve.
    c. indicate lack of pharmacologic stress hyperemia by no augmentation of MBF.
    d. identification of more severe disease with abnormal MBF reserve and single-territory MPI.

48. Assessment of left ventricular dyssynchrony by phase analysis relies on which of the following attributes of gated SPECT?
    a. High spatial resolution
    b. High temporal resolution
    c. Partial-volume effect
    d. Resolution recovery

49. A 60-year-old male patient is undergoing gated SPECT MPI for evaluation of left ventricular ejection fraction prior to implantation of a defibrillator for primary prevention. He had a prior gated SPECT MPI 6 months ago that showed a left ventricular ejection fraction of 35%. Which of the following statements is correct regarding serial evaluation of left ventricular function on gated SPECT?
    a. Since EF measurement by gated SPECT is largely automated, there is no variability on serial assessment.
    b. Biological variability of EF assessment is higher in ventricles with poor function.
    c. In the clinical situation described, only technical variability is likely to play a role in the repeatability of EF assessment on the serial studies.
    d. Many factors related to tracer dose, timing of injection, image acquisition, and processing can result in variability of EF assessment.

50. Your laboratory has moved from 8-bin ECG-gated acquisition to 16-bin data collection in keeping with current ASNC recommendations. Which of the following can be anticipated regarding ejection fraction calculation?
    a. No change in EF
    b. Increase in EF by 10%
    c. Increase in EF by 5%
    d. Drop in EF by 5%

51. A female patient undergoes a rest–stress SPECT study. Evaluation of rotating images demonstrates nonuniform breast shadow on both the rest and stress studies, with greater tissue density in the anterior portion of the heart. Images show a mild, fixed defect in the anterior wall for both rest and stress. ECG gating demonstrates normal wall motion including the anterior wall. Your interpretation?
    a. Normal. Defect consistent with attenuation artifact
    b. Abnormal. Cannot exclude CAD
    c. Equivocal. Cannot distinguish attenuation artifact from CAD
    d. Probably normal. Most likely due to attenuation artifact

52. A large perfusion defect may be defined by which of the following?
    a. A summed score of 4
    b. >17% of the left ventricle
    c. Proximal LAD distribution
    d. Six segments

53. Which of the following is *not* true regarding the raw, rotating planar images?
    a. Should be reviewed only when a technical artifact is suspected.
    b. May demonstrate an unsuspected neoplasm.
    c. Vertical patient motion may be readily detected.
    d. Assist in defining soft tissue attenuation.

54. Which of the following statements might be included in a high-quality SPECT report?
    a. Clinical correlation is suggested.
    b. There is a subtle area of questionable significance noted in the inferior wall.
    c. The mild fixed anterior wall abnormality is artifactual and related to soft tissue attenuation.
    d. Based on the current study, the risk for a perioperative cardiac event is not increased.

55. Which of the following statements is true about appropriate use criteria development for radionuclide imaging?
    a. Clinical judgment should be used when considering appropriate use.
    b. The prior terminology of "inappropriate" use meant that radionuclide imaging should never be performed for that indication.
    c. AUC are based on expert consensus opinion.
    d. The multimodality AUC strives to provide suggestions regarding the single best-testing option for a specific indication.

56. J. Smith is a 43-year-old woman with a history of hypertension who presents to her clinician with nonexertional chest pain, which started 2 weeks ago and has been relatively continuous. What would be the appropriate diagnostic strategy?
    a. Exercise ECG stress test
    b. Exercise radionuclide SPECT
    c. Exercise echocardiography
    d. CT coronary angiography

57. The category of appropriate use is selected based on which of the following:
    a. The most "appropriate" category may be selected, resulting in the highest level of categorization of appropriate use.
    b. A computer algorithm must be consulted which then designates the appropriate use category.
    c. Third-party payers ultimately decide on whether or not a test is considered appropriate.
    d. A hierarchical approach is used to select the correct table to determine the category of appropriate use.

58. Which of the following patients would be most appropriate for an exercise SPECT MPI?
    a. A 55-year-old male athlete with an LBBB on ECG.
    b. A 45-year-old male smoker with new onset chest pain and ST elevation on ECG.
    c. A 66-year-old asymptomatic male with a coronary calcium score of 80 and a normal ECG.
    d. A 55-year-old runner with exertional chest pain and a normal ECG.

59. A 65-year-old obese female presents to the clinic, with several months' history of exercise-induced chest discomfort associated with dyspnea. Baseline ECG demonstrates nonspecific ST-T changes in the lateral leads. Which one of the following is the most appropriate modality to diagnose coronary artery disease?
    a. No testing indicated
    b. Exercise tolerance test
    c. Vasodilator Tc-99m SPECT
    d. Exercise SPECT myocardial perfusion imaging

60. The overall diagnostic is best with which modality?
    a. Exercise tolerance test (ETT)
    b. Exercise SPECT myocardial perfusion imaging
    c. Vasodilator PET
    d. Vasodilator Tc-99m SPECT

61. The following are advantages of PET MPI over SPECT MPI except:
    a. increased diagnostic accuracy.
    b. improved laboratory efficiency.
    c. reduced radiation exposure.
    d. best suited for exercise PET.

62. A low risk for cardiac events:
    a. implies an annual event rate of <1% per year.
    b. is often associated with fixed perfusion defect.
    c. is an indication for repeat testing in 1 year.
    d. is present as long as there is a low Duke treadmill score.

63. Markers of patients at high risk for myocardial infarction do *not* include:
    a. transient cavity dilation.
    b. reversible perfusion defect.
    c. large, severe fixed perfusion defect.
    d. multivessel coronary disease.

64. Appropriate use criteria (AUC):
    a. define optimal use of cardiac imaging procedure.
    b. frequently deviate from practice guidelines.
    c. are based solely on medical literature.
    d. allow for clinical judgment and recognize the absence of 0% rarely appropriate threshold.

65. Which of the following statements related to cavity dilation is true?
    a. Transient cavity dilation (TID) is seen only in multivessel CAD.
    b. The presence of persistent cavity enlargement is a marker for increased risk of MI.
    c. Transient cavity dilation after dipyridamole reflects a temporary increase in left ventricular dimension.
    d. Transient cavity dilation may be seen in hypertensive patients without significant obstructive CAD.

66. Which of the following patients should be considered for preoperative evaluation with SPECT myocardial perfusion imaging?
    a. A 68-year-old woman, with a history of atypical chest pain, undergoing a breast biopsy.
    b. A 77-year-old man scheduled for a Whipple procedure with a history of diabetes and mild renal insufficiency.
    c. A 71-year-old asymptomatic man, who plays golf twice per week, scheduled for aortobifemoral bypass surgery.
    d. A 54-year-old man who is status post STEMI and had a coronary stent placement procedure 2 years ago, scheduled for elective arthroscopic knee surgery.

67. Which of the following approaches has been shown to improve outcomes with a reduction of perioperative MI and death?
    a. Beta-blocker usage in high-risk patients
    b. Clopidogrel
    c. Statins in vascular-surgery patients
    d. CABG before intermediate-risk surgery

68. Which of the following factors has been shown to increase the risk of perioperative myocardial infarction?
    a. A large fixed defect
    b. A moderately sized reversible perfusion defect
    c. A left ventricular ejection fraction of 38%
    d. Persistent ST depression after exercise stress

69. According to the 2013 multimodality AUC, which one of the following would be considered an *appropriate* post revascularization for SPECT myocardial perfusion imaging?
    a. Evaluation of atypical chest pain
    b. Asymptomatic patient <5 years post CABG
    c. Asymptomatic patient who underwent incomplete revascularization
    d. Asymptomatic patient <2 years post PCI

70. Which of the following is true regarding perfusion imaging to assess efficacy of medical therapy?
    a. Beta blockers improve myocardial perfusion mainly by increasing coronary blood flow.
    b. There is no evidence to support the use of ACE inhibitors as medical therapy for patients with known CAD.
    c. Myocardial perfusion imaging should be performed while patient is maintained on antianginal medications.
    d. Perfusion abnormalities have been shown to be significantly reduced with beta-blocker use, except when the stressing agent is a vasodilator.

71. A patient with 90% stenosis of his left anterior descending coronary artery and 70% stenosis of his left circumflex coronary artery had successful PCI with a drug-eluting stent to the left anterior descending coronary artery. The patient remains asymptomatic and comes to your clinic for a 6-month follow-up. According to current multimodality AUC, obtaining a SPECT MPI would be:
    a. Rarely appropriate
    b. May be appropriate
    c. Uncertain
    d. Appropriate

72. A 55-year-old male with hypertension and diabetes presents to the emergency room with a 2-week history of worsening dyspnea, edema, and fatigue. He denies chest pain. Chest x-ray reveals pulmonary vascular prominence, and echocardiogram shows LVEF of 25% with global hypokinesis. A diagnosis of congestive heart failure is made. Which of the following diagnostic studies is most important to complete prior to discharge?
    a. NT-proBNP
    b. Right-heart catheterization
    c. Myocardial SPECT stress test
    d. Myocardial viability testing with rest/redistribution thallium

73. A 48-year-old male, with a history of coronary artery disease and myocardial infarction in the past, presents to the hospital with signs and symptoms of heart failure. Echocardiogram reveals a dilated and dysfunctional left ventricle, with an estimated LVEF of 15%. Coronary angiography shows a patent stent in the right coronary artery (RCA) with an occluded LAD which fills via right–left collaterals (*arrows*). He undergoes a rubidium/FDG-PET viability study (image shown below). Which of the following is the most appropriate next step in his management?
    a. Surgical referral for CABG with planned LIMA-LAD bypass
    b. Continued optimization of medical therapy
    c. Cardiac MRI with gadolinium
    d. Referral for heart transplantation/left ventricular assist device (LVAD)

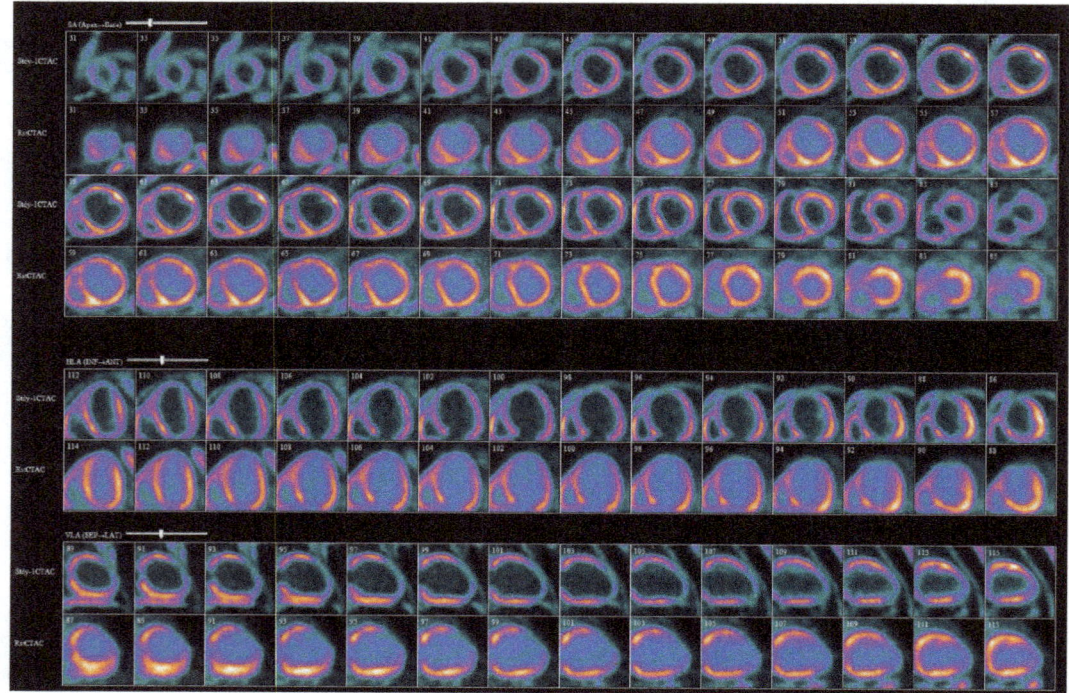

74. A 36-year-old female patient is seen in the outpatient clinic. She was diagnosed with nonischemic cardiomyopathy 3 months earlier, with LVEF of 15%. She was treated with goal-directed heart failure therapy, and clinically improved. Repeat echocardiogram in the office shows improvement of LVEF to 30%. She undergoes I-123 *m*IBG scan (image shown right) which reveals a heart-mediastinal ratio of 1.4. Which of the following is the most reasonable next step?
    a. Cardiac MRI for tissue characterization
    b. Primary-prevention ICD placement
    c. Initiation of digoxin
    d. Initiation of amiodarone

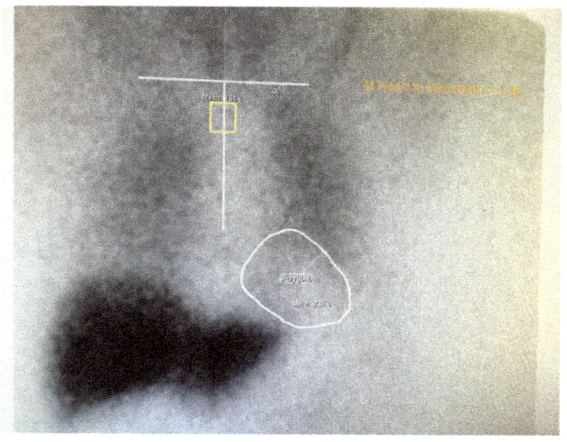

75. A 60-year-old diabetic male presented to the emergency department (ED) with chief complains of substernal chest pain while at rest. The patient was injected with Technetium-99m sestamibi during the episode of chest pain and subsequently acute rest myocardial perfusion imaging was performed. Attenuation correction (AC) was performed, and below is the AC image. Wall-motion evaluation was normal.

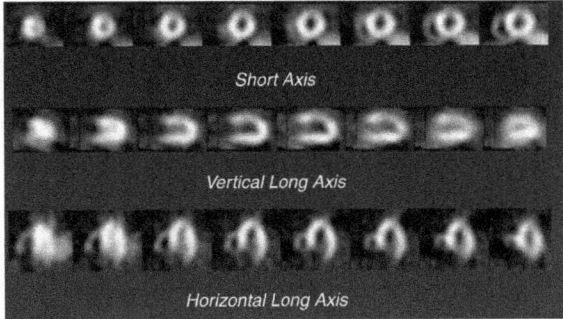

    What is the appropriate next step in the management of this patient?
    a. This is a low-risk scan, discharge patient from ED.
    b. Follow serial cardiac biomarkers for 12 to 24 hours; if negative, discharge patient home.
    c. Admit to telemetry and perform stress perfusion imaging.
    d. Admit to telemetry and schedule patient for invasive angiography.

76. A 62-year-old male with past medical history of type 2 diabetes mellitus, hypertension, dyslipidemia, and obesity presents to his primary care physician (PCP) with complaints of non-exertional chest pain for 6 weeks. The patient is unable to undergo adequate exercise and therefore receives pharmacologic stress. The resulting images are normal. What should the referring health care provider tell the diabetic patient regarding his cardiovascular outcomes and further management?
    a. Low risk of hard cardiac events (<1%) over the next 1 year.
    b. Relatively low risk of hard cardiac events (1–2%) over the next 1 year.
    c. Patient should undergo yearly nuclear stress testing, irrespective of symptoms, due to presence of diabetes.
    d. Will need referral for cardiac catheterization due to increased percentage of false-negative results in diabetic patients.

77. A 60-year-old postmenopausal woman with PMH of hypertension is referred to the cardiologist for evaluation of atypical chest pain. The patient undergoes exercise nuclear rest–stress myocardial perfusion imaging, demonstrating a moderate-sized defect involving the basal to mid-inferior and inferolateral walls. Subsequently, patient undergoes cardiac catheterization, which reveals nonobstructive CAD (45%). Which one of the following statements is true?
    a. This patient has excellent long-term prognosis.
    b. Nuclear stress testing has lower accuracy in women.
    c. Cardiovascular adverse outcomes are higher in this patient despite absence of significant epicardial coronary stenosis.
    d. Coronary microvascular dysfunction (CMD) does not play a significant role in the pathophysiology of angina in women.

78. A 55-year-old diabetic male with PMH of hypertension, dyslipidemia, and peripheral neuropathy presents for outpatients evaluation of ongoing chest pain since last 2 months. Baseline ECG reveals LVH with strain pattern. He is scheduled for a nuclear stress test. Which one of the following scenarios has the most favorable outcomes in this patient?
    a. Normal pharmacological myocardial perfusion imaging with EF >60%
    b. Normal exercise nuclear stress testing with EF >60%
    c. Normal exercise nuclear stress testing with EF <45%
    d. Normal pharmacological stress testing with EF <45%

79. When calculating "value" of a diagnostic test, which of the following factors is needed for the calculation?
    a. Quality
    b. Appropriateness
    c. Cost
    d. Both a and c

80. Quality-adjusted life year (QALY) is an important concept in cost-effectiveness. Which of the following statements is not correct?
    a. QALY is based solely on the cost of a test.
    b. Most studies have used $50,000 as a threshold for QALY.
    c. A QALY may be based on a country's gross national product.
    d. The incremental cost-effectiveness ratio is based on the cost and QALY differential between two techniques.

81. Based on the END trial, EMPIRE study, and SPECT Registry, which of the following statements is true?
    a. When scintigraphic data are used, there is a lower incidence of coronary revascularization.
    b. The costs of a strategy using radionuclide imaging study as the first procedure is greater than starting with CCTA or invasive coronary angiography.
    c. Patient outcomes were superior when using an anatomic strategy, due to the increased usage of coronary revascularization.
    d. No firm conclusions can be reached based on these trials, as they were underpowered to address cost-effectiveness.

82. What is the best definition for hibernating myocardium?
    a. A postischemic state where there is mismatch between function and flow.
    b. A state with preserved function, metabolism, and blood flow.
    c. A postischemic state where there is mismatch between flow and metabolism.
    d. Diagnosed on FDG-PET images as a match between flow tracer and metabolism.

83. A 58-year-old man with ischemic heart failure (LVEF = 32%), no angina symptoms, and with diabetes was referred for viability assessment. ECG showed sinus rhythm and no significant conduction abnormality. His coronary angiogram showed normal left main, 70% stenosis in proximal LAD, minor irregularities in LCx, and 99% proximal RCA. Based on the PET viability study shown below, what is the best option for interpretation and clinical management?
    a. Significant area of flow/metabolism mismatch in LAD/benefit from CABG.
    b. Ischemia in the anteroseptal and inferoseptal walls and apex/benefit from CABG.
    c. Significant area of mismatch in the LAD and RCA territories/benefit from CABG.
    d. FDG/perfusion match in the LAD and RCA territories/unlikely benefit from CABG.

84. Patient preparation is an important component of the ^{18}FDG-PET viability protocol. Among the options below, which one may lead to inferior image quality when used as isolated technique?
    a. Glucose loading
    b. Fasting
    c. Hyperinsulinemic–euglycemic clamp
    d. Use of acipimox

85. Which of the RBC-labeling techniques for equilibrium radionuclide angiography (ERNA) has the highest labeling efficiency?
    a. In vitro method
    b. In vivo method
    c. Modified in vivo/in vitro method
    d. All have equal efficiency

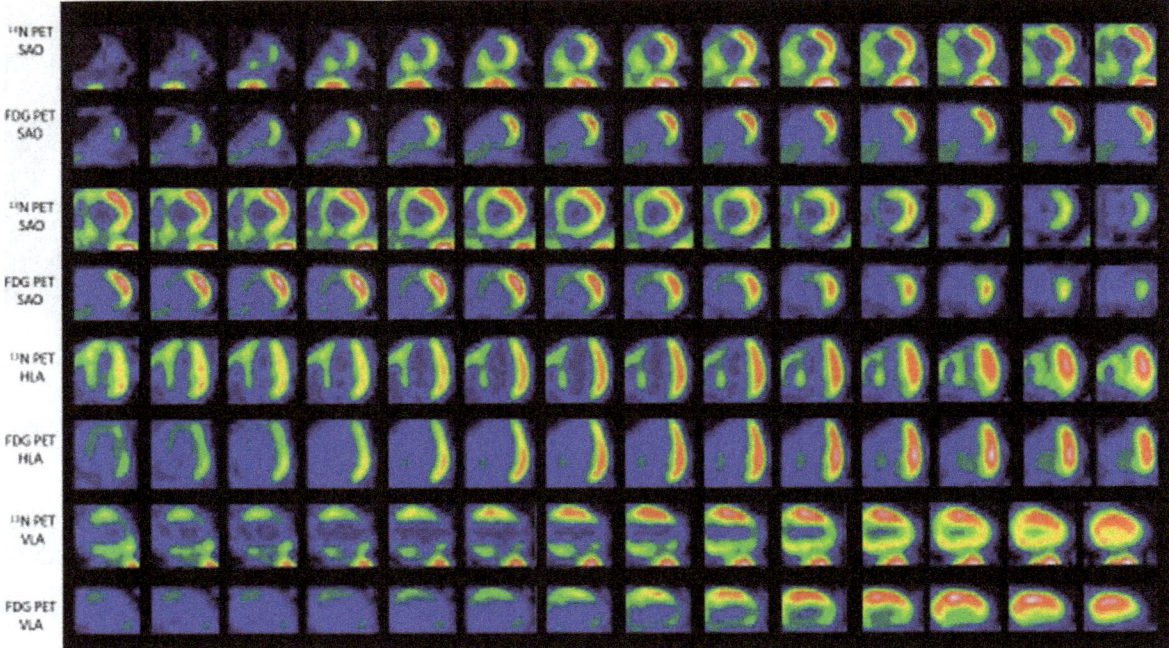

86. First-pass radionuclide angiography (FPRNA) has several distinct advantages over equilibrium radionuclide angiography. Which of these is not an advantage of FPRNA?
   a. Acquisition of data in <30 seconds
   b. Better evaluation of RV function
   c. Limited data on prognosis with FPRNA
   d. Multiple different radiopharmaceuticals can be used

87. Radionuclide angiography techniques are used clinically to assess:
   a. left ventricular systolic function.
   b. ventricular dyssynchrony.
   c. monitoring the effects of chemotherapy.
   d. all of the above.

88. Which of the radionuclide angiographic techniques is used the least these days?
   a. First-pass radionuclide angiography
   b. Gated planar equilibrium blood pool imaging
   c. Gated tomographic equilibrium blood pool imaging
   d. Gated SPECT myocardial perfusion imaging

89. ^{123}I-mIBG (meta-iodobenzylguanidine):
   a. is an analog of metoprolol and images cardiac postsynaptic receptors.
   b. is an analog of norepinephrine and images cardiac sympathetic innervation.
   c. is an analog of acetylcholine and images cardiac parasympathetic innervation.
   d. is a tracer that requires imaging using a PET camera.

90. Global myocardial uptake of ^{123}I-mIBG is customarily assessed using a/an:
   a. heart-to-mediastinum uptake ratio on planar imaging.
   b. washout of tracer.
   c. mismatching neuronal–perfusion defect on SPECT.
   d. tracer uptake in the liver.

91. Abnormalities of cardiac ^{123}I-mIBG uptake may be seen in which of the following scenarios?
   a. Severe congestive heart failure
   b. Diabetes mellitus
   c. Primary arrhythmic conditions such as arrhythmogenic right ventricular dysplasia
   d. All of the above

92. Findings in the accompanying planar ^{123}I-mIBG image (heart: mediastinum ratio [HMR] = 2.02) of a patient with HFrEF have been shown to:

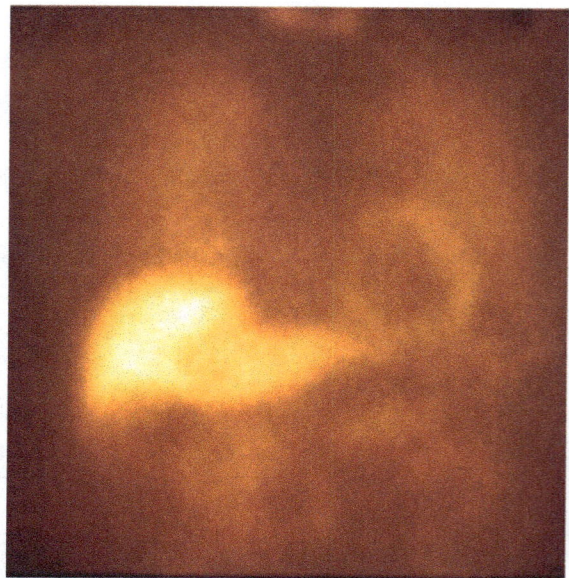

   a. have no relation to patient outcome.
   b. increase the likelihood of an acute ischemic syndrome.
   c. predict decreased risk of cardiac events, including cardiac death.
   d. increase the likelihood of a lethal arrhythmic event.

93. Dietary preparation for imaging myocardial inflammation with ^{18}F-FDG PET involves:
   a. high-fat/high-protein diet for 24 to 48 hours.
   b. prolonged fast (6–12 hours).
   c. high-carbohydrate diet for 24 to 48 hours.
   d. low-carbohydrate/high-fat diet for at least 24 hours.

94. Myocardial perfusion imaging in cardiac sarcoidosis evaluation is most helpful to distinguish:
   a. scar from normal myocardium.
   b. inflammation from scar.
   c. inflammation from normal myocardium.
   d. none of the above. Perfusion imaging is not necessary.

95. Shown below are ^{99m}Tc rest attenuation-corrected SPECT/CT myocardial perfusion images and ^{18}F-FDG PET images of a 65-year-old man with no obstructive coronary artery disease on coronary angiography. He has known focal cardiac sarcoidosis in the basal inferolateral wall, and received high-dose steroid therapy for 6 months. The scan findings are consistent with which of the following?
   a. Normal myocardium
   b. Diffuse inflammation
   c. Poor dietary preparation
   d. Basal inferolateral scar

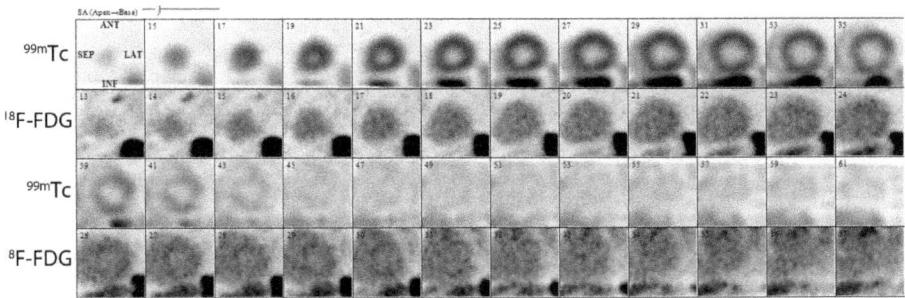
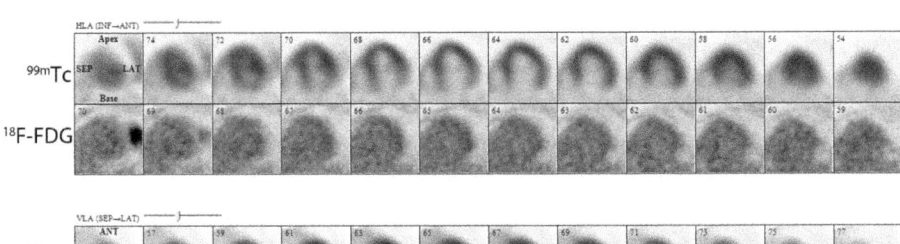
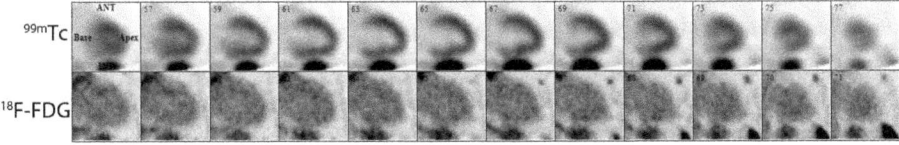

96. ^{18}F-FDG PET/CT images of a 79-year-old man with suspected ICD infection are shown below with the red arrow pointing to a focus of increased ^{18}F-FDG uptake. What is the diagnosis?

    a. No infection, normal
    b. Infected ICD leads
    c. Need more information
    d. Infected ICD device pocket

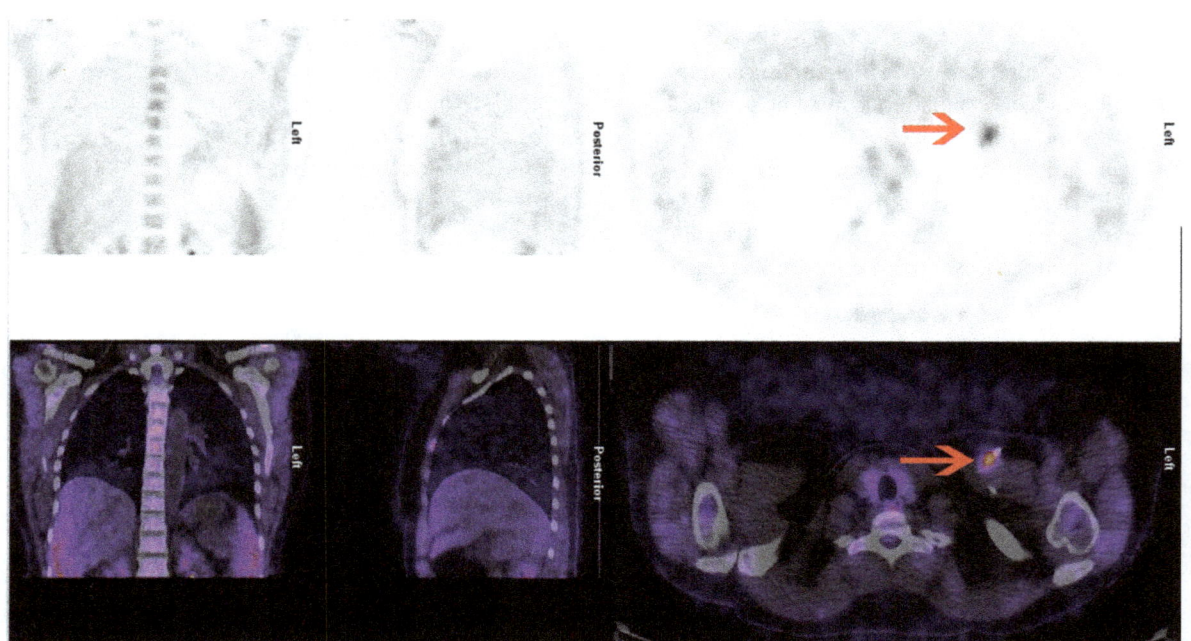

97. The primary advantage of attenuation correction (AC) includes:
    a. improved accuracy to detect coronary artery disease from higher sensitivity.
    b. ability to quantify myocardial blood flow.
    c. lower-radiation dose to the patient.
    d. improved differentiation of artifacts from real defects.

98. Which of the following statements is true about coronary artery calcification?
    a. Presence of extensive coronary artery calcification is associated with increased cardiovascular risk.
    b. Absence of coronary artery calcification excludes ischemia on myocardial perfusion imaging.
    c. Extensive coronary artery calcification is a specific marker of underlying obstructive coronary artery disease.
    d. Extensive coronary artery calcification (Agatston score >400) is of proven value to guide intensity of medical therapy.

99. A 51-year-old male with a family history of premature coronary artery disease and dyslipidemia with an intermediate-risk Framingham score has an Agatston calcium score of 1589. What is the next step in his evaluation?
    a. Coronary CTA
    b. Invasive coronary angiogram
    c. Stress testing with imaging
    d. Reassurance and no further testing

100. Which of the following statements is true regarding hybrid coronary CTA (CTA) and rest–stress PET myocardial perfusion imaging (MPI)?
    a. A CTA is a better initial test in patients with an 80% pretest likelihood of coronary artery disease.
    b. CTA may help detect multivessel disease in patients with severe ischemia.
    c. MPI is the preferred initial test in a patient with 15% pretest likelihood of coronary artery disease.
    d. Absolute myocardial blood flow assessment with PET MPI can help identify microvascular dysfunction in symptomatic patients with normal CTA.

101. Which other imaging modality in addition to echocardiography has been shown to improve accuracy of Duke criteria in diagnosis of prosthetic valve endocarditis?
    a. F^{18}-FDG-PET CT/CTA
    b. SPECT
    c. CMR
    d. Transesophageal echocardiography

102. The Guideline for the Diagnosis and Management of Patients with Stable Ischemic Heart Disease recommends stress imaging preferentially be performed rather than an exercise treadmill test in all of the following *except*:
    a. High pretest probability of CAD
    b. Left bundle branch block
    c. Elderly patients (≥70 years)
    d. Ventricular pre-excitation

103. A 57-year-old man with a history of atypical chest pain exercises 12 minutes on a Bruce protocol, achieving 90% of his maximum predicted heart rate with a normal blood pressure response. Exercise symptoms included nonlimiting angina. The electrocardiogram demonstrates 1 millimeter of horizontal ST-segment depression at peak exercise. Based on this exercise treadmill test, the patient's estimated annual cardiovascular mortality is which of the following?
    a. 0.25%
    b. 1.25%
    c. 5%
    d. 10%

104. Which of the following statements regarding standard exercise treadmill testing (ETT) and exercise SPECT imaging is true?
    a. Exercise duration is the strongest prognostic exercise test variable.
    b. Annual cardiovascular mortality in patients with an intermediate-risk Duke treadmill score is 5%.
    c. The charge for an ETT is five to seven times higher than an exercise SPECT study.
    d. Exercise SPECT is the appropriate first test in women, with an intermediate likelihood of CAD and a normal resting electrocardiogram, who are able to exercise.

105. A 56-year-old man who has been complaining of chest pain for the past 6 weeks is undergoing dobutamine stress echocardiography (DSE) for further evaluation. At peak heart rate, the patient develops severe nausea and dizziness. Echo images at that time showed an increase in LV end-systolic volume but no clear hypokinesis or akinesis of any myocardial segments.
    What is the explanation of this finding and what is the next best step?
    a. This is a normal common finding and no further evaluation is needed.
    b. This is a nonspecific finding with no clear explanation and another test is likely needed for further evaluation.
    c. This is likely an indication of underlying left ventricular hypertrophy and further evaluation for underlying cause including probable blood pressure control is needed.
    d. This patient likely has underlying multivessel or left main coronary artery disease and needs to undergo further testing, likely with a cardiac catheterization.

106. All of the following can lead to false-negative results for stress echocardiography except:
    a. Three-vessel coronary artery disease
    b. Poor image quality
    c. Significant left ventricular hypertrophy
    d. Concomitant use of beta blockers at the time of testing

107. Which of the following describes an inducible ischemic response of stress echocardiogram?
    a. A normal myocardial segment that becomes akinetic
    b. Biphasic response
    c. Decreased ejection fraction
    d. All of the above

108. Exercise echocardiography is a reasonable test choice in which of the following patients?
    a. An elderly man with symptomatic aortic stenosis
    b. A 25-year-old woman with hypertrophic cardiomyopathy and no resting pressure gradient
    c. A middle-aged woman with acute aortic dissection
    d. A 45-year-old man with chest pain and third-degree AV block

109. Which of the following statements best explains the use of contrast agents in stress echocardiography?
    a. Contrast should be used in all patients undergoing stress echocardiography.
    b. Contrast can only be used when the method of stress is a dobutamine infusion.
    c. Contrast aids in decreasing interobserver variability in stress-test interpretation.
    d. Contrast is safe to use in the presence of a large right to left intracardiac shunt.

110. Optimal evaluation of coronary arteries for atherosclerotic disease using ECG-gated CCTA is performed in which part of the cardiac cycle?
    a. Systole, as the ventricles are smallest in dimension due to myocardial contraction resulting in better visualization of coronary anatomy.
    b. Diastole, as ventricular relaxation and near-cessation of myocardial movement allows optimal visualization of plaque burden and distribution.
    c. Systole, as coronary blood flow is maximal during ventricular systole resulting in optimal visualization of the coronary arteries.
    d. Neither, as contrast enhancement of the coronary arteries during image acquisition will allow visualization of the coronary arteries regardless of the cardiac cycle.

111. The following are considered advantages of retrospective ECG-gated image acquisition, except:
    a. Reduced radiation exposure, because the projection data are acquired for short periods of the cardiac cycle.
    b. The ability to generate cine sequences that show the heart motion throughout the cardiac cycle and allow for ventricular functional assessment.
    c. The ability to examine for valvular dysfunction, especially in patients with aortic stenosis, since image acquisition spans both systole and diastole.
    d. Enhanced diagnostic value in the setting of significant cardiac motion by allowing for selection of different phases for interpretation.

112. Mr. P is a 54-year-old male with a history of coronary artery disease status post prior myocardial infarction, ischemic cardiomyopathy with left ventricular ejection fraction of 40% to 45% with inferior hypokinesis, hypertension, dyslipidemia, and tobacco abuse. He was found to have a 90% heavily calcified RCA lesion that was treated medically. He did well until the day prior to admission when he had prolonged chest pain and was found to have a low-grade elevated troponin. After being stable for 24 hours, he underwent a vasodilator stress cardiac MRI to further evaluate the cause for his chest pain. The images below are obtained. Which of the following best represents the findings seen?

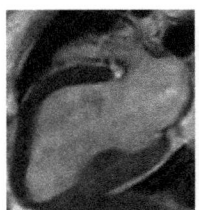
T2-weighted
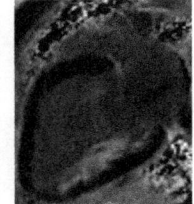
LGE

    a. Chronic inferior myocardial infarction.
    b. Acute on chronic inferior infarction.
    c. Acute myocarditis.
    d. Cardiac sarcoidosis.

113. Ms. P is a 64-year-old female with obstructive sleep apnea, dyslipidemia, chronic kidney disease, and diabetes mellitus who presented with exertional chest discomfort. She underwent a regadenoson stress cardiac MRI with the following apical perfusion images and absolute myocardial blood flow results.

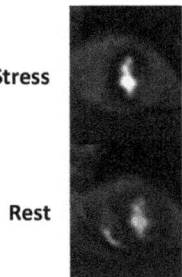

Stress

Rest

Global
Stress: 1.54 mL/g/min
Rest: 0.94 mL/g/min

Flow Reserve: 1.64

Which of the following is the most likely catheterization results?
    a. 90% left anterior descending artery stenosis.
    b. 80% left circumflex and right coronary artery stenoses.
    c. 80% left main and 70% right coronary artery stenoses.
    d. 100% right coronary artery stenosis.

114. Mr. B is a 75-year-old male with a history of coronary artery disease, diabetes mellitus, hypertension and dyslipidemia. He has an ST-elevation myocardial infarction but does not present to the hospital for 18 hours. He undergoes a cardiac MRI to assess for myocardial viability with the late gadolinium enhancement results below.

Which of the following is the likelihood of improved contractility of the inferolateral wall with coronary revascularization?
   a. 0%
   b. 10%
   c. 40%
   d. 80%

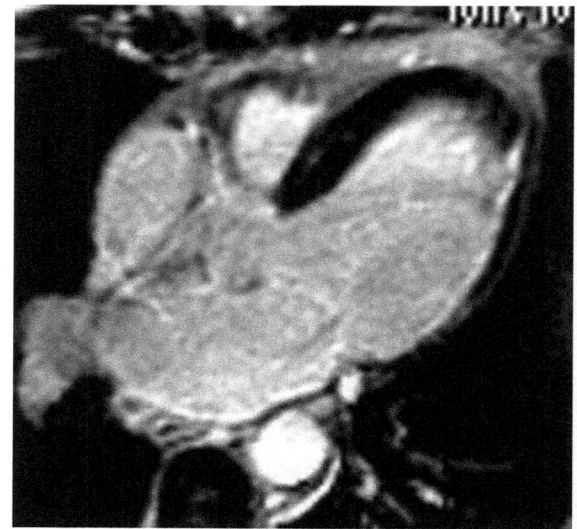

Answers and Explanations for Review Questions

SECTION 6

1. Answer **b.** The energy of characteristic x-rays are dependent on the binding energies of the shell from which they originate. Since the K and L shells have different binding energies, so will their respective characteristic x-rays.
   See Chapter 1.

2. Answer **d.** In internal conversion, the energy release from the de-excitation on the nucleus is transferred to an electron. This increase in energy will eject the electron from its shell, resulting in a particulate emission (Internal Conversion Electron).
   See Chapter 1.

3. Answer **a.** When a photon undergoes Compton scatter, it loses energy relative to its incident energy, and is therefore identifiable.
   See Chapter 1.

4. Answer **d.** As photons travel through tissue, they undergo Compton scatter, which degrades their energy.
   See Chapter 1.

5. Answer **d.** The international unit describing dose equivalent is the Sievert (Sv). The Sievert expands on the absorbed dose (Gray) and takes into account the biological burden from the type of radiation. This is accomplished by multiplying the absorbed dose by a radiation quality factor (QF).
   See Chapter 2.

6. Answer **a.** Radiation from cosmic rays as well as naturally occurring elements in the earth and human body account for approximately 3.1 mSv/yr. Radon and Thoron contribute most to this exposure. An additional 3.1 mSv is assumed from man-made products, industrial/occupational exposure, and medical radiation procedures. This additional 3.1 mSv is not considered natural background radiation.
   See Chapter 2.

7. Answer **a.** Limits to radiation are defined in Title 10, Part 20 of the Code of Federal Regulations. These include limits to the occupational worker (whole body, lens of the eye, skin, and extremity) as well as dose limitations to the public and the fetus of an occupational worker. The whole-body limit to an occupational worker is 0.05 Sv or 5 Rem.
   See Chapter 2.

8. Answer **b.** Although a facility may define its own ALARA levels, the NRC has recommendations provided in NUREG 1556 Volume 9, Revision 2. The ALARA II level is 30% of the annual dose limit and is routinely assessed on a quarterly basis. The annual whole-body dose limit is 0.05 Sv (50 mSv). An ALARA II level requires a timely investigation by the Radiation Safety Officer.
   See Chapter 2.

9. Answer **b.** Effects from radiation are either stochastic or deterministic. Deterministic effects, such as skin erythema (reddening) and cataract development will occur after a dose level (threshold) is exceeded. The severity of the effect is proportional to the radiation dose received. Stochastic effects, such as cancer, are believed to have no threshold for occurrence and the probability of occurrence increases with radiation dose.
   See Chapter 2.

10. Answer **c.**
    $I_1 \times (d_1)^2 = I_2 \times (d_2)^2$
    $20 \text{ mR/hr} \times (2 \text{ m})^2 = I_2 \times (3 \text{ m})^2$
    $20 \text{ mR/hr} \times 4 \text{ m}^2 = I_2 \times 9 \text{ m}^2$
    $I_2 = 8.9 \text{ mR/hr}$
    See Chapter 2.

11. Answer **d.** Requirements for personnel monitoring are outlined in Title 10, Part 20 Section 1502 of the Code of Federal Regulations. These include workers entering high or very high radiation areas, those likely to exceed 10% of the annual dose limits, and declared pregnant workers likely to receive 1 mSv during the entire pregnancy.
See Chapter 2.

12. Answer **c.** The decay-in-storage method requires that by-product radioactive material be disposed when the radioactivity cannot be distinguished from background levels. Prior to 2002, the NRC regulation also included a provision that waste be held for a minimum period of 10 half-lives. This provision is routinely included as a license condition as well as a requirement in many state/local health codes.
See Chapter 2.

13. Answer **a.** Radioactive packages with a surface exposure less than 0.5 mR/hr normally require a Radioactive White I label. If the package contents meet the quantity limitations specified in 49CFR173.425, an "Excepted Package Limited Quantity" label is used. The liquid form limited quantity for ^{99m}Tc is 11 mCi.
See Chapter 2.

14. Answer **c.** Radioactive packages with a surface exposure of 0.5 to 50 mR/hr are labeled with a Radioactive Yellow II label. A surface exposure of 50 to 200 mR/hr would require a Radioactive Yellow III label.
See Chapter 2.

15. Answer **c.** Upper large intestine is the target organ which receives approximately 4.5 rads/ 30 mCi administered dose.
See Chapter 3.

16. Answer **a.**
See Chapter 3.

17. Answer **b.** N-13 ammonia has the highest first-pass extraction fraction which is nearly 100% since it freely diffuses across membranes.
See Chapter 3.

18. Answer **a.** All other agents are cation (thallium-201) or cationic complexes (^{99m}Tc-agents).
See Chapter 3.

19. Answer **a.**
   b. is incorrect because attenuation correction can be performed using FBP and iterative reconstruction is also helpful when attenuation correction is not applied.
   c. is incorrect because it describes how FBP works, not iterative reconstruction.
   d. is incorrect because resolution recovery can be performed using FBP, and iterative reconstruction is useful even when resolution recovery is not used.
See Chapter 4.

20. Answer **b.**
   a. is incorrect because misregistration can be present in CT-based attenuation correction and line-source correction.
   b. is correct because line-source attenuation correction is of a similar intensity and energy, and uses the same detectors as the photopeak. This can lead to interference between the two signals.
   c. is incorrect because implanted artifacts generally do not significantly influence line-source attenuation estimates.
   d. is incorrect because line-source attenuation correction is performed in a free breathing mode, the same as the emission study.
See Chapter 4.

21. Answer **d.**
   a. is incorrect. 3D imaging generally reduces resolution.
   b. is incorrect. Both 2D and 3D modes in PET refer to tomographic techniques.
   c. is incorrect. Flow can be performed in 2D and 3D modes.
   d. is correct. The main advantage of 3D PET is that it improves the system sensitivity up to a factor of 5.
See Chapter 4.

22. Answer **a**. Daily—performed intrinsically or extrinsically with a radioactive source to check for nonuniformities in the field of view.
    See Chapter 5.

23. Answer **b**. Weekly—performed with a bar phantom to document spatial resolution over time, as well as to evaluate the detector's ability to produce straight lines.
    See Chapter 5.

24. Answer **a**. Daily—to analyze system performance and stability. The daily blank scan is the equivalent of the daily uniformity scan for SPECT and allows for detection of any sudden change in system performance such as a module malfunction.
    See Chapter 5.

25. Answer **c**. Monthly or quarterly—performed monthly or quarterly, depending on the manufacturer, to correct for variations in the sensitivity of the blocks or buckets and adjustments in the efficiency in each line of response (LOR) in the sinogram.
    See Chapter 5.

26. Answer **a**. Daily—it is necessary to acquire a reference or blank scan daily, in order to produce an appropriate attenuation map.
    See Chapter 5.

27. Answer **c**. Quality assurance and improvement programs are important for all aspects of nuclear cardiology. There is not a single part of the nuclear cardiology process including patient and test selection, radiation exposure, test performance, interpretation, and reporting that is not included.
    See Chapter 6.

28. Answer **b**. MIPPA provides that accreditation is required for reimbursement of advanced imaging studies paid for by federal programs in the United States in outpatient settings. There are multiple pathways for accreditation from four groups presently (ACR, IAC, RadSite, and TJC). Accreditation needs to be renewed every 3 years and does not require board certification of all interpreting physicians.
    See Chapter 6.

29. Answer **a**. Benchmarks when appropriately selected, allow comparison of performance to similar-type facilities regarding performance measures. If not correctly chosen, they can lead to high-risk avoidance or selection for specific studies; benchmarks need continued development and will be informed from registries and other tools. Payers may use benchmarks in the development of payment scenarios, such as "gold" versus "silver" status and associated variability in payment; however, their use is much broader in scope than this.
    See Chapter 6.

30. Answer **c**. Of the tracers listed, thallium has the greatest radiation exposure levels >20 mSv for traditional rest–stress studies. Technetium-99m sestamibi incurs approximately 12 to 15 mSv per study. The remaining two tracers, rubidium-82 and F-18 FDG, are both PET tracers which provide low levels of radiation. Current data estimate that FDG has higher-exposure levels compared to rubidium-82 (8 vs. 3.5 mSv). For these reasons, C is the correct answer.
    See Chapter 7.

31. Answer **b**. As noted throughout Chapter 7, there are many ways that radiation exposure may be reduced for traditional SPECT MPI studies. Of the techniques listed in the question, the use of Anger cameras is not associated with decrease in radiation dose. New CZT cameras allow for greater-count sensitivity, thus decreasing required count density which results in overall reduced radiation exposure. Algorithms such as OSEM provide increased-count resolution, compared with traditional filtered-back projection which decreases required dose.
    See Chapter 7.

32. Answer **d**. In a study by Jerome et al., only 1% of accredited laboratories in 2012 reported

radiation exposure of <9 mSv per patient. 10% of laboratories were still using thallium in their protocols with exposure in excess of 20 mSv.
See Chapter 7.

33. **Answer c.** A study by Rozanski et al. (*JACC* 2013) demonstrated that only 8% to 15% of nuclear cardiology studies were positive for ischemia or infarction. Radiation exposure may be reduced by performing stress-first imaging, thus eliminating the need for a second scan in the majority of studies.
See Chapter 7.

34. **Answer b.** Both theophylline and caffeine are competitive antagonists for all of the vasodilators, including dipyridamole. Beta blockers have been shown to reduce the sensitivity of dipyridamole myocardial perfusion imaging, along with underestimating the extent of disease, in a similar fashion to all of the antianginal medications. Oral dipyridamole preceding the administration of a much higher dose of IV dipyridamole for stress testing does not impact on diagnostic accuracy or safety. However, the use of oral dipyridamole prior to adenosine or regadenoson administration is contraindicated, as this will prolong and enhance the subsequent vasodilation.
See Chapter 8.

35. **Answer c.** Stress testing is contraindicated within 48 hours of an ACS. Performing SPECT myocardial perfusion imaging within 2 years of a PCI in an asymptomatic patient is inappropriate. The use of exercise MPI in patients with an LBBB is associated with a substantial false-positive rate (apparent septal ischemia); only vasodilator stress should be used. Therefore, only choice C is accurate.
See Chapter 8.

36. **Answer a.** It is incorrect, as an adenosine protocol should be at least 4 minutes in duration to allow for adequate vasodilation and extraction of the radiopharmaceutical. The other choices are supported by the medical literature and endorsed by contemporary guidelines.
See Chapter 8.

37. **Answer a.** Clinical trials support the use of regadenoson in patients with asthma or COPD, as long as these patients are not steroid-dependent or actively wheezing. While such patients may have an increased incidence of subjective dyspnea with regadenoson, no changes in spirometry or significant adverse events have been noted. Regadenoson does frequently cause headaches, usually successfully treated with caffeine or aminophylline. This agent is delivered by an IV bolus, not via an infusion pump.
See Chapter 8.

38. **Answer c,** as the other choices are all included in the calculation of the Duke treadmill score.
See Chapter 8.

39. **Answer c.** (Henzlova et al., 2016). The higher dose is necessary to offset the residual activity of the first injection. A lower dose underestimates ischemia and a higher dose than 1:3 exposes the patient to unnecessary radiation.
See Chapter 9.

40. **Answer c.**
Estimated radiation doses for a 75-kg patient are:
Tl-201: 20 to 25 mSv
Tc^{99m} sestamibi rest–stress: 11.3 to 15.5 mSv
Tl-201 rest–Tc^{99m} sestamibi stress: >20 mSv
Tc^{99m} stress-only: 7.9 mSV
See Chapter 9.

41. **Answer c.**
See Chapter 9.

42. **Answer b.** Tc^{99m} tracers are excreted by the GI tract and liver, Tl-201 is excreted by the urinary tract with minimal GI uptake. Tetrofosmin clearance from the liver is slightly faster compared to sestamibi clearance.
See Chapter 9.

43. **Answer a.** There is TID and also reversible anterior, inferior, and lateral abnormalities consistent with three-vessel ischemia. This does not represent misregistration as there are

several abnormalities. The prognosis by recent studies is higher risk than normal. More than one defect is present.
See Chapter 10.

44. Answer **b.** Currently, 95% of laboratories use the tracer Rb-82 with a half-life of 75 seconds. Therefore, exercise stress is not possible.
See Chapter 10.

45. Answer **d,** as a patient such as this should undergo ETT. For patients unable to exercise, PET is a "preferred" test according to SNMMI/ASNC Position Statement, and "recommended" for equivocal SPECT result.
See Chapter 10.

46. Answer **b,** as a strontium generator is delivered on site and available. NH-13 with a half-life of 9.8 minutes is cyclotron generated and because of short half-life requires on-site or close-proximity cyclotron.
See Chapter 10.

47. Answer **b.** Endothelial dysfunction is suggested by global MBF reserve. MBF which is normal does reduce substantially, the likelihood of obstructive CAD with normal MPI, can assist in identification of more-severe disease with single-vessel ischemia, and no augmentation of MBF strongly suggests lack of pharmacologic drug effect.
See Chapter 10.

48. Answer **c.** Phase analysis of gated SPECT relies on the principle of partial-volume effect that results in a linear relationship between myocardial thickening and myocardial count density. Fourier transformation of the count-density curve improves the inherent low temporal resolution of SPECT to generate a continuous thickening curve. Differences in the timing of myocardial thickening between various left ventricular segments allows for determination of dyssynchrony. High spatial and temporal resolutions are not attributes of SPECT, and resolution recovery does not play a direct role in phase analysis.
See Chapter 11.

49. Answer **d.** Many different factors can affect the determination of EF by gated SPECT. The normal left ventricle has a large contractile reserve, with a normal range of EF from 55% to 80%. The ventricle with systolic dysfunction has already exhausted much of this reserve. Thus, biological variability is greater in the normal left ventricle. When serial studies are separated by a long time interval, both technical and biological variability come into play. In studies performed in quick succession (separated only by minutes), technical variability is the major influence on FEF determination.
See Chapter 11.

50. Answer **c.** Data demonstrate that the change to 16-bin collection of ventricular function data increases EF calculations by approximately 5%. It is hypothesized that this is due to a better capture of maximal differences between end systole and end diastole. With 8-bin collection, either data point may be missed and therefore artificially lower the ejection fraction not consistent with the correct ventricular function. For this reason, ASNC recommends 16-bin collection.
See Chapter 11.

51. Answer **a.** ECG gating can be used to evaluate artifact from CAD, and has been carefully documented for this value. The concept is that a fixed defect with normal wall motion is consistent with attenuation artifact, while the same fixed defect with abnormal wall motion is consistent with prior MI or scar. The supportive data are very strong. Thus the reader should state the study is normally consistent with artifact and not use modifiers of "equivocal" or "probably normal" which leads to lack of confidence by the referring health care provider in the value of nuclear cardiology and may result in unnecessary catheterization.
See Chapter 11.

52. Answer **d,** as a defect that involves more than 5 segments of the 17-segment model constitutes a large defect. A is incorrect as a score of 4 defines a small (or mildly abnormal) defect. Less than 20% of the left ventricle would be a small or moderately sized defect. Finally,

proximal LAD distribution, in and of itself, is not necessarily a large defect, although this is likely as more than 4 segments will be involved. *See Chapter 12.*

53. Answer **a**, as the rotating planar (cine) images should be reviewed for every patient study. Avid uptake of Tc-99m tracers may lead to a de novo diagnosis of a malignancy. While horizontal motion is more challenging to detect and to correct, vertical patient motion is easily discernable on review of the planar images. Likewise, soft tissue attenuation may be appreciated on these cine images.
See Chapter 12.

54. Answers **c** and **d**. Choices (a) and (b) should be avoided, as these do not add to the value of the report. However, both (c) and (d) are reasonable components of a report.
See Chapter 12.

55. Answer **a**. Clinical judgment should always be included in decision making, sometimes even superseding AUC recommendations. The designation of "inappropriate" was not intended to be a never-event. The AUC are literature based, whenever possible. The multimodality AUC are designed to provide all reasonable options for care, allowing for consideration of local availability and expertise, as well as patient-specific factors.
See Chapter 13.

56. Answer **a**. As the patient is at low clinical likelihood for the presence of coronary artery disease, ECG stress testing is an appropriate option. Exercise echocardiography is considered "may be appropriate." (b) and (d) are considered "rarely appropriate."
See Chapter 13.

57. Answer **d** is the correct response, as clearly stated in all ACCF appropriate use publications. Clinicians should not simply choose a criterion based on what the result may bear, but instead follow a structured, hierarchical approach. While most of the AUC have been incorporated into computer applications and clinical-decision support tools, there is not an absolute requirement to use a computer-based assessment. Third-party payers are encouraged to use published AUC but these criteria are not intended to be used for individual payment decisions.
See Chapter 13.

58. Answer **a**. Patients with abnormal baseline ECG changes are candidates for SPECT rather than ETT alone. A patient with ST elevation should undergo catheterization, not stress testing. An asymptomatic patient with a low calcium score does not need testing. A runner should undergo ETT first.
See Chapter 14.

59. Answer **d**. Patients with abnormal ECT should undergo SPECT with exercise, not pharmacologic stress.
See Chapter 14.

60. Answer **c**. Cardiac PET has highest diagnostic accuracy, SPECT (either pharmacologic or exercise) is higher than ETT alone.
See Chapter 14.

61. Answer **d**. The first three are advantages of PET, but because of the short half-lives of current agents, pharmacologic stress is preferred over exercise for PET.
See Chapter 14.

62. Answer **a**. Choice (b) is not correct as a fixed defect is associated with an increased incidence of cardiac death. Patients without a change in symptoms should not undergo repeat testing, and a normal SPECT study usually conveys a "warranty" of at least 2 years. Finally, even patients at clinically increased (moderate or severe) risk who have a normal SPECT study still have a very annual event rate; therefore, the Duke treadmill score is not as effective a prognostic tool as SPECT imaging.
See Chapter 15.

63. Answer **c**, as a large fixed defect or reduced ejection fraction are markers of an increased

risk for a cardiac event, but are specific for cardiac death, not an ischemic event.
See Chapter 15.

64. **Answer d.** The AUC attempt to define how cardiac imaging procedures, including SPECT MPI are used, although do not specify that these tests are required. Great efforts are undertaken to ensure concordance with clinical practice guidelines. While AUC are ideally well rooted in the medical literature, certain clinical indications lack sufficient published data and hence expert opinion may be used to define appropriate use. Choice (d) is correct, as from the onset, the AUC recognized the need for patient and local factors to be considered and that a procedure deemed rarely appropriate or inappropriate is sometimes reasonable.
See Chapter 15.

65. **Answer d.** Transient cavity dilation may also be seen in the setting of severe proximal LAD disease in addition to multivessel CAD. Persistent cavity enlargement is a marker for increased risk of cardiac death, not an ischemic event such as MI. TID may be seen without an increase in LV diameter, as this is likely due to subendocardial ischemia and the loss of tracer uptake in this region, giving the appearance of cavity dilation. Choice (d) is correct.
See Chapter 15.

66. **Answer b.** This question asks the reader to not only consider the risk of the operation but the implications of test results. Answer (a) is inappropriate because the patient is undergoing a low-risk procedure and otherwise does not have any concerning clinical risk factors. Answer (c) is wrong because despite the patient undergoing a high-risk procedure, the patient's functional capacity is above 4 METs. Answer (d) is incorrect as the patient had a coronary evaluation including stent placement at the time of an acute coronary syndrome, is asymptomatic, and is not undergoing a high-risk procedure. The patient in answer (b) is older and has two cardiovascular risk factors that may increase the risk of a perioperative cardiovascular event. Furthermore, the patient is undergoing a moderate-risk (intraperitoneal) surgery, and it is otherwise unclear what the patient's functional capacity is. Although the procedure is presumably being done for cancer, which can sometimes influence the need for testing that may delay somewhat urgent surgery, in this case, a high-risk stress test result may lead to a lower-risk, more palliative procedure.
See Chapter 16.

67. **Answer c.** The data supporting beta-blocker use in the perioperative period is not as strong as it once was, as some of the studies utilizing beta blockers in this setting have been discredited. Although beta blockers may reduce the risk of perioperative MI in certain settings, some studies have shown an <u>increase</u> in mortality. Adding clopidogrel or performing CABG prior to intermediate-risk noncardiac surgery has not been shown to improve perioperative cardiac outcomes. There is evidence that statins may reduce major adverse cardiovascular events when introduced preoperatively, particularly in patients undergoing vascular surgery.
See Chapter 16.

68. **Answer b.** Several studies have shown that reversible perfusion defects on myocardial perfusion imaging increase the risk of perioperative myocardial infarction. Large fixed defects and low left ventricular ejection fraction may be predictors of cardiac death but are not as strong in predicting perioperative MI. Persistent ST depression after exercise stress increases the specificity of the test for diagnosing coronary artery disease, but has not been shown to be a predictor of perioperative MI. In older studies, functional capacity as determined by exercise testing was a strong predictor of cardiac events around the time of noncardiac surgery, which is why functional capacity determination (with or without a stress test) is a key component of the preoperative cardiac assessment.
See Chapter 16.

69. **Answer c.** However, in an asymptomatic patient, SPECT myocardial perfusion imaging

should not be performed within 2 years of PCI or within 5 years of CABG. The indication in item A may be appropriate but is not likely useful. However, for those patients who undergo incomplete revascularization, radionuclide imaging is appropriate.
See Chapter 17.

70. Answer **c**. Beta blockers function primarily by reducing myocardial oxygen consumption. There is clear evidence for the use of ACE inhibitors in the treatment of ischemic heart disease. The exception stated in choice (c), that perfusion abnormalities are NOT reduced with beta blockers is incorrect. Finally, choice (c) is correct as, in order to optimize disease detection and assess severity, antianginal medications should be withheld. However, if the test is being performed to assess therapeutic benefit, these medications should be continued.
See Chapter 17.

71. Answer **d**. As the patient underwent incomplete revascularization, the performance of SPECT MPI is appropriate or reasonable. It is not necessarily required, but would have potential value.
See Chapter 17.

72. Answer **c**. One of the most critical diagnostic steps in the evaluation of newly diagnosed heart failure is determining whether coronary artery disease is the etiology. The IMAGING study suggested that in newly diagnosed heart failure, myocardial SPECT was noninferior to coronary angiography in diagnosing coronary artery disease. NT-proBNP may provide information regarding disease severity, and longitudinal laboratory follow-up may help track response to medical therapy. Right-heart catheterization is reserved for those patients with cardiogenic shock, and viability testing is relevant in patients with established coronary artery disease in whom revascularization is being considered.
See Chapter 18.

73. Answer **d**. The viability study shows a matched perfusion/metabolism defect consistent with scar in the LAD distribution. This large vascular territory is unlikely to recover function following revascularization, and furthermore, with LVEF of 15%, he may have difficulty weaning from cardiopulmonary bypass surgery postoperatively. CABG is not recommended. Cardiac MRI may also reveal scar in the LAD distribution, but is not superior to PET imaging for viability assessment, and is unlikely to provide information that would change management. This patient should be referred for advanced heart failure consultation for transplantation/LVAD.
See Chapter 18.

74. Answer **b**. Based on findings in the ADMIRE-HF study (Jacobson et al. *JACC*. 2010;55:2212–2221).
Heart:mediastinal ratio >1.6 is associated with a more favorable prognosis, and a reduced risk of sudden cardiac death. This ratio of 1.4 is in the less favorable range. Further assessments of LVEF with other modalities may be considered, but only if the echocardiogram was of limited quality. This patient qualifies for placement of a primary prevention ICD.
See Chapter 18.

75. Answer **d**. The image is abnormal for an anterior perfusion abnormality. Since wall motion was normal, the image is consistent with ischemia. No stress imaging is necessary and the patient should go to the catheterization laboratory for treatment.
See Chapter 19.

76. Answer **b**. This is a pharmacologic stress in a diabetic patient. Thus, although normal, the post-test risk is slightly higher (1%–2%) because of both diabetes and the fact that the patient could not complete exercise. Annual nuclear studies are not recommended, and the diagnostic accuracy of nuclear imaging in diabetic patients is the same as in a nondiabetic population.
See Chapter 19.

77. Answer **c**. There is a higher risk of coronary events due to spontaneous plaque rupture and

progression of disease. The diagnostic accuracy between genders with SPECT is equivalent. CMD has been shown to have a role in angina symptoms in women.
See Chapter 19.

78. **Answer b.** Pharmacologic stress and lower ejection fraction have both been associated with higher cardiac event rates.
See Chapter 19.

79. **Answer d,** as both (a) and (c) are correct. "Value" is calculated as "quality" divided by "cost." Other metrics that indirectly impact value include selecting the right test for the right patient (appropriateness) and patient outcomes; both (b) and (c) are important for the overarching interpretation of quality as well, but do not factor in the calculation of value.
See Chapter 20.

80. **Answer a.** The cost of the test is not a component of QALY. QALY is an outcome assessment including both survival and quality of life. The other statements are correct.
See Chapter 20.

81. **Answer a.** When SPECT or PET imaging is utilized, the amount of revascularization is reduced, resulting in improved cost-effectiveness.
See Chapter 20.

82. **Answer c.** Hibernating myocardium occurs after repeated episodes of ischemia or stunning and by definition, is viable and therefore has the capacity for functional recovery after adequate revascularization. The adaptive downregulation response that occurs during the period of limited coronary flow reserve is important to prevent a "supply–demand imbalance." Myocardial glucose metabolism is preserved and is measured by PET with ^{18}Fluorodeoxyglucose (^{18}FDG), a glucose analog that is transported into the myocyte and converted to FDG-6-phosphate. Option a is the definition of stunned myocardium. Option B is incorrect because hibernating myocardium has abnormal function and flow with preserved metabolism. Option (d) describes scar/fibrosis and nonviable status.
See Chapter 21.

83. **Answer d.** The best interpretation for the ^{13}N-ammonia/FDG PET shown on the figure is a large area of scar (match) involving the anteroseptal, inferoseptal and inferior walls, and apex. There is no significant area of mismatch (hibernating myocardium) in this case. The patient's LV function is unlikely to improve with revascularization.
See Chapter 21.

84. **Answer b.** Fasting is a simple approach but can lead to inferior image quality when compared to glucose loaded. The rationale behind this approach is that the normal myocardium will consume FFA while ischemic myocardium (viable) will preferentially use ^{18}FDG and appear as a "hot spot." This approach is usually not recommended as an isolation technique but is routinely needed as a part of the preparation before one of the other three methods (glucose loading, hyperinsulinemic–euglycemic clamp or use of nicotinic acid).
See Chapter 21.

85. **Answer a.** The in vitro method is the preferred method for RBC labeling as it has the highest labeling efficiency (>97%). It is usually performed using a commercially available kit. The in vivo method is no longer recommended as it provides the lowest labeling efficiency.
See Chapter 22.

86. **Answer c.** FPRNA has some distinct advantages over ERNA. These include (1) the acquisition of data in <30 seconds; (2) the evaluation of RV function with less overlap of the activity from other chambers; (3) the use of multiple radiopharmaceuticals, including bone, renal, and myocardial scintigraphic agents; (4) a proven robust measurement of stress ventricular function at the true point of peak exercise; and (5) the presence of a wealth of prognostic information available for management of patients with ischemic heart

disease based on stratification by FPRNA exercise LVEFs.
See Chapter 22.

87. **Answer d.** All of the above. Radionuclide angiography techniques can be used clinically to assess LV size, systolic function, diastolic function, regional wall motion, and timing of mechanical activation (dyssynchrony). The most common uses clinically, these days are for LV systolic function, dyssynchrony, and for monitoring the effects of chemotherapy.
See Chapter 22.

88. **Answer a.** Although FPRNA has a wealth of prognostic data, in particular with exercise FPRNA, and is highly accurate for the assessment of LVEF, its use is limited these days as it requires a high-count rate-capable, often dedicated gamma camera. Equilibrium techniques are currently used much more widely than FPRNA.
See Chapter 22.

89. **Answer b.** ^{123}I-*m*IBG is modeled after the false-sympathetic neurotransmitter guanethidine as an analog of the sympathetic mediator norepinephrine. It is taken up into the presynaptic sympathetic terminal by a norepinephrine transporter. ^{123}I is single-photon emitter and therefore images with a SPECT camera.
See Chapter 23.

90. **Answer a.** To quantify global myocardial uptake of ^{123}I-*m*IBG, the counts per pixel in an anterior planar myocardial region of interest are divided by the counts per pixel in a region of interest (7 × 7 pixel size is recommended) in the upper mediastinum. Washout is the decrease in global cardiac tracer in an image acquired early after acquisition compared with a later (approximately 4 hours) image. SPECT is best for regional adrenergic defects.
See Chapter 23.

91. **Answer d,** as abnormalities of cardiac ^{123}I-*m*IBG uptake have been seen in all of these clinical situations.
See Chapter 23.

92. **Answer c.** A normal HMR is reported to be 2.2 ± 0.3, with a value more than 2 standard deviations below the mean, that is, <1.6, found in the ADMIRE-HF study to be associated with increased cardiac risk over a 17-month median follow-up for patients having HFrEF. The specific events monitored in the study were heart failure progression (i.e., worsening of New York Heart Association Class), arrhythmic events, cardiac death, and all-cause mortality. Thus, an HMR of 2.02 is associated with lower risk.
See Chapter 23.

93. **Answer d.**
   a. While a high-fat diet is a component of the preparation to increase fatty acid substrate for myocardial metabolism, high-protein diet alone is not.
   b. Prolonged fasting can be performed, but is not the preferred method as it has been shown to have less reliability in terms of myocardial suppression when compared to a low-carbohydrate/high-fat diet.
   c. Carbohydrates need to be avoided to shift myocardial metabolism to fatty acids and to suppress normal myocardial uptake.
See Chapter 24.

94. **Answer a.** Scar will present as a defect on myocardial perfusion imaging while normal myocardium, barring any artifacts, should have preserved perfusion.
   b. Both inflammation and scar can present as perfusion defects, depending on the degree of inflammation.
   c. Early inflammation can appear normal on myocardial perfusion images.
See Chapter 24.

95. **Answer d.** There is a focal perfusion defect at the base without corresponding FDG uptake with good myocardial suppression elsewhere, indicating that this is not inflammation but rather scar.
   a. Normal myocardium would not present as a perfusion defect.
   b. Diffuse inflammation would present as diffuse FDG uptake, which is not present in this case.

c. There is good myocardial suppression indicating good dietary preparation.
See Chapter 24.

96. Answer **c.** Need more information. While this could certainly be FDG uptake from infection, evaluation of the non–attenuation-corrected (NAC) images is necessary to exclude attenuation artifact from the device. If uptake is absent on the NAC images, then this is due to artifact.
See Chapter 24.

97. Answer **d.** After myocardial uptake of a radiotracer, the emitted photons must travel through various soft tissue structures (adipose tissue, muscle mass, bone, diaphragm, and breast tissue) before reaching the photodetectors of the gamma camera. In transit, the photons can get attenuated (absorbed or deflected by soft tissues), resulting in lower sensitivity and specificity for the detection of coronary artery disease (CAD). CT serves as an attenuation-correction tool and improves the count uniformity of the image and helps distinguish attenuation artifacts from real defects. (a) is incorrect, as the primary advantage of attenuation correction is to improve specificity to detect coronary artery disease. (b) is incorrect. Although attenuation correction is required to quantify myocardial blood flow with PET, its primary role both in SPECT and PET is to correct for attenuation artifacts and improve specificity. (c) is incorrect as radiation dose to the patient may be slightly increased.
See Chapter 25.

98. Answer **a.** Coronary artery calcification is a specific marker of underlying coronary atherosclerosis, and the association of high coronary artery calcification and increased cardiovascular risk has been well established. Statements (b), (c), and (d) are incorrect.
See Chapter 25.

99. Answer **c.** High coronary artery calcium score, even in asymptomatic individuals, has been associated with an increased risk of ischemia on SPECT or PET myocardial perfusion imaging. The frequency of ischemia on MPI in subjects with an Agatston calcium score of >400 is high (>20%). Moreover, a meta-analysis including >85,000 patients, showed that the absence of coronary artery calcification indicated very low risk with 6% prevalence of ischemia and a 99% negative predictive value to exclude acute coronary syndromes. (a) Coronary CTA may be limited in individuals with very high calcium score. (b) Invasive coronary angiogram is not indicated without objective evidence of ischemia. (d) Due to the increased risk of ischemia (see explanation for [a]), reassurance and no further testing is recommended.
See Chapter 25.

100. Answer **d.** CFR is a robust technique that assists myocardial tissue perfusion in evaluation of epicardial CAD, diffuse atherosclerosis, vessel remodeling, as well as microvascular dysfunction. In patients with normal CTA, abnormal CFR indicates microvascular dysfunction resulting in abnormal blood flow without obstructive epicardial CAD. Option (a) is incorrect, as ischemia testing, and not CTA, is a better initial test in patients with an 80% pretest likelihood of coronary artery disease. Option (b) is incorrect, as invasive coronary angiography, and not CTA, is indicated in patients with severe ischemia. Option (c) is incorrect, as CTA, and not MPI, is the preferred initial test in a patient with 15% pretest likelihood of coronary artery disease.
See Chapter 25.

101. Answer **a.** A Hybrid ^{18}FDG-PET with CT provides an incremental value to diagnose infective endocarditis in prosthetic valves and intracardiac devices where echocardiography can be inconclusive and can reclassify patients and improve the accuracy of Duke criteria. Options (b), (c), and (d) are incorrect.
See Chapter 25.

102. Answer **c.** An exercise nuclear myocardial perfusion imaging or exercise echocardiogram study is preferred in patients who have a high pretest probability of coronary artery disease

and are capable of performing at least moderate physical activity when undergoing an evaluation for suspected stable ischemic heart disease (class I recommendation). Ventricular pre-excitation is often associated with an abnormal ECG (false-positive) response and left bundle branch block makes exercise ECG uninterpretable with regard to the detection of myocardial ischemia. For elderly patients with an interpretable ECG, routine ECG exercise testing is preferred.
See Chapter 26.

103. **Answer b.** This patient's functional capacity is quite good, therefore not placing him in a high-risk category with 5% or 10% annual mortality. However, his risk is not negligible (0.25%).
See Chapter 26.

104. **Answer a.** The most important exercise treadmill test (ETT) prognostic variable is exercise capacity. The annual cardiovascular mortality in patients with a high-risk (not intermediate-risk) Duke treadmill score is 5%. One of the major advantages of ETT over stress imaging studies is the lower cost. Although diagnostic test accuracy is lower in women than in men, the ETT remains the appropriate first test in symptomatic women, at an intermediate likelihood of CAD, who are able to exercise and have a normal resting ECG.
See Chapter 26.

105. **Answer d.** The normal response to stress is a decrease in left ventricular cavity size due to a combination of reduced systemic vascular resistance and increased LV contractility. The finding of increased LV end-systolic volume during stress is the equivalent of transient ischemic dilatation of the LV on stress nuclear perfusion imaging stress and is generally indicative of extensive coronary artery disease such as three-vessel disease or left main coronary disease.
See Chapter 27.

106. **Answer a.** The primary causes for a false-negative test are inability to reach target heart rate (e.g., due to poor exercise capacity, use of a beta blocker, or delay in capturing postexercise images), poor image quality, single-vessel disease, or other pre-existing conditions such as significant LV hypertrophy or a hyperdynamic state. The sensitivity of the test is proportionally related to the number of vessels involved, being the greatest for triple-vessel disease.
See Chapter 27.

107. **Answer d.** Myocardial ischemia results from a regional mismatch between the myocardial oxygen demand and the reduced supply from arterial stenosis. This is represented on stress echocardiogram by new or worsening wall motion abnormalities, increasing left ventricular cavity size, and decreased ejection fraction. A hypokinetic segment that improves on low-dose dobutamine and worsens at peak dose, the so called biphasic response, represents viable myocardium and ischemia in this segment.
See Chapter 27.

108. **Answer b.** Exercise echocardiography can identify patients with obstructive hypertrophic cardiomyopathy if the LVOT gradient increases to above 30 mm Hg even if there is no resting gradient. Additionally, exercise testing can provide information on functional class, exercise-induced arrhythmia, and blood pressure response. Contraindications to exercise stress testing include severe symptomatic aortic stenosis, uncontrolled arrhythmias, acute aortic dissection, high-risk unstable angina, and acute pulmonary embolus.
See Chapter 27.

109. **Answer c.** Ultrasound contrast agents improve the ability to adequately visualize the endocardial borders, thus allowing the detection of LV wall motion and global systolic function, and aiding in decreasing interobserver variability in SE interpretation. Guidelines from the American Society of Echocardiography for the use of contrast for LV opacification recommend its use when two or more contiguous myocardial segments are not adequately visualized and thus, are not indicated in all stress echocardiography examinations. Contrast can be used with all

stress echocardiography modalities. However, the use of contrast is contraindicated in the presence of a large known right-to-left shunt. Recent studies have demonstrated that contrast is safe in the presence of a patent foramen ovale.
See Chapter 27.

110. Answer **b**. Patients undergoing CCTA are often given beta blockers in order to achieve a heart rate <65 beats/min. This results in prolongation of diastole, which is considered the optimal time to image coronary arteries since myocardial contraction is at a minimum, allowing for visualization of coronary arteries that run in all directions around the heart and taper in diameter along the length of the vessel. Additionally, patients (with no contraindications) are premedicated with sublingual nitroglycerin to achieve coronary vasodilation, increasing the diagnostic accuracy of CCTA and the ability to image smaller coronary side branches, while eliminating coronary spasm that may mimic stenosis.
See Chapter 28.

111. Answer **a**. The disadvantage of the retrospective gating mode is its increased radiation dose over prospective ECG triggering, because data are acquired throughout the heart cycle, even though only partial data are actually used in the final image reconstruction.
See Chapter 28.

112. Answer **b**. The patient has evidence of inferior subendocardial late gadolinium enhancement, which is consistent with an inferior myocardial infarction of unknown chronicity. However, the inferior wall increased signal on the T2-weighted images is consistent with myocardial edema from an acute process. The patient has a history of prior inferior infarction. Therefore, this is an acute on chronic myocardial infarction. Acute myocarditis could present with T2 enhancement but would have subepicardial or mid-wall late gadolinium enhancement. Cardiac sarcoid would also have subepicardial or mid-wall late gadolinium enhancement.
See Chapter 29.

113. Answer **c**. The apical perfusion images reveal a reversible anterior, septal, and inferior perfusion abnormality concerning obstructive disease in the left anterior descending territory. However, the significant reduction in global absolute myocardial blood flow suggests obstructive disease in all three major epicardial territories. The concurrent left main and right coronary stenoses are the only option that would lead to reductions in flow in all territories.
See Chapter 29.

114. Answer **c**. Mr. B has evidence of late gadolinium enhancement in the inferolateral wall. The transmural extent appears to be 26% to 50%, which is associated with a 40% likelihood of improved contractility following revascularization.
See Chapter 29.

INDEX

INDEX

Page numbers followed by f or t indicate figures or tables, respectively.

A

Absorbed dose, radiation, 15–16
Acquisition
　error, potential sources of, 72–76
　parameters for, 66
　protocols, 71–72, 139, 141, 148
　quality control (QC) process, 63–77
Acute-rest myocardial perfusion imaging, 291
Acute chest pain syndromes, 292
Adenosine/rest dual-isotope myocardial perfusion imaging, 175f
Agatston score, 431–433
Anger cameras, 97
Annihilation, 6
Aortic valve, Doppler hemodynamic assessment of, 415
Appropriate use
　categories of, 195t
　classification of, 198t
　definition, 194t
　hierarchy for, 197f
　inappropriate indications, 199t
　methodology, 195–196
　SPECT results, 200t
Arrhythmogenic right ventricular dysplasia (ARVD), 358
Artifacts image, 78t
　recognition, attenuation, 72
As Low As Reasonably Achievable (ALARA), 18
Attenuation correction, 69–70
　CT-based, 69–70, 70f
　gadolinium-153 sealed sources for SPECT systems, 69
　germanium-68 sealed sources for PET systems, 69
　techniques, 214

B

Bayes' theorem, 402
Blank scan, 66–68, 67f
Bremsstrahlung interactions, 10

C

Cadmium zinc telluride (CZT) cameras, 97, 218
Cardiac amyloid imaging, 34, 365
　evaluation algorithm, 367f
　imaging technique, 368
　indications, 366
　reporting, 369
　^{18}F-FDG PET/CT imaging, 379
Cardiac innervation
　imaging with ^{123}I-mIBG, 351–353, 357f
　iodine prophylaxis, 348
　protocol, 349–350
　radiotracer administration, 348
Cardiac positron emission tomography. See Positron emission tomography (PET)
Cardiac resynchronization therapy (CRT), 354
Cardiac sympathetic innervation, 346–347
Cardiovascular magnetic resonance
　attributes, disease conditions, 452t
　limitations/contraindications, 449–450
　methods and advantages, 349
　myocardial perfusion, 452–453
　myocardial viability, 455
　scar assessment of, 455
　sequences, 450–451
　structure and function, 450–451
　tissue characterization, 451–452, 456–457
　valvular heart disease, 459
Center of rotation (COR) evaluation, 65, 65f
Chronic kidney disease, risk stratification, 288–289
Chronotropic incompetence, 402
Clinical decision support systems (CDSS), 181–182
Coincidence timing calibration (CTC), 66, 68
Collimators, 97
Contrast agents, 426, 437
Coronary artery bypass graft (CABG), 197, 260, 322

Coronary artery calcium (CAC) scoring
  Agatston score, 431–433
  clinical utility of, 433–434
  diagnostic performance, 433
  prognostic value of, 433
  scanning protocols, 431
Coronary artery disease (CAD), 169, 209, 279
  diagnostic accuracy, 213f, 214–218
  myocardial perfusion imaging, 257–260
    acute coronary syndrome patients, 262–264
    assess efficacy of medical therapy, 264–266
    pretest probability by age, gender, and symptoms, 210t
  risk assessment of, 209–210
Coronary computed tomographic angiography, 304, 434–446
Coronary microvascular dysfunction (CMD), 283
CT-based attenuation correction, 69–70, 70f
CT myocardial perfusion, 441–442

D
Daily uniformity flood, 64, 65f
Decay, radioactive, 5–8, 7f
Deconvolution of septal penetration (DSP), 351
Defect severity, 172
Deterministic risk effects of radiation, 18–19, 19f
Displacement encoded with stimulated echoes (DENSE), 451
Dose equivalent, radiation, 15–16, 16t
DOT label, radiation exposure limits, 25t
Dual-isotope imaging, 127–128, 169f–170f, 127, 314
Duke treadmill score, 103t, 108, 402

E
ECG-gated SPECT imaging
  acquisition, 147
  evaluation of myocardial perfusion data, 149–150
  evaluation of unprocessed (raw) data, 149
  evaluation of ventricular function, 150
  interpretation procedure for, 149, 149t
  principle of, 148f
Echocardiography, 411–427
Economics of Noninvasive Diagnosis (END) study, 236, 299
Electron configuration, 4f, 6–7
Energy peaking, SPECT system, 64
ERNA techniques, 339
Exercise electrocardiography testing, 103, 105–106, 108, 211, 257, 401–408
Extracardiac activity, 74, 74f

F
Film badges, 21
Fluorine-18 (^{18}F) fluorodeoxyglucose (FDG), 37–39, 133, 271
FMEA tool, for quality improvement cycles, 82t, 83
FOCUS-PDCA model, for quality improvement cycles, 82–83, 82t
Four-quadrant phantoms, 65, 66f
FPRNA data, 332
Framingham Risk Score (FRS), 209

G
Gadolinium-153, sources for SPECT systems, 69
Gamma rays, 19
Germanium-68, sources for PET systems, 69
Gray (Gy), 16

H
Half-value thickness (HVT), for Tl, Tc, and Rb, 12t
Harmonic phase imaging (HARP), 451
Hawthorne effect, 88
Heart failure, 272–277
  molecular imaging in, 276–277
  radionuclide approaches, 274f, 275
Hibernation, 310
Hurricane sign, 168f
Hybrid imaging
  attenuation correction, 387–388
  coronary artery calcification, 388–389
  coronary CT and radionuclide imaging
    hybrid CAC score, 389–393
    hybrid coronary CTA, 393–395
  PET-CT, 387
  radiation exposure, 397
  SPECT-CT, 387
Hypertrophic cardiomyopathy (HCM), 424

I
Inverse square law, 20, 20f
Ionizing radiation, 15
  exposure, sources of, 16–17
  quality factors for, 15–16, 16t
Iterative reconstruction algorithms, 58

L

Late gadolinium enhancement (LGE), 452
LEAN model, for quality improvement cycles, 82t, 83
Left bundle branch block (LBBB), 108, 175
Left ventricular assist device (LVAD), 354, 380
Left ventricular hypertrophy (LVH), 107–108, 257
Linear non-threshold risk model, 17
Line source attenuation correction, 48–49
Linearity evaluation, 65–66
Linogram, 168f
Low-energy high-resolution (LEHR) collimators, 350

M

Medicare Payment Advisory Commission (Med-PAC), 193
Milestones model, for quality improvement cycles, 82t, 83
Myocardial deformation analysis, 426–427
Myocardial perfusion imaging (MPI), 27, 209, 279, 223–237, 452–453. *See also* SPECT myocardial perfusion imaging; Positron emission tomography (PET)
    attenuation correction, 69–70
    diabetic patients evaluation, 279–283
    display and interpretation, 77
    perfusion defects, 231f
    prognostic value of, 228–229, 226t, 235f
    quality control, *See* Quality control
    risk assessment, 223–227, 224t
    serial imaging, 233–234
    women, 283–286
Myocardial viability, 309–311, 423

N

N-13 ammonia (N-13), 36–37, 133
Non-cardiac surgery, 227–230
    ACC/AHA guidelines, 251–252
    capacity and energy requirements, 246t
    clinical evaluation, 246–248
    clinical markers of, 248f
    myocardial perfusion imaging, 248–250
    risk reduction, 252–254
Nonischemic cardiomyopathy (NICM), 271
Normalization correction, 68–69, 68f
Novel processing software, 128–129

Nuclear cardiology
    age- and sex-adjusted annual rates of, 297f
    appropriate use criteria, 298
    cost-effectiveness analysis, 298–299
        in stable ischemic heart disease, 299
        evaluation of acute chest pain, 304
    implementation, 198–202
    methodology, 195–196
    radionuclide imaging, 196–198
    use criteria of, 194, 195t
Nuclear imaging methods, 311–325
    ^{18}FDG PET imaging protocol, 317f
    ^{201}Tl rest-redistribution protocol, 312f–313f
    algorithm to guide, 324f
    flow algorithm for viability imaging approach, 325f
    imaging modalities and mechanisms for, 311t
    imaging protocols for 201-thallium SPECT, 312
    single-photon emission computed tomography, 311–312
Nuclear Regulatory Commission (NRC), 15, 63

O

Optically stimulated luminescence (OSL), 21
Ordered subsets expectation maximization (OSEM), 351
Oxygen (O)-15 water, 37

P

Patient motion, 74–75, 75f
Percutaneous coronary intervention (PCI), 197, 253, 260–262
Pharmacologic stress testing
    synthetic catecholamines, 110–112
    vasodilators, 109–110
Positron emission tomography (PET), 27, 131–132, 193, 209, 237, 265, 345, 369
    camera, 132, 132f
    cardiovascular, 131–143
    imaging, 131–132, 131f, 209
    instrumentation
        attenuation correction, 53, 54f
        basics of, 52
        PET scanners, 52, 53f
        scatter correction, 56–57
    myocardial blood flow levels and net myocardial radiotracer extraction for, 29f

Positron emission tomography (PET) (*Continued*)
  myocardial blood flow assessment, clinical value of, 138–139, 140f, 141f
  myocardial imaging, radioactive isotopes for, 132
    fluorine-18 (^{18}F) fluorodeoxyglucose, 133
    N-13 ammonia, 133
    rubidium-82, 132–133
  myocardial perfusion imaging, benefits of, 133
    diagnostic accuracy, 134–135, 134f, 135f, 136f
    improved image quality, 133–134
  myocardial viability, 142–143
  nonperfusion indications for, 142
  perfusion, patient selection for, 141–142, 142t
  protocols, 139, 141
  risk stratification, 137–138, 137f, 138f
  radiation exposure, 135–136, 136f
  radiopharmaceuticals, 27, 35, 35t–36t
    F-18 fluorodeoxyglucose (FDG), 37–38
    F-18 flurpiridaz, 38–39
    nitrogen-13 (N-13) ammonia, 36–37
    oxygen (O)-15 water, 37
    rubidium (Rb)-82, 35–36
  sarcoidosis, 143

Q

Quality control (QC) process
  before acquisition, 63
    PET system, 66–70
    solid-state SPECT systems, 66
    SPECT system, 63–66
  during acquisition, 70–71, 71t
    extracardiac activity, 74, 74f
    irregular R-R interval, 75–76
    patient motion, 74–75, 75f
    protocols and acquisition setup, 71–72
    soft tissue attenuation, 72, 72f, 73f, 74
    sources of error, 72–76
  after acquisition, 76
    display and interpretation, 76–77
    processing, 76, 76f
  gamma camera, frequency for, 63t
  PET camera, frequency for, 64t
  of positron emission tomography, 63
  single-photon emission computed tomography, 63
Quality factors, for ionizing radiation, 15–16, 16t

Quality in nuclear cardiology
  accreditation of laboratories, 84–85
  benchmarks, utilization of, 88
  certification of physician qualifications, 84–85
  cost and value of, 84
  definitions, 81–82
  evaluation of
    interpretation, 87
    patient selection, 85–86
    performance, examination of, 86–87
    quality improvement program, 87–88
    reporting, 87
  improvement cycles, 82–83, 83t

R

Rad, absorbed dose unit, 16
Radiation, 15–19
  area surveys and spill procedures, 23
  postings, 22–23, 22f
  protection principles, 19–20, 20f
  radioactive packages, shipping of, 24–26, 24f, 24t, 25f, 25t
  receiving, 24
  waste disposal, 23–24, 23t
Radioactive material
  in nuclear cardiology, limits for common isotopes, 24t
  safe use of, 26
Radioactive packages, shipping of, 24–26, 24f, 24t, 25f, 25t
Radionuclide angiography
  clinical applications, 337
    assessment of diastolic function, 338
    assessment of systolic function, 337–338
    assessment of ventricular dyssynchrony, 338–339
    chemotherapy effects, 339–340
  first-pass radionuclide angiography, 332, 332f
  functional images, 336–337
  gated planar equilibrium blood pool imaging, 333–334, 334f
  gated SPECT myocardial perfusion imaging, 335–336
  gated tomographic equilibrium blood pool imaging, 334–335, 335f
Ramp filter artifact, 169
Reverse redistribution, 173
Rubidium-82 (Rb-82), 35–36, 132–133

S

Sarcoidosis, 143, 369
   artifacts and pitfalls, 377–378
   diagnostic algorithm for, 372f
   image interpretation and repression, 374, 378
   imaging technique, 372–374
   sensitivity and specificity of, 371t
Semi-quantitative metrics of standardized uptake value (SUV), 376
Six-Sigma, for quality improvement cycles, 82t, 83
Sodium iodide (NaI) cameras, 97
Soft tissue attenuation, 72, 72f–73f
Solid state cameras, 66, 128
SPECT instrumentation, 43–48
SPECT myocardial perfusion imaging
   analysis of tomographic slices, 171
   attenuation correction, 179–180
   clinical decision support systems, 181–182
   gated SPECT, 175–178
   interpretation, 163–166, 163t
   perfusion defect, 172
   prone imaging, 180–181
   quantitative analysis, 174
   reporting, 182–186
   semiquantitative defect analysis, 173t
   TID cutoffs, 173t
Stochastic risk effects of radiation, 18–19, 19f
Stress echocardiography techniques, 417–418
Stunning, 309–310
Subsets expectation maximization (OSEM), 351
System spatial resolution, 65–66

T

Tc-99m-isonitrile, 31
Tc-99m-labeled MPI agents, 30–34
   biodistribution, 32–33
   dosimetry, 32–33
   physiologic characteristics, 31–32
Tc-99m pyrophosphate, 34–35
Tc-99m sestamibi, 19t, 31–33
Tc-99m-tetrofosmin, 33–34
Thallium-201, 28–30
Thermo luminescent device (TLD), 21
"Time-of-flight" (TOF), 58
Transient ischemic cavity dilation (TID), 128, 230–233, 232t

U

Useful fields of view (UFOV), 64

V

Valvular heart disease, 459
Vascular grafts, 381
Viability, 309–311, 423

W

Waste disposal, for radiation protection, 23–24, 23t
Well counter correction (WCC), 69
Wide-beam reconstruction (WBR), 97

CPSIA information can be obtained
at www.ICGtesting.com
Printed in the USA
LVHW05s0744160418
573212LV00001B/1/P